AF182245

Breast Cancer Radiation Therapy

Orit Kaidar-Person • Icro Meattini
Philip Poortmans
Editors

Breast Cancer Radiation Therapy

A Practical Guide for Technical Applications

Springer

Editors
Orit Kaidar-Person
Radiation Oncology Unit
Sheba Medical Center
Ramat Gan, Israel

Sackler School of Medicine
Tel-Aviv University
Tel-Aviv, Israel

GROW-School for Oncology and
Developmental Biology (Maastro)
Maastricht University
Maastricht, The Netherlands

Icro Meattini
Radiation Oncology Unit
Oncology Department
Azienda Ospedaliero-Universitaria
Careggi
Florence, Italy

Philip Poortmans
Faculty of Medicine and Health Sciences
University of Antwerp
Antwerp, Belgium

Department of Radiation
Oncology Iridium Netwerk
Antwerp, Belgium

ISBN 978-3-030-91169-0 ISBN 978-3-030-91170-6 (eBook)
https://doi.org/10.1007/978-3-030-91170-6

© The Editor(s) (if applicable) and The Author(s), under exclusive license to Springer Nature Switzerland AG 2022
This work is subject to copyright. All rights are solely and exclusively licensed by the Publisher, whether the whole or part of the material is concerned, specifically the rights of translation, reprinting, reuse of illustrations, recitation, broadcasting, reproduction on microfilms or in any other physical way, and transmission or information storage and retrieval, electronic adaptation, computer software, or by similar or dissimilar methodology now known or hereafter developed.
The use of general descriptive names, registered names, trademarks, service marks, etc. in this publication does not imply, even in the absence of a specific statement, that such names are exempt from the relevant protective laws and regulations and therefore free for general use.
The publisher, the authors and the editors are safe to assume that the advice and information in this book are believed to be true and accurate at the date of publication. Neither the publisher nor the authors or the editors give a warranty, expressed or implied, with respect to the material contained herein or for any errors or omissions that may have been made. The publisher remains neutral with regard to jurisdictional claims in published maps and institutional affiliations.

This Springer imprint is published by the registered company Springer Nature Switzerland AG
The registered company address is: Gewerbestrasse 11, 6330 Cham, Switzerland

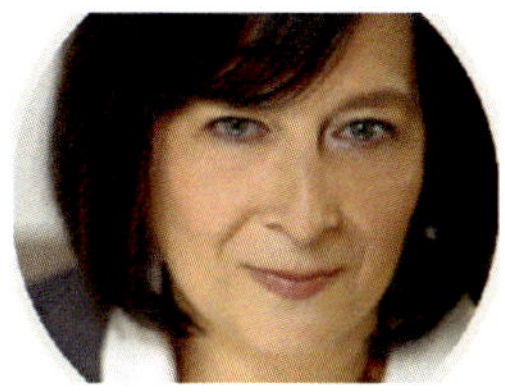

In loving memory of our dear friend and colleague
Professor Bella Kaufman (1956–2021)

Joshua the son of Perachia Jewish sage, second century BCE, would say: "Appoint for yourself a master, acquire for yourself a friend, and judge every man to the side of merit" (Ethics of the Fathers, Chapter 1)

We had the great privilege to have Bella as a master and mentor, as well as a friend and role model, who judged all favourably and with great kindness. Bella was a passionate clinician and researcher, a mentor to many young oncologists, and a beloved friend to her colleagues. She combined the highest levels of professionalism with uncompromising compassion and humanitarianism. The cruel irony, of having the disease for which she was an expert, did not stop her for even one moment, from continuing her work as a devoted breast oncologist and researcher. She lived with her breast cancer with great courage and grace—her loss is a painful reminder to all of us of our responsibility to support and pursue further research to find a cure.

May her memory be a blessing,

Shani Paluch-Shimon & Einav Nili Gal-Yam

Preface

Please find hereby your copy of *Breast Cancer Radiation Therapy*. In contrast to what the classical title suggests, this is an unconventional textbook, consisting of several sections, each of them written by dedicated specialists with distinct expertise on a very specific topic.

This way, we have many contributors with different expertise, writing completely within their current topic of interest. The editors subsequently assembled sections and chapters into a philharmonic final product. As such, our book is mainly dedicated to our patients, and it is aimed to improve breast cancer care by merging evidence-based facts, experiences, and expertise of excellent professionals who are intensively involved in cancer patients treatment.

Radiation therapy (RT) for breast cancer rapidly evolved from 2D (2-dimensional, field-based) to 3D (3-dimensional, volume-based), and from there gradually to more sophisticated intensity-modulated radiation therapy (IMRT) and volumetric-based IMRT techniques. However, centres are often currently working with "volumes" but continue thinking and reasoning in terms of "fields," including adapting the volumes to the RT fields instead of the other (correct) way around.

For years, we took part in several educational programmes to implement the use of volume-based planning in breast RT, for which we based the volumes on anatomical and clinic-pathological regions at risk. Much of the work was done in cooperation with the European SocieTy for Radiotherapy and Oncology (ESTRO) Breast Courses team. Together, we aim that RT planning will be based on the concept that target volumes come first, adapted per case based on patient- and tumour-related risk factors. Next comes the defining of clear dose objectives for target volumes and dose constraints for organs at risk. Therefore, we should not any longer be "looking "at the breast or lymph node "fields," like we used to do previously for conventional simulator-based breast RT planning. The latter should be urgently referred to as obsolete, as it is formerly done for most other RT indications.

The impact of modern and new systemic therapies on current implications and radiation therapy synergistic interactions has been also assessed, with crucial contributions from experts in the clinical oncology field.

The increasing body of literature makes it difficult, if not impossible, to keep track with everything, thereby opening doors for misconceptions and misunderstandings concerning modern breast RT. New technologies and innovative radiation planning should be carefully evaluated and supervised, as it involves a large population of patients, in which the outcomes are to be evaluated up to many years after treatment (e.g. cardiac toxicity; cosmesis; low dose bath from volumetric-IMRT technique). Although a high burden of brand-new literature exists, it is very scattered and difficult to compile all together in order to cover the full scope of the breast cancer world of modern radiation oncology. Literature is too often directed at one of the multidisciplinary groups that together compose the field of radiation oncology: medical doctors, medical physicists, dosimetrists, radiation therapists, radiobiologists, again making the information scattered rather than harmonised.

Finally, we are extremely happy that much data deriving from clinical trials, several led by our co-authors of the book, allowed us to progressively tailor RT with respect to volumes, doses, and techniques, according to each individual patient and tumour features.

In this special book, result of many years of friendship and professional collaboration between editors and contributors, we tried to bring together all the components of radiation oncology for breast cancer, in a handy applicable and useable format, bridging textbook information with hands-out teaching-styled modules, favouring tables and illustrations above plain text.

The authors were selected based on their knowledge, experience, and expertise. Some have contributed to a lifelong education radiation oncology and key trial that changed the management of breast cancer patients, while others were identified as future leaders in the field.

We are delighted and proud that so many highly esteemed colleagues from the entire multidisciplinary field of breast cancer oncology contributed to this work! We would also want to thank the many other wonderful and inspiring colleagues that were not included in this book and continue to contribute to the care of our patients.

We hope you enjoy the reading of our book as much we enjoyed working on it.

I would like to thank my family for their support. I thank those who did not believe in me, as you made me want to improve. I am grateful for those who supported and believed in me, many of them are collaborators in this book, as you gave me the strength and knowledge to power through. A special appreciation to the Israel Cancer Association for their endless support to our dear patients.

Orit Kaidar-Person

I feel truly privileged to have had the opportunity to work with two of the most respected experts in the field of breast cancer who represent for me dearest friends, mentors, and a great source of inspiration at the same time. I am grateful to my family, my daughter Alice and my wife Livia, for the inexhaustible support that make every aspect of my life sustainable. I thank my patients, an essential component of my learning curve, constant inspiration, and motivation, to always improve my human and professional skills.

Icro Meattini

It feels like a great privilege to working together with so many young talented colleagues, including Orit and Icro, as well as many who contributed to the composition of this book. We are together on a travel to further improving multidisciplinary diagnostic and therapeutic paradigms such as they can be optimised for every single patient. The future is bright, for us as "breast cancer specialists," and even more for our patients!

Philip Poortmans

Ramat Gan, Israel — Orit Kaidar-Person
Florence, Italy — Icro Meattini
Wilrijk-Antwerp, Belgium — Philip Poortmans

Contents

Part IX Specific Disease Topics

Part X Risk Assessment and Radiation Quality Assurance

Abbreviations

3D	3-Dimensional
3DCRT	3-Dimensional conformal radiotherapy
4D	4-Dimensional
4DCRT	4-Dimensional conformal radiotherapy
5-FU	5-Fluorouracil
AAPM	American Association of Physicists in Medicine
Ab	Antibody
ABMT	Autologous bone marrow transplant
ABS	American Brachytherapy Society
ACOSOG	American College of Surgeon Oncology Group
ACS	American Cancer Society
ADL	Activity of daily living
ADM	Acellular dermis matrix
ADR	Adverse drug reaction
ADT	Androgen deprivation treatment
AE	Adverse event
AIRO	Associazione Italiana di Radioterapia ed. Oncologia Clinica
AJCC	American Joint Committee on Cancer
ALL	Acute lymphocytic leukaemia
ALND	Axillary lymph node dissection
ALT	Alanine aminotransferase
AP	Anterior-posterior
APBI	Accelerated partial breast irradiation
ASCO	American Society of Clinical Oncology
ASTRO	American Society for Therapeutic Radiology and Oncology
AUC	Area under the curve
b.i.d	Twice a day (bis in die)
BCS	Breast-conserving surgery
BCT	Breast-conserving treatment (lumpectomy and radiotherapy)
BED	Biological effective dose
BEV	Beam-eyes view
BUN	Blood urea nitrogen
Bx	Biopsy
CALGB	Cancer and Leukemia Group B
CBC	Complete blood count
CBCT	Cone beam CT
cc	Cubic centimetre

cCR	Clinical complete response
cGy	CentiGray
Chemo	Chemotherapy
CI	Conformity index
cm	Centimetre
CPAP	Continuous positive airway pressure
CR	Complete response
Cr	Creatinine
CRT	Chemo-radiotherapy
CSF	Cerebrospinal fluid
CSI	Craniospinal irradiation
CSS	Cause-specific survival
CT	Computed tomography
CTCAE	Common Toxicity Criteria for Adverse Events
CT-SIM	CT simulation
CTVn	Clinical target volume of regional nodes
CTVp	Clinical target volume primary—chest wall/breast
CTV_X	Clinical target volume $x = 1, 2, 3, \ldots$
Cu	Copper
CXR	Chest X-ray
CY	Cyclophosphamide
CyK	CyberKnife
DBCG	Danish Breast Cancer Group
DCIS	Ductal carcinoma in situ
DEGRO	German Society of Radiation Oncology
DES	Diethylstilbestrol
DFS	Disease-free survival
DIBH	Deep inspiration breath hold
DIR	Deformable image registration
dL	Deciliter
DLBCL	Diffuse large B cell lymphoma
DLCO	Diffusing capacity
Dmax	Maximum dose
DRR	Digitally reconstructed radiograph
DSS	Disease-specific survival
DVH	Dose-volume histogram
EBCTCG	Early Breast Cancer Trialists' Collaborative Group
EBRT	External beam radiation therapy
ECE	Extracapsular extension
ECOG	Eastern Cooperative Oncology Group
EFRT	Extended field radiotherapy
EFS	Event-free survival
EORTC	European Organisation for Research and Treatment of Cancer
EPID	Electronic portal imaging device
ER	Oestrogen receptor
ERBB	Epidermal growth factor
ESO	European School of Oncology
ESR	Erythrocyte sedimentation rate

ESTRO	European Society for RadioTherapy
EtOH	Alcohol
EUA	Exam under anaesthesia
EUS	Endoscopic ultrasound
F/U	Follow up
FALCON	Fellowship in Anatomic deLineation and CONtouring
FDA	Food & Drug Administration
FDG	Fludeoxyglucose
FiF	Field-in-field
FISH	Fluorescence in situ hybridization
FNA	Fine needle aspiration
FOV	Field of view
FSRT	Fractionated stereotactic radiotherapy
FSU	Functional subunit
fx	Fraction(s)
GaK	Gamma Knife
GTV	Gross tumour volume
Gy	Gray
H&E	Haematoxylin and Eosin
H&P	History and physical exam
Hb	Haemoglobin
hCG	Human chorionic gonadotropin
HCV	Hepatitis C virus
HDR	High dose rate
HER2	Human epidermal growth factor receptor 2
HIV	Human immunodeficiency virus
HPV	Human papilloma virus
HRT	Hormone replacement therapy
HT	Helical tomotherapy
HTN	Hypertension
HVL	Half-value layer
Hx	History
IBR	Immediate breast reconstruction
IBTR	Ipsilateral breast tumour recurrence
ICRU	International Commission of Radiation Units and Measurements
ICS	Intercostal space
ICU	Intensive care unit
IDC	Invasive ductal carcinoma
IDL	Isodose line
IGRT	Image-guided radiotherapy
IHC	Immunohistochemical staining
IJROBP	International Journal of Radiation Oncology Biology Physics
ILC	Invasive lobular carcinoma
IM	Internal margin
im	Intramuscular
IMN	Internal mammary nodes
IMRT	Intensity-modulated radiotherapy
IOeRT	Intraoperative electron radiation therapy

IORT	Intraoperative radiation therapy
ITV	Internal target volume [ITV = CTV + IM]
iv	Intravenous
IVC	Inferior vena cava
JCO	Journal of Clinical Oncology
KPS	Karnofsky Performance Status
LABC	Locally advanced breast cancer
LCIS	Lobular carcinoma in situ
LDH	Lactate dehydrogenase
LDR	Low dose rate
LET	Linear energy transfer
LFTs	Liver function tests
LINAC	Linear accelerator
LN	Lymph node(s)
LND	Lymph node dissection
LR	Local recurrence/relapse
LRC	Local-regional control
LRF	Local-regional failure
LVEF	Left ventricular ejection fraction
LVSI	Lymphovascular space invasion
m	Metre
MDT	Multidisciplinary teams
mg	Milligram
MHD	Mean heart dose
MLC	Multileaf collimator
MLD	Mean lung dose
mm	Millimetre
mOS	Median overall survival
MRC	Medical Research Council
MRI	Magnetic resonance imaging
MRSI	Magnetic resonance spectroscopy imaging
MSKCC	Memorial Sloan Kettering Cancer Center
MTD	Maximal tolerated dose
MUGA	Multiple-gated acquisition scan
N+	Node positive
N0	Node negative
NAC	Nipple-areola complex
NCCN	National Comprehensive Cancer Network
NCI	National Cancer Institute
NCIC	National Cancer Institute of Canada
NED	No evidence of disease
NEJM	New England Journal of Medicine
NHL	Non-Hodgkin's lymphoma
NPV	Negative predictive value
NSABP	National Surgical Adjuvant Breast and Bowel Project
NSCLC	Non-small cell lung cancer
NSM	Nipple sparing mastectomy
NTCP	Normal tissue complication probability

OAR	Organ at risk
OS	Overall survival
PA	Posterior-anterior
Pb	Lead
PBI	Partial breast irradiation
pCR	Pathologic complete response
PET	Positron emission tomography
PMRT	Postmastectomy irradiation
PNI	Perineural invasion
Post-op	Postoperative
PPV	Positive predictive value
PR	Partial response
PR	Progesterone receptor
Pre-op	Preoperative
prn	as required
PROMs	Patient-reported outcomes measures
PRV	Planning organ at risk volume [PRV = OAR + IM + SM]
PS	Performance status
PST	Primary systemic therapy
PTVx	Planning target volume $x = 1,2\ldots$
q.d	Once daily
q.i.d	Four times a day (quater in die)
q.o.d	Every other day
QALY	Quality-adjusted life year
QoL	Quality of life
RBE	Relative biological effectiveness
RCT	Randomised clinical trials
RFS	Relapse-free survival
RIP	Radiation-induced pneumonitis
RNI	Regional node irradiation
ROW	Regional node irradiation
RT	Radiation therapy
RTOG	Radiation Therapy Oncology Group
RTT	Radiation therapist
s/p	Status post
SBRT	Stereotactic body radiotherapy
SCLC	Small cell lung cancer
SCV	Supraclavicular
SEER	Surveillance, Epidemiology, and End Results
SGOT	Serum glutamic oxaloacetic transaminase
SGPT	Serum glutamic pyruvic transaminase
SIB	Simultaneous integrated boost
SLNB	Sentinel lymph node biopsy
SPECT	Single-photon emission computed tomography
SPEP	Serum protein electrophoreses
SqCC	Squamous cell carcinoma
SRS	Stereotactic radiosurgery
SSM	Skin sparing mastectomy

START	UK Standardisation of Breast Radiotherapy Trial
SWOG	Southwest Oncology Group
t.i.d	Three times a day (ter in die)
TG101	AAPM Task Force Group 101
TNBC	Triple negative breast cancer
TNM	Tumour node metastasis
UCSF	University of California, San Francisco
UKCCCR	United Kingdom Coordinating Committee on Cancer Research
US	Ultrasound
USA	United States of America
vm	Voluntary moderate (vmDIBH)
VMAT	Volumetric arc radiotherapy
WART	Whole abdominal radiotherapy
Wbc	White blood cell count
WBI	Whole breast irradiation
WBRT	Whole brain radiotherapy
WHO	World Health Organization
WLE	Wide local excision

Part I

Introduction

Epidemiology

1

Toral Gathani and David Dodwell

1.1 Background

Breast cancer is an important public health challenge accounting for one in four cancers diagnosed in women and almost one in seven cancer-related deaths in women globally. In 2020, 2.25 million incident breast cancers and 685,000 breast cancer-related deaths were recorded, and these estimates are projected to rise to 3.2 million incident cases and over a million deaths by 2040. Although historically considered a "disease of the west", it should be noted that in 2018 roughly 50% of all incident cases and almost 70% of all breast cancer-related deaths occurred in less developed regions of the world [1].

Breast cancer incidence rates are highly correlated to *human development*. The *human development index* (HDI) is a composite measure taking into account health (measured by life expectancy), education (measured by years of schooling) and standard of living (measured by gross national income per capita) and is considered to be a fairer comparator of countries/regions than the use of income level alone [2]. Breast cancer mortality rates are also correlated with development, with the most unfavourable outcomes from the disease seen in the lowest resource settings [3]. There have been significant gains made in breast cancer survival in more developed countries largely achieved through early detection and diagnosis and access to comprehensive cancer care [4]. The reasons for disproportionate poorer survival in lower resource settings are multifactorial and complex but include low levels of cancer awareness, delays in presentation and variable levels of treatment provision [5].

The global age-standardised annual incidence rate for breast cancer is 47.8/100,000 but varies from an average of 75.6/100,000 in countries with a very high HDI to 36.1/100,000 in countries with a low HDI. Although the incidence rates of breast cancer are higher in more developed countries, the absolute burden of disease is almost equal in less developed countries due to their larger population numbers. Over 80% of the world population live in less developed regions, and as these countries develop, their breast cancer incidence rates will increase largely as a result of increasing life expectancy, but also due to changing reproductive patterns and lifestyles within these populations.

Age is the most important risk factor for breast cancer. In the UK, 80% of breast cancer occurs in women over the age of 50 years, and one third in women over the age of 70 years, with the highest

T. Gathani
Cancer Epidemiology Unit, Nuffield Department of Population Health, University of Oxford, Oxford, UK
e-mail: toral.gathani@ndph.ox.ac.uk

D. Dodwell (✉)
Nuffield Department of Population Health, University of Oxford, Oxford, UK
e-mail: david.dodwell@ndph.ox.ac.uk

© The Author(s), under exclusive license to Springer Nature Switzerland AG 2022

O. Kaidar-Person et al. (eds.), *Breast Cancer Radiation Therapy*,
https://doi.org/10.1007/978-3-030-91170-6_1

age-specific risks seen in the oldest of women [6]. In comparison, only half of breast cancer occurs in women over the age of 50 years in poorer countries which is largely explained by their younger populations [7]. Female global life expectancy from birth varies by almost two decades, with an average of 81 years in Europe and 63 years in Africa [8] and explains in part the lower incidence of breast cancer in less developed regions of the world. However, the increase in life expectancy that is associated with development will contribute significantly to the expected increase in breast cancer incidence globally.

The other risk factors of importance for the development of breast cancer can be classified into reproductive and non-reproductive. There is a large body of evidence supporting the role of hormones, and in particular exposure to endogenous and exogenous oestrogens in the subsequent development of breast cancer. An increased breast cancer risk is associated with earlier menarche and later menopause but with differing magnitudes of effect. The excess risk associated with lengthening a woman's reproductive years by 1 year at menarche is greater than the excess associated with 1 year's lengthening at menopause [9]. Childbearing reduces the risk of breast cancer and the higher the number of full-term pregnancies, the greater the protection. There is no effect of breast cancer risk associated with loss of pregnancy either as a result of spontaneous or induced abortion [10]. The risk of breast cancer reduces by 7% with each full-term pregnancy, and overall women who have had children have a 30% lower risk than nulliparous women. Women who breastfeed reduce their risk of developing breast cancer compared with women who do not breastfeed, and there is a dose-dependent effect as breast cancer risk reduces by 4% for every 12 months of breastfeeding [11]. The use of exogenous hormones in reproductive life, in the form of the contraceptive pill, is associated with a small increased risk of breast cancer [12], as is the use of hormone replacement therapy in non-reproductive life [13].

Non-reproductive factors for breast cancer of importance include alcohol consumption and obesity and should be considered modifiable risk factors for the disease. Alcohol consumption increases breast cancer risk in women who consume 2–3 units of alcohol daily [14, 15]. Postmenopausal obesity is associated with increased breast cancer risk probably due to increased circulating oestrogens [16], and taller women are also at an increased risk [17]. There is little evidence to show that vegetarian diets are protective [18, 19].

Up to 5% of breast cancer in Western countries may be a result of a genetic predisposition to the disease, such as the *BRCA1* and *BRCA2* gene mutations. High-risk allele mutations probably account for most of the families with four or more cases of breast cancer, and for around 20–25% of the familial breast cancer risk overall, but for only 5% of all breast cancers [20]. Women who have a positive history of breast cancer are at a two-fold increased relative risk of breast cancer; however, most of these women will never develop breast cancer and most who do will do so after the age of 50 years [21].

1.2 Summary

The epidemiology of breast cancer is complex but understanding differences in the epidemiology of breast cancer in different countries will underpin the development of effective breast cancer care and control policies which have utility in different resource settings and are relevant to the needs of local populations and translate to improved outcomes from the disease.

References

1. Globocan. Cancer Today. 2020. https://gco.iarc.fr/today/home. Accessed Mar 2022.
2. United Nations Development Programme. Human development reports. 2020. http://hdr.undp.org/en/content/humandevelopment-index-hdi. Accessed Mar 2022.
3. Ferlay J, Ervik M, Lam F, Colombet M, Mery L, Piñeros M, et al. Global cancer observatory: cancer today. Lyon: International Agency for Research on Cancer; 2018. https://gco.iarc.fr/today. Accessed Mar 2022.
4. Beral V, Peto R. UK cancer survival statistics. BMJ. 2010;341:c4112.

5. Anderson BO, Cazap E, El Saghir NS, Yip C, Khaled H, Otero I, et al. Optimisation of breast cancer management in low-resource and middle-resource countries: executive summary of the Breast Health Global Initiative consensus, 2010. Lancet Oncol. 2011;12:387–98.
6. Cancer Research UK. Breast cancer statistics. 2020 https://www.cancerresearchuk.org/health-professional/cancer-statistics/statistics-by-cancer-type/breast-cancer. Accessed Mar 2022.
7. Gupta S. Breast cancer in India: a continuing challenge. Indian J Cancer. 2010;47(1):1–2.
8. World Health Organisation. The global health observatory. 2020. https://www.who.int/data/gho/data/indicators/indicator-details/GHO/lifeexpectancy-at-birth-(years). Accessed Mar 2022.
9. Collaborative Group on Hormonal Factors in Breast Cancer. Menarche, menopause and breast cancer risk: individual participant meta-analysis including 118964 women with breast cancer from 117 epidemiological studies. Lancet Oncol. 2012;13:1141–51.
10. Beral V, Bull D, Doll R, Peto R, Reeves G, Collaborative Group on Hormonal Factors in Breast Cancer. Breast cancer and abortion: collaborative reanalysis of data from 53 epidemiological studies, including 83000 women with breast cancer from 16 countries. Lancet. 2004;363(9414):1007–16.
11. Collaborative Group on Hormonal Factors in Breast Cancer. Breast cancer and breastfeeding: collaborative reanalysis of individual data from 47 epidemiological studies in 30 countries, including 50302 women with breast cancer and 96973 women without the disease. Lancet. 2002;360(9328):187–95.
12. Collaborative Group on Hormonal Factors in Breast Cancer. Breast cancer and hormonal contraceptives: collaborative reanalysis of individual data on 53 297 women with breast cancer and 100 239 women without breast cancer from 54 epidemiological studies. Lancet. 1996;347(9017):1713–27.
13. Collaborative Group on Hormonal Factors in Breast Cancer. Type and timing of menopausal hormone therapy and breast cancer risk: individual participant meta-analysis of the worldwide epidemiological evidence. Lancet. 2019;394(10204):1159–68.
14. Collaborative Group on Hormonal Factors in Breast Cancer. Alcohol, tobacco and breast cancer—collaborative reanalysis of individual data from 53 epidemiological studies, including 58,515 women with breast cancer and 95,067 women without the disease. Br J Cancer. 2002;87(11):1234–45.
15. Allen NE, Beral V, Casabonne D, Kan SW, Reeves GK, Brown A, et al. Moderate alcohol intake and cancer incidence in women. J Natl Cancer Inst. 2009;101(5):296–305.
16. Key T. Endogenous oestrogens and breast cancer risk in premenopausal and postmenopausal women. Steroids. 2011;76(8):812–5.
17. Green J, Cairns BJ, Cassabonne D, Wright FL, Reeves G, Beral V. Height and cancer incidence in the Million Women Study: prospective cohort, and meta-analysis of prospective studies for height and total cancer risk. Lancet Oncol. 2011;12(8):785–94.
18. Gathani T, Barnes I, Ali R, Arumugham R, Chacko R, Digumarti R, et al. Lifelong vegetarianism and breast cancer risk: a large multicentre case control study in India. BMC Womens Health. 2017;17(1):6.
19. Key T, Appleby P, Rosell M. Health effects of vegetarian and vegan diets. Proc Nutr Soc. 2006;65:35–41.
20. Key T, Verkasalo P, Banks E. Epidemiology of breast cancer. Lancet Oncol. 2001;2:133–40.
21. Collaborative Group on Hormonal Factors in Breast Cancer. Familial breast cancer: collaborative reanalysis of individual data from 52 epidemiological studies including 58,209 women with breast cancer and 101,986 women without the disease. Lancet. 2001;358(9291):1389–99.

General Management

2

Riccardo Alberto Audisio, Philip Poortmans, and Gabriel Hortobagyi

2.1 Background

Substantial progress has been made in the conceptual approach and clinical management of breast cancer over the past decades. Much of the progress was the result of hypothesis-driven research, with stepwise improvements in all aspects of diagnosis and treatment of the various stages of the disease. Improved three-dimensional imaging of the primary lesion and regional lymph nodes resulted in improved surgical and RT planning. BCT has largely supplanted mastectomy, and sentinel lymph node biopsy has replaced axillary lymph node dissection in most patients. Technical progress ensures the delivery of maximally effective RT to the target area, while limiting the dose to surrounding normal tissues. Well-designed and powered clinical trials have defined the respective roles and the interaction between surgery and RT, while the youngest discipline in the armamentarium against breast cancer, the use of systemic therapies, simultaneously made major strides. Targeted hormonal interventions and cytotoxic chemotherapy are now important tools for the management of breast cancer, both for metastatic disease and as an adjuvant treatment, to further improve outcomes. More recently, the introduction of newer targeted agents has revolutionised the management of several subtypes of breast cancer.

As for much of the first 70 years of the twentieth century, radical mastectomy was the only treatment for non-metastatic disease, patients with suspected breast abnormalities were first seen and evaluated by a surgeon who, upon completing the assessment, proceeded to an incisional (or sometimes excisional) biopsy, followed by a radical mastectomy, often within hours after the diagnosis. Other disciplines were not involved or consulted, and the patient was only referred to other specialists in case the surgical treatment failed, or if the surgeon feared his treatment would be insufficient to control the tumour. By the mid-century, a few courageous radiation oncologists proposed combinations of limited surgical excisions with comprehensive RT, causing much controversy. It was only in the 1960s that, by force, these two fields of science were brought together, leading to increased discussions about joint decision-making to define the best sequence and com-

R. A. Audisio
Institute of Clinical Sciences, Sahlgrenska University Hospital, Göteborg, Sweden
e-mail: raudisio@doctors.org.uk

P. Poortmans (✉)
Faculty of Medicine and Health Sciences, University of Antwerp, Antwerp, Belgium

Department of Radiation Oncology, Iridium Netwerk, Antwerp, Belgium
e-mail: philip.poortmans@gza.be

G. Hortobagyi
Department of Radiation Oncology, Iridium Netwerk, Antwerp, TX, Belgium
e-mail: ghortoba@mdanderson.org

© The Author(s), under exclusive license to Springer Nature Switzerland AG 2022

O. Kaidar-Person et al. (eds.), *Breast Cancer Radiation Therapy*,
https://doi.org/10.1007/978-3-030-91170-6_2

bination of therapies. In the 1970s, the emerging role of systemic therapies led to the practice of sequential consultations in the management of primary breast cancer, followed by the development by leading cancer centres of multidisciplinary planning clinics, where all relevant diagnostic and therapeutic specialist met and discussed the optimal combination and sequence of therapies. These improved interactions led to better planning and, ultimately, better long-term outcomes. At this point, the direct communication and two-way discussion took place between the therapeutic specialists (breast surgeon, radiation oncologist and medical oncologist) and the diagnostic team (imaging and pathology), in such a way that they all had the opportunity to assess the patient before any treatment was given; this allowed contributing a complete and accurate information to the multispecialty team. Equally important, the results of these discussions could be shared with the patient and her family, the existing options were explained, recommendations were made and the patient's choice of therapy implemented. What a dramatic change! No longer did the patient wake up from anaesthesia for a biopsy not knowing whether she had had a mastectomy or not; diagnosis, staging and treatment planning were now completed in a systematic manner, leading to better decision-making and improved outcomes. This process did not develop overnight and required concessions from all therapeutic team members. It also led to hypothesis-based multidisciplinary clinical trials to resolve clinical controversies.

Today, all patients with malignant breast disease have the right, as described in the recent update of "The requirements of a specialist breast centre" by the European Society of Breast Cancer Specialists (EUSOMA) and endorsed by the European Cancer Organisation as part of Essential Requirements for Quality Cancer Care (ERQCC) programme, and by ESMO, to be treated according to the following infrastructure and organisation [1]:

- Patients should be treated in a breast centre, including all services, from genetics and prevention, over diagnosis, through the treatment of the primary tumour, to care of advanced disease, supportive, palliative and psychosocial care, and follow-up.
- The multidisciplinary team (MDT) consists of dedicated breast cancer specialists working together in the breast centre, with access to all facilities required to deliver high-quality care throughout the breast cancer pathway.
- Breast cancer management entails knowledge of state-of-the-art literature; availability of guidelines, protocols, recommendations and minimal standards; clearly defined local policies and available resources and organise regular quality control including au breast data audits and formal internal review meetings.
- All new diagnoses and changes of treatment plans have to be discussed during a breast multidisciplinary meeting (MDM), where the core MDT members meet to evaluate and plan patient care at any step of the diagnostic and treatment process.
- If indicated, but not routinely involved for every patient, supplementary specialists are to be consulted during the multidisciplinary meeting to discuss and participate in breast cancer care and treatment: psycho-oncologists, geriatric oncologists, oncology pharmacists, nuclear medicine physicians, physiotherapists, plastic surgeons, interventional radiologists, self-image professionals, palliative care specialists, clinical geneticists and prevention specialists.
- A breast centre must be of sufficient size to manage at least 150 newly diagnosed cases of early breast cancer and at least 50 cases of metastatic breast annually [2]. This minimum number is necessary to maintain expertise for each team member and to ensure cost-effective working of the breast centre [3]. Moreover, there is good quality data that shows that breast cancer survival is related to the number of cases treated per annum [4]. As such, the

minimum caseload for core MDT members is clearly advised as well.
- The process of conforming to structured guidelines by obtaining a "Breast Centres Certification" is ongoing and rapidly growing [5].

Finally, the work in a breast centre has to be patient-centred [6]. It is now mandatory to prioritise, incorporating important factors including patient's aims and expectations; patient's fitness, frailty, life expectancy and cognition; patient's compliance to treatment; patient's social and familial network; alongside with elements of rather logistic nature including geography and access to health care and the availability of caregivers. In this light, it is time to capitalise on the enormous number of real-time information collected and to get patient-reported outcomes into the game—this would give unsustainable approaches a reason to disappear, while poorly recognised but well-appreciated treatments room to become more broadly available.

References

1. Biganzoli L, Cardoso F, Beishon M, Cameron D, Cataliotti L, Coles CE, et al. The requirements of a specialist breast centre. Breast. 2020;51:65–84.
2. Biganzoli L, Marotti L, Hart CD, Cataliotti L, Cutuli B, Kühn T, et al. Quality indicators in breast cancer care: an update from the EUSOMA working group. Eur J Cancer. 2017;86:59–81.
3. Grilli R, Minozzi S, Tinazzi A, Labianca R, Sheldon TA, Liberati A. Do specialists do it better? The impact of specialization on the processes and outcomes of care for cancer patients. Ann Oncol. 1998;9:365–74.
4. Roohan PJ, Bickell NA, Baptiste MS, Therriault GD, Ferrara EP, Siu AL. Hospital volume differences and five-year survival from breast cancer. Am J Public Health. 1998;88:454–7.
5. https://www.breastcentrescertification.com/
6. Fayanju OM, Mayo TL, Spinks TE, Lee S, Barcenas CH, Smith BD, et al. Value-based breast cancer care: a multidisciplinary approach for defining patient-centered outcomes. Ann Surg Oncol. 2016;23:2385–90.

Part II

Quality Management

3 Education and Training

Sandra Turner, Zvi Symon, and Jesper Grau Eriksen

3.1 Introduction

The links between health professional education and training, patient outcomes and organisational quality and safety within health systems are well established [1–3]. Consequently, ensuring high-quality evidence-based education for all radiation oncology professionals is crucial in optimising cancer patient care, particularly for those undergoing radiation therapy.

Supplementary Information The online version contains supplementary material available at [https://doi.org/10.1007/978-3-030-91170-6_3].

S. Turner (✉)
Western Sydney Radiation Oncology Network, Westmead Hospital, Westmead, NSW, Australia
e-mail: sandra.turner1@optusnet.com.au

Z. Symon
Chair Radiation Oncology, Sheba Medical Center, Tel Hashomer, Ramat Gan, Israel
e-mail: symonz@sheba.health.gov.il

J. Grau Eriksen
Department of Experimental Clinical Oncology, Aarhus University Hospital, Aarhus N, Denmark

Department of Oncology, Research 2, Aarhus University Hospital, Aarhus N, Denmark
e-mail: jesper@oncology.au.dk

3.2 Theoretical Background

Explicit competency- (or learning outcome-) based curricula are a recognised requirement for effective health professional learning [4, 5]. Such curricula must be supported by structured training programmes providing the full scope of opportunities for learning, appropriate supervision and assessment of progression and competence. Curriculum frameworks such as CanMEDS (Canadian Medical Education Directives for Specialists) support the design of such curricula [6], including for radiation oncology training [7, 8]. Modern curriculum frameworks serve to highlight the multiple overlapping roles of health professionals in addition to their core expertise, e.g. medical expertise for doctors, physics knowledge and skills for medical physicists, and so on (Fig. 3.1).

By way of example, some skills to be mastered by training radiation oncologists in managing breast cancer and the links to the CanMEDS Medical Expert and other ('Intrinsic') roles are shown in Table 3.1.

It is important to recognise that education is an on-going commitment for all health professionals in order to maintain currency and expertise. Life-long learning is of utmost relevance to the field of radiation oncology due to its rapid and continual evolution.

© The Author(s), under exclusive license to Springer Nature Switzerland AG 2022

O. Kaidar-Person et al. (eds.), *Breast Cancer Radiation Therapy*,
https://doi.org/10.1007/978-3-030-91170-6_3

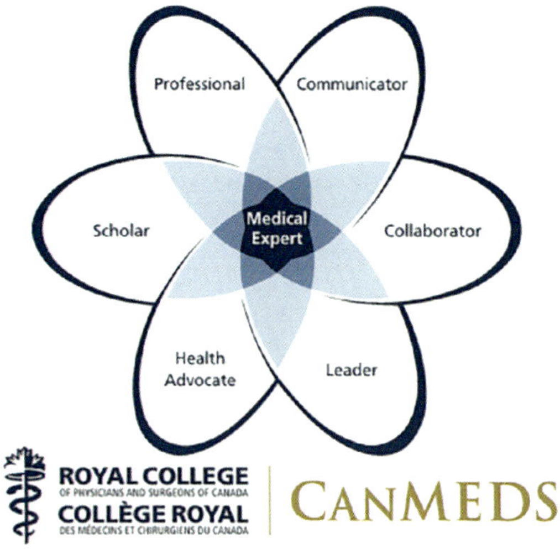

Fig. 3.1 CanMEDS diagram showing the multiple roles of the medical specialist. (Copyright © 2015 The Royal College of Physicians and Surgeons of Canada. http://www.royalcollege.ca/rcsite/canmeds/canmeds-framework-e. Reproduced with permission)

Table 3.1 Example radiation oncologist competencies and corresponding CanMEDS roles

Competence	CanMEDS role/s
Assessing a new patient for breast radiation therapy	Medical expert, communicator
Presenting a patient & actively participating in a breast cancer multidisciplinary meeting	Medical expert, collaborator, advocate, scholar
Contouring target volumes & organs/structures at risk for a course of breast radiation therapy	Medical expert
Recruiting & consenting a woman with breast cancer to a clinical trial	Medical expert, communicator, scholar
Managing psychosocial/sexual &/or cultural issues relating to change in body image following breast cancer treatment	Medical expert, communicator, professional
Participating in a quality improvement project (e.g. to streamline bookings for breast radiation therapy at your centre)	Collaborator, leader

3.3 Foundational Oncology Sciences

All radiation oncology professionals require education in the sciences underlying the safe practice of oncology including planning and delivery of radiation therapy. The different radiation oncology professional team members need varying levels of expertise across the subjects of cancer/radiation biology, radiation physics, oncological anatomy including imaging techniques and pathology.

3.4 Core Requirements for Training Institutions/Departments

Training institutions should be accredited in accordance with national and/or international regulations. The training institution, either alone or in cooperation with other regional departments, must be adequately equipped to support both the workload and range of radiation oncology services required for training professionals in state-of-the-art breast radiation oncology. If such minimum requirements cannot be met by a single institution, several training institutions should offer an integrated programme that meet the minimum requirements.

For standardising work-place-based training and ensuring that minimum competences are reached, the programme should be founded on a nationally or internationally recognised core curriculum (or both). Training departments must also facilitate access to a formal programme of theoretical learning and provide resources to ensure trainees gain the knowledge they require. International courses dealing with clinical and/or technical skills in the management of breast cancer may add value to the local radiation oncology breast cancer curriculum [9].

The human resources necessary for high-quality education are vitally important. Qualified trainers (radiation oncologists, radiation physicists and radiation therapists) that educate trainees should be sufficient in number to provide continuous training and easy access to supervision. It is advised that medical trainees are exposed to several radiation/clinical oncologists that have different perspectives on the content being learned. Furthermore, it is recommended that trainers themselves undergo ongoing training in supervision and teaching methods in order to maintain a high pedagogical level of training delivery [9].

3.5 Requirements for Work-Place-Based Clinical and Technical Education

In order to receive comprehensive training, the radiation oncology trainee should be exposed to an adequate case-mix and a sufficient number of breast cancer patients to mirror the full spectrum of disease. Thus, trainees must have access to patients at all stages of cancer—from early diagnosis to completion of follow-up as well as in terminal care. It is important that the trainee requires the hands-on experience in all practical procedures that is required to work independently as a future specialist. Such skills are wide-ranging, for example, the ability to lead a breast cancer multidisciplinary team conference, mastering difficult conversations with patients, being aware of acute and late morbidities and how to manage these, as well as having the appropriate technical skills in delineation and planning of breast cancer radiation therapy. Preferably, training should take place in departments that actively participate in breast cancer research in order that trainees be exposed to practical challenges of acquiring scientific data and to facilitate skills in critical appraisal of the scientific literature [9].

3.6 Assessment of Learning

Although summative evaluation (e.g. formal examinations) has value in driving learning, it cannot stand alone in modern work-place-based education. Formative assessment that evaluates progression in line with curriculum competencies (knowledge, skills and attitudes) is even more important and allows timely and repeated feedback to the trainee. In addition, formative assessments help determine if the trainee can be granted additional responsibility in their daily work. Milestones and Entrusted Professional Activities (EPAs) have developed as useful tools to ascertain such progress, i.e. does the trainee have the required competencies to be entrusted to work more independently or to aim at acquiring higher level skills? [10]. An example of an EPA for breast cancer radiation oncology is shown in Table 3.2.

Formative evaluation can be achieved in a variety of ways, for instance direct observation during a work procedure with structured feedback from a supervisor, audit of learning portfolios and applying multisource feedback tools. These assessment methods are very reliable for testing practical skills and other competencies. Such evaluations need to be performed regularly throughout training in order to be most effective. Formative work-place-based evaluation and summative assessment are complementary and can supplement each other when applied in a balanced way [11].

3.7 Effective Educational Methods

A central challenge in educating members of any team is to address both the lack of knowledge and skill of the novice and the, sometimes misguided, assuredness of the experienced mem-

Table 3.2 Example of an entrusted professional activity (EPA) for breast cancer management

Milestone: The trainee can independently evaluate a radiation treatment plan for breast cancer
EPA: Independent plan evaluation
Assessed by direct structured observation by a supervisor including discussion of (but not limited to): • Indication for radiation therapy, dose and fractionation • Previous radiotherapy or contraindications • Is positioning appropriate for the target in question? • Evaluation of target volumes (TV) and organs at risk (OAR) delineation. Sufficient number of OARs? • Evaluation of dose levels, homogeneity and dose distribution • Evaluation of constraints met or not met—median doses vs. max dose and use of dose–volume histograms (DVH) • Discuss the balance between TV coverage and OAR involvement • If compromises are made—why, where and possible consequences

bers. Team-based education initiatives are highly valuable as they improve understanding of how, if performed incorrectly, steps of a process can cascade into a sequence of errors that could otherwise go unrecognised and have major consequences. For example, a tense painful shoulder girdle during the planning CT in a woman who has recently undergone breast and axillary surgery, compounded by a cold bunker and a non-empathic caregiver, can result in an unreproducible set-up for treatment delivery which if uncorrected, could under-dose the target or deposit unnecessary dose in normal tissues.

Some useful approaches to engage learners include:

- *Peer-Based Comparisons*. For example, a peer-based comparison of how different radiation therapists/technologists deal empathetically with an anxious patient [12], or how different radiation oncologists contour treatment volumes, or how different dosimetrists deal with hotspots, are helpful platforms on which the trainer can build their discussion and teaching.
- *Blended Learning*. Combining interactive live (or virtual) learning with computer-assisted learning (including exercises, quizzes and videos) such as for contouring workshops, is an engaging approach to learning. National and international societies (e.g. ASTRO, ESTRO, IAEA) hold contouring and treatment planning workshops and refresher courses. It is especially enriching to connect with professionals at other centres to learn how they approach the same challenges. For example, ESTRO's FALCON programme (Fellowship in Anatomic Delineation and Contouring) is an online multifunctional Educase® platform for contouring and delineation. FALCON workshops are held for different disease sites and/or organs at risk contouring. The workshops are aimed at all radiation oncology professionals and trainees wanting to improve their contouring skills or to refresh knowledge. Workshops provide direct participant feedback and contouring comparisons under supervision from FALCON teaching faculty.
- *Simulation-Based Training*. To err is human. Virtual breast cancer RT environments allow trainees to make mistakes safely. The Virtual Education in Radiation Therapy (VERT) platform (www.vertual.co.uk) [13] is a sophisticated RT simulation system used mainly for radiation therapist technical training. Another example of simulation in training radiation oncology professionals is the use of role-playing actors for building communication skills. Audio-visual recording, debriefing and constructive feedback are central components of simulation-based training. Collaboration with experienced existing medical simulation and training facilities and the IAEA "Train the Trainers" initiative are useful in establishing a tailored programme [14].
- *Error-Based Learning*. Identifying and learning from common mistakes is a useful approach and easily implemented without sophisticated equipment. The inability to recognise an error is associated with a complete gap or an incomplete understanding of necessary core knowledge components comprising the entirety of the process. For example, in Fig. 3.2, the knowledge necessary to detect and correct the error includes an understanding of isodose plots, hotspots, the impact of varying separations, depth dose curves of different photon energies, wedges and the use of segments or the "field within field" concept.

3.8 Summary

In summary, there is a wealth of evidence-based techniques and tools for effective learning in radiation oncology as it applies to the treatment of breast cancer, as well as other tumour sites. These methods are not only valuable to novice learners in the field but should be used as part of life-long learning for all our professionals. It is the responsibility of the individual (regardless of seniority) as well as training institutions and treatment departments to ensure that knowledge

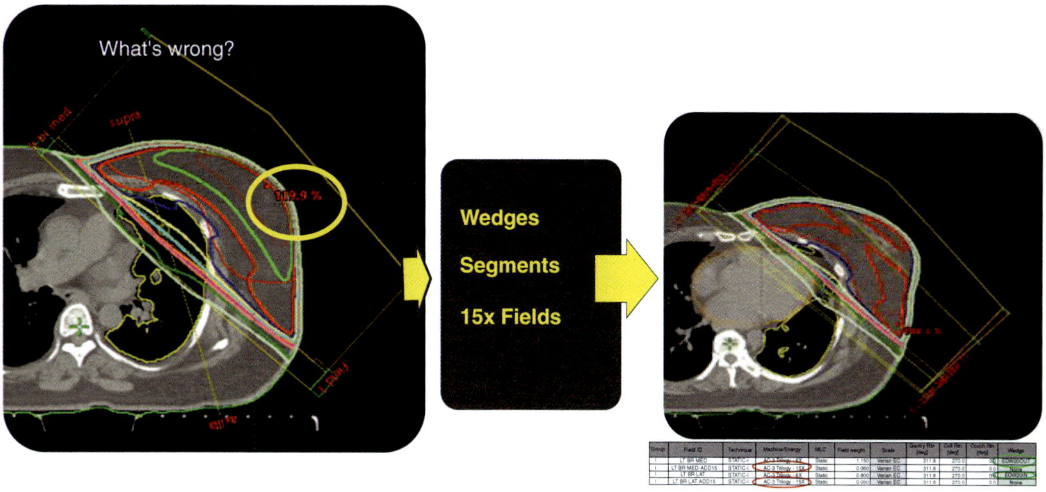

Fig. 3.2 Summary figure demonstrating error-based learning. Supervisor notes: Ask the trainee to review the plan and identify the error. Note the high hotspot (119.9%). Discuss the cause of the hotspot including the large separation and use of 6MV beams only. Discuss how to correct the plan with the use of higher energy photons, wedges and/or segments (field within field). Discuss the corrected plan. For the full teaching slide set, go to link: https//etc

and skills are up to date, and "old ways" are constantly challenged. These goals could not be more important in our rapidly evolving discipline. Finally, compliance with the known evidence supporting high-quality education programmes should underpin all radiation oncology professional training, not be considered an optional extra. Optimal education is thus a foundation to optimal care for patients undergoing RT for breast cancer.

References

1. Asch D, et al. Evaluating obstetrical residency programs using patient outcomes. JAMA. 2009;302:1277–83.
2. Kerfoot B, et al. Durable improvements in prostate cancer screening from online spaced education. Am J Prev Med. 2010;39(5):472–8.
3. Barker J. Error reduction through team leadership: what surgeons can learn from the airline industry. Clin Neurosurg. 2007;54:195.
4. Iobst WF, Sherbino J, Cate OT, Richardson DL, Dath D, Swing SR, Harris P, Mungroo R, Holmboe ES, Frank JR. Competency-based medical education in postgraduate medical education. Med Teach. 2010;32(8):651–6. https://doi.org/10.3109/0142159X.2010.500709. PMID: 20662576.
5. Rosenblatt E, Prajogi G, Barton M, Fidarova E, Eriksen J, Hafty B, et al. Need for competency-based radiation oncology in developing countries. Creat Educ. 2017;8:66–80.
6. Frank J, Snell L, Sherbono J. CanMEDS 2015 physican competency framework. Ottawa: Royal College of Physicians and Surgeons of Canada; 2015.
7. Benstead K, Lara PC, Andreopoulos D, Bibault JE, Dix A, Eller YG, Franco P, Guiliani M, Jaal J, Juretic A, Kozma E, Lumsden G, Maddalo M, Magrini S, Mjaaland I, Pfeffer R, de Sousa de Sa Pinto OMT, Spalek M, Vozenin MC, Verfaillie C, Van Egten V, Eriksen JG. Recommended ESTRO core curriculum for radiation oncology/radiotherapy 4th edition. Radiother Oncol. 2019;141:1–4. https://doi.org/10.1016/j.radonc.2019.08.013. Epub 2019 Sep 5. PMID: 31495514
8. Turner S, Seel M, Berry M. Radiation Oncology Training Program Curriculum developments in Australia and New Zealand: design, implementation and evaluation—what next? J Med Imaging Radiat Oncol. 2015;59:728–35.
9. Eriksen JG, Beavis AW, Coffey MA, Leer JW, Magrini SM, Benstead K, Boelling T, Hjälm-Eriksson M, Kantor G, Maciejewski B, Mezeckis M, Oliveira A, Thirion P, Vitek P, Olsen DR, Eudaldo T, Enghardt W, François P, Garibaldi C, Heijmen B, Josipovic M, Major T, Nikoletopoulos S, Rijnders A, Waligorski M, Wasilewska-Radwanska M, Mullaney L, Boejen A, Vaandering A, Vandevelde G, Verfaillie C, Pötter R. The updated ESTRO core curricula 2011 for clinicians, medical physicists and RTTs in radiotherapy/radiation oncology. Radiother

Oncol. 2012;103(1):103–8. https://doi.org/10.1016/j.radonc.2012.02.007. Epub 2012 Mar 21. PMID: 22444243.

10. Dewey CM, Jonker G, Ten Cate O, Turner TL. Entrustable professional activities (EPAs) for teachers in medical education: has the time come? Med Teach. 2017;39(8):894–6. https://doi.org/10.1080/0142159X.2016.1270447. Epub 2016 Dec 27. PMID: 28027689.
11. Hawkins RE, Welcher CM, Holmboe ES, Kirk LM, Norcini JJ, Simons KB, Skochelak SE. Implementation of competency-based medical education: are we addressing the concerns and challenges? Med Educ. 2015;49(11):1086–102. https://doi.org/10.1111/medu.12831. PMID: 26494062.
12. Riess H, Kraft-Todd G. E.M.P.A.T.H.Y.: a tool to enhance nonverbal communication between clinicians and their patients. Acad Med. 2014;89(8):1108–12. https://doi.org/10.1097/ACM.0000000000000287. PMID: 24826853.
13. Leong A, Herst P, Kane P. VERT, a virtual clinical environment, enhances understanding of radiation therapy planning concepts. J Med Radiat Sci. 2018;65(2):97–105. https://doi.org/10.1002/jmrs.272. Epub 2018 Mar 8. PMID: 29516649; PMCID: PMC5986053.
14. Katzman T, Symon Z, Shelly E, Luxenburg O. Case report: a novel model for educating radiation therapists in small countries: case study of the "Train the Trainer" initiative in Israel. Tech Innov Patient Support Radiat Oncol. 2018;8:10–2. https://doi.org/10.1016/j.tipsro.2018.09.004. PMID: 32095582; PMCID: PMC703379.

4 International Criteria for Excellence Breast Centres

Lorenza Marotti, Isabel Teresa Rubio, and Luigi Cataliotti

4.1 Background

The Manifesto, following the 1st European Breast Cancer Conference (EBCC) [1], held in Florence in 1998, had drawn the attention of health professionals, advocacy, institutions at national and European level to the urgent need of setting up all over Europe dedicated Units for Breast Cancer Care. Therefore, Eusoma took the commitment and the challenge to define the requirements for such dedicated Breast Cancer Units [2], first published in 2000.

During the last 20 years, a lot has been done to achieve the difficult aim of harmonising quality breast cancer care in Europe, but not enough, as highlighted in the 2016 EBCC manifesto [3], which claimed that the 2016 deadline set by the 2006 European Parliament resolution [4] has not been met: in Europe still too many patients do not have access to Breast Units or Breast Centres, as they are also called today.

In the last 20 years, following the first publication of the position paper, Eusoma has regularly updated the requirements, to make sure that these indications are constantly aligned with the advances in breast cancer care.

This document has become a milestone for the implementation of Breast Centres, not only for health professionals but also for hospital management and local/national and international authorities.

In 2020, Eusoma has published the last updating of the requirements, a completely revised document, which has seen the collaboration and endorsement of ECCO as part of the Quality Cancer Care programme and ESMO [5].

"*The requirements of a specialist breast centre*" gives indication on the different aspects that have to be taken into consideration for the management of breast cancer care, defining detailed requirements on how a breast centre has to be organised in terms of:

L. Marotti (✉)
European Society of Breast Cancer Specialists (EUSOMA), Florence, Italy
e-mail: lorenza.marotti@eusoma.org

I. T. Rubio
Breast Surgical Oncology, Clinica Universidad de Navarra, Madrid, Spain
e-mail: irubior@unav.es

L. Cataliotti
Breast Centres Certification, Florence, Italy

© The Author(s), under exclusive license to Springer Nature Switzerland AG 2022
O. Kaidar-Person et al. (eds.), *Breast Cancer Radiation Therapy*,
https://doi.org/10.1007/978-3-030-91170-6_4

- Case load, both in the early and metastatic setting
- Core and extended team
- Multidisciplinary approach
- Services and equipment that have to be available
- Patient pathway from diagnosis to follow-up including advanced disease, palliative care and end of live
- Research and education
- Data collection and quality control

The principle, linking together the different aspects involved in breast cancer care, is the multidisciplinary approach, which is the base for building up a cohesive team and for ensuring an integrated patient care.

A retrospective, comparative interventional cohort study on 13,722 women has demonstrated that after multidisciplinary care was introduced, breast cancer mortality was 18% lower in the intervention area than in the non-intervention area [6]. Another national cohort study comparing patients with multidisciplinary treatment with those without has shown a significant increase of survival rate in the multidisciplinary intervention group [7].

Expertise and dedication is another important element that contributes to the delivery of optimal patient care, as it makes sure that health professionals have received the adequate training, have reached and keep the necessary expertise in terms of procedures delivered per annum, and time dedicated to all those other activities that build up a dedicated specialist, i.e. participation in multidisciplinary and audit meeting, outpatient clinics, research, scientific work, attendance at courses and conferences. In literature, evidence on specialist volume is partially based on breast surgery. A study found that a high hospital and surgeon volume predicted lower subsequent re-operation following breast conservative surgery [8]. A systemic review on the relation volume–outcome in breast surgery has highlighted that improved survival was associated with high volume providers [9].

Within the concept of continuum of care and multidisciplinary approach, primary care plays an important role also in the frame of breast cancer care [10].

Excellence goes together with quality. Only through a rigorous quality control of performance and outcomes, a team can demonstrate the quality and the level of excellence they are offering to breast cancer patients.

For this reason, Eusoma has defined a set of Quality Indicators in Breast Cancer Care [11] that each Breast Centre has to monitor to make sure they are offering to their patients a quality standard of care.

To do that, it is essential that Breast Centres collect in a database the data for each patient through the pathway from diagnosis to follow-up and advanced disease.

The analysis of data compared with the target standard set by Eusoma, and/or any other referring societies, gives to the Breast Centre team the state of the art about the level of their patient care.

Eusoma has created a Datacentre, which in compliance with the European Regulation on privacy, includes data on patients treated in the European breast centres that undergo the certification process based on Eusoma requirements and wish to participate in benchmarking activity (see Fig. 4.1). The datacentre makes the analysis on the compliance with quality indicators and for each Breast Centre issues a data report detailing the performance for each quality indicator, which is used for internal audit and quality indicator evaluation within the certification process.

This represents an important tool for discussion among the health professionals to find solutions to raise the bar and make all efforts to improve their performance to the benefit of the patients.

But internal audits represent only one piece of a comprehensive quality control.

To improve quality of care, it is important that Breast Centre measures with defined standard at national and or international level and that their compliance to these is evaluated by an external audit.

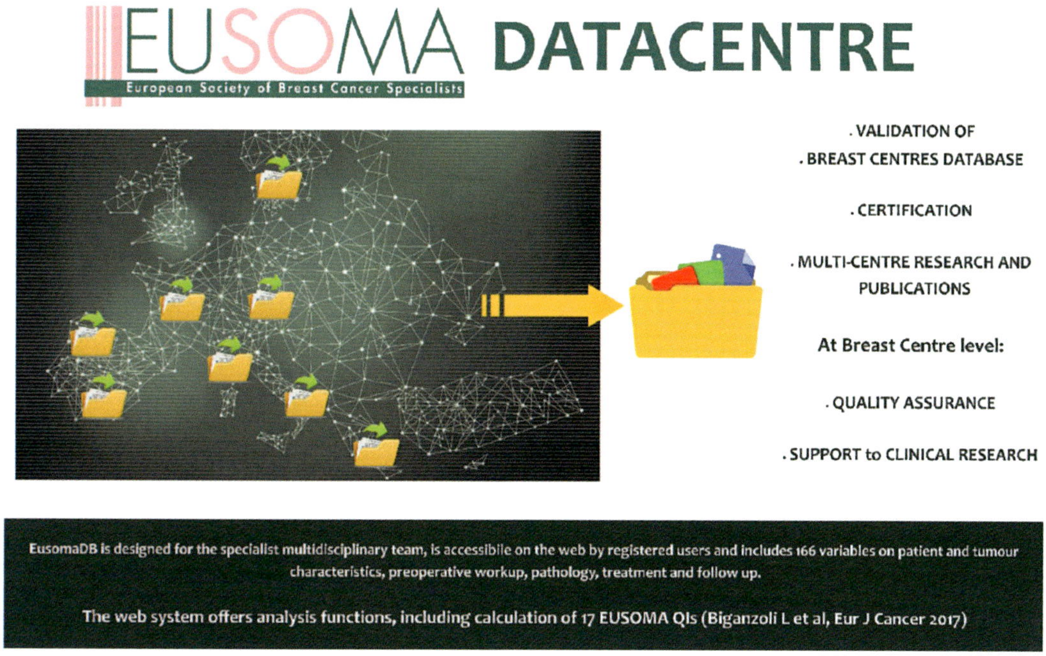

Fig. 4.1 Requirements for EUSOMA accreditation Eusoma Datacentre

Looking with external eyes, through a defined quality scheme, i.e. certification processes or accreditation helps in highlighting all the issues that can be improved or need intervention and make sure that the Breast Centre takes formal commitment in finding solutions, taking action and showing compliance with the defined standards.

In Europe, there are several national projects on quality control, i.e. certification processes, accreditation or peer review programmes such as the German Cancer Society voluntary certification system [12], the National Accreditation programme of Breast Centre (NAPBC) run by the America College of surgery [13], The NABON Breast Cancer Audit in the Netherlands [14].

The European Commission has also developed an initiative on Breast Cancer (ECIBC), to develop the new edition on screening and diagnosis guidelines and the quality assurance scheme to develop a set of quality and safety requirements for Breast Centres in Europe [15].

A European voluntary certification process, "Breast Centres Certification" (see Fig. 4.2), with an accredited scheme, has been developed [16] based on the Eusoma requirements and Quality Indicators.

4.2 Summary

It is now more than 20 years that Eusoma has published the first version of the requirements of a specialist Breast Centre, but steps forward still need to be made to ensure that breast cancer patients has equitable access to Breast Centres in Europe regardless the country where they live. This can be achieved only with a common action among health professionals, policy makers and patients' advocates. This is another challenge to show that only joining efforts and competencies we can make it, for the benefit of the entire society as women play a pivotal role in the family, the working and social context.

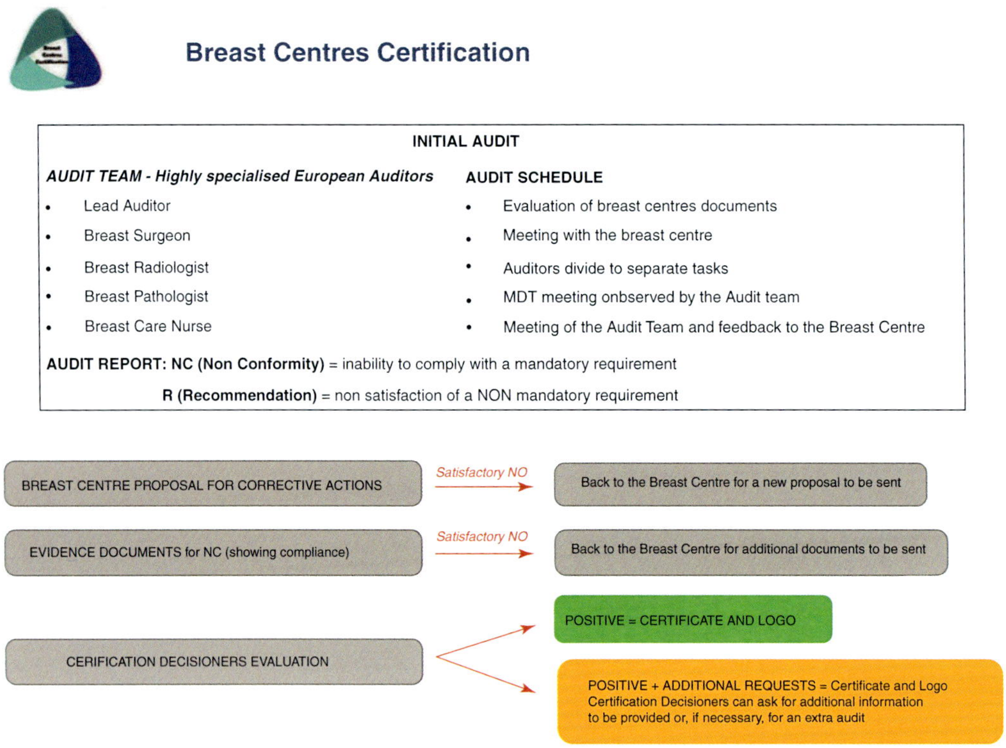

Fig. 4.2 "Breast Centres Certification" based on the EUSOMA requirements and quality indicators

References

1. Cataliotti L, Costa A, Daly PA, et al. Florence statement on breast cancer, 1998 forging the way ahead for more research on and better care in breast cancer. Eur J Cancer. 1999;35:14–5.
2. Blamey RW, et al. The requirements of a specialist breast unit. Eur J Cancer. 2000;36:2288–93.
3. Cardoso F, Cataliotti L, Costa A, et al. European breast cancer conference manifesto on breast Centre/breast units. Eur J Cancer. 2017;72:244–50.
4. European Parliament resolution on breast cancer in the enlarged European Union B6-0528/2006.
5. Biganzoli L, Cardoso F, Beishon M, et al. The requirements of a specialist breast Centre. The Breast. 2020;51:65–84.
6. Kesson EM, Allardice GM, George WD, et al. Effects of multidisciplinary team working on breast cancer survival: retrospective, comparative, interventional cohort study of 13,722 women. BMJ. 2012;433 https://doi.org/10.1136/bmj.e2718.
7. Kung P-T, et al. Effects of multidisciplinary care on survival of breast cancer: results from a national cohort study. Eur J Cancer. 2014;50(Suppl 4):e69. https://doi.org/10.1016/j.ejca.2014.03.257.
8. de Camargo Cancela M, Comber H, Sharp L. Hospital and surgeon caseload are associated with risk of re-operation following breast-conserving surgery. Breast Canc Res Treat. 2013;140:535–44.
9. Gooiker GA, van Gijn W, Post PN, et al. A systematic review and meta-analysis of the volume-outcome relationship in the surgical treatment of breast cancer. Are breast cancer patients better off with a high volume provider? Eur J Surg Oncol. 2010;36(suppl1):S27–35.
10. Banks I, Weller D, Ungan M, et al. ECCO essential requirements for quality cancer care: primary care. Crit Rev Oncol Hematol. 2019;142:187–99.
11. Biganzoli L, Marotti L, Hart CD, et al. Quality indicators in breast cancer care: an update from the EUSOMA working group. Eur J Cancer. 2017;86:59–81.
12. https://www.krebsgesellschaft.de/gcs/german-cancer-society/certification.html
13. https://www.facs.org/quality-programs/napbc
14. https://www.dica.nl/nbca
15. https://ecibc.jrc.ec.europa.eu
16. www.breastcentrescertification.com

5 Organisational Quality Assurance: Certification and Accreditation

Simon Oberst

5.1 Background

However good individual breast RT teams are, and however good the overall breast multidisciplinary teams (MDT), it is also important to see how the breast MDT sits within the overall cancer institution or network, and how it can draw upon the resources, quality systems, and research integration, which the institution and wider environment can supply.

This discussion is complicated by countries having different health systems in which breast MDTs operate, which either promote or sustain:

1. Specialist cancer hospitals aligned with research (for instance, France and Italy); or
2. Centres based around general University Hospitals and Universities (for instance, the UK, the Netherlands and the Nordic countries); or
3. Mixed health economies where private or insurance-funded specialist Breast Units can flourish, in addition to those within larger oncology centres (e.g. Germany and Switzerland).

S. Oberst (✉)
The Organisation of European Cancer Institutes (OECI, Brussels), The Cancer Research UK Cambridge Center, Cambridge, UK
e-mail: simon.oberst@improvingcancerservices.net

A further challenge is posed by the imperative to fully leverage the benefits and knowledge of molecular medicine as it applies to RT. Inevitably, this will be more feasible in larger institutional units—free-standing Comprehensive Cancer Centres, or Comprehensive Cancer Centres between a University Hospital and a University [1]. These will tend to have the resources and multi-professional breadth to apply molecular profiling analyses and interpretations on particular patients from multiple diagnostic sources to the breast MDT meeting [2], as well as having broad access to basic and translational research [3].

This more recent challenge increases the importance of the institutional environment in which the breast MDT sits. Although because of the incidence and prevalence of breast cancer, the breast MDT is often the largest team within a cancer centre, it is nonetheless dependent on leveraging the full benefits of organisation-wide resources, quality systems, and scientific knowledge. For instance, how does the breast MDT interact with: histopathology services; radiology services; nursing and nurse training; operational management for aspects such as waiting times, outpatient appointments, RT and systemic therapy delivery units; patient trackers/case managers; electronic patient records, data management and analysis; and supportive, psychological, and palliative care?

There is therefore a vital place for organisational quality assurance in cancer. This is complementary to specific practice requirements for

© The Author(s), under exclusive license to Springer Nature Switzerland AG 2022

O. Kaidar-Person et al. (eds.), *Breast Cancer Radiation Therapy*,
https://doi.org/10.1007/978-3-030-91170-6_5

breast RT (such as outlined in the previous and following sections), and it leverages the institutional quality systems to ensure that a breast cancer patient has the best possible outcomes and experience. Indeed, there is emerging evidence that patients treated within a comprehensive environment have better outcomes (not simply related to volume/quality relationships [4, 5]). Every clinical team knows that they operate within a framework where resources and operational issues require reliance on wider processes; these management and quality assurance processes of the centre need to be stress-tested at an institutional level. Examples of institutional quality assurance processes will include procedures for recording Suspected Unexpected Serious Adverse Reactions (SUSARs); monitoring of waiting times at key points in the patient pathway; recording deviations in clinical decision-making from approved clinical guidelines; and checking calibrations and functioning of key machines, together with comprehensive maintenance contracts. Cross-cutting processes which should be embedded in the centre include patient involvement and empowerment.

Any independent quality assurance accreditation process essentially requires four steps:

1. Evidence-based sets of standards or requirements which are both qualitative (standards) and quantitative (indicators);
2. A self-assessment process by the centre;
3. An external independent process with auditors or peer reviewers and an independent Accreditation Board; and
4. An agreed improvement action plan to remedy any processes or structures which were not fully compliant with the standards.

A number of international cancer accreditation systems use this methodology in cancer and concentrate on an institutional approach. A notable example is that of the American College of Surgeons (ACS). The Commission on Cancer [6] has been established for many decades, beginning with a surgical focus, but since the 1970s it has embraced more broadly all forms of diagnosis, treatment, and survivorship, with a particular concentration on the centrality of MDTs (referred to as Cancer Committees). Despite the huge coverage of this accreditation programme (estimated to cover 70% of all cancer patients diagnosed in the USA), the standards not related to surgery are surprisingly general in nature. Furthermore, the only references to research concern the required percentages of patient accrual to clinical trials (between 2 and 6%, except for paediatric cancers). Specific standards related to radiation oncology are lacking, but each centre providing RT is required to have a quality assurance programme in place for RT [5]. In 2018, the ACS also launched the National Accreditation Program for Breast Centres [7] which stands independently of the Commission on Cancer (Cancer Centre/Network) programme. The standard on breast RT requires a subsidiary accreditation by relevant US RT accreditation bodies [8]. Regarding clinical trials (all modalities and all forms of trial), the required percentage accrual is a very modest 2% of patients. In summary, the US accreditation systems do little to seriously challenge the fault-lines between cancer research (evaluated by the National Cancer Institute (NCI) [9]) and clinical delivery.

In Europe, there are only two bodies which embrace an institutional-wide approach to quality assurance and accreditation in cancer. These are the Organisation of European Cancer Institutes (OECI) and the German Cancer Society (GCS). These bodies take different approaches to accreditation. The GCS essentially takes a bottom-up approach based on organ-specific accreditation programmes/units (including Breast Cancer, as referred to in the section above). Only once an oncology centre has achieved accreditation of the required percentage of organ-specific accreditations (more than 70% of the cancers treated) can the centre be further accredited and recognised as an "Oncology Centre". At the end of 2020, 132 such oncology centres have been accredited by GCS in Germany, 8 in Switzerland and 2 in Austria [10]. Regarding research, as with the ACS programme, the "catalogue of requirements" for the GCS Oncology Centres focusses only on clinical studies, the requirements for personnel managing those studies, and an overall requirement that 5% of newly managed patients in the oncology centre should be recruited to such studies. However, for the dozen or so Spitzenzentren/Interdisciplinary Comprehensive Cancer Centres in Germany competitively selected for funding every 5 years by Deutsche Krebshilfe, a minimum of 10% clinical trials accrual is expected, and a demanding set of research criteria are required to be met [11].

The Organisation of European Cancer Institutes, however, takes an organisation-wide and truly comprehensive view of quality assurance in cancer and focusses only on cancer centres or Comprehensive Cancer Centres which have a minimum of 1500 (Comprehensive Cancer Centres 2500) new patients per year [12]. It is the only organisation worldwide whose standards encompass diagnosis, treatment, aftercare, and research integration in all its forms. OECI takes the view that improvements in cancer treatment are going to come principally from a bench to bedside and back approach. Whilst not aspiring to evaluate scientific excellence in depth (such as the European Academy of Cancer Sciences' Designation of Research Excellence [13, 14]), the OECI standards do test research infrastructure, and key processes, to ensure the scientific research in cancer is efficiently and effectively translated into changes to clinical practice. Fifty-three of Europe's largest cancer centres and Comprehensive Cancer Centres are part of the OECI accreditation programme at the time of writing, distributed in 18 European countries. Together, these centres have treated more than one million cancer patients since their accreditations.

The OECI standards [15] are set out in nine chapters (see Table 5.1) which encompass governance processes and then follow the common patient pathway, also embracing all forms of education, and research. Of these, 100 Core Quality Standards have been published as a European consensus for cancer centres [16]. Because they are focussed on the activities within cancer centres and cancer networks, the standards do not include many activities of prevention and screening which are uncommon within secondary or tertiary centres. However, oncogenetics services, stop smoking programmes, and exercise and other programmes in prevention of cancer recurrence, such as that commonly provided in centres, are included within the standards.

Table 5.1 Organisation of European Cancer Institutes (OECI) standards in Manual 3.0; chapter subjects

Chapter	Domain	Number of standards
1	Governance of the cancer centre	11
2	Organisation of quality systems	49
3	Patient involvement and empowerment	38
4	Multidisciplinary	28
5	Prevention and early detection	13
6	Diagnosis	36
7	Treatment and care	97
8	Research	53
9	Education and training	18

Of relevance to breast RT, the OECI standards and accreditation programme ensure that MDTs are properly constituted to include radiation (or clinical) oncologists at all times; that decisions are taken by consensus and appropriately recorded; that all patients have a case manager or contact nurse to ensure their continuity of care; and that patients are structurally screened for eligibility within clinical trials (including RT trials). And within the wider cancer centre or Comprehensive Cancer Centres, standards evaluate whether clinicians (including radiation oncologists) are able to have protected time for research and trials (remunerated by university or research programmes); that the centre has a robust MD PhD programme; and that there are structured and regular colloquia and seminars where clinicians and scientists can interact, disseminating scientific and technological advances on the one hand, and sharing the latest clinical challenges on the other. Comprehensive Cancer Centres are also evaluated on the structure of their research programmes (including radio-genomics); infrastructure and staffing for research; and their output in terms of peer-reviewed publications, especially those of high impact.

5.2 Summary

Breast RT teams, and the MDTs of which they form part, should endeavour to be fully aligned with larger cancer infrastructures to leverage all aspects of comprehensiveness: exercising full multidisciplinarity; being embedded within systematic quality and management systems; and being integrated with translational cancer science as well as clinical research. This comprehensiveness should be evaluated by a recognised accreditation system such as OECI, thus demonstrating that the breast RT service is benefiting from the latest research and technology and is capable of providing the best outcomes and experience for patients.

References

1. Oberst S. Bridging research and clinical care—the comprehensive cancer centre. Mol Oncol. 2019;13:614–8. https://doi.org/10.1002/1878-0261.12442.
2. De Mattos-Arruda L, Caldas C. Cell-free circulating tumour DNA as a liquid biopsy in breast cancer. Mol Oncol. 2016;10:464–74.
3. Celis J, Pavalkis D. A mission-orientated approach to cancer in Europe. Mol Oncol. 2017;11:1661–72.
4. Pfister DG, et al. Risk adjusting survival outcomes in hospitals that treat patients with cancer without information on cancer stage. JAMA Oncol. 2015;1(9):1303–10. https://doi.org/10.1001/jamaoncol.2015.3151.
5. Wolfson JA, et al. Impact of care at comprehensive cancer centres on outcome: results from a population-based study. Cancer. 2015;121(21):3885–93. https://doi.org/10.1002/cncr.29576.
6. https://www.facs.org/-/media/files/quality-programs/cancer/coc/optimal_resources_for_cancer_care_2020_standards.ashx. Accessed 15 Nov 2020.
7. https://accreditation.facs.org/accreditationdocuments/NAPBC/Portal%20Resources/2018NAPBCStandardsManual.pdf. Accessed 15 Nov 2020.
8. ibid, page 42. American College of Radiology Radiation Oncology Practice Accreditation (ACR-ROPA), the American Society for Radiation Oncology Accreditation Program for Excellence (ASTRO-APEx), the American College of Radiation Oncology (ACRO).
9. NIH NCI. Cancer Center Support Grants (CCSGs) for NCI-designated cancer centers, NIH funding opportunities and notices; 2020.
10. https://www.oncomap.de/cnetworks/cnoncos. Accessed 15 Nov 2020.
11. https://www.krebshilfe.de/fileadmin/Downloads/PDFs/Foerderung/CCCs_7th_call/Ausschreibung_Leitfaden_7._Call__08_Sep_2017.pdf. Accessed 15 Nov 2020.
12. https://www.oeci.eu/accreditation/Page.aspx?name=BACKGROUND. Accessed 16 Nov 2020.
13. Ringborg U, Celis J, Eggermont A, Berns A. European Academy of Cancer Sciences-designation of comprehensive cancer centres of excellence. Eur J Cancer. 2018;93:138–9. https://doi.org/10.1016/j.ejca.2018.01.003. Epub 2018 Feb 14. PMID: 29454744.
14. Rajan A, et al. Excellent translational research in oncology: a journey towards novel and more effective anti-cancer therapies. Mol Oncol. 2016;10:645–51.
15. https://www.oeci.eu/accreditation/Page.aspx?name=MANUAL_3. Accessed 16 Nov 2020.
16. Oberst S. 100 European core quality standards for cancer care and research centres. Lancet Oncol. 2020;21(8):2009–1011. https://doi.org/10.1016/S1470-2045(20)30318-1.

Quality Assurance Programmes in Radiation Oncology

6

Lawrence B. Marks, Shekinah N. C. Elmore, and Abraham Kuten

6.1 Introduction

Radiation therapy plays an important role in the treatment of breast cancer—increasing both local control and overall survival in both the post-lumpectomy and post-mastectomy settings [1, 2]. The close proximity of the target tissues (e.g. breast, chest-wall, regional nodes) to critical normal tissues (e.g. lung, heart, brachial plexus, spinal cord) mandates care in the planning and delivery of RT. Indeed, the therapeutic ratio of RT in some settings is narrow, and modest errors in planning/set-up can meaningfully impact this ratio (e.g. reduce target coverage and/or increase normal tissue risks). Nevertheless, this is the case for many disease types; radiation is a potent agent, and this "need for care and attention to detail" is largely ubiquitous within our field.

We herein briefly review the numerous initiatives throughout our field aimed to ensure quality care for all patients (i.e. not specific for breast cancer) and highlight several issues that are more-specific to assuring quality in patients receiving RT for breast cancer. Broadly speaking, strategies to assure quality can be considered to be technology—vs. human-based and (inter)-national vs. local (Table 6.1), and these are mutually reinforcing and interdependent.

L. B. Marks (✉)
Department of Radiation Oncology, and Lineberger Comprehensive Cancer Center, University of North Carolina, Chapel Hill, NC, USA
e-mail: marks@med.unc.edu

S. N. C. Elmore
Department of Radiation Oncology, University of North Carolina, Chapel Hill, NC, USA
e-mail: shekinah_elmore@med.unc.edu

A. Kuten
Israel Cancer Association, Department of Oncology, Rambam Campus, Technion University, Haifa, Israel

6.2 Broad Quality Assurance/Improvement Initiatives

Overall, modern RT applications are generally very safe. The founding members of our field recognised the risks of RT and instilled within our field's fabric the need for precision and careful oversight. Having physicists, engineers and other technically/quantitatively minded individuals integral to our practice has facilitated an objective and systematic approach to quality assurance.

Our professional societies (e.g. ESTRO, AAPM, ASTRO) have done an excellent job generating guidance documents to facilitate the safe practice of radiation oncology. For example, there are multiple "best-practice" statements to guide physician's clinical decisions and contouring atlases to guide image segmentation—for multiple diseases, including breast cancer [3–5]. For dosimetry/physics, there are multiple reports addressing things such as machine calibration,

© The Author(s), under exclusive license to Springer Nature Switzerland AG 2022
O. Kaidar-Person et al. (eds.), *Breast Cancer Radiation Therapy*,
https://doi.org/10.1007/978-3-030-91170-6_6

Table 6.1 Quality assurance strategies in radiation oncology

	Technology-based	Human-based
(Inter)-National	1. Guidance documents 2. Standards for nomenclature, prescription, and other items 3. Programmes to assess and assure interoperability of technologies 4. Tools embedded into planning and delivery software 5. Integrating the Healthcare Enterprise-Radiation Oncology (IHE-RO)	1. Incident Learning Systems (e.g. RO-ILS, ROSEIS, SAFRON) 2. Central review of plans (e.g. as part of clinical trials, QARC [Quality Assurance Review Center]) 3. Peer Review opportunities (ChartRounds, IAEA AFRONET)
Local (i.e. institutionally-based)	1. Local adoption of recommendations from professional societies 2. Accreditation 3. Machine learning and artificial intelligence-based initiatives	1. Creating culture supportive of QA/QI 2. Local incident reporting 3. Time-outs, checklists 4. Standardisation where able 5. Peer review 6. Huddles to promote clear communication 7. Safety rounds 8. Training 9. Involvement of all stakeholders (including physicians)

NB: Assignment is somewhat arbitrary for some items as they may straddle different zones. Accreditation programmes touch all four zones

RO-ILS Radiation Oncology Incident Learning System, *ROSEIS* Radiation Oncology Safety Education and Information System, *SAFRON* Safety in Radiation Oncology, *IAEA* International Atomic Energy Agency

machine/software QA, interconnectivity between various soft/hardwares, dose calculation and IMRT/patient-specific QA (e.g. see https://www.aapm.org/QualitySafety/default.asp and https://www.estro.org/Library). The value of real-time peer review was recognised decades ago and persists today [6, 7].

Nevertheless, errors do occur, and indeed the risks as well as impact of errors within radiation oncology appear to have perhaps increased over the last one to two decades related (at least in part) to the increased complexity of advanced techniques. For example, technologies such as IMRT, image guidance, radiosurgery/SBRT have fundamentally altered the way that RT is planned and delivered. In many settings, with the transition from field- to volume-based RT, light fields or portal films are not suitable any more as useful as an "end of the line checks" of the accuracy of the upstream work. The number of monitor units for a beam/arc/plan are no longer readily intuitive or representative of anything clinically meaningful. And, the use of fewer fractions, with higher-doses-per-fraction (e.g. with SBRT/SRS), make it critical to "get it right the first time". Newer technologies require increased efforts for many members of the radiation oncology team; e.g. for image segmentation, iterative dose calculations, patient-specific QA, image acquisition/review, treatment delivery. Individual's tasks are more interdependent, with more hand-offs, thus increasing opportunities for delay and sub-optimal information transfer; e.g. dosimetrist image segmentation → MD image segmentation and specification of dose/volume constraint → dosimetrist planning → MD review → dosimetrist re-plan → iterate → physics check → etc. As an illustration, IMRT planning and treatment initiation requires ≈54 discrete tasks to be performed by various team members, with ≈15 hand-offs [8, 9].

Public awareness of radiation delivery errors in the USA increased after a number of high-profile reports in *The New York Times* in 2010 [10]. In the USA, professional societies responded by publishing additional quality and safety publications (e.g. the ASTRO-sponsored "Safety is no Accident") have held several safety-focused meetings, expanded accreditation options and created a new AAPM/ASTRO-sponsored national error reporting system (ROILS: Radiation Oncology Incident

Learning System) [11, 12]. Similarly, serious accidents were reported in the 1990s in the United Kingdom, triggering a strong response by the National Health Service (NHS), as well as in the early 2000s in France, causing similar severe interventions. The European Radiation Oncology Safety Information System (ROSIS) project was started in the early 2000s to gather information about errors to promote safety through systematic incident reporting and analysis [13]. Similar initiatives have been implemented elsewhere as well (e.g. IAEA SAFRON) [14, 15]. Incident reporting systems are particularly helpful to us, as a field, in order to help create and promote a culture of quality/safety; i.e. emphasising that this cannot be achieved if we rely on technical considerations alone. Many quality/safety challenges arise due to suboptimal interactions of people with each other and with our workflows/environment, etc. (i.e. medicine is a human endeavour). However, as artificial intelligence and machine learning (AI/ML) approaches become more integrated into radiation oncology, there will be increasing opportunities to augment human expertise in error prevention and detection [16, 17].

6.3 Several Quality-Related Issues Somewhat Unique to Patients with Breast Cancer

1. Target volume delineation: patients receiving RT for breast cancer are typically being treated for possible residual microscopic disease, and target volumes are essentially CTVs. Target definition is thus somewhat imprecise as, for example, we use blood vessels and soft tissue borders to define at-risk nodal regions. The borders of the chest-wall or breast are similarly somewhat ambiguous. Imaging and physical examination (e.g. visualisation of scars, skin folds and palpation) are complementary; the physical assessment of the patient (e.g. at the simulator and treatment machine) remains important in assuring quality despite our modern imaging. There are differences between the contouring instructions provided by different professional groups that can lead to meaningful variation in doses delivered to CTVs [18]. Quality can suffer if these guidance documents are interpreted too literally. For example, if the breast tissue is contoured erroneously extending to the midline, simple tangents would need to extend well-across the midline to provide full dosimetric coverage to this area which may or may not be appropriate depending on the location of the tumour bed and other clinical factors (i.e. midline tangents were used in the most of the foundational studies demonstrating the utility of breast RT and the added dosimetric coverage may not improve the therapeutic ratio in a patient with a laterally located tumour). On the other hand, one does need to be sure that the "key target tissues" are covered for any individual patient. Particular care is needed when defining in the tumour bed (for a boost or for definitive treatment during APBI). Optimally, the surgeon can leave some radiologic markers to help target delineation. In the absence of markers, the surgical cavity is usually readily visible, albeit sometimes a poor representation of the true target, i.e. the tissue surrounding the original tumour which rarely coincides with the margins around the cavity. Moreover, the increasing use of "cosmetically friendly" approaches means that the radiologic or palpable/visible scar tissue may not accurately represent the tumour bed. As an extreme example, "oncoplastic tissue rearrangement surgery" makes identification of the post-op tumour bed virtually impossible, thus eliminating the possibility of boosting this site and the associated anti-tumour benefits. Communication with surgical colleagues is critically important, especially as surgical techniques evolve. Additionally, AI/ML or other algorithmic approaches may improve consistency and quality of target delineation.
2. Immobilisation and positioning. Accurate and reproducible positioning of the patient on the simulation/treatment table (including of the torso, arm, head, etc.) is required to assure consistent set-up. Small changes can be clinically meaningful in the deformable breast (especially with the use of smaller RT fields

and/or in the prone or decubitus positions). Immobilisation cradles and image/surface guidance methods are useful for the breast. Further, positioning can alter the location of the target breast tissue relative to surrounding normal tissues, so care is needed during simulation to define the "optimal" position. For example, when supine, a large breast might tend to fall superiorly towards the neck (due to gravity) and the use of an angled board to elevate the shoulders/head can displace the breast inferiorly (thus facilitating tangents that cover the breast without delivering dose to the neck and shoulder region).

Prone positioning is an effective manner to move much of the breast tissue away from the chest wall and internal normal organs and may improve the therapeutic ratio in cases where only the breast is being targeted. However, if the deep breast/chest wall are part of the target, the heart is displaced anteriorly when prone, and this might *negatively* impact the therapeutic ratio [19]. Further, set-up reproducibility may be reduced when treating prone (vs supine), though this issue perhaps can be obviated with pre-treatment imaging.

3. Respiratory control, like DIBH, is a useful method to move the heart away (i.e. inferior, medial and posterior) from the chest wall. This is particularly useful when treating the left breast, but can also be useful when treating the right breast in some patients. AAPM TG 76 provides guidance specific to DIBH [20].
4. Narrow therapeutic ratio. While RT is a very effective modality for patients with breast cancer, optimising the therapeutic ratio is critical since the absolute benefits are often modest, and there are many nearby radiosensitive structures. Thus, small differences in item such as positioning, target volume delineation, and daily localisation can have meaningful clinical impacts (i.e. small differences may matter).
5. Plethora of treatment approaches: Traditional beam arrangements (e.g. tangents to the breast, chest-wall, ±the IMNs, enface electrons to the chest-wall ± IMNs, "AP" or "APPA" beams to the supraclavicular ± axilla) have been used successfully for decades. While certainly not ideal and nowadays to be considered as obsolete, their benefit is that its utility and shortcomings are largely recognised. Newer treatment approaches (e.g. IMRT via an arc of photon beams or protons), all based on contemporary target-volume based RT [21], afford exciting opportunities to improve the therapeutic ratio of RT and should be aggressively considered. Further, within each of these approaches, there are many options (e.g. an infinite number of IMRT plans are indeed possible, and perhaps reasonable, for any given geometry). However, the unknowns associated with these new approaches should be acknowledged and further study is needed. For example, especially volumetric photon IMRT generally might, depending on the approach, increase the integral dose (i.e. by increasing the volume exposed to a low doses outcomes) and the possible effects of this are not known.

6.4 Concluding Remarks

Radiation oncology is a highly technical field and QA/QI efforts aimed at these technical issues are critical. Nevertheless, the practice of radiation oncology is a human endeavour, and most errors are linked to human-based aspects (e.g. workflows, communication, human–machine interactions). Thus, quality must be assured by addressing both the technical and non-technical aspects of our practice. Creating a culture of safety, in which leaders and workers together openly address these issues, is critical. However, we should refrain from well-intended measures that freeze the current state and slow down or even fully block the introduction of improvements in treatment preparation or delivery.

References

1. Early Breast Cancer Trialists' Collaborative Group (EBCTCG), Darby S, McGale P, Correa C, Taylor C, Arriagada R, et al. Effect of radiotherapy after breast-conserving surgery on 10-year recurrence and 15-year breast cancer death: meta-analysis of

individual patient data for 10,801 women in 17 randomised trials. Lancet. 2011;378:1707–16. https://doi.org/10.1016/S0140-6736(11)61629-2.
2. EBCTCG (Early Breast Cancer Trialists' Collaborative Group), McGale P, Taylor C, Correa C, Cutter D, Duane F, et al. Effect of radiotherapy after mastectomy and axillary surgery on 10-year recurrence and 20-year breast cancer mortality: meta-analysis of individual patient data for 8135 women in 22 randomised trials. Lancet. 2014;383:2127–35. https://doi.org/10.1016/S0140-6736(14)60488-8.
3. Smith BD, Bellon JR, Blitzblau R, Freedman G, Haffty B, Hahn C, et al. Radiation therapy for the whole breast: executive summary of an American Society for Radiation Oncology (ASTRO) evidence-based guideline. Pract Radiat Oncol. 2018;8:145–52. https://doi.org/10.1016/j.prro.2018.01.012.
4. White JT, Arthur D, Buchholz T. Breast cancer atlas for radiation therapy planning: consensus definitions. RTOG. http://www.rtog.org/LinkClick.aspx?fileticket ZvzJFhPaBipEZ.
5. Offersen BV, Boersma LJ, Kirkove C, Hol S, Aznar MC, Biete Sola A, et al. ESTRO consensus guideline on target volume delineation for elective radiation therapy of early stage breast cancer. Radiother Oncol. 2015;114:3–10. https://doi.org/10.1016/j.radonc.2014.11.030.
6. Glicksman AS, Wasserman TH, Bjarngard B, Laurie F. The structure for a radiation oncology protocol. The Committee of Radiation Oncology Group Chairmen. Int J Radiat Oncol Biol Phys. 1992;23:1079–82. https://doi.org/10.1016/0360-3016(92)90916-6.
7. Meet the Chartrounds Team. In: Chartrounds [Internet]. [cited 20 Oct 2020]. https://ind.chartrounds.org/Meet-the-Chartrounds-Team.aspx.
8. Moran JM, Dempsey M, Eisbruch A, Fraass BA, Galvin JM, Ibbott GS, et al. Safety considerations for IMRT: executive summary. Pract Radiat Oncol. 2011;1:190–5. https://doi.org/10.1016/j.prro.2011.04.008.
9. Marks LB, Jackson M, Xie L, Chang SX, Burkhardt KD, Mazur L, et al. The challenge of maximizing safety in radiation oncology. Pract Radiat Oncol. 2011;1:2–14. https://doi.org/10.1016/j.prro.2010.10.001.
10. Bogdanich W. Radiation offers new cures, and ways to do harm. The New York Times. 23 Jan 2010. https://www.nytimes.com/2010/01/24/health/24radiation.html. Accessed 16 Nov 2020.
11. Safety is no accident. American Society for Radiation Oncology. 2019. https://www.astro.org/ASTRO/media/ASTRO/Patient%20Care%20and%20Research/PDFs/Safety_is_No_Accident.pdf.
12. RO-ILS-American Society for Radiation Oncology (ASTRO)—American Society for Radiation Oncology (ASTRO). [cited 16 Nov 2020]. https://www.astro.org/Patient-Care-and-Research/Patient-Safety/RO-ILS.
13. Radiation Oncology Safety Education and Information System (ROSEIS). [cited 16 Nov 2020]. https://www.estro.org/Advocacy/ROSEIS.
14. Safety in Radiation Oncology (SAFRON). International Atomic Energy Agency. [cited 16 Nov 2020]. https://www.iaea.org/resources/rpop/resources/databases-and-learning-systems/safron.
15. Quality and Standards. In: The Royal Australian and New Zealand College of Radiologists (RANZCR) [Internet]. [cited 16 Nov 2020]. https://www.ranzcr.com/our-work/quality-standards.
16. Thompson RF, Valdes G, Fuller CD, Carpenter CM, Morin O, Aneja S, et al. Artificial intelligence in radiation oncology: a specialty-wide disruptive transformation? Radiother Oncol. 2018;129:421–6. https://doi.org/10.1016/j.radonc.2018.05.030.
17. Huynh E, Hosny A, Guthier C, Bitterman DS, Petit SF, Haas-Kogan DA, et al. Artificial intelligence in radiation oncology. Nat Rev Clin Oncol. 2020;17(12):771–81. https://doi.org/10.1038/s41571-020-0417-8.
18. Gee HE, Moses L, Stuart K, Nahar N, Tiver K, Wang T, Ward R, Ahern V. Contouring consensus guidelines in breast cancer radiotherapy: comparison and systematic review of patterns of failure. J Med Imaging Radiat Oncol. 2019;63:102–15. https://doi.org/10.1111/1754-9485.12804.
19. Chino JP, Marks LB. Prone positioning causes the heart to be displaced anteriorly within the thorax: implications for breast cancer treatment. Int J Radiat Oncol Biol Phys. 2008;70:916–20. https://doi.org/10.1016/j.ijrobp.2007.11.001.
20. American Association of Physicists in Medicine. The management of respiratory motion in radiation oncology: report of AAPM Task Group 76. 7/2006.
21. Offersen BV, Boersma LJ, Kirkove C, Hol S, Aznar MC, Biete Sola A, Kirova YM, Pignol JP, Remouchamps V, Verhoeven K, Weltens C, Arenas M, Gabrys D, Kopek N, Krause M, Lundstedt D, Marinko T, Montero A, Yarnold J, Poortmans P. ESTRO consensus guideline on target volume delineation for elective radiation therapy of early stage breast cancer. Radiother Oncol. 2015;114(1):3–10. https://doi.org/10.1016/j.radonc.2014.11.030. Epub 2015 Jan 24. PMID: 25630428.

Surgery

7

Maria-Joao Cardoso, Oreste Gentilini, and Thorsten Kuehn

7.1 Introduction

Breast cancer surgery has advanced immensely in the last two decades. The concept of cure through radical mutilating operations has been replaced successfully by BCT with identical OS [1, 2]. Furthermore, the substitution of ALND by SLNB, in negative axilla reduced the serious associated morbidities to almost no impact in upper limb functionality [3].

For almost 20 years now BCS and SLNB turned into routine practice. But progression in knowledge did not stop there, and the concept of replacing an ALND by an SLNB in axilla with less than three nodes positive became current practice even before the results of the trials proving non-inferiority of ALND to regional node irradiation (RNI) [4, 5].

M.-J. Cardoso (✉)
Breast Unit, Champalimaud Clinical Center, Champalimaud Foundation, Lisbon, Portugal

Nova Medical School Lisbon, Lisbon, Portugal
e-mail: maria.joao.cardoso@fundacaochampalimaud.pt

O. Gentilini
Breast Surgery Unit, San Raffaele University and Research Hospital, Milan, Italy
e-mail: gentilini.oreste@hsr.it

T. Kuehn
Interdisciplinary Breast Center, Klinikum Esslingen, Esslingen, Germany

By 2015 and according to the analyses derived from very large retrospective databases [6], BCT outdated mastectomy (without PMRT) not only in DFS but also in OS, in early breast cancer. This gain being most likely the consequence of not only better locoregional approaches but also improved systemic treatments.

Locoregional treatment, previously driven mainly by burden of disease/staging, is nowadays primarily directed by tumour biology in early breast cancer stages. This knowledge of tumour biology pushed neo-adjuvant treatments (primary systemic therapy, PST) to replace upfront surgery in all triple-negative and HER2-positive stage II and III breast cancer and in many countries even in some Stage 1 (T1c) tumours. The use of PST allows not only less extensive surgery but, based on disease response, also the possibility of testing tumour sensitivity in vivo, and better tailoring postoperative systemic treatments in patients without pCR.

With the increment of responses after PST, mainly with chemotherapy but also with hormone therapy in post-menopausal women, again BCS became even more conservative and axillary approaches changed further from ALND to SLNB, not only in clinically negative axilla (usually clinic examination and US, and biopsy if suspicious) before primary systemic treatment but also in women with a clinically positive axilla before treatment that turned out into a clinically negative axilla before surgery.

© The Author(s), under exclusive license to Springer Nature Switzerland AG 2022
O. Kaidar-Person et al. (eds.), *Breast Cancer Radiation Therapy*,
https://doi.org/10.1007/978-3-030-91170-6_7

Along with all this progress came the introduction and nowadays routine use of all the techniques of plastic and reconstructive breast surgery into the available armamentarium of breast surgeons [7]. Again therapeutic mammaplasties, partial local flaps added potentially more solutions to the classic BCS with better aesthetic outcomes without compromising the oncologic result [8].

And last but not least when mastectomy still is the choice, the use of skin sparing techniques with immediate reconstruction whenever possible also changed dramatically the outcome for all those women that were previously offered a total mastectomy without reconstruction [9]. All these improvements were obtained without affecting oncologic outcomes, as long as careful presurgical evaluation and multidisciplinary discussion to consider the pros and cons of each approach according to disease stage and patient's wishes [10].

Importantly, this evolutional pathway with so many new possibilities that will ultimately lead to optimal breast cancer care are mainly acquired and sustained within a trained multidisciplinary environment and the access to the necessary technologic armamentarium [11].

7.2 Quality Criteria in Surgery

With all the before mentioned evolution, there are however important endpoints that need to be addressed to obtain the best possible outcome for the patient in all fronts. The best possible locoregional control of the disease, the best systemic treatment that will give the patient the maximum OS and the best possible QoL.

In 2010, the first paper by EUSOMA was published on the quality indicators in breast cancer care in which a set of benchmark quality indicators (QIs) were described to be adopted by breast centres to allow standardised auditing and quality assurance, and to establish an agreed minimum standard of care [12]. An updated EUSOMA paper was published in 2017 [13] in order to incorporate new scientific knowledge in the field, to evaluate the experience acquired in more than 80,000 primary cases treated in European Breast Centres undergoing certification procedures, and to encourage ongoing improvement in the level of care by upgrading minimum standards.

As a general concept, the quality of surgical approach is widely dependent on the multidisciplinary management adopted in a certain Breast Unit. The more appropriate path for the single patient is better determined within the multidisciplinary board especially for borderline situations or to determine indications to primary systemic treatments. Furthermore and just to mention some, other issues might be better defined if discussed in a multidisciplinary environment like the participation to clinical trials to increase treatment options or the possible management outside of standard indications to avoid overtreatment in niches of patients (e.g. elderly or frail patients).

In the following paragraphs, we summarised the main quality indicators (QI) concerning different procedures in breast cancer surgery.

7.3 Breast Conserving Surgery

As previously pointed out [6], there is level I evidence of at least equivalence of BCT compared to modified radical mastectomy (MRM) for early breast cancer. Therefore, BCT should be the first option in early sporadic breast cancer patients undergoing primary surgery also considering that preservation of the breast has an important impact on life quality and mastectomy plus breast reconstruction (primary or secondary, implant or autologous) is associated with additional risks and costs. Oncoplastic techniques or primary systemic treatments are important tools to increase breast conservation rates, even in patients with an unfavourable breast/tumour relation or tumour site. There is also evidence from meta-analyses that 'no ink on tumour' can be accepted as sufficient margin width in invasive disease [14]. In the EUSOMA recommendations, the proportion of patients (BRCA1 and BRCA2 patients excluded) with invasive breast cancer not greater than 3 cm (total size, including DCIS component) who underwent BCT as primary treatment should be 70% as minimum standard, with a target of 85%.

However, it is well known that significant variability occurs in re-operation after initial wide excision for breast cancer. Rates of re-operation can vary from less than 10% to more than 50%, being far from acceptable figures and adversely affecting cosmetic outcome posing additional stress for patients and families. In the EUSOMA requirements, the proportion of patients with invasive cancer who received a single breast operation for the primary tumour (excluding reconstruction) should be 80% as minimum standard and 90% as target. This QI encompasses not only the level of surgical performance but also reflects the proper use of preoperative imaging, preoperative and intraoperative handling, use of onco-plastic techniques and optimal pathological examination.

Considerable work still has to be done in order to increase BCT rates after PST, which is increasingly used in the treatment of patients with early stage breast cancer. Few guidelines specifically address optimal loco-regional therapies and identify quality indicators in this setting. An international consortium was established to discuss clinical evidence and to provide expert advice on technical management of patients with early stage breast cancer. A recent paper was published to provide physicians with a toolbox addressing all major clinical questions [15].

7.4 Mastectomy

Mastectomy is still performed in 30–40% of breast cancer patients. The availability of breast reconstructive techniques largely reflects patient demand and should be a key consideration in the multidisciplinary management of breast cancer. In the EUSOMA recommendations, the proportion of patients receiving immediate reconstruction at the same time of mastectomy should be at least 40% as minimum standard with a target defined as not applicable. However, these figures need to be extensively discussed, aiming that the number of women not receiving breast reconstruction should be in our opinion very limited.

Modern evaluation of QI in the breast cancer surgery setting should be updated beyond the already available indicators (e.g. rate of breast conservation; rate of immediate reconstruction; reinterventions for insufficient margins) (Table 7.1) taking into consideration the fundamental dimension of cosmetic outcome and patient' satisfaction. For instance, one of the easily evaluated variables that can help define the quality of the performance offered is the number of patients in whom photos have been taken prior to surgery and after a proper follow-up (6–12 months) [16].

7.5 Axillary Approach

The process of surgical de-escalation has been extremely effective in the field of axillary surgery due to the motivation change, from treatment to staging purposes, of the procedure. SLNB is clearly regarded as the gold standard to assess the axillary lymph node status in clinically node-negative patients and the proportion of patients with invasive cancer and clinically negative axilla who undergo SLNB only (excluding patients who received PST) should be 90% as minimum standard and 95% as a target. A further continuous reduction in axillary lymph node dissection is ongoing especially after the publication of milestone randomised trials like Z-0011 and AMAROS [4, 5].

Another QI concerning axillary surgery is the proportion of patients with DCIS only who do not undergo axillary clearance. DCIS is a non-invasive disease, and tumour cells cannot spread to the lymph nodes in cases of pure DCIS. Therefore, axillary staging is rarely required. In some patients (1–2%), the histological assessment of the surgical specimen reveals unexpected invasive disease. A secondary SLNB is feasible and reliable after BCT and should be recommended in these patients. When mastectomy is performed, a secondary SLNB is sometimes technically not feasible because the efferent lymphatic vessels are destroyed by the primary surgery. Upfront SLNB is therefore still an option in patients who are scheduled for mastectomy [17]. Therefore, the minimum standard is set at 97% with the target being 99%.

Table 7.1 EUSOMA quality indicators: breast cancer surgery [13]

Quality indicator	LOE	Mand/Recom	Minimum standard	Target
Waiting time				
5—Time interval ≤6 weeks from the date of first diagnostic examination within the breast centre to the date of surgery or first treatment	IV	R	80%	90%
Multidisciplinary approach				
8—Proportion of patients to be discussed pre and post operatively by a multidisciplinary team	III	M	90%	99%
Appropriate surgical approach				
9a—Proportion of patients (invasive cancer only) who received a single (breast) operation for the primary tumour (excluding reconstruction)	II	M	80%	90%
9b—Proportion of patients (DCIS only) who received just one operation (excluding reconstruction)	II	M	70%	90%
9c—Proportion of patients receiving immediate reconstruction at the same time of mastectomy	III	R	40%	NA
Surgery and quality of life: avoidance of overtreatment				
11a—Proportion of patients with invasive cancer and clinically negative axilla who underwent sentinel lymph node biopsy (SLNB) only (excluding patients who received PST)	I	M	90%	95%
11b—Proportion of patients with invasive cancer who underwent sentinel lymph node biopsy with no more than 5 nodes excised	I	R	90%	95%
11c—Proportion of patients (BRCA1 and BRCA2 patients excluded) with invasive breast cancer not greater than 3 cm (total size, including DCIS component) who underwent BCT as primary treatment	I	M	70%	85%
11d—Proportion of patients with non-invasive breast cancer not greater than 2 cm who underwent BCT	II	M	80%	90%
11e—Proportion of patients with DCIS only who do not undergo axillary clearance	II	M	97%	99%

LOE level of evidence, *Mand* mandatory, *Recom* recommended

7.6 Quality Indicators

Although globally we see the improvements in surgical treatment of breast cancer, we also understand that these improvements need to be evaluated routinely in every unit/centre dedicated to the treatment of breast cancer patients. In Europe, EUSOMA is dedicated to the creation and auditing of quality indicators in breast cancer treatment [13]. Although the before-mentioned criteria are not applied in all countries in the world, there is a consistence among the most important and several initiatives at the national level are worth mentioning. In UK, the National Health Service (NHS) system operates the National Cancer Peer Review (currently renamed as Quality Surveillance Programme QSP), a quality assurance programme for NHS services, including breast cancer [18]. In the Netherlands, the NABON Breast Cancer Audit has been established as a systemic audit of breast cancer services, collecting data from all Dutch hospitals with the aims of nationwide evaluation of quality parameters, evaluation of guidelines adherence and weekly feedback to participating institutions [19]. In Germany, the vast majority of hospitals treating Breast Cancer have joined the certification system developed by the Breast Cancer Society and the German Society for Breast Disease. This system includes requirements and quality indicators collected during the certification process. Annually, anonymised results are reported to the public for all breast cancer centres through benchmarking reports [20]. In Italy, some regions like Lombardia have adopted EUSOMA criteria that need to be fulfilled in order to qualify for the list of Breast Units and have subsequent access to DRG reimbursement for breast cancer procedures.

Of note, ICHOM (The International Consortium for Health Outcomes Measurement) Initiative to develop a standard set of value-based patient-centred outcomes for breast cancer. The standard set encompasses survival and cancer control, and disutility of care outcomes, to be collected through patients' reports and administrative and/or clinical records (A Standard Set of Value-Based Patient-Centred Outcomes for Breast Cancer, The International Consortium for Health Outcomes Measurement (ICHOM) Initiative) [21].

Recently, another initiative has been launched in Europe in order to set the requirements for breast surgeons. The BRESO project represents a Breast Surgical Oncology platform for the certification of breast surgeons (www.breastsurgeoncertification.com). In fact, currently, training across Europe in Breast Surgery appears to be very heterogeneous. Most often, a general surgical training certification is achieved after 4–6 years of residency training. Consequently, many surgeons will have spent very little time doing breast surgery but will be able to undertake breast surgery, despite lack of specific and dedicated training in this discipline. BRESO aims to promote accredited specialist breast surgical care for breast cancer patients and women at high risk of breast cancer by offering a dedicated certification programme in breast cancer surgery [22].

Last but not least, it is very interesting to realise that patients, when questioned about the existing quality indicators, do not value them in the same order as health professionals, underlying the significance of including in the auditing criteria what patients value as important [23].

7.7 Summary

Breast cancer surgery has advanced immensely in the last two decades. The concept of cure through radical mutilating operations has been replaced successfully by breast conserving surgery, breast oncoplastic surgery and new types of skin sparing and nipple sparing mastectomies and reconstructive procedures. Additionally, de-escalation of axillary surgery allows to reduce the risk for arm morbidity. Working together with a multidisciplinary team with specialties such as breast radiologist, pathologists, medical, clinical and radiation oncologists and setting standards according to excellence criteria such as EUSOMA will assure a comprehensive treatment that will benefit the patient in oncological and quality of life outcomes.

References

1. Fisher B, Anderson S, Bryant J, Margolese RG, Deutsch M, Fisher ER, et al. Twenty-year follow-up of a randomised trial comparing total mastectomy, lumpectomy, and lumpectomy plus irradiation for the treatment of invasive breast cancer. N Engl J Med. 2002;347(16):1233–41.
2. Veronesi U, Cascinelli N, Mariani L, Greco M, Saccozzi R, Luini A, et al. Twenty-year follow-up of a randomised study comparing breast-conserving surgery with radical mastectomy for early breast cancer. N Engl J Med. 2002;347(16):1227–32.
3. Giuliano AE, Haigh PI, Brennan MB, Hansen NM, Kelley MC, Ye W, et al. Prospective observational study of sentinel lymphadenectomy without further axillary dissection in patients with sentinel node-negative breast cancer. J Clin Oncol. 2000;18(13):2553–9.
4. Donker M, van Tienhoven G, Straver ME, Meijnen P, van de Velde CJ, Mansel RE, et al. Radiotherapy or surgery of the axilla after a positive sentinel node in breast cancer (EORTC 10981-22023 AMAROS): a randomised, multicentre, open-label, phase 3 non-inferiority trial. Lancet Oncol. 2014;15(12):1303–10.
5. Giuliano AE, Ballman K, McCall L, Beitsch P, Whitworth PW, Blumencranz P, et al. Locoregional recurrence after sentinel lymph node dissection with or without axillary dissection in patients with sentinel lymph node metastases: long-term follow-up from the American College of Surgeons Oncology Group (Alliance) ACOSOG Z0011 randomised trial. Ann Surg. 2016;264(3):413–20.
6. Gentilini OD, Cardoso MJ, Poortmans P. Less is more. Breast conservation might be even better than mastectomy in early breast cancer patients. Breast. 2017;35:32–3.
7. Association of Breast Surgery at B, Association of Breast Surgery at B, Training Interface Group in Breast S, Baildam A, Bishop H, Boland G, et al. Oncoplastic breast surgery—a guide to good practice. Eur J Surg Oncol. 2007;33(Suppl 1):S1–23.

8. Kosasih S, Tayeh S, Mokbel K, Kasem A. Is oncoplastic breast conserving surgery oncologically safe? A meta-analysis of 18,103 patients. Am J Surg. 2020;220(2):385–92.
9. Fang SY, Shu BC, Chang YJ. The effect of breast reconstruction surgery on body image among women after mastectomy: a meta-analysis. Breast Cancer Res Treat. 2013;137(1):13–21.
10. Zhang P, Li CZ, Wu CT, Jiao GM, Yan F, Zhu HC, et al. Comparison of immediate breast reconstruction after mastectomy and mastectomy alone for breast cancer: a meta-analysis. Eur J Surg Oncol. 2017;43(2):285–93.
11. Biganzoli L, Cardoso F, Beishon M, Cameron D, Cataliotti L, Coles CE, et al. The requirements of a specialist breast centre. Breast. 2020;51:65–84.
12. Del Turco MR, Ponti A, Bick U, Biganzoli L, Cserni G, Cutuli B, et al. Quality indicators in breast cancer care. Eur J Cancer. 2010;46(13):2344–56.
13. Biganzoli L, Marotti L, Hart CD, Cataliotti L, Cutuli B, Kuhn T, et al. Quality indicators in breast cancer care: an update from the EUSOMA working group. Eur J Cancer. 2017;86:59–81.
14. Houssami N, Macaskill P, Marinovich ML, Morrow M. The association of surgical margins and local recurrence in women with early-stage invasive breast cancer treated with breast-conserving therapy: a meta-analysis. Ann Surg Oncol. 2014;21(3):717–30.
15. Dubsky P, Pinker K, Cardoso F, Montagna G, Ritter M, Denkert C, et al. Breast conservation and axillary management after primary systemic therapy in patients with early-stage breast cancer: the Lucerne toolbox. Lancet Oncol. 2021;22(1):e18–28.
16. Serra M, Li AQ, Cataliotti L, Cianchetti E, Corsi F, De Vita R, et al. Aesthetic results following breast cancer surgery: a prospective study on 6515 cases from ten Italian Senonetwork breast centers. Eur J Surg Oncol. 2020;46(10 Pt A):1861–6.
17. Pyfer BJ, Jonczyk M, Jean J, Graham RA, Chen L, Chatterjee A. Analysis of surgical trends for axillary lymph node management in patients with ductal carcinoma in situ using the NSQIP database: are we following national guidelines? Ann Surg Oncol. 2020;27(9):3448–55.
18. NACRAS. National Cancer Registry and Analysis Service 2020. http://www.ncin.org.uk/cancer_type_and_topic_specific_work/topic_specific_work/cancer_outcome_metrics.
19. NABON. NABON Breast Cancer Audit 2019. https://dica.nl/nbca/home.
20. Onkologie L. Leitlinienbasierte Qualitätsindikatoren im Leitlinienprogramm Onkologie (OL) 2019. https://www.leitlinienprogramm-onkologie.de/qualitaetsindikatoren/.
21. Ong WL, Schouwenburg MG, van Bommel ACM, Stowell C, Allison KH, Benn KE, et al. A standard set of value-based patient-centered outcomes for breast cancer: the International Consortium for Health Outcomes Measurement (ICHOM) initiative. JAMA Oncol. 2017;3(5):677–85.
22. Kovacs T, Rubio IT, Markopoulos C, Audisio RA, Knox S, Kuhn T, et al. Theoretical and practical knowledge curriculum for European Breast Surgeons. Eur J Surg Oncol. 2020;46(4 Pt B):717–36.
23. Salampessy BH, Bijlsma WR, van der Hijden E, Koolman X, Portrait FRM. On selecting quality indicators: preferences of patients with breast and colon cancers regarding hospital quality indicators. BMJ Qual Saf. 2020;29(7):576–85.

8 Pathology Report

Trine Tramm and Farid Moinfar

8.1 Background

The pathology report should provide diagnostic accuracy and completeness of clinically relevant prognostic and predictive information extracted from tissue and cells in the pre- or postoperative setting and should be completed with agreed timeliness.

Through the pathological examination, individual tumours of varying biology are separated into a number of evidence-based categories for which a likely clinical outcome and treatment response can be predicted. With the development of molecular pathology, the biological information of the tumour is getting increasingly nuanced and complex, and the diagnostic and predictive categories more specific.

The preoperative pathology reports should basically verify, if the lesion detected clinically or by image analysis is benign or malignant, and if a lymph node is positive or negative for metastasis. The postoperative report should, on the other hand, deliver extensive information on T- and N-stage, histological type, malignancy grade, ER- and HER2 status, possible treatment response, etc.

The pathology report is often considered to be providing the "truth". However, though striving to describe and quantify all parameters meticulously, pathological examination including molecular analysis cannot capture the comprehensive picture of the multifaceted tumour biology. Instead of the "truth", it provides the best possible estimation of the tumour's true nature, upon which the current treatment is based.

8.2 Turnaround Time for the Pathology Report

Cytology is the science of interpreting morphological changes in cells obtained through, e.g. aspiration (FNA) or exfoliation. Cytological specimens need little processing before staining, and the cytological material is immediately smeared on glass slides and sprayed with alcohol for fixation to preserve the appearance of the cells. The unstained material needs subsequent staining to enhance contrast and differentiate between cellular components, before it can be used for diagnostic purposes. The turnaround time of FNAs is, nevertheless, short, and a

Supplementary Information The online version contains supplementary material available at [https://doi.org/10.1007/978-3-030-91170-6_8].

T. Tramm (✉)
Department of Pathology, Aarhus University Hospital, Aarhus N, Denmark
e-mail: tramm@clin.au.dk

F. Moinfar
Department of Pathology, Ordensklinikum, Barmherzige Schwestern, Linz, Austria
e-mail: farid.moinfar@pathologieverbund.at

© The Author(s), under exclusive license to Springer Nature Switzerland AG 2022
O. Kaidar-Person et al. (eds.), *Breast Cancer Radiation Therapy*,
https://doi.org/10.1007/978-3-030-91170-6_8

diagnosis can be provided within hours to few days. If sediment is available from the aspiration, this may be processed into paraffin blocks (cell blocks) similar to histological material as described below. This allows for sections to be cut from the cell block, which increases the possibilities for further analysis.

Histological specimens need a longer tissue-processing procedure than FNAs. Histology is the science of studying morphological and architectural changes in tissue, and the material provided is more abundant (e.g. core needle biopsies or surgical specimens). After fixation and gross examination, the histological specimens pass specific steps of dehydration before paraffin embedding, sectioning of the paraffin-blocks and staining of the slides. The tissue-processing steps are largely dependent on automated tissue processors, and the turnaround time can usually not be accelerated.

For some specimen types, there is a constant prolonged turnaround time (e.g. bone biopsies need decalcification prolonging the processing time). For individual specimens, the turnaround time may be prolonged due to unexpected findings, need to repeat suboptimal analysis or to do supplemental molecular analysis. Inappropriate expectations of turnaround times that cannot be met by the laboratory may create understandable frustrations among physicians and patients waiting for the pathology report. Communication from the pathologist to the clinician on general or individual turnaround time, as well as the clinician's appreciation of the processing time supports a successful interdisciplinary teamwork and may prevent unnecessary concerns for the patient.

8.3 Choice of Biopsy Method Important for Usability of Pathology Report

In general, core needle biopsies are preferred to FNA from lesions in the breast, since it offers better possibilities of an accurate diagnosis. Cytology is associated with diagnostic limitations, since it relies on quantitative and cytomorphological features without architectural characteristics. The cytological material is further limited (3–6 slides) and performing additional tests including immunohistochemical (IHC) staining's or molecular analysis is restricted, rendering FNA for some purposes unsuitable—unless a cell block is available (Table 8.1).

In an FNA, it is not possible to determine whether atypical cells showing unusual, but not evidently malignant, features are reactively changed (due to e.g. inflammation or irradiation) or part of a neoplastic proliferation. Therefore, FNA is often not useful for ruling out whether a mass in a previous irradiation field is a local recurrence or not, and the result may end up inconclusive. Based on the cytomorphological features alone, the distinction between invasive carcinoma versus DCIS is also not possible. To answer the above-mentioned questions, a core needle biopsy is more appropriate.

Histological material is further required if subsequent IHC analysis e.g. hormone receptor status or multigene testing is requested.

FNA is, on the other hand, well-suited for verifying metastasis to lymph nodes. The sensitivity of FNA in detecting a lymph node metastasis has been reported to be around 63% with a specificity of 99% [1], meaning that a positive FNA provides a very reliable basis for axillary management. A negative FNA followed by an involved sentinel node biopsy may be due to sampling but also to interpretation of the cells in the FNA. The false-negative rate may vary according to procedure in the pathology lab, where addition of IHC testing with an epithelial marker on a single glass may increase diagnostic accuracy.

In general, discrepancies between preoperative (from both FNA and core needle biopsies) and post-operative findings may primarily be related to sampling and to a minor degree to interpretation of the cyto-/histopathological findings on the more limited biopsy material. For instance, approximately 26% of patients with pre-operatively diagnosed DCIS on core needle biopsies are likely to be upgraded to invasive carcinoma on the surgical specimen [2].

Table 8.1 Appropriate choice of biopsy method

Examples of clinical questions	Fine-needle aspiration, smear only	Fine-needle aspiration, with cell block[a]	Core-needle biopsy
Breast			
Malignant tumour: Yes/no	x	x	xx
Invasive/carcinoma in situ: Yes/no	Not suited	Not suited	xx
Paget's disease of the nipple: Yes/no	Not suited	Not suited	xx (punch biopsy)
Local recurrence in irradiated area: Yes/no	Not suited	x	xx
Secondary angiosarcoma: Yes/no	Not suited	x	xx
Metastasis			
Metastasis to lymph nodes: Yes/no	xx	xx	(x)
Metastasis to internal organs: Yes/no	x	x	xx
Verification of primary origin of cancer	Not suited	x	xx
Evaluation of predictive factors			
Determination of ER/HER2 status	Not suited	x	xx
Determination of PD-L1 status	Not suited	Not suited	xx
Gene expression profiling	Not suited	Not suited	xx

xx: optimal choice of biopsy; x: may be used, if core-needle biopsy cannot be obtained; (x): core-needle biopsy can be used, but not necessary

ER Oestrogen receptor

[a]Fine-needle aspiration with cell block renders possibility of supplementing the cytological evaluation with immunocytochemical stainings, which is not a possibility with smears only

8.4 Aiming to Capture "the Truth" of Multifaceted Tumour Biology in a Snapshot

The pathological examination of the tumour especially in the postoperative setting is challenged by trying to (1) visualise a 3D structure in a 2D setting, (2) give an exhaustive description of the tumour from representative "snapshots" and by (3) biology not always fitting into interpretable and pre-constructed diagnostic/predictive categories. According to national and international guidelines (e.g. CAP (College of American Pathologists), DBCG (Danish Breast Cancer Group)), the pathologist selects through a systematic grossing procedure sections of the tumour to answer clinically relevant questions (i.e. tumour size, distance to margins) (Fig. 8.1a–d). The following paragraph does not provide a description of the pathological examination but exemplifies some of the challenges, when trying to describe multifaceted tumour biology.

8.4.1 Measuring distance to the margin

The measurement of tumour distance to the margin is offered substantial attention by the pathologist in order to provide a precise measurement for decisions on e.g. subsequent re-resection and RT indications including addition of a boost dose. However, tumours are often not well-circumscribed, and the surface of a lumpectomy may be highly irregular (Fig. 8.1e). The true distance of the tumour to the margins are as such not just six distinct measurements (towards the lateral, medial, cranial, caudal, anterior (skin-side) and posterior (chest-wall side)) but a high number of measurements in all possible directions (Fig. 8.1f, g). Furthermore, even if the tumour is completely embedded, and all possible relations potentially encompassed in the paraffin-blocks, only a 3 μm thick section per 2–3 mm slice from each paraffin block will be evaluated in the microscope. The measurement of margin distance may seem to be very exact (e.g. 1 mm) in the actual section presented for microscopy, but a large part of the

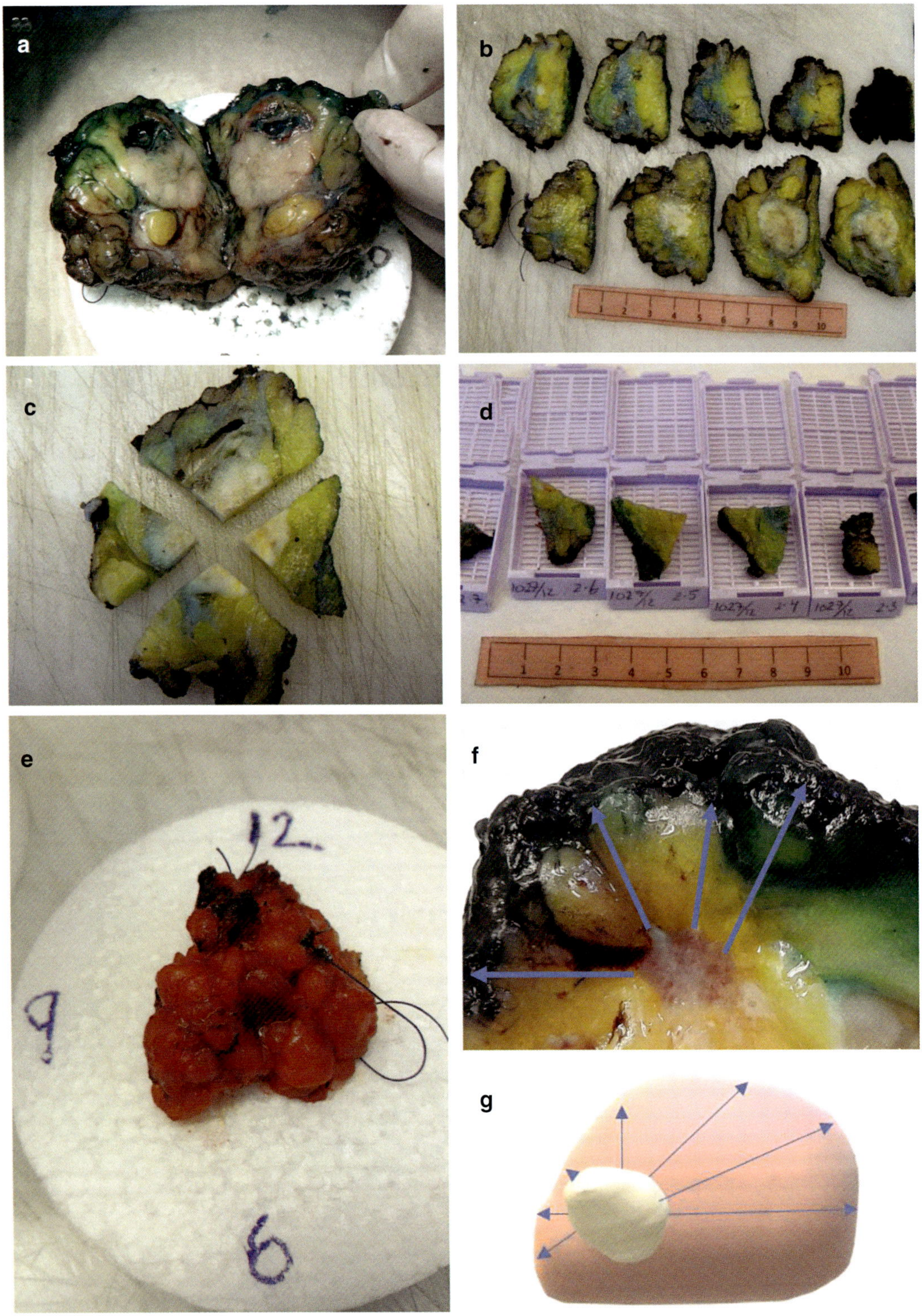

Fig. 8.1 (**a–d**) During grossing, the specimen is cut into 2–3 mm thick slices and representative sections are selected for embedding in paraffin. Here showing tumour relation to margins in four directions. (**e**) The surface of a lumpectomy may be highly irregular, and measurement of a similarly irregular, three-dimensional tumour may lead to a high number of margin distances (**f**, **g**)

tumour will always remain unexamined. Reported margin distance in the pathology reports used in daily clinical practice as well as in large clinical trials is, therefore, based on the pathologist's best estimate of the closest distance. In cases with reported "negative" but close margins (<2 mm), residual disease (primarily DCIS) may be present in re-excisional breast surgery in a substantial fraction of patients (20–30%) [3]. Following oncological treatments, the risk of residual disease is, however, not translated into increased local recurrence rates. Report of histopathological "negative margins", therefore, indicate but can not guarantee complete removal of the cancer either [4].

8.4.2 Biomarker Evaluation

Biomarker analysis is most often based on a semiquantitative estimate using a single slide, and clinical implementation of potentially promising markers may be limited due to intratumour heterogeneity as well as intra- and interobserver variability.

For instance, Ki-67 is associated with significant prognostic value in large population-based clinical studies, but may be, due to inferior analytical validity, of limited value for the individual patient [5, 6]. The suboptimal analytical validity of Ki-67 relates to pre-analytical issues (e.g. appropriate collection, fixation and processing of tissue) as well as analytical issues (e.g. intra- and interobserver variation in interpretation and scoring). The International Ki67 Working Group (IKWG) has since 2011 strived to standardise methods for determining and interpreting Ki67. The IKWG has suggested that Ki-67 may have prognostic relevance in a limited number of patients with favourable disease (T1N0, ER+/HER2), when using 5 and 30% as cut-off points to identify patients that may benefit from adjuvant chemotherapy [7]. In general, Ki-67 is, however, not internationally recommended as the only predictor of chemotherapy treatment. Digital image analysis may assist the pathologist in delivering a more precise estimate [8], though still based on only one or a couple of slides.

Discordance rates between hormone-receptor and HER2 status in primary and recurrent/metastatic lesions can potentially be related to technical issues but have been reported to be in the range of 10–16% for ER, 24–40% for PR and 3–10% for HER2 in studies with centralised pathological review reducing potential analytical variations [9, 10]. In general, a biologically "true" discordance with positive-to-negative changes is more likely than negative-to-positive changes for ER and PR [10], whereas a negative-to-positive change is more likely for HER2 [11]. The discordance rate is higher for metachronous than synchronous pairs, and between primary tumour and paired distant metastasis in comparison to paired primary tumour and lymph node metastases [9–11]. This discordance may be due to spatial tumour intra-heterogeneity, where tumour subclones display differences in mutational load and structural alterations. Through selective pressure during the metastatic process, this may lead to metastasis of a subclone different from the dominant clone of the primary tumour [12] and to possible discordance in ER/PR and/or HER2 status. Discordances have been described not only in metachronous metastasis but also in treatment-naïve, synchronous metastasis and their corresponding primary tumour, indicating a non-therapy-related cause [13]. A discordance may, however, also be due to mutational driven switches due to systemic treatment, and a reduction in ER expression can be found with treatment with Taxanes and Aromatase inhibitors [9], whereas a reduction in HER2 expression may be found with Trastuzumab.

Technical issues may also affect biomarker evaluation; decalcification of a bone biopsy carries for instance a risk of false-negative results, especially for HER2, and a core needle biopsy from an extraskeletal metastasis is to be preferred, if obtainable, to secure optimal biomarker analysis (see also Table 8.1).

8.4.3 Evaluation of Treatment Response

Neoadjuvant chemotherapy (NACT) reduces microvessel density on MRI, and tumour enhancement decreases, but only 30–50% patients with clinical complete response on MRI will have a pathological complete response (pCR), and 20% with clinical residual disease have pCR [14]. Pathological complete response is described as a robust prognosticator (surrogate marker) for overall survival, but no globally agreed definition of pCR exists. Different, often categorical, systems have been used to describe treatment response varying in, for instance, whether complete absence of carcinoma in *both* breast *and* axilla or only in the breast is considered a pCR, and if DCIS in the prior tumour bed is allowed or not. Most recently, the Residual Cancer Burden (RCB) has gained acceptance as a reproducible system to evaluate treatment response. The RCB delivers a continuous score that can be categorised into four groups of residual tumour burden (pCR, minimal, moderate, extensive). The RCB takes the extent of residual tumour in both breast and axilla into account as well as the fraction of residual invasive carcinoma in comparison to residual in situ component [15]. Examining surgical specimens for treatment response relies heavily on a high-quality histopathological examination with extensive sampling of the prior tumour bed, particularly when no macroscopical residual tumour is observed or when the residual tumour is diffusely scattered. Tumours shrink differently under NACT, and especially ER+/HER2− tumours are associated with a diffuse, heterogeneous shrinkage pattern, whereas ER−/HER2− (triple negative) and HER2+ tumours are associated with a more concentric shrinkage [16, 17]. Estimation of the extent of the former may be challenging and may require a large number of sections for microscopy. When no residual tumour is observed macroscopically, identification of the radiopaque marker and microscopical evidence of a treatment response should be clearly stated in the pathology report to secure that the relevant area has been examined. Treatment response in the prior tumour bed is characterised by distortion of the normal architecture and replacement of glandular tissue with loosely cohesive, fibrous tissue with scattered chronic inflammatory cells and macrophages. This is normally easily identifiable, whereas treatment response in lymph nodes may be associated with a larger degree of diagnostic uncertainty. The histopathological appearance of a treatment response is basically a healing process with scar-tissue and subsequent regeneration, and the histopathological findings are unspecific and appear the same regardless of the injury. Larger areas of fibrosis after NACT in a patient with pretreatment cN+ disease may as such indicate a treatment response, but fibrotic areas in lymph nodes may also be present as a consequence of prior biopsy. Since the determination of a treatment response in the lymph nodes may influence the decision of subsequent axillary irradiation, the pathologist should clearly state how many lymph nodes show certain treatment response, and any uncertainty should be discussed with the radiation oncologist.

8.4.4 Molecular Pathology

In general, molecular pathology and digital image analysis are expected to assist conventional histopathology in providing more refined diagnostic, predictive and/or prognostic classification of tumours, providing an increasingly precise estimate of the true tumour biology. These modalities remain, nevertheless, still limited to evaluation of only part of the tumour (a sample/slice/biopsy), delivering a "snapshot" of the tumour, though in a "higher resolution". Several multigene tests are now commercially available and render prognostic information especially in women with ER+/HER2−, early stage breast cancer (Table 8.2). The outcome of these molecular analysis is generally categorical and not personalised.

Determination of molecular subtype by PAM50 is, for instance, based on correlation to the nearest centroid (expression of 50 genes in the patient's tumour is correlated to a prefixed "mean"/centroid of the same 50 genes) determining the four subtypes (Luminal A, Luminal B, HER2-enriched and Basal-like). The patient's tumour is categorised according to the highest correlation with one of these four centroids; a categorisation that cannot fully capture tumour heterogeneity and does not provide information

Table 8.2 Assays for multigene testing

	OncotypeDX Breast recurrence score	MammaPrint	Prosigna Breast Cancer Prognostic Gene Signature Assay (PAM50)	Breast Cancer Index	EndoPredict
Assay	Genomic Health	Agendia	Veracyte	Biotheranostics	Myriad Genetics, Inc.
	21-gene recurrence score	70-gene assay	50-gene assay	11-gene assay	12-gene assay
Methods	RT-PCR	DNA microarray	Nanostring nCounter	RT-PCR	RT-PCR
Tissue requirements	FFPE	FFPE or frozen tissue	FFPE	FFPE	FFPE
Output	Recurrence score (1–100) *Separated into 4 groups related to risk of recurrence*	Low or high risk of recurrence	4 molecular subtypes (Luminal A, Luminal B, HER2-enriched, Basallike) ROR score (0–100) in combination with T and N stage	Low, intermediate or high risk of recurrence	EPclin Risk Score (1.1–6.2) *Separated into low or high risk of recurrence*
Level of evidence	1A (5 years)	1A (5 years)	1B	1B	1B
Prospective trials	TAILORx RxPONDER ADAPT	MINDACT	OPTIMA PRECISION NEOPAL	Extended endocrine treatment	ADENDOM

Prognostic gene expression tests for predicting clinical in patients with ER-positive, HER2-negative, N0–1, early stage breast cancer

FFPE formalin-fixed paraffin-embedded tissue, *RT-PCR* reverse transcriptase-polymerase chain reaction, *ER* oestrogen receptor, *ROR* risk of recurrence

on whether two distinct subtypes are present in the tumour.

Molecular pathology adds to the histopathological information but may also deliver information of unknown significance or information that seems diverging or confusing. For example, only up to 65% of tumours with a HER2-enriched subtype, as determined by PAM50, are HER2 positive by IHC/FISH. The reason being that the tumour may show highest correlation with the HER2-enriched molecular centroid due to high expression of other genes than *ERBB2*. An example of another kind is that HER2-positive tumours (determined from IHC) by gene-expression profiling can be found not only within the HER2-enriched molecular subtype but also within the Luminal B, Basal-like and Luminal A molecular subtypes in approximately 20%, 14% and 7%, respectively [18]. Gene-expression-based subtypes and IHC delivers complementary information, but the biological information arises from mRNA/DNA and protein level, respectively, and cannot be expected to be fully interchangeable. The clinical value of using a combination of IHC and gene-expression-based determination of, e.g. HER2 status is not clear. Therefore, multigene tests are currently not recommended for determining ER- and HER2 status.

Of special note, the commercially available multigene tests (Oncotype Dx, MammaPrint; Prosigna (PAM50), EndoPredict, etc.) show similar prognostic ability on a population-based level, but lack of consistency in risk prediction of the individual patient with 30–40% disagreement between tests [19]. The discordance is highly likely related to the gene signatures being driven by different pathways (ER pathway or proliferation pathway) [20] or having varying capability of predicting late recurrences [21]. Furthermore, the prediction of patients with intermediate-risk tumours may represent a considerable source of variation between the signatures [22]. In general, the multigene tests show the greatest accuracy for detecting low-risk patients in whom chemotherapy may be safely omitted but show low specificity and low positive predictive value among patients in the high-risk molecular groups [23–25].

The Declaration of Molecular Pathology as agreed on by the European Union of Medical Specialists (UEMS) 2013 [26] states that molecular pathology must be performed under the authority of and as part of the responsibility of the pathologist and provided in an integrated form in the pathology report. This emphasises the pathologist's growing responsibility for interpreting and presenting the combined biological information with careful consideration and understanding of clinical implications.

8.5 The Pathologist's Responsibility for Securing the Analytical Validity

The clinical utility of a given treatment is dependent not only on the clinical validity as determined from clinical studies but also of the analytical validity securing reliable and reproducible tests, overcoming variations within and between labs and pathologists. Increasingly, clinical trials testing new drugs may use specific biomarkers associated with specific assays (and technical platforms) to identify patients that might respond to the drug, and approval of the drug may be dependent on the use of the specific assay. This procedure may unfortunately lead to the selection of suboptimal assays and scoring systems, compromising the analytical validity and the intention of providing individualised treatment may lead to "unintended imprecision medicine". For instance, many PD-L1 assays are FDA-approved in different cancer types, including breast cancer. The PD-L1 staining patterns, scoring methods and cut-off values are, however, highly different, and the assays are not interchangeable though aiming to predict response to the same type of drugs. Furthermore, the PD-L1 IHC assays are associated with substantial inter- and intraobserver variation. Though clinical evidence from studies have proven significant disease-free survival benefits for eligible patients treated with PD-L1 inhibitors according to their PD-L1 expression, the analytical validity of the associated PD-L1 assays is not consolidated.

8.6 A Document for All Members of the Multidisciplinary Team

The pathology report should, above all, deliver a diagnosis and provide prognostic/predictive information, but it also serves other purposes for the different members of the multidisciplinary team. First of all, it may serve as quality assurance and as a tool for continuous education e.g. for the radiologist by comparing the pathological diagnosis with the interpretation of an infiltrate on a mammogram. The report also presents information on morphology (study of form and structure), often in more descriptive phrases. This serves to "hand over" essential information to other pathologists and may contribute to discriminate in the future whether a second neoplastic event in a breast is to be considered a new primary tumour or a true recurrence. Besides describing evidence-based prognostic/predictive parameters, the pathology report may also include observations empirically known to be related with high-risk disease (Table 8.3). Since the reports are also being read by the patient, careful contemplation of the wording is needed to avoid creating unnecessary concern, especially regarding areas/questions of doubt.

Table 8.3 Histopathological indicators of high-risk disease[a]

Invasive carcinoma	Ductal carcinoma in situ
• High nuclear grade • High Ki-67 • Widespread lymphovascular invasion	• High nuclear grade • Comedo necrosis • Periductal fibrosis and lymphocytic infiltration • Ki-67-positive cells scattered throughout the neoplastic proliferation

[a] Not encompassing conventional prognostic and predictive factors as TNM stage, malignancy grade, ER- and HER2 status and resection margins

8.7 Summary

The pathology report should provide accurate diagnostic, prognostic and predictive information and should be provided within timeliness determined by tissue-processing. It should deliver unambiguous communication between the pathologist and the rest of the multidisciplinary team, but should also emphasise unusual or biologically divergent findings. The output and extent of the obtained information must be related to the material provided and can reveal biology not "fitting" into current diagnostic/prognostic categories.

The conditions of pathological examination are challenged by the attempt to capture the essence of highly individual tumours, which with the addition of molecular pathology is getting increasingly precise, but never exhaustive. Current treatment strategies are, however, based on these estimates.

For novel biomarkers to be clinically implementable, clinical as well as analytical validity needs to be confirmed, and though showing prognostic/predictive information in population-based studies, some biomarkers including multigene tests may not yet be sufficiently reliable for categorising individual patients.

The pathologist is responsible for staying up-to-date with optimal evaluation of cytological and histological material, for interpreting the increasingly complex, combined biological picture, and for presenting it as precisely as possible to the clinicians in order to provide a basis for subsequent therapeutic decisions.

References

1. Yu YH, Mo QG, Zhu X, et al. Axillary fine needle aspiration cytology is a sensitive and highly specific technique for the detection of axillary lymph node metastasis: a meta-analysis and systematic review. Cytopathology. 2016;27:59–69.
2. Brennan ME, Turner RM, Ciatto S, et al. Ductal carcinoma in situ at core-needle biopsy: meta-analysis of underestimation and predictors of invasive breast cancer. Radiology. 2011;260:119–28.
3. Garvey EM, Senior DA, Pockaj BA, et al. Rates of residual disease with close but negative margins in breast cancer surgery. Breast. 2015;24:413–7.
4. Houssami N, MacAskill P, Marinovich ML, et al. Meta-analysis of the impact of surgical margins on local recurrence in women with early-stage invasive breast cancer treated with breast-conserving therapy. Eur J Cancer. 2010;46:3219–32.
5. Denkert C, Budczies J, von Minckwitz G, Wienert S, Loibl S, Klauschen F. Strategies for developing Ki67 as a useful biomarker in breast cancer. Breast. 2015;24:S67–72.
6. Denkert C, Budczies J, Regan MM, et al. Clinical and analytical validation of Ki-67 in 9069 patients from IBCSG VIII + IX, BIG1-98 and GeparTrio trial: systematic modulation of interobserver variance in a comprehensive in silico ring trial. Breast Cancer Res Treat. 2019;176:557–68.
7. Nielsen TO, Leung SCY, Rimm DL, et al. Assessment of Ki67 in breast cancer: updated recommendations from the International Ki67 in Breast Cancer Working Group. J Natl Cancer Inst. 2021;113(7):808–19.
8. Stålhammar G, Fuentes Martinez N, Lippert M, et al. Digital image analysis outperforms manual biomarker assessment in breast cancer. Mod Pathol. 2016;29:318–29.
9. Ongaro E, Gerratana L, Cinausero M, et al. Comparison of primary breast cancer and paired metastases: biomarkers discordance influence on outcome and therapy. Future Oncol. 2018;14:849–59.
10. Sighoko D, Liu J, Hou N, Gustafson P, Huo D. Discordance in hormone receptor status among primary, metastatic, and second primary breast cancers: biological difference or misclassification? Oncologist. 2014;19:592–601.
11. Houssami N, Macaskill P, Balleine RL, Bilous M, Pegram MD. HER2 discordance between primary breast cancer and its paired metastasis: tumour biology or test artefact? Insights through meta-analysis. Breast Cancer Res Treat. 2011;129:659–74.
12. Yates LR, Gerstung M, Knappskog S, et al. Subclonal diversification of primary breast cancer revealed by multiregion sequencing. Nat Med. 2015;21:751–9.
13. Ng CKY, Bidard F-C, Piscuoglio S, et al. Genetic heterogeneity in therapy-naïve synchronous primary breast cancers and their metastases. Clin Cancer Res. 2017;23:4402–15.
14. Viale G. Characterization and clinical impact of residual disease after neoadjuvant chemotherapy. Breast. 2013;22(Suppl 2):S88–91.
15. Symmans WF, Wei C, Gould R, et al. Long-term prognostic risk after neoadjuvant chemotherapy associated with residual cancer burden and breast cancer subtype. J Clin Oncol. 2017;35:1049–60.
16. Namura M, Tsunoda H, Yagata H, et al. Discrepancies between pathological tumour responses and estimations of complete response by magnetic resonance imaging after neoadjuvant chemotherapy differ by breast cancer subtype. Clin Breast Cancer. 2018;18:128–34.
17. Ballesio L, Gigli S, Di Pastena F, et al. Magnetic resonance imaging tumour regression shrinkage patterns after neoadjuvant chemotherapy in

patients with locally advanced breast cancer: correlation with tumour biological subtypes and pathological response after therapy. Tumour Biol. 2017;39:101042831769454.
18. Prat A, Carey LA, Adamo B, et al. Molecular features and survival outcomes of the intrinsic subtypes within Her2-positive breast cancer. J Natl Cancer Inst. 2014;106.
19. Bartlett JMS, Bayani J, Marshall A, et al. Comparing breast cancer multiparameter tests in the OPTIMA prelim trial: no test is more equal than the others. J Natl Cancer Inst. 2016;108(9):djw050.
20. Buus R, Sestak I, Kronenwett R, et al. Molecular drivers of Onco *type* DX, Prosigna, EndoPredict, and the Breast Cancer Index: a TransATAC study. J Clin Oncol. 2021;39(2):126–35.
21. Sestak I, Buus R, Cuzick J, et al. Comparison of the performance of 6 prognostic signatures for estrogen receptor–positive breast cancer a secondary analysis of a randomized clinical trial. JAMA Oncol. 2018;4:545–53.
22. Vallon-Christersson J, Häkkinen J, Cecilia H, et al. Cross comparison and prognostic assessment of breast cancer multigene signatures in a large population-based contemporary clinical series. Sci Rep. 2019;9:12184.
23. Paik S, Shak S, Kim C, et al. A multigene assay to predict recurrence of tamoxifen-treated, node-negative breast cancer. N Engl J Med. 2004;351:2817–26.
24. Buyse M, Loi S, van't Veer L, et al. Validation and clinical utility of a 70-gene prognostic signature for women with node-negative breast cancer. J Natl Cancer Inst. 2006;98:1183–92.
25. Van de Vijver M, He YD, van't Veer LJ, et al. A gene-expression signature as a predictor of survival in breast cancer. N Engl J Med. 2002;347:1999–2009.
26. Cuvelier C, President B, Maillet B, et al. UEMS specialists section of pathology declaration on molecular pathology. 2013.

Breast Imaging

9

Kristina Lång and Miri Sklair Levy

9.1 Background

Imaging is an integral part of breast cancer diagnosis, staging and follow-up. Breast imaging is also important for RT planning. The radiation oncologist needs to review patient's imaging (e.g. mammography) to evaluate the extent of disease (for RT planning, not for diagnostic purposes) and for treatment planning. Pre-treatment imaging is the key for planning RT volumes, especially the RT tumour bed boost if indicated and regional nodal irradiation. For radiation treatment planning, the radiation oncologist needs to be familiar with patient anatomy as seen on imaging done for treatment planning (e.g. CT simulation, MRI simulation). Therefore, participating in a multidisciplinary meeting with breast radiologist experts, learning how to read/understand breast imaging, and consulting with a breast radiologist expert if there is any doubt, is essential for proper breast radiation planning.

The current chapter will review breast imaging for screening, preoperative evaluation and provide tools for the radiation oncologist to review breast imaging in clinical practice.

9.1.1 Breast Cancer Screening

The aim of breast cancer screening is early cancer detection in asymptomatic women to improve patient outcome. Breast cancer screening is typically performed with biennial mammography for women between 50 and 69 years of age, but could also be considered for an extended age interval (age 45–74 years) [1]. The benefit of mammography screening was initially assessed in several large RCTs, performed for over 30 years ago and showed a relative reduction of breast cancer specific mortality of about 20% [2]. Adding case–control studies, the estimated breast cancer mortality reduction for women attending screening is about 40% [3]. The effect of mammography screening in the current era of targeted therapies is, however, likely less pronounced [4, 5]. Importantly, the benefit of screening has to be balanced with the harms, false positives and overdiagnosis [6]. Experiencing a false-positive recall is stressful and can lead to anxiety that can endure for up to 3 years [7]. It is therefore important to have a

K. Lång (✉)
Unilabs Mammoraphy Unit/Skane University Hopsital, Malmö, Sweden

Division of Diagnostic Radiology, Departement of Translational Medicine, Lund University, Malmö, Sweden
e-mail: kristina.lang@med.lu.se

M. Sklair Levy
Breast Imaging Center, Department of Diagnostic Imaging, Meirav Breast Center, Chaim Sheba Medical Center, Ramat Gan, Israel

Tel Aviv University, Tel Aviv, Israel
e-mail: miri.sklairlevy@sheba.health.gov.il

© The Author(s), under exclusive license to Springer Nature Switzerland AG 2022
O. Kaidar-Person et al. (eds.), *Breast Cancer Radiation Therapy*,
https://doi.org/10.1007/978-3-030-91170-6_9

reasonably low recall rate in screening. The rate of overdiagnosis has been a matter of intense debate but is estimated to be about 10–20% [6, 8].

Ways to improve the sensitivity of breast cancer screening are currently being investigated on a broad front [9, 10]. Both digital breast tomosynthesis, ultrasound and MRI, have been shown to increase the cancer-detection rate in screening compared with mammography [11–14]. However, no study has so far measured the effect of supplementary screening on reducing breast cancer mortality [1, 15].

9.1.2 Tumour Appearance

Heterogeneity of breast cancer disease is reflected in its various presentations in breast imaging. Breast composition also varies from the fatty involuted breast to the extremely dense breast. Put together, the combination of anatomy and tumour morphology poses different challenges in breast imaging.

The radiologic appearance of breast cancer can be characterised in four major groups: mass, microcalcifications, asymmetry and associated features (such as nipple retracement, unilateral oedema). Masses can further be described based on their shape, margins and density. The most common invasive tumour appearance is the spiculated mass. The spicules radiating out from the mass periphery are part of a desmoplastic reaction with productive fibrosis that contribute to the symptom of a palpable lump even at rather small tumour sizes. The most common type of cancer, IDC, often presents as a spiculated mass, which in general is easily detectable with mammography and ultrasound. However, mammographic sensitivity declines significantly with increasing breast density [10, 16], which is a problematic limitation particularly in the screening setting. Women with extremely dense breasts also have a relative increase in breast cancer risk of 2.1 compared with the average woman [10].

A cancer type with a subtle growth pattern, less prone to incite desmoplasia, is the ILC. Due to its indistinct growth pattern, it can be a challenging task to detect and to further evaluate tumour extent. Lack of associated calcifications and low tumour density are contributing factors to the higher false-negative rate of ILC compared to other invasive cancers [17]. ILC can present as a spiculated mass but also with the more elusive radiographic pattern of architectural distortion and focal asymmetry. The difficulties in detecting ILC is reflected in the fact that they are often larger and multifocal at diagnosis compared with IDC [18]. The size of ILC can be underestimated at preoperative imaging with mammography and ultrasound [19]. As a result, BCS of ILC is more often converted to mastectomy compared with IDC [18]. When BCS is under consideration, MRI can therefore be useful to determine tumour extent, especially in women with dense breasts and/or when there is not a clear focal mass on conventional imaging [19–22]. The morphologic appearance of ILC on MRI can be both mass and non-mass like. The most common manifestation of a mass-like lesion is a heterogeneously enhancing irregular mass with spiculated border. The non-mass like lesion appears as an asymmetric enhancement and are more difficult to recognise. ILC can also be missed at MRI due to the sometimes diffuse and slow tumour growth pattern that does not require extensive neovascularization which in turn impedes contrast enhancement.

Another challenge in breast imaging are breast cancer types that can have a benign mass appearance. Fibroadenomas and cysts are by far the most common imaging finding, and they typically present as a well-circumscribed mass. Both triple negative, medullar and mucinous carcinomas can present as benign looking circumscribed masses. A scrutinised ultrasound evaluation and a biopsy can however easily solve the issue. The challenge is to determine a threshold to recall a circumscribed mass from mammography screening when the vast majority of lesions with this appearance are benign.

Calcifications are a very common finding in mammography and are most often of a benign aetiology. Calcifications are evaluated for morphology and distribution. Benign calcifications

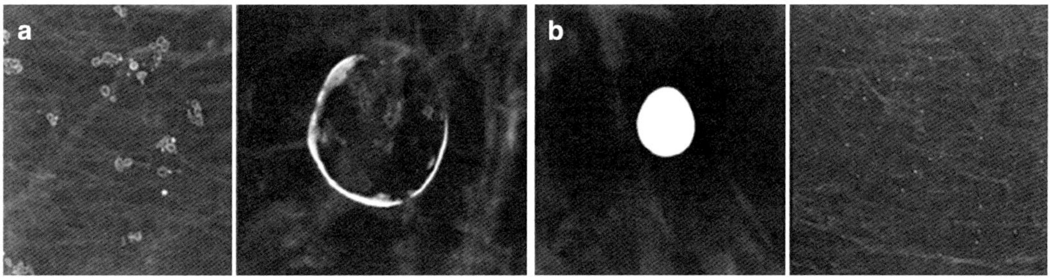

Fig. 9.1 (**a**) Benign calcifications with lucent-centred (left) and rim-like (right) morphology. (**b**) Benign calcifications with round (left) and punctate (right) morphology

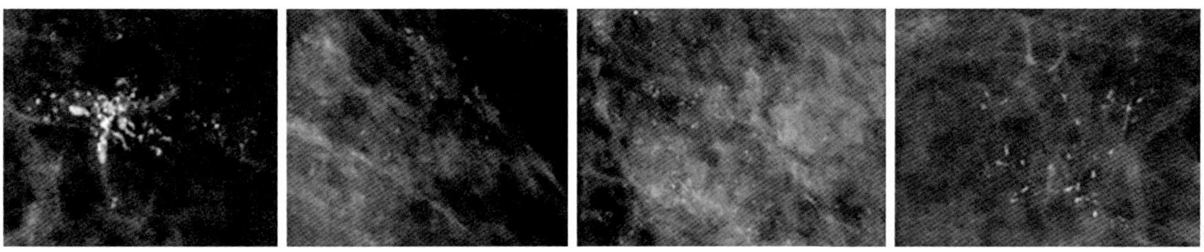

Fig. 9.2 Calcifications with suspicious morphology. Digital zoom mammographic projection images show calcifications with increasing risk for malignancy: coarse heterogeneous (far left), amorphous (second from left), fine pleomorphic (second from right), and fine linear or fine linear branching (far right)

can have a variety of appearances, for example, coarse, dystrophic, rim, round or rod-like and often have a diffuse/scattered or regional distribution (Fig. 9.1a, b). Suspicious calcifications can be amorphous, coarse heterogeneous, fine pleomorphic, fine linear or fine linear branching and often have a clustered or segmental distribution (Fig. 9.2).

A unilateral mammographic finding of a fibroglandular density that cannot be clearly identified as a true mass may raise suspicion of malignancy if it is visible on two mammographic views, so-called focal asymmetry, or if it is new or more conspicuous over time, so-called developing asymmetry.

Associated features are used to further characterise masses, calcifications, and asymmetries. The most worrisome are skin retraction, nipple retraction, skin thickening, and axillary adenopathy (Fig. 9.3).

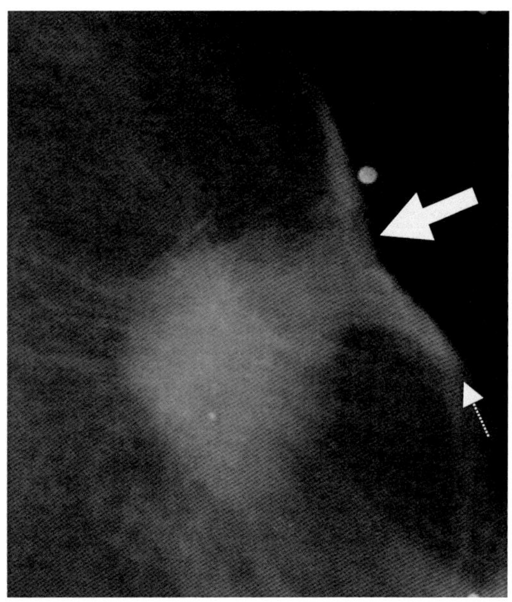

Fig. 9.3 A malignant mass with associated skin retraction (arrow) and skin thickening (dashed arrow)

9.2 Hands on Guide/Tips and Tricks to View Breast Imaging

A diagnostic mammography examination typically consists of three projections per breast (craniocaudal, mediolateral oblique and lateral view). The radiologist checks for suspicious findings by analysing each quadrant and by comparing the left and right breast, and, importantly, with prior examinations. Lesion localisation by quadrant is determined by combining the position of the finding on the different mammographic views. The presence of a suspicious finding invokes further work-up with at least ultrasound (see Preoperative assessment). Lesion localisation at ultrasound is typically determined by clock position and distance from the nipple. It can be a challenge to correlate the location and size of a lesion on different modalities. On mammography, women are in standing position, and the breast is compressed in different angles. On ultrasound, women are in a supine position, and the breasts are collapsed. On MRI, women are in a prone position with the breast hanging freely. On CT-simulations, women are again in a supine position with collapsed breasts.

Imaging findings and breast composition are reported in a standardised way according to the Breast Imaging Reporting and Diagnosis System [23], or similar classification systems [24]. Findings are typically reported on a 5-level scale from normal to highly suspicious, and breast density is reported on a 4-level scale from fatty involuted breasts to extremely dense breasts.

9.2.1 Preoperative Assessment

For the majority of cases, triple assessment with conventional imaging (mammography, and/or tomosynthesis, and ultrasound) and core-needle biopsy is sufficient to obtain diagnosis and to determine tumour extent. The axilla is assessed with ultrasound, and suspicious lymph nodes undergo fine-needle aspiration or core needle biopsy.

A contrast-enhanced method could be considered in the evaluation of tumour extent and to determine synchronous lesions. Contrast-enhanced MRI is the breast imaging modality with the highest sensitivity, regardless of breast density [25]. MRI enables an analysis of lesion morphology and contrast-enhancement dynamics. Malignant lesions typically show a rapid enhancement followed by an early wash-out as a result of tumour angiogenesis [26].

Despite considerable research, the routine use of preoperative MRI still remains a controversial topic [27, 28]. MRI has the highest sensitivity to determine tumour extent [29–31] and has been shown to detect clinically and mammographically occult contralateral disease in about 3% of women recently diagnosed with breast cancer [32]. While some studies show a benefit of preoperative MRI in terms of positive surgical margins and a reduction of reoperations [33, 34], others, including RCTs, show no such benefits but rather that MRI leads to more extensive surgery with higher mastectomy rates [35–41]. The question is whether additionally MRI-detected tumour foci have an impact on patient outcome (survival and recurrence). In a recent study comparing premenopausal women with and without preoperative MRI, no difference was found in local or distant recurrence [42]. The low recurrence rate after BCS without preoperative MRI could be explained by additional foci being eliminated by adjuvant therapy [43, 44].

Nevertheless, preoperative MRI could enable a more careful tailored surgical planning [27], including the possibility to treat contralateral disease at the same session as the index cancer [32]. This have to be weighed against the increase in false-positive biopsies after MRI, increased cost, and with a possible delay in treatment [27]. Even if current evidence advice against a routine use, preoperative MRI can still be of value in certain subgroups; women at high risk, at clinical and conventional imaging discrepancy, suspicion of multifocal disease unconfirmed on conventional imaging, mammographically occult breast cancer, and patients with Paget's disease or ILC planned to undergo BCS [20–22, 36, 37].

9.2.2 Metastasis Screening

Screening for metastatic disease should be performed according to national/international guidelines. It is routinely performed at T3 and T4 disease, at large axillary burden (>4 abnormal lymph nodes) or at the presence of signs or symptoms [22]. The first choice for visceral screening is contrast-enhanced CT of thorax and abdomen, and a bone scan (scintigraphy) to assess skeletal engagement. If available, FDG PET/CT can be used for evaluating metastatic disease, e.g. in case of inconclusive conventional CT findings (if a biopsy is not planned) or to confirm oligometastatic disease if radical treatment is considered. FDG PET/CT is less sensitive for ILC and low-grade tumours, as well as for sub-centimetre lesions (due to limited spatial resolution) [45]. The reconstructed spatial resolution of clinical PET is about 4–6 mm full width at half maximum, which corresponds to a lower detection threshold of a 7-mm-large tumour (0.2 ml; $2*10^8$ cells). Therefore, PET has limited value in the assessment of early stage disease including early axillary node involvement and micrometastases [45, 46].

9.2.3 Residual Disease and Surveillance

It is important to not only localise surgical clips post-BCS but also correlate the preoperative imaging to that of the simulated CT in the planning of RT (Fig. 9.4). Postoperative and radiation changes such as architectural distortion can mask tumours at conventional imaging. If there is an indication to exclude residual disease due to positive margins or multifocal disease, MRI can be performed as early as 1 month post lumpectomy [47].

Image surveillance after breast cancer treatment is typically performed with annual

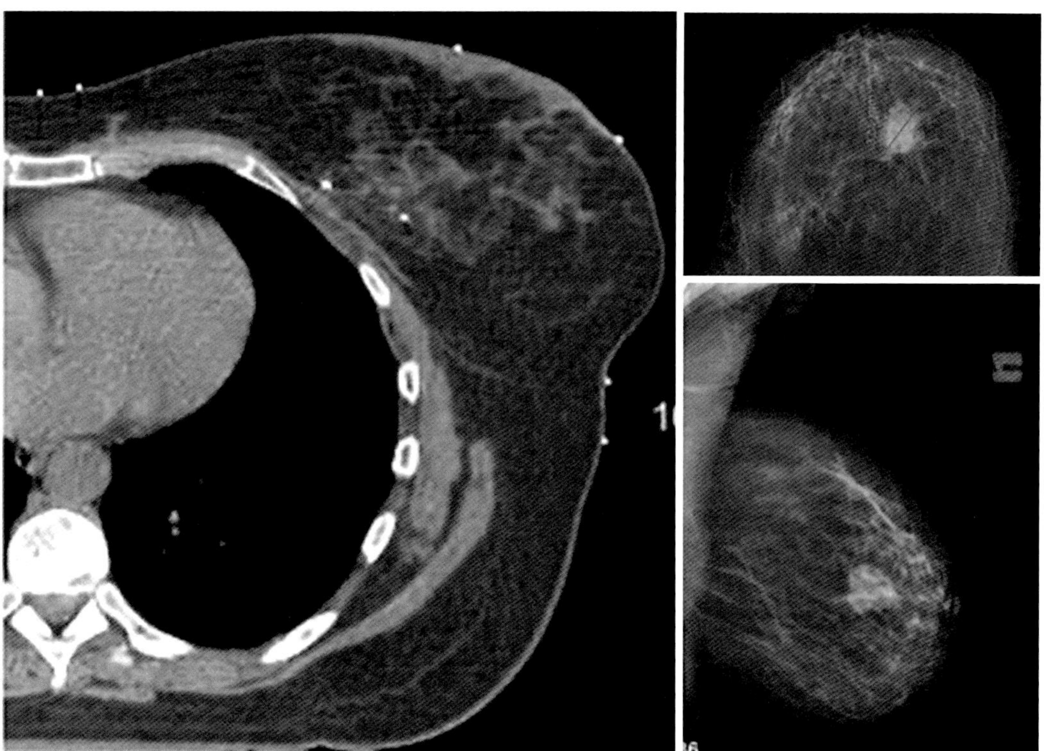

Fig. 9.4 Surgical clips on postoperative CT simulation are not on the site of the tumour bed when correlated to preoperative mammography in this case after oncoplastic surgery

mammography for 5–10 years, depending on age and on national/international guidelines [26]. The sensitivity of surveillance mammography of the ipsilateral breast is about 67% [48]. The risk of primary contralateral metachronous disease is increased for up to 20 years after BCS [48].

MRI is the most accurate imaging method to detect recurrence after BCS, since it can discriminate scar tissue from recurrence due to the latter showing contrast enhancement [49]. Post-treatment surveillance with MRI could be considered for young women, women with dense breasts and/or with a history of mammographically occult breast cancer [50].

9.2.3.1 Post Mastectomy Imaging and Surveillance

With the increase in the rate of mastectomy and post mastectomy radiation raises the question regarding the approach to surveillance. Risk reducing mastectomy in high-risk BRCA women reduces the risk of subsequent breast cancer by 85–95%. And in standard-risk females, it reduces the risk of subsequent breast cancer by approximately 28%. Patients and physicians assume that there is no residual fibroglandular tissue post mastectomy.

Therefore, the current guidelines do not recommend imaging surveillance.

However, in a study by Kaidar-Person et al. [47], residual glandular breast tissue after mastectomy is not a rare event, reported in up to 100%. MRI was found to be the most accurate method to evaluate residual breast tissue which was located mostly at the outer quadrants and/or the NAC in case of NSM [47]. The skin envelope thickness of the native breast in SSM/NSM may range from 5 to 14 mm and thicker.

This information is essential, since some of these patients after mastectomy are not referred to PMRT. The role of the multidisciplinary team and a breast specialised radiologist is to evaluate the preoperative MRI with special attention for areas of skin involvement, or DCIS/invasive lesion that is near the skin or subcutis that will not allow for a safe SSM/NSM. Thus, the assessment of preoperative images can assist in the surgical planning to identify patients eligible for NSM/SSM and those in need of removal of skin and subcutis over the lesion to assure a clear anterior margin. Importantly, in most cases, the anterior margins in case of mastectomy, including SSM/NSM, are not reported in the pathology report, thus the preoperative assessment of these patients by a breast radiologist is essential.

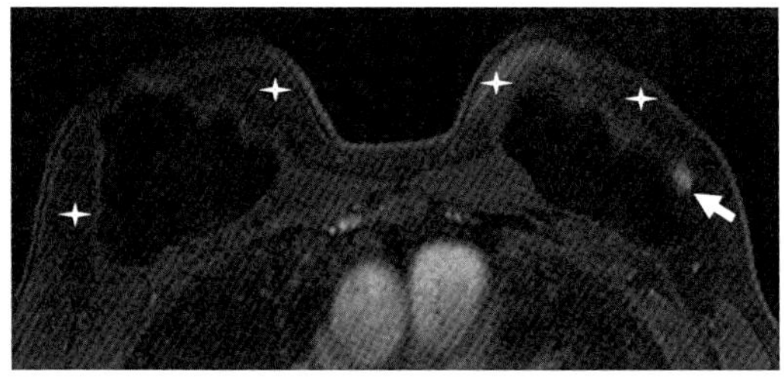

Fig. 9.5 Bilateral post mastectomy with silicon reconstruction, left breast recurrence (arrow). Of note is the large bilateral residual breast glandular tissue (stars)

Since residual breast glandular tissue is not rare, and in patients after mastectomy who are followed up with MRI (or any other imaging), we suggest to consider reporting the location of the residual breast glandular tissue and the amount. This could assist the radiation oncologist in individually planning PMRT according to these "high-risk" volumes (Fig. 9.5).

9.2.4 New Imaging Methods

Breast imaging is a constantly evolving field, and new methods to improve the performance of both screening and diagnostics are continually being investigated [9]. A modality of particular interest is contrast-enhanced spectral mammography. The method is based on the use of intravenous iodinated contrast agent and dual energy exposure mammography, taking advantage of contrast enhancement in neovascularised tissue, and has been shown to have a high sensitivity [51–54] (Fig. 9.6). The sensitivity and specificity levels are suggested to be comparable to MRI [53, 55, 56], but specificity has also been reported to be low in a systematic review [51]. Suggested indications include those currently considered for MRI [21]. Contraindications are known allergy to iodine, abnormal renal function, pregnancy and lactation. Serious adverse contrast reactions are

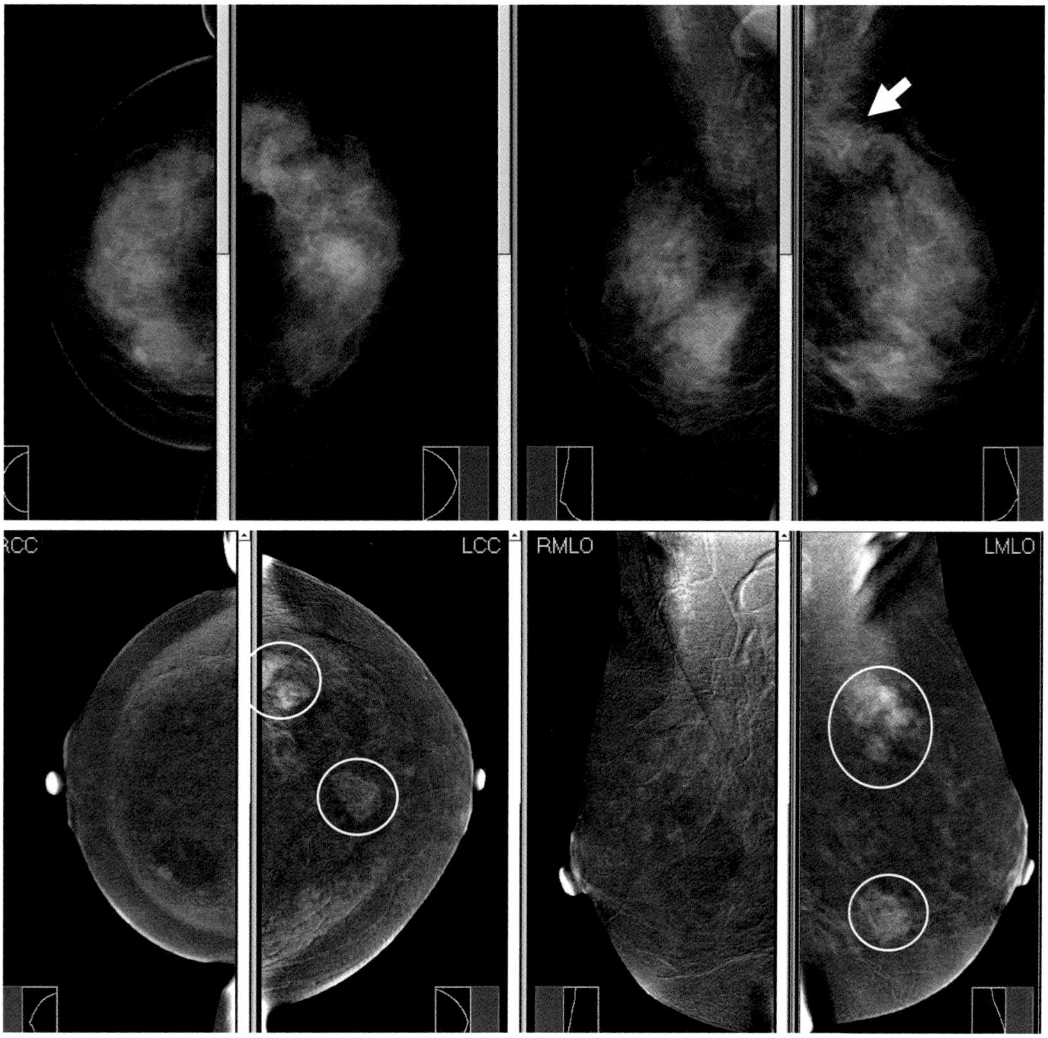

Fig. 9.6 A 41-year-old woman with a palpable lump in her left breast. With contrast-enhanced spectral mammography, two sets of images are acquired; below and above the k-edge of iodine. An image-processing algorithm subtracts the two exposures (low- and high-energy images) into a subtracted image displaying areas of contrast enhancement. An indistinct mass in the upper part of the left breast is apparent (arrow), but due to dense breasts additional lesions are not visualised on the low-energy image (comparable to a standard mammogram). Subtracted images reveal multiple enhancing lesions in the left breast (circle). Biopsy confirms multifocal IDC

rare [57]. Compared to MRI, contrast-enhanced spectral mammography is less expensive, easier to implement in clinical practice, and might therefore provide greater accessibility.

Abbreviated MRI refers to a shortening of a standard breast MRI protocol and has been suggested to have similar sensitivity compared with a conventional full-length protocol [58–60]. Abbreviated MRI could therefore increase the availability of breast MRI with better patient tolerance, higher efficiency, and lower cost. Of special interest is its potential use in a screening setting for women with dense breasts [58, 61].

Diffusion-weighted imaging is a MRI technique that measures the movement of water molecules, where solid lesions typically demonstrate restricted movement. The method has been shown to be useful as part of multiparametric MRI [62]. In recent years, concerns regarding the long-term use of gadolinium-based contrast agents [63] have propelled the interest of using diffusion-weighted imaging as a non-contrast alternative to contrast-enhanced MRI, especially in the screening setting [64]. Even if promising [65, 66], diffusion-weighted imaging used as stand-alone does not reach the sensitivity level to that of contrast-enhanced MRI [63, 66].

Recent development of computer-aided detection with artificial intelligence, especially for mammography interpretation, presents exciting possibilities for improving breast cancer screening. Retrospective studies have shown that deep-learning-based artificial intelligence systems can reach human level performance in terms of accuracy [67–71]. Artificial intelligence tools can be used both as a decision support for radiologists [72, 73] and as a mean to triage examinations according to the risk of malignancy [74–77]. The impact of artificial intelligence in screening has not yet been investigated in a prospective trial, but several studies are initiated.

9.3 Summary

Breast radiologists are an essential part of the multidisciplinary team. The main tasks of the radiologist are to detect asymptomatic cancers at screening and to diagnose and evaluate manifest disease. Additionally, the input of the breast radiologist is essential to determine the most appropriate surgical procedure. The variation of tumour appearance and breast anatomy poses different challenges for the radiologist and requires the use of different imaging methods. Contrast-enhanced imaging methods can be used to increase the sensitivity compared with conventional imaging, especially for women with dense breasts and for certain breast cancer subtypes. ILC can be challenging to detect and to determine disease extent, for which preoperative MRI can be of value.

It is recommended to consult breast imaging colleagues in the event of uncertainties in the RT planning such as suspicion of residual disease, or residual tissue after mastectomy, at the finding of suspicious lymph nodes at CT simulations or for difficulties in boost delineation.

References

1. European guidelines on breast cancer screening and diagnosis. 2020. https://healthcare-quality.jrc.ec.europa.eu/european-breast-cancer-guidelines. Accessed 1 Nov 2020.
2. The benefits and harms of breast cancer screening: an independent review. Lancet. 2012;380:1778–86. https://doi.org/10.1016/S0140-6736(12)61611-0.
3. Lauby-Secretan B, Scoccianti C, Loomis D, et al. Breast-cancer screening—viewpoint of the IARC working group. N Engl J Med. 2015;372:2353–8. https://doi.org/10.1056/NEJMsr1504363.
4. Sebuødegård S, Botteri E, Hofvind S. Breast cancer mortality after implementation of organized population-based breast cancer screening in Norway. J Natl Cancer Inst. 2020;112:839–46. https://doi.org/10.1093/jnci/djz220.
5. Trimboli RM, Giorgi Rossi P, Battisti NML, et al. Do we still need breast cancer screening in the era of targeted therapies and precision medicine? Insights Imaging. 2020;11:105. https://doi.org/10.1186/s13244-020-00905-3.
6. Marmot MG, Altman DG, Cameron DA, Dewar JA, Thompson SG, Wilcox M. The benefits and harms of breast cancer screening: an independent review. Br J Cancer. 2013;108:2205–40. https://doi.org/10.1038/bjc.2013.177.
7. Bond M, Pavey T, Welch K, et al. Systematic review of the psychological consequences of false-positive screening mammograms. Health Technol Assess. 2013;17:1–170. , v–vi. https://doi.org/10.3310/hta17130.
8. Zackrisson S, Andersson I, Janzon L, Manjer J, Garne JP. Rate of over-diagnosis of breast cancer 15 years after end of Malmö mammographic screening trial: follow-up study. BMJ. 2006;332:689–92. https://doi.org/10.1136/bmj.38764.572569.7C.
9. Mann RM, Hooley R, Barr RG, Moy L. Novel approaches to screening for breast cancer. Radiology. 2020;297:266–85. https://doi.org/10.1148/radiol.2020200172.
10. Freer PE. Mammographic breast density: impact on breast cancer risk and implications for screening. Radiographics. 2015;35:302–15. https://doi.org/10.1148/rg.352140106.
11. Marinovich ML, Hunter KE, Macaskill P, Houssami N. Breast cancer screening using tomosynthesis or mammography: a meta-analysis of cancer detection and recall. J Natl Cancer Inst. 2018;110(9):942–9. https://doi.org/10.1093/jnci/djy121.
12. Bakker MF, de Lange SV, Pijnappel RM, et al. Supplemental MRI screening for women with extremely dense breast tissue. N Engl J Med. 2019;381:2091–102. https://doi.org/10.1056/NEJMoa1903986.
13. Ohuchi N, Suzuki A, Sobue T, et al. Sensitivity and specificity of mammography and adjunctive ultrasonography to screen for breast cancer in the Japan Strategic Anti-cancer Randomized Trial (J-START): a randomised controlled trial. Lancet. 2016;387:341–8. https://doi.org/10.1016/s0140-6736(15)00774-6.

14. Houssami N, Turner RM. Rapid review: estimates of incremental breast cancer detection from tomosynthesis (3D-mammography) screening in women with dense breasts. Breast. 2016;30:141–5. https://doi.org/10.1016/j.breast.2016.09.008.
15. Melnikow J, Fenton JJ, Whitlock EP, et al. Supplemental screening for breast cancer in women with dense breasts: a systematic review for the U.S. Preventive Services Task Force. Ann Intern Med. 2016;164:268–78. https://doi.org/10.7326/m15-1789.
16. Kolb TM, Lichy J, Newhouse JH. Comparison of the performance of screening mammography, physical examination, and breast US and evaluation of factors that influence them: an analysis of 27,825 patient evaluations. Radiology. 2002;225:165–75. https://doi.org/10.1148/radiol.2251011667.
17. Krecke KN, Gisvold JJ. Invasive lobular carcinoma of the breast: mammographic findings and extent of disease at diagnosis in 184 patients. AJR Am J Roentgenol. 1993;161:957–60. https://doi.org/10.2214/ajr.161.5.8273634.
18. Yeatman TJ, Cantor AB, Smith TJ, et al. Tumor biology of infiltrating lobular carcinoma. Implications for management. Ann Surg. 1995;222:549–59; discussion 559–61. https://doi.org/10.1097/00000658-199522240-00012.
19. Mann RM, Hoogeveen YL, Blickman JG, Boetes C. MRI compared to conventional diagnostic work-up in the detection and evaluation of invasive lobular carcinoma of the breast: a review of existing literature. Breast Cancer Res Treat. 2008;107:1–14. https://doi.org/10.1007/s10549-007-9528-5.
20. Mann RM, Loo CE, Wobbes T, et al. The impact of preoperative breast MRI on the re-excision rate in invasive lobular carcinoma of the breast. Breast Cancer Res Treat. 2010;119:415–22. https://doi.org/10.1007/s10549-009-0616-6.
21. Sardanelli F, Boetes C, Borisch B, et al. Magnetic resonance imaging of the breast: recommendations from the EUSOMA working group. Eur J Cancer. 2010;46:1296–316. https://doi.org/10.1016/j.ejca.2010.02.015.
22. The Royal College of R. Guidance on screening and symptomatic breast imaging, 4th ed.; 2019.
23. D'Orsi CJ, Sickles EA, Mendelson EB, Morris EA. ACR BI-RADS® atlas, breast imaging reporting and data system. Reston, VA: American College of Radiology; 2013.
24. Maxwell AJ, Ridley NT, Rubin G, Wallis MG, Gilbert FJ, Michell MJ. The Royal College of Radiologists Breast Group breast imaging classification. Clin Radiol. 2009;64:624–7. https://doi.org/10.1016/j.crad.2009.01.010.
25. Mann RM, Cho N, Moy L. Breast MRI: state of the art. Radiology. 2019;292:520–36. https://doi.org/10.1148/radiol.2019182947.
26. Taylor JS, Tofts PS, Port R, et al. MR imaging of tumor microcirculation: promise for the new millennium. J Magn Reson Imaging. 1999;10:903–7. https://doi.org/10.1002/(sici)1522-2586(199912)10:6<903::aid-jmri1>3.0.co;2-a.
27. Sardanelli F. Additional findings at preoperative MRI: a simple golden rule for a complex problem? Breast Cancer Res Treat. 2010;124:717–21. https://doi.org/10.1007/s10549-010-1144-0.
28. Morrow M. Magnetic resonance imaging in breast cancer: one step forward, two steps back? JAMA. 2004;292:2779–80. https://doi.org/10.1001/jama.292.22.2779.
29. Houssami N, Hayes DF. Review of preoperative magnetic resonance imaging (MRI) in breast cancer: should MRI be performed on all women with newly diagnosed, early stage breast cancer? CA Cancer J Clin. 2009;59:290–302. https://doi.org/10.3322/caac.20028.
30. Bluemke DA, Gatsonis CA, Chen MH, et al. Magnetic resonance imaging of the breast prior to biopsy. JAMA. 2004;292:2735–42. https://doi.org/10.1001/jama.292.22.2735.
31. Braun M, Pölcher M, Schrading S, et al. Influence of preoperative MRI on the surgical management of patients with operable breast cancer. Breast Cancer Res Treat. 2008;111:179–87. https://doi.org/10.1007/s10549-007-9767-5.
32. Lehman CD, Gatsonis C, Kuhl CK, et al. MRI evaluation of the contralateral breast in women with recently diagnosed breast cancer. N Engl J Med. 2007;356:1295–303. https://doi.org/10.1056/NEJMoa065447.
33. Kuhl CK, Strobel K, Bieling H, et al. Impact of preoperative breast MR imaging and MR-guided surgery on diagnosis and surgical outcome of women with invasive breast cancer with and without DCIS component. Radiology. 2017;284:645–55. https://doi.org/10.1148/radiol.2017161449.
34. Obdeijn IM, Tilanus-Linthorst MM, Spronk S, et al. Preoperative breast MRI can reduce the rate of tumor-positive resection margins and reoperations in patients undergoing breast-conserving surgery. AJR Am J Roentgenol. 2013;200:304–10. https://doi.org/10.2214/ajr.12.9185.
35. Houssami N, Turner RM, Morrow M. Meta-analysis of pre-operative magnetic resonance imaging (MRI) and surgical treatment for breast cancer. Breast Cancer Res Treat. 2017;165:273–83. https://doi.org/10.1007/s10549-017-4324-3.
36. Vos EL, Voogd AC, Verhoef C, Siesling S, Obdeijn IM, Koppert LB. Benefits of preoperative MRI in breast cancer surgery studied in a large population-based cancer registry. Br J Surg. 2015;102:1649–57. https://doi.org/10.1002/bjs.9947.
37. Fortune-Greeley AK, Wheeler SB, Meyer AM, et al. Preoperative breast MRI and surgical outcomes in elderly women with invasive ductal and lobular carcinoma: a population-based study. Breast Cancer Res Treat. 2014;143:203–12. https://doi.org/10.1007/s10549-013-2787-4.
38. Weber JJ, Bellin LS, Milbourn DE, Verbanac KM, Wong JH. Selective preoperative magnetic resonance imaging in women with breast cancer: no reduction in the reoperation rate. Arch Surg. 2012;147:834–9. https://doi.org/10.1001/archsurg.2012.1660.

39. Peters NHGM, van Esser S, van den Bosch MAAJ, et al. Preoperative MRI and surgical management in patients with nonpalpable breast cancer: the MONET—randomised controlled trial. Eur J Cancer. 2011;47:879–86. https://doi.org/10.1016/j.ejca.2010.11.035.
40. Turnbull L, Brown S, Harvey I, et al. Comparative effectiveness of MRI in breast cancer (COMICE) trial: a randomised controlled trial. Lancet. 2010;375:563–71. https://doi.org/10.1016/S0140-6736(09)62070-5.
41. Houssami N, Turner R, Macaskill P, et al. An individual person data meta-analysis of preoperative magnetic resonance imaging and breast cancer recurrence. J Clin Oncol. 2014;32:392–401. https://doi.org/10.1200/jco.2013.52.7515.
42. Zeng Z, Amin A, Roy A, et al. Preoperative magnetic resonance imaging use and oncologic outcomes in premenopausal breast cancer patients. NPJ Breast Cancer. 2020;6:49. https://doi.org/10.1038/s41523-020-00192-7.
43. Holland R, Veling SHJ, Mravunac M, Hendriks JHCL. Histologic multifocality of tis, T1–2 breast carcinomas implications for clinical trials of breast-conserving surgery. Cancer. 1985;56:979–90. https://doi.org/10.1002/1097-0142(19850901)56:5<979::AID-CNCR2820560502>3.0.CO;2-N.
44. Darby S, McGale P, Correa C, et al. Effect of radiotherapy after breast-conserving surgery on 10-year recurrence and 15-year breast cancer death: meta-analysis of individual patient data for 10,801 women in 17 randomised trials. Lancet. 2011;378:1707–16. https://doi.org/10.1016/s0140-6736(11)61629-2.
45. Groheux D, Espié M, Giacchetti S, Hindié E. Performance of FDG PET/CT in the clinical management of breast cancer. Radiology. 2013;266:388–405. https://doi.org/10.1148/radiol.12110853.
46. Erdi YE. Limits of tumor detectability in nuclear medicine and PET. Mol Imaging Radionucl Ther. 2012;21:23–8. https://doi.org/10.4274/Mirt.138.
47. Kaidar-Person O, Boersma LJ, Poortmans P, et al. Residual glandular breast tissue after mastectomy: a systematic review. Ann Surg Oncol. 2020;27:2288–96. https://doi.org/10.1245/s10434-020-08516-4.
48. Robertson C, Arcot Ragupathy SK, Boachie C, et al. The clinical effectiveness and cost-effectiveness of different surveillance mammography regimens after the treatment for primary breast cancer: systematic reviews registry database analyses and economic evaluation. Health Technol Assess. 2011;15:v–vi, 1–322. https://doi.org/10.3310/hta15340.
49. Walstra CJEF, Schipper R-J, Winter-Warnars GA, et al. Local staging of ipsilateral breast tumor recurrence: mammography, ultrasound, or MRI? Breast Cancer Res Treat. 2020;184:385–95. https://doi.org/10.1007/s10549-020-05850-9.
50. Lehman CD, Lee JM, DeMartini WB, et al. Screening MRI in women with a personal history of breast cancer. J Natl Cancer Inst. 2016;108. https://doi.org/10.1093/jnci/djv349.
51. Tagliafico AS, Bignotti B, Rossi F, et al. Diagnostic performance of contrast-enhanced spectral mammography: systematic review and meta-analysis. Breast. 2016;28:13–9. https://doi.org/10.1016/j.breast.2016.04.008.
52. Sung JS, Lebron L, Keating D, et al. Performance of dual-energy contrast-enhanced digital mammography for screening women at increased risk of breast cancer. Radiology. 2019;293:81–8. https://doi.org/10.1148/radiol.2019182660.
53. Patel BK, Lobbes MBI, Lewin J. Contrast enhanced spectral mammography: a review. Semin Ultrasound CT MRI. 2018;39:70–9. https://doi.org/10.1053/j.sult.2017.08.005.
54. Houben IPL, Van de Voorde P, Jeukens CRLPN, et al. Contrast-enhanced spectral mammography as work-up tool in patients recalled from breast cancer screening has low risks and might hold clinical benefits. Eur J Radiol. 2017;94:31–7. https://doi.org/10.1016/j.ejrad.2017.07.004.
55. Fallenberg EM, Schmitzberger FF, Amer H, et al. Contrast-enhanced spectral mammography vs. mammography and MRI—clinical performance in a multi-reader evaluation. Eur Radiol. 2017;27:2752–64. https://doi.org/10.1007/s00330-016-4650-6.
56. Lee-Felker SA, Tekchandani L, Thomas M, et al. Newly diagnosed breast cancer: comparison of contrast-enhanced spectral mammography and breast MR imaging in the evaluation of extent of disease. Radiology. 2017;285:389–400. https://doi.org/10.1148/radiol.2017161592.
57. Zanardo M, Cozzi A, Trimboli RM, et al. Technique, protocols and adverse reactions for contrast-enhanced spectral mammography (CESM): a systematic review. Insights Imaging. 2019;10:76. https://doi.org/10.1186/s13244-019-0756-0.
58. Kuhl CK, Schrading S, Strobel K, Schild HH, Hilgers R-D, Bieling HB. Abbreviated breast magnetic resonance imaging (MRI): first postcontrast subtracted images and maximum-intensity projection—a novel approach to breast cancer screening with MRI. J Clin Oncol. 2014;32:2304–10. https://doi.org/10.1200/JCO.2013.52.5386.
59. Leithner D, Moy L, Morris EA, Marino MA, Helbich TH, Pinker K. Abbreviated MRI of the breast: does it provide value? J Magn Reson Imaging. 2018;49:e85–e100. https://doi.org/10.1002/jmri.26291.
60. Pham R, Marshall H, Plecha D. Abbreviated protocol breast MRI. Am J Roentgenol. 2020;215:765–9. https://doi.org/10.2214/AJR.19.22292.
61. Comstock CE, Gatsonis C, Newstead GM, et al. Comparison of abbreviated breast MRI vs digital breast tomosynthesis for breast cancer detection among women with dense breasts undergoing screening. JAMA. 2020;323:746. https://doi.org/10.1001/jama.2020.0572.
62. Shi R-y, Yao Q-y, Wu L-m, Xu J-r. Breast lesions: diagnosis using diffusion weighted imaging at 1.5T and 3.0T—systematic review and meta-analysis.

Clin Breast Cancer. 2018;18:e305–20. https://doi.org/10.1016/j.clbc.2017.06.011.
63. Baltzer P, Mann RM, Iima M, et al. Diffusion-weighted imaging of the breast—a consensus and mission statement from the EUSOBI International Breast Diffusion-Weighted Imaging working group. Eur Radiol. 2020;30:1436–50. https://doi.org/10.1007/s00330-019-06510-3.
64. Amornsiripanitch N, Bickelhaupt S, Shin HJ, et al. Diffusion-weighted MRI for unenhanced breast cancer screening. Radiology. 2019;293:504–20. https://doi.org/10.1148/radiol.2019182789.
65. Partridge SC, Demartini WB, Kurland BF, Eby PR, White SW, Lehman CD. Differential diagnosis of mammographically and clinically occult breast lesions on diffusion-weighted MRI. J Magn Reson Imaging. 2010;31:562–70. https://doi.org/10.1002/jmri.22078.
66. McDonald ES, Hammersley JA, Chou S-HS, et al. Performance of DWI as a rapid unenhanced technique for detecting mammographically occult breast cancer in elevated-risk women with dense breasts. Am J Roentgenol. 2016;207:205–16. https://doi.org/10.2214/AJR.15.15873.
67. McKinney SM, Sieniek M, Godbole V, et al. International evaluation of an AI system for breast cancer screening. Nature. 2020;577:89–94. https://doi.org/10.1038/s41586-019-1799-6.
68. Rodriguez-Ruiz A, Lång K, Gubern-Merida A, et al. Stand-alone artificial intelligence for breast cancer detection in mammography: comparison with 101 radiologists. J Natl Cancer Inst. 2019;111(9):916–92. https://doi.org/10.1093/jnci/djy222.
69. Schaffter T, Buist DSM, Lee CI, et al. Evaluation of combined artificial intelligence and radiologist assessment to interpret screening mammograms. JAMA Netw Open. 2020;3:e200265. https://doi.org/10.1001/jamanetworkopen.2020.0265.
70. Wu N, Phang J, Park J, et al. Deep neural networks improve radiologists' performance in breast cancer screening. IEEE Trans Med Imaging. 2020;39:1184–94. https://doi.org/10.1109/tmi.2019.2945514.
71. Kim H-E, Kim HH, Han B-K, et al. Changes in cancer detection and false-positive recall in mammography using artificial intelligence: a retrospective, multireader study. Lancet Digital Health. 2020;2:e138–48. https://doi.org/10.1016/S2589-7500(20)30003-0.
72. Wu N, Phang J, Park J, et al. Deep neural networks improve radiologists' performance in breast cancer screening. IEEE Trans Med Imaging. 2019;39(4):1184–94. https://doi.org/10.1109/TMI.2019.2945514.
73. Rodríguez-Ruiz A, Krupinski E, Mordang J-J, et al. Detection of breast cancer with mammography: effect of an artificial intelligence support system. Radiology. 2018;290:305–14. https://doi.org/10.1148/radiol.2018181371.
74. Rodriguez-Ruiz A, Lång K, Gubern-Merida A, et al. Can we reduce the workload of mammographic screening by automatic identification of normal exams with artificial intelligence? A feasibility study. Eur Radiol. 2019;29(9):4825–32. https://doi.org/10.1007/s00330-019-06186-9.
75. Yala A, Schuster T, Miles R, Barzilay R, Lehman C. A deep learning model to triage screening mammograms: a simulation study. Radiology. 2019;293:38–46. https://doi.org/10.1148/radiol.2019182908.
76. Kyono T, Gilbert FJ, van der Schaar M. Improving workflow efficiency for mammography using machine learning. J Am Coll Radiol. 2020;17:56–63. https://doi.org/10.1016/j.jacr.2019.05.012.
77. Lång K, Dustler M, Dahlblom V, Åkesson A, Andersson I, Zackrisson S. Identifying normal mammograms in a large screening population using artificial intelligence. Eur Radiol. 2020;31(3):1687–92. https://doi.org/10.1007/s00330-020-07165-1.

Management and Workflow

10

Jana Jaal, Philip Poortmans,
and Orit Kaidar-Person

10.1 Background

Radiation therapy (RT) is an important modality in the treatment of cancer patients. It is estimated that up to 87% of breast cancer patients will be treated with RT for different indications [1]. It is well recognised that postoperative RT decreases LRR and cancer-specific mortality for early stage disease [2]. In addition to curative indications, RT is a major modality for palliation or symptom control and recently, used as an ablative non-invasive treatment to oligometastatic patients or in case of oligo-progression (see section about oligometastatic and oligo-progressive disease). In this setting, RT has been shown to significantly increase 5-year survival rates in oligometastatic patients [3]. New protocols with a limited number of fractions (e.g. FAST or FAST FORWARD protocols, APBI-FLORENCE protocol or SBRT for metastatic lesions) allow for RT to the breast or metastatic site associated with minimal morbidity and minimal interference with quality of life (QoL) and other cancer treatments. There are a number of RT techniques (e.g. EBRT, brachytherapy, IORT), and different RT doses and fractionation, which are used according to the clinical indication. In some cases, concomitant treatment of systemic therapy and RT is indicated (see section about inoperable breast cancer). These new indications for RT, together with exciting new protocols for adjuvant RT and in the metastatic setting, along with the global increase in cancer incidence and higher need for RT, put much higher demands on efficient treatment management and workflow. While the indications for RT and volumes to be irradiated are often a matter of discussion at multidisciplinary meetings that include surgeons, medical oncologists, pathologists and breast radiologists, management of RT itself is complex. Its application needs the involvement of the RT multidisciplinary team which includes radiation oncologists, nurses, RTTs, dosimetrists and physicists to plan and apply treatments. A proper predefined workflow, adapted to each institution according to the resources available, will secure quality care for

J. Jaal (✉)
Hematology and Oncology Clinic, Tartu University Hospital, Tartu, Estonia
e-mail: Jana.Jaal@kliinikum.ee

P. Poortmans
Faculty of Medicine and Health Sciences, University of Antwerp, Antwerp, Belgium

Department of Radiation Oncology, Iridium Netwerk, Antwerp, Belgium
e-mail: philip.poortmans@gza.be

O. Kaidar-Person
Radiation Oncology Unit, Sheba Medical Center, Ramat Gan, Israel

Sackler School of Medicine, Tel-Aviv University, Tel-Aviv, Israel

GROW-School for Oncology and Developmental Biology (Maastro), Maastricht University, Maastricht, The Netherlands
e-mail: Orit.kaidarperson@sheba.health.gov.il

© The Author(s), under exclusive license to Springer Nature Switzerland AG 2022
O. Kaidar-Person et al. (eds.), *Breast Cancer Radiation Therapy*,
https://doi.org/10.1007/978-3-030-91170-6_10

breast cancer patients. This chapter focusses on workflow adjustment and optimisation and gives additionally some practical hints that are based on experience at several radiation oncology departments.

10.2 Adjusting the Workflow

RT management and workflow are highly dependent on the services the RT department provides. These include the RT tertiary facility that patients are also referred from other institutions, RT department that only serves patients that are treated in-house or/and RT facility without other department (such as surgery/medical oncology) services.

Regardless of the setting, it is recommended to establish a working relationship with other disciplines and departments and that the radiation oncologists will be involved with the management of the patient from the time of diagnosis. As shown within the different sections of this book, advances in RT allow for new innovative approaches in the treatment of breast cancer that might not be known to other experts; therefore, the input of radiation experts at initial management discussion can be crucial to determine further management.

The RT department workflow has become quite complex. Although the use of workflow management software programmes (e.g. ARIA®, MOSAIQ®, RayCare®) has been shown to significantly improve overall efficiency and organisational ergonomics [4], the whole process is complex and thereby at risk for having several "bottlenecks" (Fig. 10.1), varying in different departments and countries. Different regions and countries have distinct availability of resources and needs for radiation oncology [5]. These include significant heterogeneity in the access to modern imaging as well as RT equipment. In some countries, PET-CT is often done for locally advanced breast cancer and metastatic setting and is used for RT planning by fusing the images with the CT simulation, while in other countries PET-CT is not used even in the metastatic setting. These differences were discussed in the 2020 EBCC manifesto dedicated to inappropriate reimbursement and funding rules and regulations that act as disincentives to best breast cancer care [6]. Additionally, significant differences are noted between high-income European countries, especially in Northern-Western Europe, that are well served with RT resources, whereas other countries are facing shortages of both equipment in general and especially machines capable of delivering high precision conformal treatments (IMRT, IGRT) [5].

Moreover, a considerable variation in available personnel and delivered courses per year exists between countries with highest and lowest staffing levels [7]. This is even more complicated by the variation in cancer incidence and socio-economic status of different countries, but also by different professional roles and responsibili-

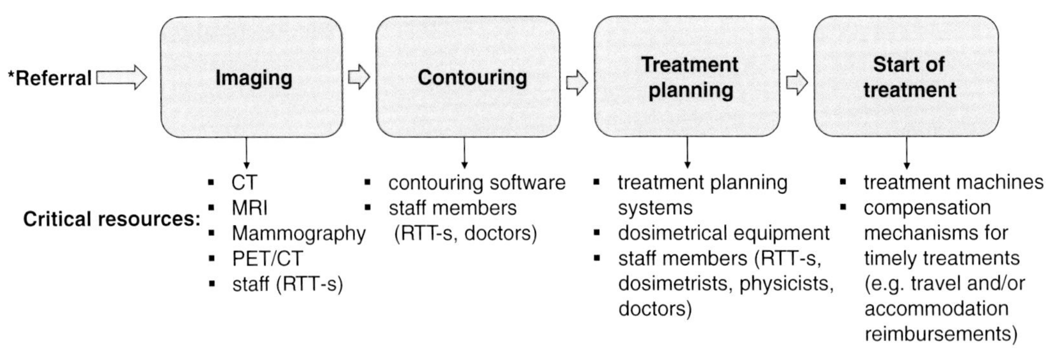

Fig. 10.1 Critical resources in radiation oncology workflow. *All relevant clinical data should be available at time of referral

ties. Importantly, the optimally required number of medical physicists, RTTs, dosimetrists, nurses and others depend highly on the tasks assigned to each of them, such as delineation of OARs (in some departments, it is done by the radiation oncologist while in others by the RTT, dosimetrists, etc.), treatment planning activities, quality assurance, maintenance of the technical infrastructure and accompaniment of patients [7–9]. Furthermore, RT workflow can also be influenced by the availability of optimal healthcare budgets [10] and other resources, such as travel and/or accommodation compensations, especially in areas with low population density.

Even more in view of this variability of technical, human and health service resources needed for proper RT planning and delivery, it is critical to systematically evaluate and analyse the RT workflow in every single department and facility. The latter is extremely important for further workflow optimisation processes. Therefore, each department should create a workflow that will be adjusted to the human and equipment resources but allow for quality care.

10.3 Workflow Optimisation

Workflow optimisation is the improvement of an existing workflow to ensure that it performs as efficiently as possible with the main goal to reduce waiting times and maximise patient throughput. For this, four steps are important to follow (to be repeated with a constructive evaluation) (Fig. 10.2).

The workflow starts with patient referral to the RT department to first visit by the radiation oncologists. The initial task is to clearly define a list for the secretary team to verify that all medical information is available prior to the patient's visit. These include original pathology reports (from biopsy, surgery, etc.), operative report, genomic testing, genetic consultation and results, and all relevant imaging reports and imaging scans (e.g. mammography, CT, PET-CT, MRI) uploaded to a picture archiving and communication system (PACS), any other relevant information. This will allow the radiation oncologist or a dedicated team of nurse/physician assistant to review the information prior to the patient visit if needed. In some cases, the patient can be referred to additional evaluation prior to RT consultation. For example, if there were diffuse microcalcification on preoperative mammography, without a postoperative imaging, the radiation oncologist can decide to refer the patient to additional mammography to exclude residual microcalcifications/residual disease prior to the first visit.

Organising the medical record with all essential information can save significant time at the time of patient's visit.

At the time of patient's visit and RT planning, the radiation oncologist needs to carefully view all dedicated imaging (e.g. mammography, CT, MRI, PET-CT), to allow for correct determination of target volumes and treatment protocol

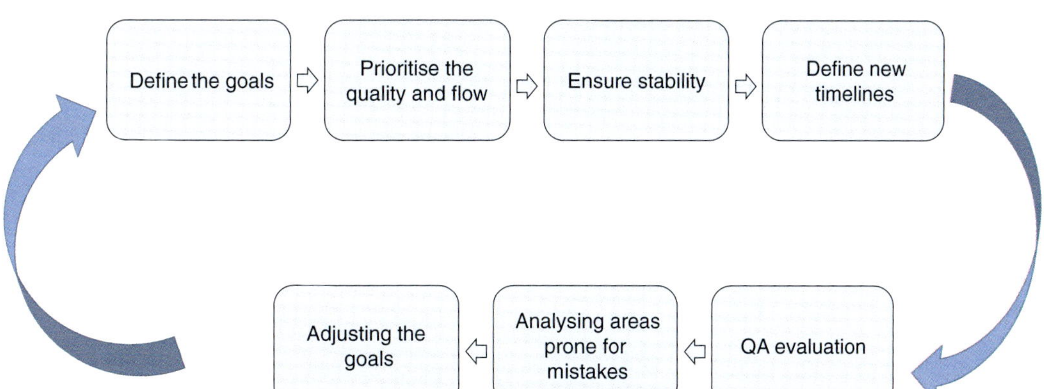

Fig. 10.2 Radiation therapy workflow optimisation steps

(e.g. a PET-avid IMN). Dedicated imaging will allow for correct contouring the target volumes and the relevant OARs, treatment planning, and quality assurance [8].

When there is no other workup that needs to be completed prior to RT, **the first goal should be to avoid delays in RT** and to reach acceptable throughput times. Although every country might have different resource-driven possibilities, it is reasonable to set target RT waiting times to a maximum of 4 weeks. Indeed, previously published meta-analysis showed that every 4 weeks of waiting time for postoperative RT was associated with an 8% relative increase in the risk of breast cancer LRR [11]. Even as this argument, for breast cancer, might not be valid anymore in the setting of a well-organised multidisciplinary approach [12], it remains of great importance, both for several other (faster proliferating) tumour types as for the setting up of the workflow as such.

Secondly, it is important to prioritise process **quality and flow**. Every radiation oncology facility must have quality assurance protocols and quality management [10]. In line with the best available quality control, every department has to set up optimal flow of different components of radiation therapy pre-treatment processes that help to avoid radiation therapy delays. As described earlier, resources differ from country to country; therefore, there are no common guidelines that would fit to all. Instead, local and currently available technical and human resources should be used in creating suitable workflow settings. Acceptable time frames for completing each pre-treatment task should be agreed. It is also highly recommended to make optimal use of the software programmes (e.g. ARIA®, MOSAIQ®, RayCare®) to generate automated timestamps upon completion of each critical workflow task, as well as reminders if a task is not completed [13].

Thirdly, after creating the local radiation therapy workflow, it is important to ensure its **stability**. For example, in the whole process, there should not be components that rely only on a single machine or individual. Together with strategic staffing activities, the need for department investments should be equally assessed and items prioritised to guarantee workflow stability.

Fourthly, subsequent activities are required to increase the overall workflow **speed**, since even a 4-week delay in cancer treatment has been shown to be associated with increased mortality in several tumour types, including breast cancer [14]. Therefore, policies on minimising system delays to cancer treatment initiation are the first tool to improve survival outcomes on population level. As a good example, maximum waiting time targets defined by the Dutch Society for Radiation Oncology state that **acute patients** should be treated within **1 day**, **subacute patients** should start treatment **within 7 days**, and **regular patients** should start treatment **within 21 days** [15].

10.4 A Personal Viewpoint Based on Experience at Several Radiation Oncology Departments

- In the past, similar to other medical specialties, the link between the single patient and the single doctor was "untouchable". Notwithstanding the advantage of the importance of an optimal patient–doctor relationship, its pitfalls lie in missing specific expertise, fluctuation in workload, availability for performing timewise every single step in the workflow at the best moment, and presence or absence. All this seriously limits flexibility and availability, and thereby optimal workflow management. Therefore, the workflow should ideally be organised per team, each consisting of several professionals that will handle assigned tasks not on a personal but on a team base.
- The ideal workflow should be as such that all steps should be manageable within the shortest timeframes as possible, why not within 24 h, infrastructure and staffing permitting. However, it has to be accepted that setting up an idealistic workflow creates also margins in time, offering equalising the tides of high- and low-workloads.

- Several organisations offer professional support in setting up workflow management systems, both in medical and in non-medical settings. Of particular interest is the use of the "lean management" principles in a radiation oncology department, as it will not only improve the workflows themselves but also give insight to all healthcare providers in their role in the daily setting up of activities, allow improved monitoring of performances, increase involvement of all staff members and, very importantly, improve safety for both patients and organisations [16–21].
- An interesting note lies in forward versus backwards planning within the workflow management. When switching to backwards planning, improved adaptation of the stepwise scheduling allows better adaptation to availability of resources and staff: for example, if a breast cancer patient is to be started within 21 days from her discussion at the MTB, the first RT-fraction can be set, from which backwards all preparatory steps should be planned respecting the time required for each of them.
- Medical doctors traditionally struggle to accepting standardisation of medical processes, claiming that every single patient is unique and presents with a unique challenging disease. As such, the medical professionals needed to acquire the skills of team playing, which is clearly influenced by cultural background. It is not by pointing to individual flaws, but by demonstrating the advantages of optimised multidisciplinary team-based workflows that we can keep all essential healthcare workers on board. As derived from the Pareto Principle, stating that 20% of the activities will account for 80% of the results and, conversely, that 80% of impact stems from just 20% of potential causes, standardising for the 80% will not only limit strongly the risks for errors but simultaneously allow to spend significantly more time on the 20% who require an individually adapted approach [22, 23].
- Indeed, optimising a workflow is tightly connected to people management. The transition from an archaic workflow based on an endless combination of options for each individual to a well-structured organisation for the entire workload (patients and activities) takes time and costs. During this period, all staff members need to be kept onboard, preferably by involving them actively in the transition process.

10.5 Future Perspectives

Recently, artificial intelligence has emerged to improve and optimise radiation therapy workflow and quality of care [24]. There are several ways where artificial intelligence can be used throughout the radiation therapy workflow components, including image reconstruction and registration, image segmentation and analysis, risk modelling and profiling, treatment planning and quality assurance [25, 26]. Currently, it is not yet clear to which extent automation and artificial intelligence will help to increase radiation therapy utilisation in countries with remarkable shortages in technical and human radiation therapy resources. Nevertheless, it is hoped that all these technical advances will foster integrated care that is centred around the needs of the patient and not of the system. Additionally, artificial intelligence cannot overcome a disorganised workflow and cannot be of aid without the intellect of the treating team.

References

1. Borras JM, Barton M, Grau C, Corral J, Verhoeven R, Lemmens V, et al. The impact of cancer incidence and stage on optimal utilization of radiotherapy: methodology of a population based analysis by the ESTRO-HERO project. Radiother Oncol. 2015;116:45–50.
2. Darby S, McGale P, Correa C, Taylor C, Arriagada R, Clarke M, et al. Effect of radiotherapy after breast-conserving surgery on 10-year recurrence and 15-year breast cancer death: meta-analysis of individual patient data for 10,801 women in 17 randomised trials. Lancet. 2011;378:1707–16.
3. Palma DA, Olson R, Harrow S, Gaede S, Louie AV, Haasbeek C, et al. Stereotactic ablative radiotherapy for the comprehensive treatment of oligometastatic cancers: long-term results of the SABR-COMET phase II randomized trial. J Clin Oncol. 2020;38:2830–8.
4. Miriyala R, Thakur P, Singh A, Gupta A, Yadav B, Kumar N, et al. Workflow management in radiation

oncology: the impact on a high volume department. Br J Health Care Manag. 2018;24:302–7.
5. Grau C, Defourny N, Malicki J, Dunscombe P, Borras JM, Coffey M, et al. Radiotherapy equipment and departments in the European countries: final results from the ESTRO-HERO survey. Radiother Oncol. 2014;112:155–64.
6. EBCC. EBCC-12 Manifesto. EBCC-12 European Breast Cancer Conference. Virtual 2020. https://conferences.eortc.org/ebcc12/.
7. Lievens Y, Defourny N, Coffey M, Borras JM, Dunscombe P, Slotman B, et al. Radiotherapy staffing in the European countries: final results from the ESTRO-HERO survey. Radiother Oncol. 2014;112:178–86.
8. Vieira B, Demirtas D, van de Kamer JB, Hans EW, van Harten W. Improving workflow control in radiotherapy using discrete-event simulation. BMC Med Inform Decis Mak. 2019;19:199.
9. Willmann J, Poortmans P, Monti AF, Grant W, Clementel E, Corning C, et al. Development of staffing, workload and infrastructure in member departments of the European Organisation for Research and Treatment of Cancer (EORTC) radiation oncology group. Radiother Oncol. 2020;155:226–31.
10. Zubizarreta E, Van Dyk J, Lievens Y. Analysis of global radiotherapy needs and costs by geographic region and income level. Clin Oncol (R Coll Radiol). 2017;29:84–92.
11. Gupta S, King WD, Korzeniowski M, Wallace DL, Mackillop WJ. The effect of waiting times for postoperative radiotherapy on outcomes for women receiving partial mastectomy for breast cancer: a systematic review and meta-analysis. Clin Oncol (R Coll Radiol). 2016;28:739–49.
12. van Maaren MC, Bretveld RW, Jobsen JJ, Veenstra RK, Groothuis-Oudshoorn CG, Struikmans H, et al. The influence of timing of radiation therapy following breast-conserving surgery on 10-year disease-free survival. Br J Cancer. 2017;117:179–88.
13. Manyam BV, Yu N, Meier T, Suh JH, Chao ST. A review of strategies for optimizing workflow, quality improvement, and patient safety within radiation oncology departments. Appl Radiat Oncol. 2018:7–12.
14. Hanna TP, King WD, Thibodeau S, Jalink M, Paulin GA, Harvey-Jones E, et al. Mortality due to cancer treatment delay: systematic review and meta-analysis. BMJ. 2020;371:m4087.
15. NVRO. Waiting times. https://www.nvro.nl/kwaliteit/indicatoren.
16. Kim CS, Spahlinger DA, Kin JM, Coffey RJ, Billi JE. Implementation of lean thinking: one health system's journey. Jt Comm J Qual Patient Saf. 2009;35:406–13.
17. Simons PA, Houben R, Benders J, Pijls-Johannesma M, Vandijck D, Marneffe W, et al. Does compliance to patient safety tasks improve and sustain when radiotherapy treatment processes are standardized? Eur J Oncol Nurs. 2014;18:459–65.
18. Simons PA, Houben R, Vlayen A, Hellings J, Pijls-Johannesma M, Marneffe W, et al. Does lean management improve patient safety culture? An extensive evaluation of safety culture in a radiotherapy institute. Eur J Oncol Nurs. 2015;19:29–37.
19. Simons P, Backes H, Bergs J, Emans D, Johannesma M, Jacobs M, et al. The effects of a lean transition on process times, patients and employees. Int J Health Care Qual Assur. 2017;30:103–18.
20. Al-Balushi MM, Al-Mandhari Z. Implementing lean management techniques at a radiation oncology department. Sultan Qaboos Univ Med J. 2018;18:e362–e6.
21. Nabelsi V, Plouffe V. Breast cancer treatment pathway improvement using time-driven activity-based costing. Int J Health Plann Manag. 2019;34:e1736–e46.
22. Koch R. The 80/20 principle: the secret to success by achieving more with less. Nicholas Brealey Publishing; 2017.
23. Harvey HB, Sotardi ST. The Pareto principle. J Am Coll Radiol. 2018;15:931.
24. Pillai M, Adapa K, Das SK, Mazur L, Dooley J, Marks LB, et al. Using artificial intelligence to improve the quality and safety of radiation therapy. J Am Coll Radiol. 2019;16:1267–72.
25. Poortmans PMP, Takanen S, Marta GN, Meattini I, Kaidar-Person O. Winter is over: the use of artificial intelligence to individualise radiation therapy for breast cancer. Breast. 2020;49:194–200.
26. Korreman S, Eriksen JG, Grau C. The changing role of radiation oncology professionals in a world of AI—just jobs lost—or a solution to the under-provision of radiotherapy? Clin Transl Radiat Oncol. 2021;26:104–7.

Part III

Essential Knowledge

Breast and Lymph Node Anatomy 11

Petra Steyerova and David Kachlik

11.1 Background

The female breast is a complex organ with rich vascular, lymphatic and nerve supply and many relations to the thoracic wall, axilla and other neighbouring structures. A precise knowledge of anatomy is crucial for diagnosis, treatment and follow-up of breast cancer. As there are also numerous variants of anatomy of the breast tissue, blood and lymphatic vessels and nerves, these can be important for understanding the treatment guidelines, research and clinical issues that arise during management of patients with breast cancer.

11.2 Key Information for Clinical Practice

11.2.1 Breast Anatomy

Breast is a paired organ located on the thoracic wall at the level of the second to the sixth intercostal spaces. While anatomically it is delineated medially by the parasternal line and extending laterally to the anterior axillary line, for the purpose of irradiation its medial aspect is located lateral to the medial perforating mammary vessels and its lateral aspect is situated anterior to the lateral thoracic vessels. Posteriorly it overlays muscles of the thoracic wall—the pectoralis major muscle (clinically referred to as the major pectoral muscle), the serratus anterior muscle and cranial portions of the abdominal muscles. It consists of the mammary gland and surrounding connective and adipose (fat) tissues and is situated in the subcutaneous tissue, within the superficial thoracic fascia.

The size of the breast depends on the amount of adipose and glandular tissues. The relative proportions of the glandular tissue and the fat determines the so-called density, which is important for detection of cancer in mammography. Patients with dense breasts (breasts with high amount of glandular parenchyma and low amount of fat) benefit less from mammography screening [1]. The body of the breast can be divided into two parts: circular body and axillary tail. Accessory breast tissue appears in 2–6% of women and is located along the developmental milk line, typically in the axilla [2]. At the centre of the breast, there is the elevated nipple with ductal openings, surrounded by the areola, a pigmented area of the skin containing numerous apocrine glands and a few hair follicles.

P. Steyerova (✉)
Breast Cancer Screening and Diagnostic Centre, Department of Radiology, First Faculty of Medicine, Charles University and General University Hospital, Prague, Czech Republic
e-mail: petra.steyerova@vfn.cz

D. Kachlik
Department of Anatomy, Second Faculty of Medicine, Charles University, Prague, Czech Republic
e-mail: david.kachlik@lfmotol.cuni.cz

© The Author(s), under exclusive license to Springer Nature Switzerland AG 2022

O. Kaidar-Person et al. (eds.), *Breast Cancer Radiation Therapy*,
https://doi.org/10.1007/978-3-030-91170-6_11

The mammary gland is an exocrine apocrine milk-producing gland consisting of a complex of tubo-alveolar glands formed by 15–20 individual coned-shaped lobes (each of 1–2 mm in size) [3], arranged in a radial pattern and separated by fibrous interlobular bundles. Lobular anatomy determines the distribution and location of ductal carcinoma in situ, which tends to have lobular/segmental distribution following the radial arrangement and extending along the course of the ducts. This pattern is one of the features that helps diagnosing the disease in imaging [4]. Each lobe is associated with its own lactiferous duct extending to the nipple. Some authors state that the number of openings on the nipple does not always correlate with the number of ducts, the number of openings drop to as few as 5–9, indicating that larger areas may have a common duct and opening [5], or that more ducts can share the same opening as they join behind the nipple [6]. This has to be taken into account in the evaluation of patients with bloody discharge from the nipple or patients with Paget's disease of the nipple.

The glandular parenchyma is supported by connective tissue called the suspensory ligaments/retinacula of the breast (ligaments of Cooper) which penetrate the gland from the pectoralis major muscle towards the skin and provide support for the parenchyma. The mammary gland is delineated posteriorly by the posterior layer of the superficial thoracic fascia [7]. The space between the pectoralis major muscle and the posterior layer is called the retromammary bursa (of Chassaignac). Ventrally, the parenchyma is encased by the anterior layer of the superficial thoracic fascia, which reaches various distances from the skin of the nipple and areola. Both these spaces and fascial planes are important for surgical approaches in cancer surgery and reconstruction [8]. Caudally, the breast is supported by strong inframammary fold ligament, which ensures a fixed position of the breast during its changes and ageing. A centrally located fibrous septum (of Würinger) is located horizontally at the level of the fifth rib, extending towards the nipple and containing neurovascular structures. The lower portion of the breast is divided vertically by the septum of Awad [9] which can sometimes be visible in a MRI of the breast (Fig. 11.1).

11.2.2 Blood Supply and Innervation

The arterial blood supply to the breast is provided by the anterior intercostal arteries (from the internal thoracic artery), posterior intercostal arteries (directly from the aorta), lateral thoracic, superior thoracic and thoraco-acromial arteries (from the axillary artery). The medial part of the breast is supplied by the medial mammary branches, and the perforating branches of the second to fourth anterior intercostal arteries (from the internal thoracic artery), which constitute the major supply to the nipple-areolar complex and have major influence of the vitality of the nipple in surgery [10]. Laterally, the breast receives blood from the lateral thoracic artery. The upper part of the breast is supplied by the pectoral branch of the thoraco-acromial artery. The deep portion of the lateral breast is supplied by the lateral mammary branches, and the perforating branches of the second to sixth posterior intercostal arteries. The venous system of the breast has a larger superficial and a smaller deep group and gathers towards the axillary, internal thoracic and intercostal veins. A major venous subareolar plexus (of Haller) is located under the nipple and areola.

The sensory innervation of the breast is provided by a number of small nerves, mainly the anterior (medial part of the breast) and lateral (lateral part of the breast) cutaneous branches of the second to sixth intercostal nerves. The largest branch to the nipple usually arises from the deep branch of the lateral branch of the fourth intercostal nerve [11]. The upper part of the breast is innervated by the supraclavicular nerves from the cervical plexus. The intercostobrachial nerve usually originates from the lateral cutaneous branch of the second intercostal nerve and innervates the axilla and a small part of the adjacent lateral thoracic wall and of the proximal medial part of the

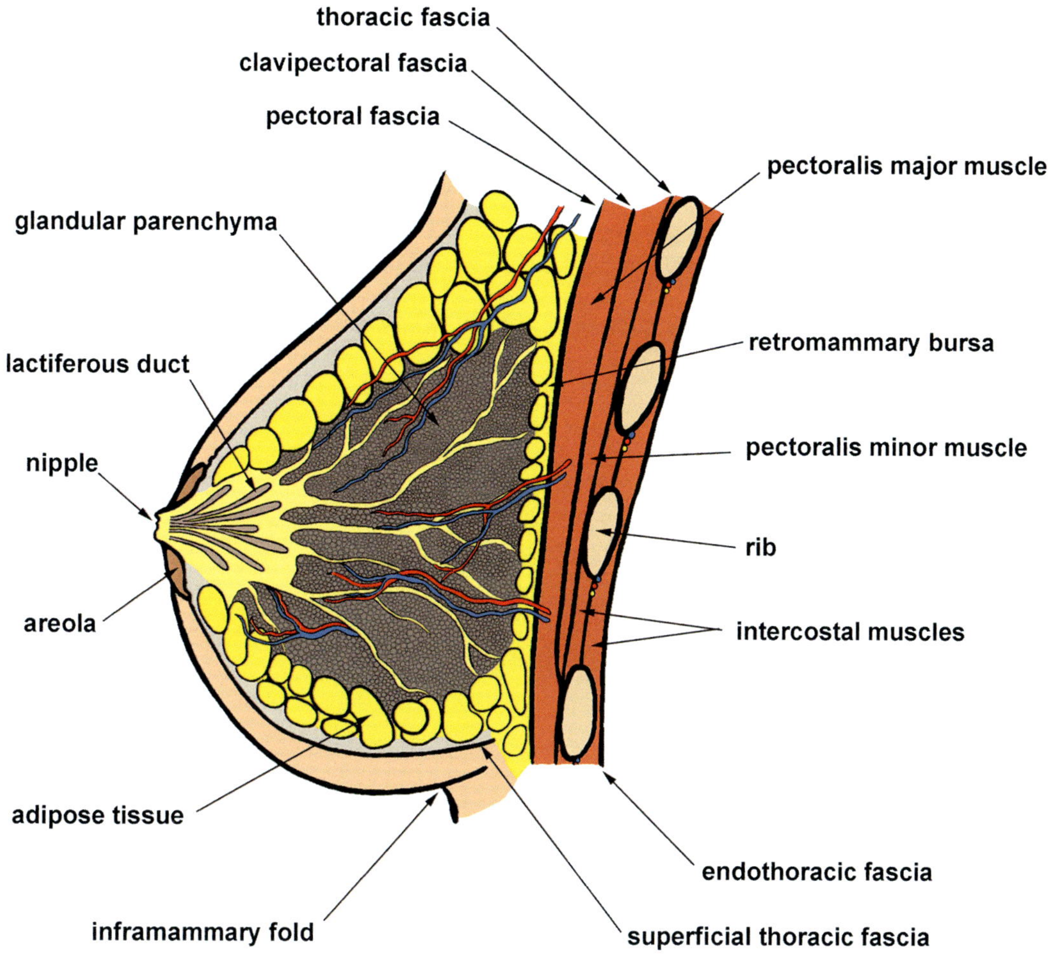

Fig. 11.1 Anatomy of the breast

arm. It is at risk for injury during operative procedures and its lesioning has been associated with postoperative sensory loss and neuropathic pain, decreasing quality of life of breast cancer survivors [12]. Less frequently, the second (accessory) intercostobrachial nerve can be present in 61% of cases, originating from the lateral cutaneous branch of the third intercostal nerve [13, 14].

11.2.3 Anatomy of Axilla

The axilla is a pyramidal space with an apex cranially, a base caudally, and four walls. It is surrounded by the pectoral muscles (anteriorly), latissimus dorsi and teres major muscles (posteriorly), serratus anterior muscle, the thoracic wall and its muscles (medially), humerus and its muscles (laterally). The apex is located at the junction of the clavicle, the superior border of the scapula, and the first rib. The base is formed by the axillary fascia. The axilla contains the axillary artery (with its branches) and vein (with its tributaries), the brachial plexus with its three fascicles, thoracodorsal, long thoracic, pectoral and subscapular nerves, and the axillary lymphatic plexus featuring multiple axillary lymph nodes, surrounded by adipose tissue (Fig. 11.2).

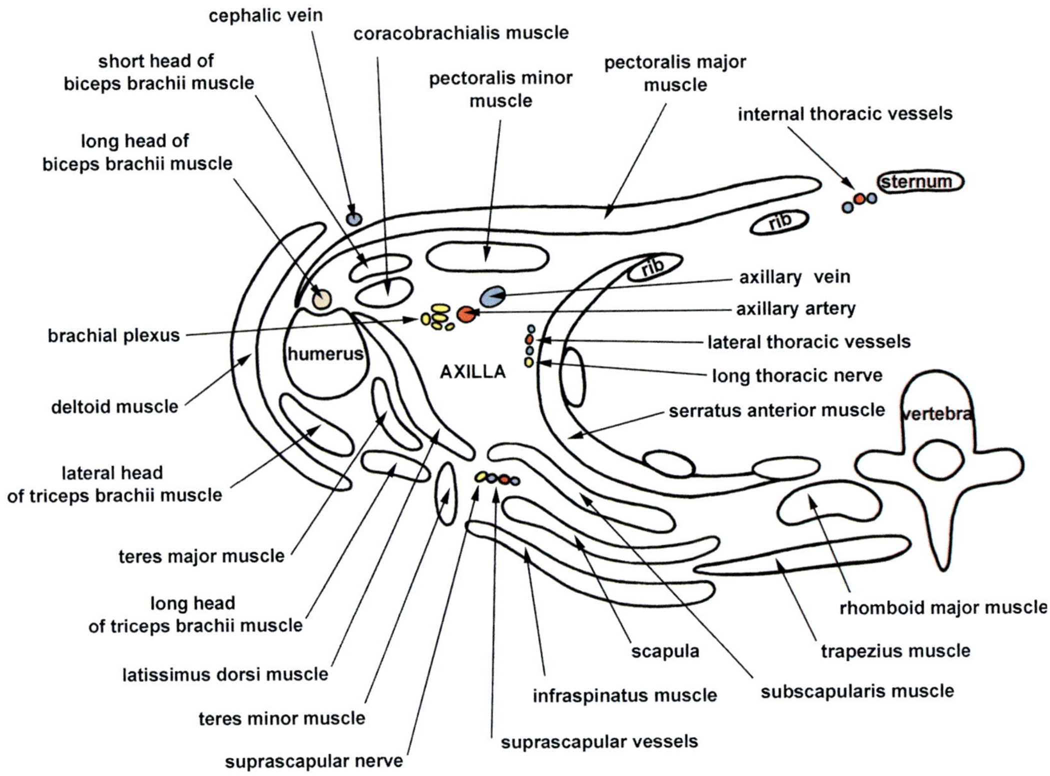

Fig. 11.2 Cross-sectional anatomical schema of the axilla

11.2.4 Lymphatic Drainage of the Breast

The lymphatic system of the breast is rich and complex and consists of superficial (cutaneous and subcutaneous), deep (glandular and fascial) and perforating systems [15]. The richest lymphatic network is located under the nipple-areolar complex in the subcutaneous layer and is called the subareolar plexus (of Sappey). All the other networks are connected to the subareolar plexus through perforating branches and branches in the connective tissue and along the ducts (Fig. 11.3).

Primary lymphatic drainage direction of the breast comprising approximately 75% of the lymphatic drainage is to the axilla via 4–6 lymphatic vessels called collectors [16, 17]. There are several groups of lymph nodes in the axilla named according to their anatomical location. The most caudal axillary lymph node is called the pectoral node of Sorgius, located on the second/third digitation of the serratus anterior muscle, at the crossing of the lateral thoracic vessels and intercostobrachial nerve [18]. The lymph nodes in axilla are grouped and named according to their location (Table 11.1).

Surgically, the axilla can be divided into three levels [19]:

- Level I: Lymph nodes inferolateral to the pectoralis minor muscle.
- Level II: Lymph nodes behind the pectoralis minor muscle.
- Level III: Lymph nodes superomedial to the pectoralis minor muscle.

For tissue of the lower inner quadrant of the breast, lymphatic drainage to the parasternal lymph nodes (in clinical terminology usually called "internal mammary chain/lymph nodes") is more significant [20, 21], but also it can be an important lymphatic drainage pathway for tumours of the lateral part of the breast [22]. There is a number of parasternal lymph nodes

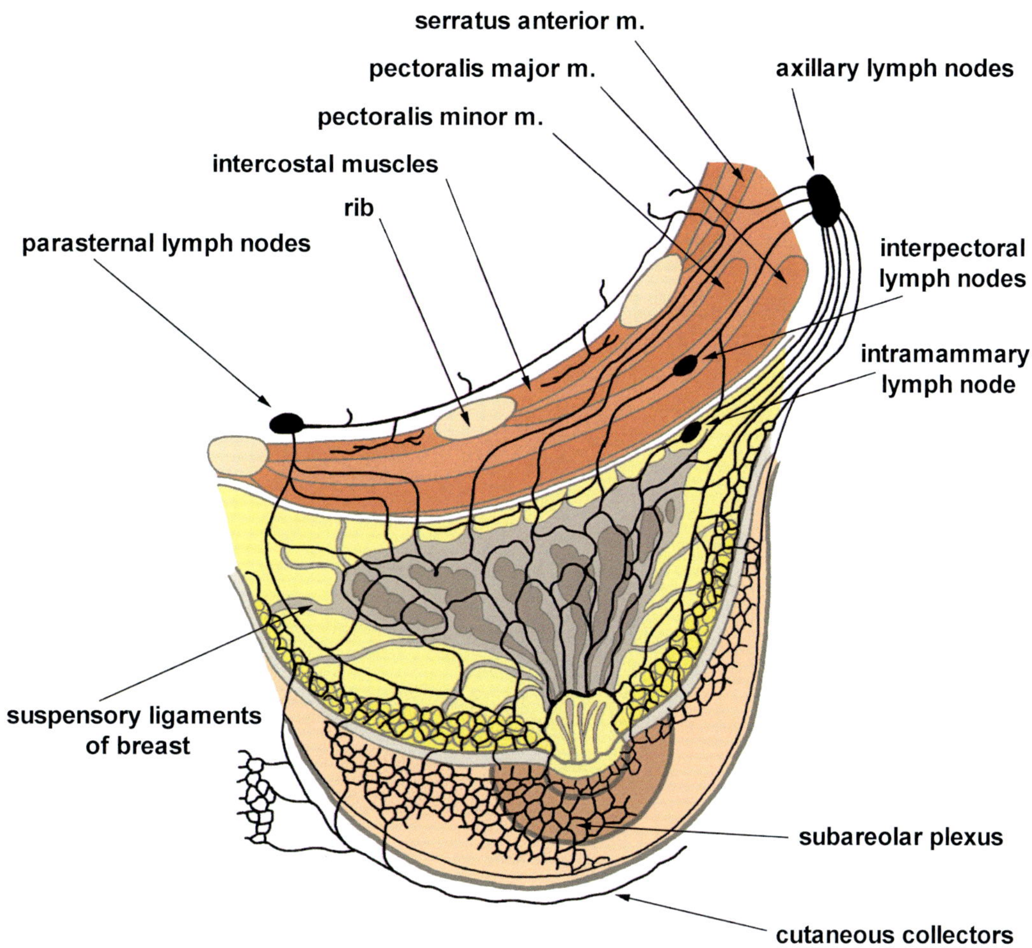

Fig. 11.3 Lymphatic drainage of the breast

Table 11.1 Axillary lymph node groups

Group	Location	Lymphatic drainage
Pectoral (anterior) group	Behind pectoralis major muscle, along inferior border of pectoralis minor muscle and lateral thoracic vessels	Lateral quadrants of breast, upper abdominal wall
Subscapular (posterior) group	In front of subscapular muscle, posterior axillary wall	Posterior and inferior trunk wall
Humeral (lateral) group	Along medial side of axillary vein	Arm
Central group	Axillary fat in centre of axilla	Drainage of above listed three groups
Deltopectoral (infraclavicular) group	Between deltoid and pectoralis major muscles	Lateral side of arm
Apical group	Apex of axilla, lateral border of first rib	Drainage of all above listed groups

located along the course of the internal thoracic vessels between the endothoracic fascia and the thoracic wall near the margin of the sternum located in the first to sixth intercostal space. Besides these two main directions, there are several more lymphatic drainage pathways. In some cases, the lymph flows upwards, piercing the pectoralis major muscle and draining directly to the interpectoral lymph nodes (of Rotter) or supraclavicular lymph nodes. The interpectoral lymph nodes, described by Rotter and Grossman [23], are affected in a minority of patients and the likelihood of their metastatic involvement increases mainly with the size of the primary tumour and axillary tumour burden [24]. A lymphatic drainage to the supraclavicular lymph nodes has been described by Mornard [25] and pathological involvement of these lymph nodes importantly affects the patient's prognosis [26]. There are also pathways directly to the deep inferior cervical lymph nodes [27], or downwards along the branches of the superior epigastric artery to prepericardiac lymph nodes or even contralaterally across the midline, especially when the primary ways are closed [17]. Sporadically, a retrosternal lymphatic drainage can occur to the contralateral parasternal lymph nodes or a subcutaneous drainage to the contralateral axilla is possible, occurring in patients where ipsilateral drainage is compromised by lymphatic obstruction caused by scarring, irradiation or tumour involvement [28]. These lymphatic pathways might contribute to the cancer spread beyond the locoregional treated area. In the case of metastatic involvement of lymph nodes the pattern of spread in the axilla is usually progressive, however also discontinuous ("skip") metastases can occur in 1–5% of cases [29] (Fig. 11.4).

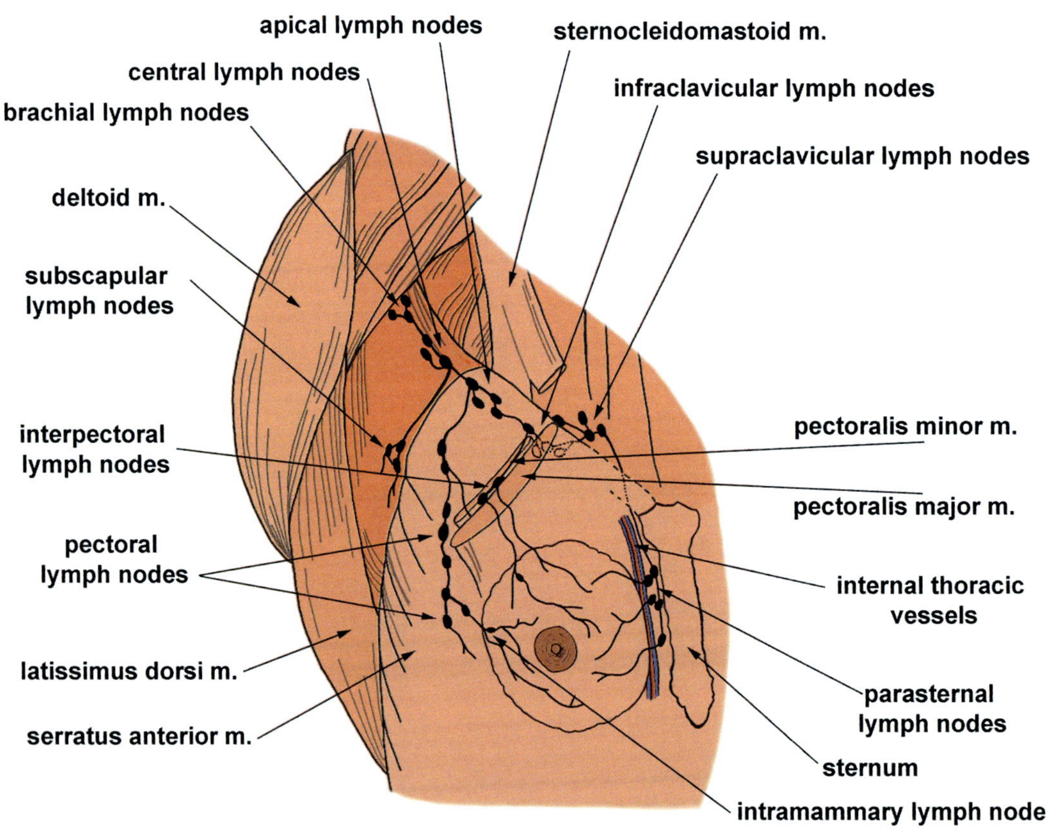

Fig. 11.4 Anatomy of the locoregional lymphatic vessels and lymph nodes

11.2.5 Intramammary Lymph Nodes

Some lymph nodes can be located within the breast tissue and are then called the intramammary lymph nodes. According to the literature, their incidence varies between 0.7% and 48% of cases [30]. In the TNM classification, these lymph nodes are coded as axillary lymph nodes level I [31]. In patients with breast cancer, it has been shown that a metastatic involvement of the intramammary lymph node predicts metastatic involvement of the axillary lymph nodes, but in some cases, the intramammary lymph nodes can be the only lymph nodes affected with no further tumour burden within the axilla [30].

At the time of diagnosis of the breast cancer, ultrasound is a reliable and available tool for lymph node staging. Axillary imaging by ultrasound is mandatory, and infraclavicular, supraclavicular, cervical and even parasternal lymph nodes are also easily reachable and identifiable (especially when pathological) [32], however not always a part of every examination. Advanced imaging modalities such as PET/CT, PET/MRI, SPECT/CT can add important information regarding lymphatic spread in locations mainly outside the axilla. These modalities could bring important information, which might affect planning of the treatment but the clinical value of these imaging methods and the impact on further management of the patient and survival are still to be studied [33] (Fig. 11.5a, b).

For the purpose of target volume delineation, a cross-sectional anatomy is essential. Different volume areas are delineated by anatomical structures, which are visible on planning CT. For orientation, see Fig. 11.6. Note that the CT scan is obtained with arms raised over the patient's head, so the anatomy might be shifted from the position in anatomy atlases, the vascular and nerve bundles are displaced cranially, muscles around the axilla rotated.

11.2.6 Thoracic Wall Muscles and Fasciae

The pectoralis major muscle, forming the base for the breast, originates from the medial half of the clavicle, lateral half of the sternum, the first to seventh costal cartilage and abdominal muscles aponeuroses, inserts on the crest of the greater tubercle of the humerus and is covered by the pectoral fascia. The underlying pectoralis minor muscle originates from the third to fifth rib, inserts on the coracoid process of the scapula and is enveloped by the clavipectoral fascia. The serratus anterior muscle originates usually from the first to ninth rib, inserts on the medial border of the scapula and its adjacent angles and is enveloped by the clavipectoral fascia as well. The latissimus dorsi muscle originates from the back (vertebrae, thoracolumbar fascia, iliac crest, 10th to 12th rib), inserts on the crest of the lesser tubercle of the humerus and is covered by the fascia dorsi. The deltoid muscle originates from the lateral one-third of the clavicle, acromion and lateral two-thirds of the scapular spine, inserts on

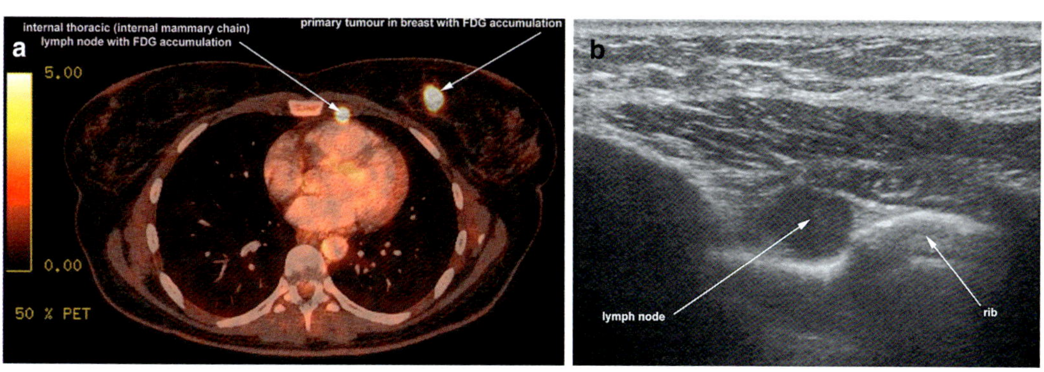

Fig. 11.5 Parasternal lymph nodes in (**a**) PET/CT and in (**b**) ultrasound

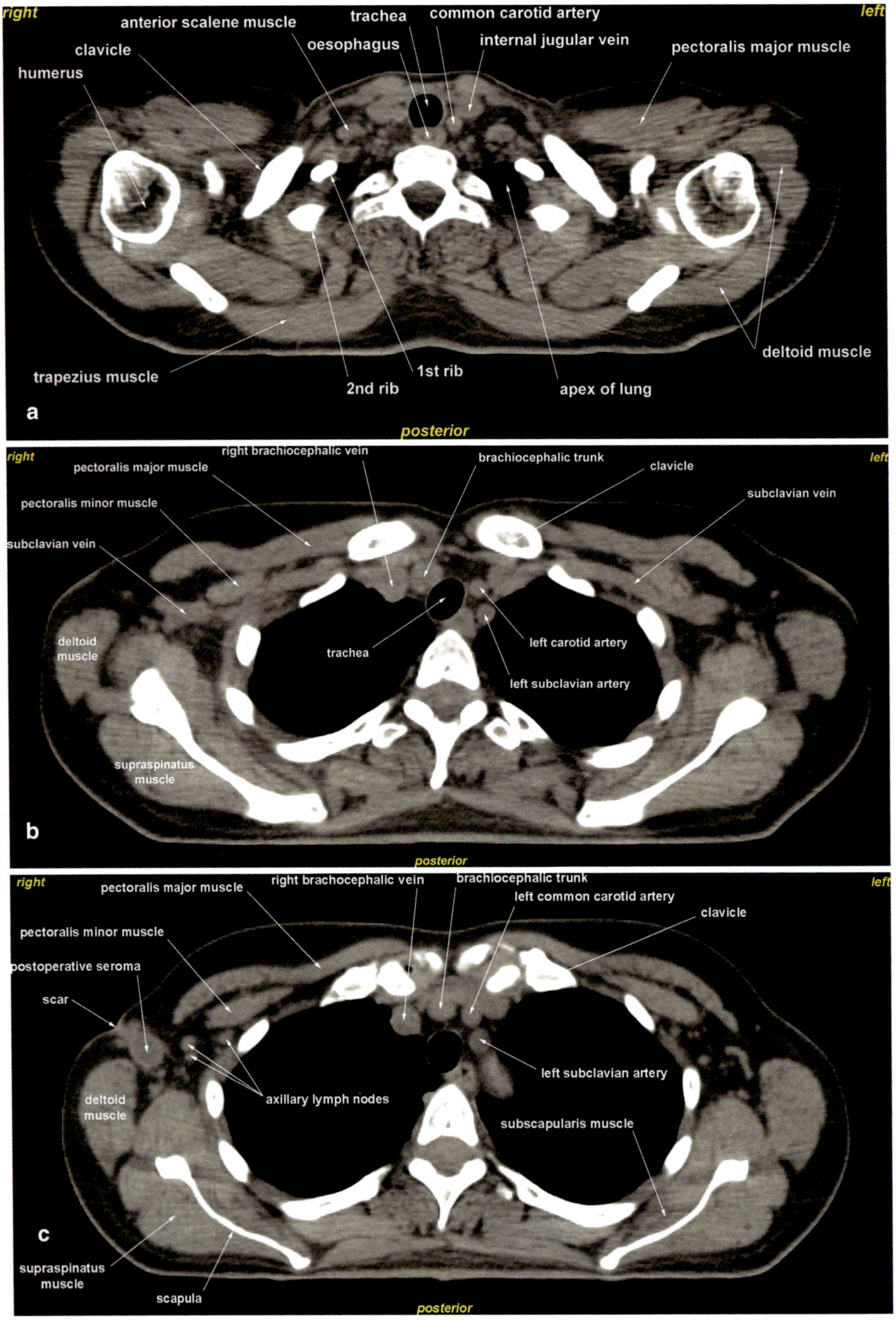

Fig. 11.6 Axial non-contrast CT scans at different levels of the thorax. (**a**) Level of the superior thoracic aperture. (**b**) Level of the subclavian vessels. (**c**) Level of the centre of axilla. (**d**) Level of the aortic arch. (**e**) Level of the nipple. (**f**) Level of the apex of the heart

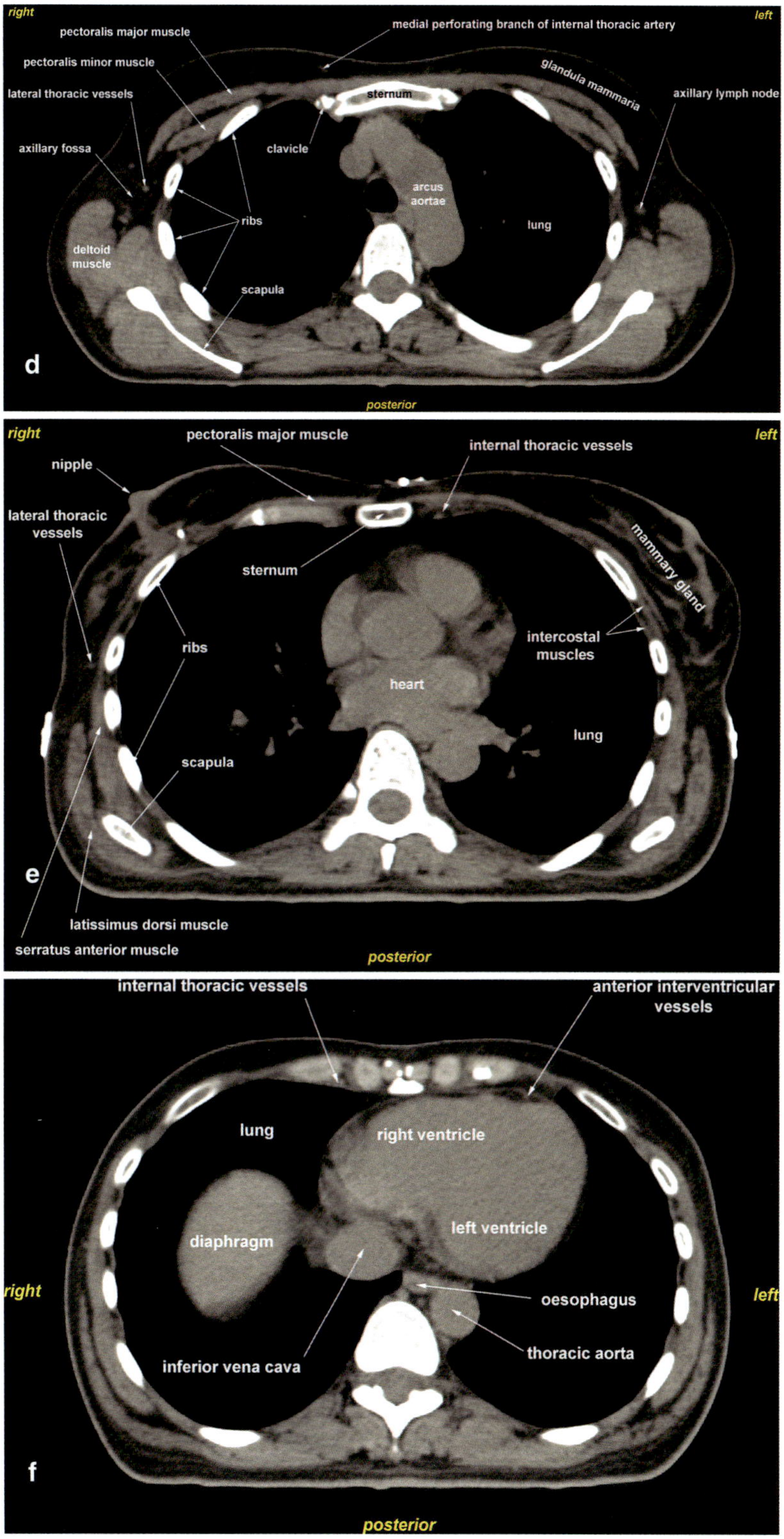

Fig. 11.6 (continued)

the deltoid tuberosity of the humerus and is enveloped by the deltoid fascia. The subscapularis muscle originates from the costal surface of the scapula and inserts on the lesser tubercle of the humerus, covered by the homonymous fascia. The subclavius muscle is hidden between the clavicle and the first rib, covered by the clavipectoral fascia. Finally, the scalenus anterior and medius muscles originate from the transverse processes of the cervical vertebrae, insert on the superior surface of the first rib, forming a slit (scalenic fissure) for the subclavian artery, lymphatic subclavian trunk and brachial plexus. In less than 10%, there can exist a transverse muscular band, called the axillary arch (of Langer), extending between the anterior aspect of the latissimus dorsi muscle and the posterior aspect of the pectoralis major muscle (or the proximal arm muscles/tendons/fasciae).

The superficial thoracic fascia is thickened between the clavicle and the mammary gland as the suspensory ligament (of Giraldés), providing suspension for the breast and forming its shape. The clavipectoral fascia attaches to the clavicle, envelopes the subclavius muscle, descends as the coracoclavicular fascia (its lateral margin extending between the coracoid process and the first costal cartilage, called the costocoracoid ligament, separates the axillary space from the anterior thoracic wall), envelops the pectoralis minor and serratus anterior muscles and dorsally continues to the rhomboid muscles. The axillary floor (inferior wall) is formed by the thin superficial axillary fascia, and the thick quadrangular deep axillary fascia, continuing laterally to the brachial fascia, medially to the clavipectoral fascia of the serratus anterior muscle, ventrally to the pectoral fascia and dorsally to the fascia dorsi of the latissimus dorsi. It is attached to the lateral part of the clavipectoral fascia, called the axillary suspensory ligament (of Gerdy). The axillary fascia supports the contents of the axilla, including the fat pad, and is pierced by superficial veins and lymphatic vessels from the breast.

11.3 Summary

The anatomy of thorax, axilla, breast and its lymphatic drainage is complex. A thorough knowledge of anatomy including cross-sectional and topographical anatomy is essential for target volume delineation as well as for understanding various anatomical aspects that affect breast cancer diagnosis, surgery and possible pathways of spread of the disease within and beyond the irradiation fields.

Acknowledgements Special thanks to Barbora Vyhnankova M.D., Department of Surgery, University Hospital Kralovske Vinohrady, Prague, Czech Republic, for original drawings and schemas.

References

1. Chiu SY, Duffy S, Yen AM, Tabár L, Smith RA, Chen HH. Effect of baseline breast density on breast cancer incidence, stage, mortality, and screening parameters: 25-year follow-up of a Swedish mammographic screening. Cancer Epidemiol Biomark Prev. 2010;19(5):1219–28.
2. Lesavoy MA, Gomez-Garcia A, Nejdl R, Yospur G, Syiau TJ, Chang P. Axillary breast tissue: clinical presentation and surgical treatment. Ann Plast Surg. 1996;36(6):661–2.
3. Parks AG. The micro-anatomy of the breast. Ann R Coll Surg Engl. 1959;25(4):235–51.
4. D'Orsi CJ. Imaging for the diagnosis and management of ductal carcinoma in situ. J Natl Cancer Inst Monogr. 2010;2010(41):214–7.
5. Love SM, Barsky SH. Anatomy of the nipple and breast ducts revisited. Cancer. 2004;101(9):1947–57.
6. Rusby JE, Brachtel EF, Michaelson JS, Koerner FC, Smith BL. Breast duct anatomy in the human nipple: three-dimensional patterns and clinical implications. Breast Cancer Res Treat. 2007;106(2):171–9.
7. Stecco L. Functional atlas of the human fascial system. London: Churchill Livingstone; 2014.
8. Palhazi P. Gross anatomy of the breast and axilla. In: Wyld L, Markopoulos C, Leideius M, Senkus-Konefka E, editors. Breast cancer management for surgeons' book. New York: Springer; 2018.
9. Awad MA, Sherif MM, Sadek EY, Helal HA, Hamid WR. A new septum in the female breast. Arch Plast Surg. 2017;44(2):101–8.

10. Michelle le Roux C, Kiil BJ, Pan WR, Rozen WM, Ashton MW. Preserving the neurovascular supply in the Hall-Findlay superomedial pedicle breast reduction: an anatomical study. J Plast Reconstr Aesthet Surg. 2010;63(4):655–62.
11. Sarhadi NS, Shaw Dunn J, Lee FD, Soutar DS. An anatomical study of the nerve supply of the breast, including the nipple and areola. Br J Plast Surg. 1996;49(3):156–64.
12. Henry BM, Graves MJ, Pękala JR, Sanna B, Hsieh WC, Tubbs RS, Walocha JA, Tomaszewski KA. Origin, branching, and communications of the intercostobrachial nerve: a meta-analysis with implications for mastectomy and axillary lymph node dissection in breast cancer. Cureus. 2017;9(3):e1101.
13. Gray H. Anatomy of the human body. Philadelphia: Lea & Febiger; 1918.
14. Soares EW. Anatomical variations of the axilla. Springerplus. 2014;24(3):306.
15. Suami H, Pan WR, Mann GB, Taylor GI. The lymphatic anatomy of the breast and its implications for sentinel lymph node biopsy: a human cadaver study. Ann Surg Oncol. 2008;15(3):863–71.
16. Turner-Warwick RT. The lymphatics of the breast. Br J Surg. 1959;46:574–82.
17. Földi M, Földi E, Kubik S. Lehrbuch lymfologie. Munich: Elsevier; 2005. p. 119–22.
18. Földi M, Földi E, Kubik S. Lehrbuch lymfologie. Munich: Elsevier; 2005. p. 123.
19. Berg JW. The significance of axillary node levels in the study of breast carcinoma. Cancer. 1955;8(4):776–8.
20. Vendrell-Torné E, Setoain-Quinquer J, Doménech-Torné FM. Study of normal mammary lymphatic drainage using radioactive isotopes. J Nucl Med. 1972;13(11):801–5.
21. Hultborn KA, Larsson LG, Ragnhult I. The lymph drainage from the breast to the axillary and parasternal lymph nodes, studied with the aid of colloidal Au198. Acta Radiol. 1955;43(1):52–64.
22. Estourgie SH, Nieweg OE, Olmos RA, Rutgers EJ, Kroon BB. Lymphatic drainage patterns from the breast. Ann Surg. 2004;239(2):232–7.
23. Grossman F. Ueber die axillaren Lymphdrusen. Inaug. Dissert. Berlin, 1896. Rotter J. Zur topographie des Mammacarcinoms. Arch Klin Chir. 1899;58:346.
24. Cody HS, Egeli RA, Urban JA. Rotter's node metastases. Therapeutic and prognostic considerations in early breast carcinoma. Ann Surg. 1984;199(3):266–70.
25. Mornard P. Étude anatomique des lymphatiques de la mammelle au point de vue de l'extension lymphatique des cancers. Rev Chir. 1916;11(5-6):492–501.
26. Grotenhuis BA, Klem TM, Vrijland WW. Treatment outcome in breast cancer patients with ipsilateral supraclavicular lymph node metastasis at time of diagnosis: a review of the literature. Eur J Surg Oncol. 2013;39(3):207–12.
27. Ellis H, Colborn GL, Skandalakis JE. Surgical embryology and anatomy of the breast and its related anatomic structures. Surg Clin North Am. 1993;73(4):611–32.
28. Perre CI, Hoefnagel CA, Kroon BB, Zoetmulder FA, Rutgers EJ. Altered lymphatic drainage after lymphadenectomy or radiotherapy of the axilla in patients with breast cancer. Br J Surg. 1996;83(9):1258.
29. Rosen PP, Lesser ML, Kinne DW, Beattie EJ. Discontinuous or "skip" metastases in breast carcinoma. Analysis of 1228 axillary dissections. Ann Surg. 1983;197(3):276–83.
30. Troupis T, Michalinos A, Skandalakis P. Intramammary lymph nodes: a question seeking for an answer or an answer seeking for a question? Breast. 2012;21(5):615–20.
31. Brierley JD, Gospodarowicz MK, Wittekind C. TNM classification of malignant tumours. Hoboken: Wiley; 2017.
32. Fornage BD. Local and regional staging of invasive breast cancer with sonography: 25 years of practice at MD Anderson Cancer Center. Oncologist. 2014;19(1):5–15.
33. Marino MA, Avendano D, Zapata P, Riedl CC, Pinker K. lymph node imaging in patients with primary breast cancer: concurrent diagnostic tools. Oncologist. 2020;25(2):e231–42.

Risk Assessment: Calculating the Benefit of RT for Individual Patients

12

Marissa C. van Maaren and Nina Bijker

12.1 Background

The primary aim of RT treatment for breast cancer is to reduce the risk of local-regional failure (LRF) [1]. Following BCS, post-operative RT gives a 70% reduction in the risk of LRF [2–4], and it additionally has proven its benefit in node-positive disease treated with mastectomy [5]. Although the proportional benefits are substantial, the absolute benefits may be very small in specific patient groups [2, 5], especially when considering the fact that recurrence risks are largely based on clinical trials executed decades ago, and absolute risks of LRF have continued to drop since [6]. On top of that RT comes with not only a potential risk of cardiac morbidity [7, 8] and secondary cancer [9], but also a risk of health effects such as arm morbidity and fibrosis [10, 11]. These RT-related complications are reduced with volume-based planning and dose-homogeneity, but especially in early-stage breast cancer or in older patients with a lower health condition, the benefits in terms of reduced risks of LRF may not outweigh the harms in terms of treatment burden of RT [12]. In the current era of treatment de-escalation, it is therefore crucial to weigh the efficacy of RT against its potential side effects.

12.2 Key Information for Clinical Practice

Tumour characteristics such as tumour size, nodal stage, grade and receptor status play a key role in breast cancer prognosis and thus in RT decision-making. As breast cancer is a very heterogeneous disease and different combinations of tumour characteristics largely influence prognosis, a wide range of clinical prediction tools have been developed incorporating these factors. Examples of prediction tools are models that estimate the risk of local or regional failure and/or survival outcomes following BCS [13–16] or mastectomy [17, 18], models that predict the risk of nodal metastasis [19, 20] or a model that predicts the risk of mastectomy-free interval following BCS [21]. Such models can be very useful to assist RT treatment decision-making. However, they do not take into account the patient's general health condition and the

M. C. van Maaren (✉)
Department of Research and Development, Netherlands Comprehensive Cancer Organisation (IKNL), Utrecht, The Netherlands

Department of Health Technology and Services Research, Faculty of Behavioural, Management and Social Sciences, Technical Medical Centre, University of Twente, Enschede, The Netherlands
e-mail: m.vanmaaren@iknl.nl

N. Bijker
Department of Radiation Oncology, Amsterdam University Medical Center, Amsterdam, The Netherlands
e-mail: n.bijker@amsterdamumc.nl

© The Author(s), under exclusive license to Springer Nature Switzerland AG 2022
O. Kaidar-Person et al. (eds.), *Breast Cancer Radiation Therapy*,
https://doi.org/10.1007/978-3-030-91170-6_12

expected risk on side effects, making RT treatment decision-making a complex matter. Besides, a general limitation of such prediction tools is that they are always based on patients diagnosed and treated many years ago—while treatment strategies are continuously evolving—which makes it difficult to translate predicted risks to current individual patients. Table 12.1 summarises some of the available risk assessment tools. Using two case descriptions the complexities and possibilities of RT are discussed in light of recent developments.

Table 12.1 Available online risk assessment tools

Prediction tool	Population	Type of RT	Predictors	Outcome	Reference (PMID)
MD Anderson Cancer Center: breast cancer nomogram to predict benefit of radiation for older patients with breast cancer treated with conservative surgery	Women 66–79 years with primary nonmetastatic epithelial ductal breast cancer treated with BCS	Yes/no, as given in daily practice	• Age • Race • Tumour size • Oestrogen receptor status • Nodal status	5- and 10-year mastectomy-free survival	22734034
IBTR! Version 2.0	Breast cancer patients treated with BCS	Yes/no, as given in daily practice	• Age • Tumour size • Tumour grade • Margin status • Lymphovascular invasion • Chemotherapy • Endocrine therapy	10-year ipsilateral breast tumour recurrence risk	17921706
Sichuan University nomogram predicting locoregional recurrence to assist decision-making of postmastectomy radiation therapy in patients with T1-2N1 breast cancer	Breast cancer patients with T1-2N1 breast cancer treated with mastectomy, T1-2N1-3	Post-mastectomy radiation therapy	• Tumour size • Number of positive nodes • Oestrogen receptor status • TNM stage • Lymphovascular invasion	5-year locoregional recurrence risk, 5-year distant recurrence risk and 5-year breast cancer mortality.	30419307
Memorial Sloan Kettering Cancer Center: sentinel lymph node metastasis	SLN biopsy procedures	Not intended to estimate effect of RT but to estimate general risks that help in decision-making RT treatment	• Age • Tumour size • Special type (tubular, mucinous or medullary carcinoma) • Tumour located in upper inner quadrant • Lymphovascular invasion • Multifocality • Tumour type and grade (ductal + grade or lobular) • Oestrogen receptor status • Progesterone receptor status	Risk of positive SLN	17664461

Table 12.1 (continued)

Prediction tool	Population	Type of RT	Predictors	Outcome	Reference (PMID)
Memorial Sloan Kettering Cancer Center: additional nodal metastasis	Patients who underwent complete ALND	Not intended to estimate effect of RT but to estimate general risks that help in decision-making RT treatment	• Frozen section performed? • Tumour size • Tumour type and grade (ductal + grade or lobular) • Number of positive SLNs • SLN Method of detection • Number of negative SLNs • Lymphovascular invasion • Multifocality • Oestrogen receptor status	Risk of additional nodal metastasis in case of a positive SLN biopsy	14654469
Memorial Sloan Kettering Cancer Center: ductal carcinoma in situ recurrence	Patients treated with BCS for DCIS	Not intended to estimate effect of RT but to estimate general risks that help in decision-making RT treatment	• Age • Family history • Clinical or radiologic presentation • Radiotherapy • Endocrine therapy • Tumour grade • Presence of necrosis • Surgical margins • Number of surgical excisions • Year of surgery	5- and 10-year risk of ipsilateral breast cancer recurrence	20625132
Nomogram for predicting the risk of locoregional recurrence in patients treated with accelerated partial-breast irradiation	Patients treated with BCS followed by APBI for early stage breast cancer	Accelerated partial breast irradiation (APBI) Not intended to estimate effect of RT but to estimate general risks that help in decision-making RT treatment	• Age <50 or ≥50 • Menopausal status • Margin status • Oestrogen receptor status • Tumour grade	5-year risk of locoregional recurrence	25446607
A prediction model for the presence of axillary lymph node involvement in women with invasive breast cancer: a focus on older women	Patients diagnosed with clinically node-negative invasive breast cancer who underwent ALN sampling	Not intended to estimate effect of RT but to estimate general risks that help in decision-making RT treatment	• Tumour size • Lymphovascular invasion • Menopausal status	Risk of ALN metastases	24475876

(continued)

Table 12.1 (continued)

Prediction tool	Population	Type of RT	Predictors	Outcome	Reference (PMID)
IEO and MSKCC nomogram for prediction of local relapse after surgery for invasive breast carcinoma	Patients with primary invasive breast cancer	Not intended to estimate effect of RT but to estimate general risks that help in decision-making RT treatment	• Age • Histology • Tumour size • Nodal stage • Tumour grade • Peritumoural vascular invasion • Subtype • Endocrine therapy • Chemotherapy • Radiotherapy (external, intraoperative or none)	1-, 5- and 10-year ipsilateral breast tumour recurrence risks	31965372
Radiotherapy for older women (ROW): a risk calculator for women with early-stage breast cancer	Older women with breast cancer	Yes vs no	• Age • BMI • Smoking status • COPD • Other cancer • Congestive heart failure • Diabetes • Difficulty walking several blocks • Difficulty managing finances • Difficulty bathing • Difficulty pushing/pulling large objects • Tumour grade • Tumour size • Oestrogen receptor status • Margin status • Nodal stage • Additional health conditions (neutral, more favourable, less favourable) • Additional breast cancer factors (neutral, more favourable, less favourable)	10-year local recurrence risk, 10-year all-cause mortality risk	31899199

Table 12.1 (continued)

Prediction tool	Population	Type of RT	Predictors	Outcome	Reference (PMID)
Individualised prediction of survival benefit from postmastectomy radiotherapy for patients with breast cancer with one to three positive axillary lymph nodes	Women with N1-3 breast cancer treated with mastectomy	PMRT	• Age • Histology • Tumour grade • Tumour size • Oestrogen receptor status • Progesterone receptor status • Number of positive nodes	5- and 10-year overall and disease-specific survival	31315963
Nomogram to predict ipsilateral breast relapse based on pathology review from the EORTC 22881-10882 boost versus no boost trial	Patients treated with BCS+whole breast RT	RT boost yes/no after BCS+RT	• Tumour size • Age • Tamoxifen • Chemotherapy • Boost • DCIS • Tumour grade	10-year proportion IBR free	21821304
Fibrosis prediction model based on the EORTC Trial 22881-10882 'boost versus no boost'	Patients treated with BCS+whole breast RT	RT boost yes/ not after BCS+RT	In patients treated with a boost • Age • Haematoma • Oedema • Tamoxifen • Concomitant chemotherapy • Radiation quality • Type of boost • If electron boost, energy (MeV) • Maximum dose (if known) In patients NOT treated with boost • Age • Concomitant chemotherapy • Maximum dose	Risk of moderate/severe fibrosis at 10 year	18757193

Response to preoperative radiation therapy can be predicted by gene expression patterns [38, 39]
[a] It might be that some of the avilable tools are missing

12.2.1 Case 1

Mrs. X is a 57-year-old woman with a non-palpable mass in the upper-outer quadrant of the left breast detected during population-based screening. She is married, has two children, and works three days a week as a receptionist. She has hypertension, a BMI of 31 kg/m^2 and smokes with 30 pack-years. She failed several attempts to quit smoking. She underwent an iodine seed-guided excision and SLNB. Histology revealed an invasive carcinoma of no special type (NST), grade 2, diameter 1.5 cm, without LVI. The tumour was removed with clear surgical margins (≤3 mm). Oestrogen (ER, 100%) and progesterone receptor (PR, 20%) positive, HER2 negative. TNM staging pT1c N0 (sn) Mx.

Mrs. X was discussed in both a pre- and post-operative multidisciplinary breast meeting where referral to both the radiation oncologist and medical oncologist was advised to discuss post-operative breast RT and endocrine therapy.

According to the IBTR! tool [22], which can be accessed via https://www.tuftsmedicalcenter.org/ibtr/, RT will result in a 70% relative risk reduction of local failure (LF) (10% risk without RT, 3% risk with RT) at 10 years in this patient. In case of treatment with endocrine therapy, the risks are reduced to 7.3% and 2.2%, without and with RT, respectively. It should be noted that this IBTR! tool may not be directly applicable to all populations, as validation studies give mixed results, and thus results should be interpreted with care. The tool only includes general prognostic parameters, and no factors related to tumour biology. Furthermore, the IBTR! tool presents risks for whole breast irradiation (WBI), while our patient X is eligible for partial breast irradiation (see partial breast irradiation section) according to both European (ESTRO) [23] and American (ASTRO) guidelines [24]. In addition, the introduction of hypofractionation has reduced the number of necessary visits to the RT department from 25 times in five weeks to fractionation schedules of as low as five times in one week, with equal effectiveness and similar low risk of side effects (see dose & fractionation section) [25, 26]. Thus, the burden for the patient is much less when it comes to time investment and might have an impact on family life, fatigue caused by travelling, and work-return. Further, the possible long-term risk of fibrosis, affecting cosmesis and causing discomfort and pain, is proven to occur less and of lower toxicity grade in patients treated with PBI as compared to patients treated with WBI [27]. Also, with modern 3DCRT planning and breath-hold techniques we are able to minimise the risk of cardiac morbidity [8], which is therefore not a reason to refrain from treatment with RT. However, it has been shown that women who continue to smoke during breast RT have an increased risk of developing lung cancer [28]. One could easily argue that, if Mrs. X—having low risk breast cancer and excellent expected breast cancer-specific survival rates—continues to smoke, her already substantial risk of lung cancer will be further increased due to RT. This risk may outweigh the benefit in terms of local control. We advise that this information will be clearly communicated to the patient and appropriate measures should be taken to promote health-related behaviours, such as referring the patient to smoking cessation programmes.

Something that could additionally be taken into account to estimate prognosis is Ki-67 status. This was not measured here, due to substantial heterogeneity in methods of assessment and limited clinical utility [29]. However, when (automated) Ki-67 scoring will be further developed, this may be a relevant factor in the future.

12.2.2 Case 2

Mrs. Y is a 45-year-old woman with a palpable mass in her right breast. Tomosynthesis (density category C) showed a 2.3 cm mass in the lower outer quadrant. On the axillary ultrasound one lymph node with a cortex width of 0.28 cm was seen. The biopsy revealed an invasive carcinoma of NST, grade 3, ER and PR negative, HER2 positive (score 3+). The fine needle aspiration of the axilla was positive. Breast MRI showed three additional satellite lesions extending in a total area of 5.3 cm. A PET-CT showed uptake in all four breast lesions and in one axillary lymph node, without any evidence of other regional or distant metastases. TNM cT2 mc N1 M0.

Mrs. Y is a healthy woman without comorbidity, non-smoker, no medication use. BMI 27 kg/m^2. She is divorced and has two teenage children, she is self-employed.

Mrs. Y was counselled for preoperative systemic therapy including a dual blockade anti-HER2 treatment and a MRI showed a breast and nodal clinical complete response. Because of the extent of the lesions, she underwent a skin-sparing mastectomy with excision of the marked axillary lymph node and SLNB followed by direct reconstruction with a tissue expander. Histologic analysis showed a pathologic complete response (pCR) in both the breast and the removed lymph node (marker node same as sentinel node). TNM ypT0 N0. Because of the initial stage II disease and no complete axillary treatment, it was advised to counsel her for locoregional RT (reconstructed breast and regional lymphatics).

In stage III breast cancer, PMRT is generally accepted as treatment strategy as it causes a substantial absolute reduction in risk of LRF which also results in survival benefit [30], while in stage I or low risk (node negative) stage II disease current LRF risks are so low that the benefit of RT may not outweigh its harms. However, for intermediate risk—mostly stage II such as for Mrs. Y—the decision on RT is more difficult. One can rely even less on prediction tools such as the one developed by Luo et al. [17], as it does not include women treated with modern (preoperative) systemic therapy with dual anti-HER2 treatment. Mrs. Y shows a pCR, which has been shown to be correlated with a low risk of LRF [31]. However, we are still awaiting results of randomised trials comparing PMRT with no RT in intermediate risk breast cancer [32], and especially in the primary systemic situation many answers are still to be given. In patients such as Mrs. Y there is a debate on whether the axilla has been treated sufficiently, with some physicians preferring a safe option and offering her RT to the axilla [33] or even an ALND. A review to identify factors that may permit PMRT omission in a selected group of patients after PST confirmed the positive contribution of PMRT to reduce the risk of LRF and increase OS in patients with locally advanced breast cancer treated with PST and mastectomy, irrespective of the tumour response to PST. In the case of patients with earlier stage disease, PMRT omission could be considered in patients over the age of 40 years, with clinical stage II tumours (except for cT3N0 tumours), luminal A subtype, and those who achieve a pCR in the breast and lymph nodes (ypN0), without LVI or ECE [34]. However, the impact of the type of mastectomy (skin or nipple sparing versus total mastectomy) on the rate of LR is not fully understood. Additionally, in patients with HER2-type tumours with 1–3 involved lymph nodes, an analysis of the HERA trial showed that PMRT decreases the risk of LRR, albeit with a magnitude of benefit which is lower than historic studies [35]. Lastly, although not applicable to our case, presence of BRCA mutations [36] and presence of residual breast tissue and dermal lymphatics after skin-sparing procedures are described to increase the risk of LRR [37].

12.2.3 The Shared Decision-Making Process: Current State of the Art and Future Perspectives

Regarding Mrs. X and Mrs. Y, the shared decision-making process resulted in the following: Mrs. X was convinced of the beneficial health effects of smoking cessation, and she was advised to contact her general practitioner to guide her in this. She decided to aim for maximal local control and to be treated with hypofractionated PBI, also because of the low burden of five treatments in one week. Mrs. Y has chosen for a direct breast reconstruction. Chest wall RT (PMRT) will increase her risk of complications, fibrosis and capsular contractures, resulting in an increased risk of poor cosmetic outcome and pain around the reconstructed area [40]. The pCR following PST helped her in the decision to forego RT.

As the case descriptions show, the RT decision-making process can be very complex. Existing prediction tools do not cover all the aspects, making it difficult to discuss the outcomes with individual patients. Predicted risks of LRF are discussed in the context of tumour- and treatment-related characteristics as well as the patient's personal situation and wish. Ideally, multigene assays developed and proved to guide selective use of adjuvant chemotherapy [41], could also be used to assess a patient's individual risk of LRF, and hence to better predict the benefit of RT than the current classic clinical and histopathological factors. So far, studies investigating this gave conflicting results and therefore these multigene assays are not yet used for this purpose [42]. Also, studies have shown that side effects are largely dependent on each patient's intrinsic susceptibility to radiation-induced side effects [43–45], which is subject of ongoing research. However, we should not neglect the benefits of advances in RT preparation and delivery that led to a strong decrease of its burden to the patients including the frequency and severity of side effects.

In order for patients to understand the predicted risks, uncertainties around the estimates should be taken into account as well. One can imagine that all of this information can be overwhelming, and that prediction tools on its own are not sufficient. Patient decision aids, such as developed in the BRASA study [NCT03375801] [46], may improve patient's understanding of LRF risks with or without RT as well as the estimated side effects. This decision aid includes information on both benefits and harms of RT including uncertainties and presents textual as well as visualised risks, which is shown to improve patients' understanding of risk estimations [47].

12.3 Summary

Here, we described two cases in which both the complexities and possibilities of RT risk assessment are clarified. The key message is that besides tumour characteristics, the personal situation and wish of the patient have to be part of the shared decision-making process concerning RT treatment. Prediction tools on its own are not always adequate due to the inclusion of patients diagnosed and treated many years ago. In order for patients to interpret all the information well, decision aids can be very helpful. Future research should include the use of multigene assays and patient's intrinsic susceptibility to radiation-induced side effects in the assessment of LRF risks, which can help further personalise the benefits and risks of RT.

References

1. Poortmans P. Optimal approach in early breast cancer: radiation therapy. EJC Suppl. 2013;11(2):27–36.
2. Speers C, Pierce LJ. Postoperative radiotherapy after breast-conserving surgery for early-stage breast cancer: a review. JAMA Oncol. 2016;2(8):1075–82.
3. Darby S, Correa C, Taylor C, Arriagada R, et al. Effect of radiotherapy after breast-conserving surgery on 10-year recurrence and 15-year breast cancer death: meta-analysis of individual patient data for 10,801 women in 17 randomised trials. Lancet. 2011;378(9804):1707–16.
4. Vinh-Hung V, Verschraegen C. Breast-conserving surgery with or without radiotherapy: pooled-analysis for risks of ipsilateral breast tumor recurrence and mortality. J Natl Cancer Inst. 2004;96(2):115–21.
5. Recht A, Comen EA, Fine RE, Fleming GF, Hardenbergh PH, Ho AY, et al. Postmastectomy radiotherapy: an American Society of Clinical Oncology, American Society for Radiation Oncology, and Society of Surgical Oncology focused guideline update. Pract Radiat Oncol. 2016;6(6):219–34.
6. van Maaren MC, de Munck L, Strobbe LJA, Sonke GS, Westenend PJ, Smidt ML, et al. Ten-year recurrence rates for breast cancer subtypes in the Netherlands: a large population-based study. Int J Cancer. 2019;144(2):263–72.
7. van den Bogaard VAB, van Luijk P, Hummel YM, van der Meer P, Schuit E, Boerman LM, et al. Cardiac function after radiation therapy for breast cancer. Int J Radiat Oncol Biol Phys. 2019;104(2):392–400.
8. Loap P, Kirov K, Kirova Y. Cardiotoxicity in breast cancer patients treated with radiation therapy: from evidences to controversies. 2020. https://doi.org/10.1016/j.critrevonc.2020.103121.
9. Grantzau T, Overgaard J. Risk of second non-breast cancer among patients treated with and without postoperative radiotherapy for primary breast cancer: a systematic review and meta-analysis of population-based studies including 522,739 patients. Radiother Oncol. 2016;121(3):402–13.
10. Gregorowitsch ML, Verkooijen HM, Houweling A, Fuhler N, Koelemij R, Schoenmaeckers EJP, et al. Impact of modern-day axillary treatment on patient reported arm morbidity and physical functioning in breast cancer patients. Radiother Oncol. 2019;131:221–8.
11. Collette S, Collette L, Budiharto T, Horiot JC, Poortmans PM, Struikmans H, et al. Predictors of the risk of fibrosis at 10 years after breast conserving therapy for early breast cancer: a study based on the EORTC Trial 22881-10882 'boost versus no boost'. Eur J Cancer. 2008;44(17):2587–99.
12. Poortmans PMP, Arenas M, Livi L. Over-irradiation. Breast. 2017;31:295–302.
13. Sanghani M, Balk E, Cady B, Wazer D. Predicting the risk of local recurrence in patients with breast cancer:

an approach to a new computer-based predictive tool. Am J Clin Oncol. 2007;30(5):473–80.
14. Rudloff U, Jacks LM, Goldberg JI, Wynveen CA, Brogi E, Patil S, et al. Nomogram for predicting the risk of local recurrence after breast-conserving surgery for ductal carcinoma in situ. J Clin Oncol. 2010;28(23):3762–9.
15. Corso G, Maisonneuve P, Massari G, Invento A, Pravettoni G, De Scalzi A, et al. Validation of a novel nomogram for prediction of local relapse after surgery for invasive breast carcinoma. Ann Surg Oncol. 2020;27(6):1864–74.
16. van Werkhoven E, Hart G, Tinteren H, Elkhuizen P, Collette L, Poortmans P, et al. Nomogram to predict ipsilateral breast relapse based on pathology review from the EORTC 22881-10882 boost versus no boost trial. Radiother Oncol. 2011;100(1):101–7.
17. Luo C, Zhong X, Deng L, Xie Y, Hu K, Zheng H. Nomogram predicting locoregional recurrence to assist decision-making of postmastectomy radiation therapy in patients with T1-2N1 breast cancer. Int J Radiat Oncol Biol Phys. 2019;103(4):905–12.
18. Zhang N, Zhang J, Zhang H, Liu Y, Zhao W, Wang L, et al. Individualized prediction of survival benefit from postmastectomy radiotherapy for patients with breast cancer with one to three positive axillary lymph nodes. Oncologist. 2019;24(12):e1286–e93.
19. Van Zee KJ, Manasseh DM, Bevilacqua JL, Boolbol SK, Fey JV, Tan LK, et al. A nomogram for predicting the likelihood of additional nodal metastases in breast cancer patients with a positive sentinel node biopsy. Ann Surg Oncol. 2003;10(10):1140–51.
20. Greer LT, Rosman M, Charles Mylander W, Liang W, Buras RR, Chagpar AB, et al. A prediction model for the presence of axillary lymph node involvement in women with invasive breast cancer: a focus on older women. Breast J. 2014;20(2):147–53.
21. Albert JM, Liu DD, Shen Y, Pan IW, Shih YC, Hoffman KE, et al. Nomogram to predict the benefit of radiation for older patients with breast cancer treated with conservative surgery. J Clin Oncol. 2012;30(23):2837–43.
22. Sanghani M, Truong PT, Raad RA, Niemierko A, Lesperance M, Olivotto IA, et al. Validation of a web-based predictive nomogram for ipsilateral breast tumor recurrence after breast conserving therapy. J Clin Oncol. 2010;28(5):718–22.
23. Polgar C, Van Limbergen E, Potter R, Kovacs G, Polo A, Lyczek J, et al. Patient selection for accelerated partial-breast irradiation (APBI) after breast-conserving surgery: recommendations of the Groupe Europeen de Curietherapie-European Society for Therapeutic Radiology and Oncology (GEC-ESTRO) breast cancer working group based on clinical evidence. Radiother Oncol. 2010;94(3):264–73.
24. Kirby AM. Updated ASTRO guidelines on accelerated partial breast irradiation (APBI): to whom can we offer APBI outside a clinical trial? Br J Radiol. 2018;91(1085):20170565.
25. Murray Brunt A, Haviland JS, Wheatley DA, Sydenham MA, Alhasso A, Bloomfield DJ, et al. Hypofractionated breast radiotherapy for 1 week versus 3 weeks (FAST-Forward): 5-year efficacy and late normal tissue effects results from a multicentre, non-inferiority, randomised, phase 3 trial. Lancet. 2020;395(10237):1613–26.
26. Brunt AM, Haviland JS, Sydenham M, Agrawal RK, Algurafi H, Alhasso A, et al. Ten-year results of FAST: a randomized controlled trial of 5-fraction whole-breast radiotherapy for early breast cancer. J Clin Oncol. 2020;38(28):3261–72.
27. Strnad V, Ott OJ, Hildebrandt G, Kauer-Dorner D, Knauerhase H, Major T, et al. 5-year results of accelerated partial breast irradiation using sole interstitial multicatheter brachytherapy versus whole-breast irradiation with boost after breast-conserving surgery for low-risk invasive and in-situ carcinoma of the female breast: a randomised, phase 3, non-inferiority trial. Lancet. 2016;387(10015):229–38.
28. Taylor C, Correa C, Duane FK, Aznar MC, Anderson SJ, Bergh J, et al. Estimating the risks of breast cancer radiotherapy: evidence from modern radiation doses to the lungs and heart and from previous randomized trials. J Clin Oncol. 2017;35(15):1641–9.
29. Nielsen TO, Leung SCY, Rimm DL, Dodson A, Acs B, Badve S, et al. Assessment of Ki67 in breast cancer: updated recommendations from the International Ki67 in Breast Cancer Working Group. J Natl Cancer Inst. 2020;113(7):808–19.
30. Overgaard M, Jensen MB, Overgaard J, Hansen PS, Rose C, Andersson M, et al. Postoperative radiotherapy in high-risk postmenopausal breast-cancer patients given adjuvant tamoxifen: Danish Breast Cancer Cooperative Group DBCG 82c randomised trial. Lancet. 1999;353(9165):1641–8.
31. Asaoka M, Narui K, Suganuma N, Chishima T, Yamada A, Sugae S, et al. Clinical and pathological predictors of recurrence in breast cancer patients achieving pathological complete response to neoadjuvant chemotherapy. Eur J Surg Oncol. 2019;45(12):2289–94.
32. Kunkler IH, Canney P, van Tienhoven G, Russell NS. Elucidating the role of chest wall irradiation in 'intermediate-risk' breast cancer: the MRC/EORTC SUPREMO trial. Clin Oncol. 2008;20(1):31–4.
33. Donker M, van Tienhoven G, Straver ME, Meijnen P, van de Velde CJ, Mansel RE, et al. Radiotherapy or surgery of the axilla after a positive sentinel node in breast cancer (EORTC 10981-22023 AMAROS): a randomised, multicentre, open-label, phase 3 non-inferiority trial. Lancet Oncol. 2014;15(12):1303–10.
34. Montero A, Ciervide R, Poortmans P. When can we avoid postmastectomy radiation following primary systemic therapy? Curr Oncol Rep. 2019;21(12):95.
35. Abi Jaoude J, de Azambuja E, Makki M, Tamim H, Tfayli A, Geara F, et al. Post-mastectomy radiation therapy in human epidermal growth factor receptor 2 positive breast cancer patients: analysis

of the HERA trial. Int J Radiat Oncol Biol Phys. 2020;106(3):503–10.
36. Bernstein-Molho R, Laitman Y, Galper S, Jacobson G, Boursi B, Gal-Yam EN, et al. Locoregional treatments and ipsilateral breast cancer recurrence rates in BRCA1/2 mutation carriers. Int J Radiat Oncol Biol Phys. 2020;109(5):1332–40.
37. Kaidar-Person O, Boersma LJ, Poortmans P, Sklair-Levy M, Offersen BV, Cardoso MJ, et al. Residual glandular breast tissue after mastectomy: a systematic review. Ann Surg Oncol. 2020;27(7):2288–96.
38. Bosma SCJ, Hoogstraat M, van der Leij F, de Maaker M, Wesseling J, Lips E, et al. Response to preoperative radiation therapy in relation to gene expression patterns in breast cancer patients. Int J Radiat Oncol Biol Phys. 2020;106(1):174–81.
39. Tanic M, Krivokuca A, Cavic M, Mladenovic J, Plesinac Karapandzic V, Beck S, et al. Molecular signature of response to preoperative radiotherapy in locally advanced breast cancer. Radiat Oncol. 2018;13(1):193.
40. Rozen WM, Ashton MW. Radiotherapy and breast reconstruction: oncology, cosmesis and complications. Gland Surg. 2012;1(2):119–27.
41. Markopoulos C, Hyams DM, Gomez HL, Harries M, Nakamura S, Traina T, et al. Multigene assays in early breast cancer: Insights from recent phase 3 studies. Eur J Surg Oncol. 2020;46(4):656–66.
42. Mamounas EP, Mitchell MP, Woodward WA. Molecular predictive and prognostic markers in locoregional management. J Clin Oncol. 2020;38(20):2310–20.
43. Rosenstein BS. Identification of SNPs associated with susceptibility for development of adverse reactions to radiotherapy. Pharmacogenomics. 2011;12(2):267–75.
44. Russell NS, Knaken H, Bruinvis IA, Hart AA, Begg AC, Lebesque JV. Quantification of patient to patient variation of skin erythema developing as a response to radiotherapy. Radiother Oncol. 1994;30(3):213–21.
45. West CM, Barnett GC. Genetics and genomics of radiotherapy toxicity: towards prediction. Genome Med. 2011;3(8):52.
46. Raphael DB, Russell NS, Immink JM, Westhoff PG, Stenfert Kroese MC, Stam MR, et al. Risk communication in a patient decision aid for radiotherapy in breast cancer: How to deal with uncertainty? Breast. 2020;51:105–13.
47. Klein KA, Watson L, Ash JS, Eden KB. Evaluation of risk communication in a mammography patient decision aid. Patient Educ Couns. 2016;99(7):1240–8.

13 Organs at Risk Delineation

Filipe Cidade de Moura and Mirjam Mast

13.1 Background

Accurate delineation of organs at risk (OARs) became crucial in the 3D planning era. With the implementation of CT simulation in the RT process, slowly volumetric delineation for both target volumes and OARs turned mandatory for improving treatment outcome and reducing toxicity. Quantitative analysis of normal tissue effects in the clinic (QUANTEC) is the latest reference for most of the OARs. 3D dose/volume/outcome data were reviewed and synthetized for better risk prediction and therapeutic ratio optimisation [1]. Concerning the delineation of target volumes and OARs, the American Association of Physicists in Medicine (AAPM) Task Group 263 (2018) [2] published a report for standardisation of nomenclatures in radiation oncology.

Recently, the RT Quality Assurance (RTQA) Global Harmonization Group (GHG) defined the consensus guidelines for OAR delineation for RT clinical trials, along with AAPM TG263 and the American Society for Radiation Oncology (ASTRO) [3]. Together with peer-reviewed, the anatomically defined contouring guidance, intent to be integrated into future clinical trial protocols independent of the RT delivery technique.

Standardised names for the treatment planning processes will allow for quality improvement of communication inside departments and within departments at national and international levels. Standardisation of terminology would facilitate scripting and automated processes and reports. It also enables better data collection and registries, which would be of benefit for the routine clinical care, population-based studies and clinical trials. Within the scope of this chapter, the adoption of AAPM TG263 and RTQA GHG OAR WG will be recommended when defining OARs for breast RT.

Supplementary Information The online version contains supplementary material available at [https://doi.org/10.1007/978-3-030-91170-6_13].

F. C. de Moura (✉)
Escola Superior de Tecnologia da Saúde de Lisboa, Instituto Politécnico de Lisboa, Lisboa, Portugal
e-mail: Filipe.moura@estesl.ipl.pt

M. Mast
Haaglanden Medical Center, Leidschendam, The Netherlands
e-mail: m.mast@haaglandenmc.nl

13.2 Treatment Planning: From 3DCRT to IMRT/VMAT

Targeting breast cancer tissues avoiding surrounding tissues is a major goal for EBRT. The radiation team should be aware that the OARs that might be exposed to RT dose can be significantly different if IMRT or VMAT (volumetric-modulated arc therapy or vIMRT) is used. Therefore, care should be given to delineate all

© The Author(s), under exclusive license to Springer Nature Switzerland AG 2022
O. Kaidar-Person et al. (eds.), *Breast Cancer Radiation Therapy*,
https://doi.org/10.1007/978-3-030-91170-6_13

organs that might be exposed to radiation, otherwise treatment might result in increased or unexpected toxicity [4].

If IMRT/VMAT will be used for breast only and/or regional node irradiation, extra requirements should be adopted for volumes of interest (VOIs) definition, see chapter treatment planning. In this section all relevant OARs are described. Finally the adoption of OARs models, atlas based auto-segmentation, and artificial intelligence for planning are now being used to fasten the generation of a reliable structure set, but human visual inspection still needs to be done for structure validation and approval [3].

13.3 Visualisation of OARs on a CT Simulation Scan

Hounsfield number described as units (HU) or more commonly mentioned as CT numbers, is being used for planning purposes applied on Treatment Planning System (TPS) for an accurate conversion to electronic densities (ED). The so-called CT to ED curves allow for treatment beam dose attenuation at TPS for specific CT equipment under calibrated conditions. Displayed CT numbers will then result in different attenuations between tissues. Visualisation and organ recognition are possible under a specified window width (WW) and window level (WL). The transition of dark to light structures would require a narrow window width (<350 HU) and a wide window width (>1000 HU) would result in lower recognition between tissues, mainly soft tissues, which would become unclear. The WL, also referred as window centre, is the midpoint of the WW. When WL is increased, the CT image would become darker and vice versa.

13.4 Delineation of Organs at Risk

Heart (TG 263: Heart)

Modalities: 3DCRT/IMRT/VMAT

CT Contouring recommendation: WW:500, WL:50

Heart three-dimensional anatomy should be checked prior delineation. Coronal planes visualisation is essential to recognise and set the superior and inferior (CC) and lateral borders for discrimination of substructures such as the great vessels as well as the coronary arteries. For a global definition, the heart contour should encompass the outer surface of the pericardial sac [5]. The cranial border should be delineated from the point at which the pulmonary trunk and right pulmonary artery are seen as separate structures [3]. The contour should extend inferiorly to the apex of the heart, where the left ventricle touches the diaphragm [6].

Great vessels should be contoured separately from the heart namely the aorta, vena cava, and pulmonary vessels.

Left Anterior Descending Coronary Artery (LADCA)

(TG 263: A_LAD)

Modalities: 3DCRT/IMRT/VMAT

CT Contouring recommendation: WW:150, WL:50

The LADCA originates from the left main coronary artery (LMCA), on the top left of the heart, between the pulmonary trunk and the left auricle, and extends all way to the apex [7]. Additionally LAD become a small round structure descending in the anterior interventricular groove in close relation to the pericardium [6].

Where the LAD is not visible, the interventricular groove should be used as a surrogate.

Heart and LAD are shown in Fig. 13.1.

Great Vessels

(TG 263: GreatVes)

Modality: IMRT/VMAT

CT Contouring recommendation: WW:350, WL:40

Great vessels around the heart, for breast treatment planning, may encompass the superior vena cava, aorta, and the pulmonary arteries/veins. The delineation of great vessels can be contoured separately or as a single volume. The branches of the aortic arch: the brachiocephalic artery, the left common carotid artery, and the left subclavian

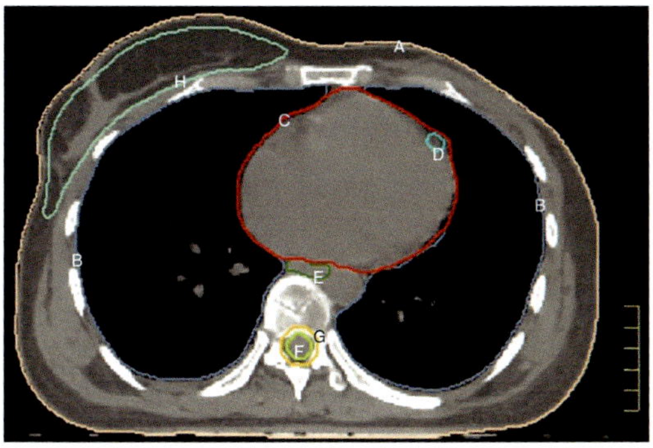

Fig. 13.1 *A* BODY, *B* Lungs, *C* Heart, *D* A_LAD, *E* Esophagus, *F* SpinalCord, *G* SpinalCord_PRV3, *H* Breast_R

artery may be included. Cranial great vessels extended from the top heart, inferiorly, to the superior aspect of aorta, approximately at the level of T2/T3 vertebra. Attention must be paid to avoid delineation of central structures such as trachea, main bronchus, and oesophagus.

Lung/Lungs (TG 263: Lung_L, Lung_R, Lungs)

Modalities: 3DCRT/IMRT/VMAT

CT Contouring recommendation: CT WW:1500 WL: −600|WW:1600 WL: −600

The right and left lungs should be contoured separately. One single structure (Lungs) should be generated from individual Lung_R and Lung_L summation, for evaluation and reporting purposes. Contour the whole lung from apex to diaphragm, including all air-inflated parenchyma, excluding trachea and the proximal bronchus, fluid and atelectasis [8].

Spinal Cord

(TG 263: SpinalCord/SpinalCord~ (partial organ))

Modalities: 3DCRT/IMRT/VMAT

CT Contouring recommendation: CT WW:350, WL:40

The spinal cord should be delineated as the true spinal cord, not the spinal canal. It has slightly higher density than the surrounding cerebrospinal fluid and ligaments. The spinal cord extends from the cranial cervical junction, after the brainstem, to the cauda equina at the inferior border of L2 vertebral body [8]. For planning purposes, the spinal cord should be contoured at least 5 cm extra lenght, in the longitudinal plane, from cranial and caudal PTV borders. For dosimetric evaluation and dose optimisation, a PRV margin applied to the spinal cord would be necessary (SpinalCord_PRV). When deemed necessary for standardisation reasons the PRV margin could be included in the nomenclature, according to AAPM TG 263, as SpinalCord_PRVxx.

Trachea

(TG 263: Trachea)

Modalities: 3DCRT/IMRT/VMAT

CT Contouring recommendation: CT WW:350, WL:40

The trachea should be fully contoured (including lumen) to the outer boundary of the cartilage and trachealis muscle, from the caudal edge of the cricoid cartilage to approximately 2 cm superior to the carina.

Oesophagus

(TG 263: Oesophagus/Oesophagus~ (partial organ))

Modalities: 3DCRT/IMRT/VMAT

CT Contouring recommendation: CT WW:350, WL:40

The oesophagus contour should include all muscle layers out to the fatty adventitia, superiorly at the level of the cricoid cartilage to the caudal edge of the gastroesophageal junction, usually at the level of the diaphragm [8]. Oesophagus lies close to the anterior border of vertebral bodies, behind heart and trachea, with a round/oval axial shape. Contour in visible slices and interpolate when possible.

Larynx

(TG 263: Larynx)

Modalities: 3DCRT/IMRT/VMAT

CT Contouring recommendation: CT WW:350, WL:40

The larynx should be contoured from the tip of epiglottis to the inferior aspect of the thyroid cartilage, near the caudal limit of the cricoid cartilage [9]. The anterior and lateral borders are the outer aspect of the thyroid cartilage. Posteriorly, the contour should include the arytenoid cartilages and extend to the edge of the pharyngeal constrictor muscles.

Thyroid
(TG 263: Glnd_Thyroid)
Modalities: 3DCRT/IMRT/VMAT
CT Contouring recommendation: CT WW:350, WL:100

The thyroid gland is located inferiorly to the thyroid cartilage. Thyroid has two lobes, connected in its anterior and lower portion. Thyroid is recognised by slightly high density than the adjacent soft tissues [10]. It extends and surrounds the thyroid and cricoid cartilages. Common carotid arteries border the lateral aspects.

Liver
(TG 263: Liver)
Modality: IMRT/VMAT
CT Contouring recommendation: CT WW:450, WL:40

The liver should be contoured as a single structure, excluding the gallbladder, and the inferior vena cava when clearly separated to the liver. It should be outlined from the diaphragm to the bottom of the right lobe.

Contralateral Breast
(TG 263: Breast_L, Breast_R)
Modality: IMRT/VMAT
CT Contouring recommendation: CT WW: 350, WL: 40

For evaluation purposes, the contralateral breast should be contoured for an accurate dose determination. When IMRT/VMAT is the chosen technique, the contralateral breast should be outlined as part of the inverse planning optimisation process. The cranial limit is at the upper border of visible breast tissue, normally up to the caudal edge of the sternoclavicular joint. The breast extends inferiorly to the intermammary sulcus, where breast shape is still visible. Medially the breast extends to the ipsilateral edge of the sternum, close to the medial mammary branches [11]. The lateral border may be defined using breast tissue lateral fold and, when visible, relate to the lateral thoracic artery as lateral/posterior anatomic reference.

Anteriorly the contralateral breast should be contoured 5 mm under the skin surface. Posteriorly should be delineated to the anterior border of the pectoralis major and where is not perceived, it should be contoured around the rib cage and intercostal muscles [12].

Humerus
(TG 263: Humerus_L, Humerus_R)
CT Contouring recommendation: CT WW:2000, WL:350

The ipsilateral humeral head is delineated for treatment optimisation and evaluation. It should be contoured from the top head to the full PTV extension plus margin, according to the technique field entrance and length.

To avoid inclusion of the glenohumeral joint and the connective tissues, a PRV of 1 cm around the humeral head may be generated [12].

Brachial Plexus
(TG 263: BrachialPlex_L, BrachialPlex_R)
Modality: IMRT/VMAT
CT Contouring recommendation: CT WW:350, WL:40

The brachial plexus (BP) is a neural network composed by 5 roots spinal nerves (SNs) started at the neural foramina:

1. Vertebral bodies C4-C5 (SN: C5)
2. Vertebral bodies C5-C6 (SN: C6)
3. Vertebral bodies C6-C7 (SN: C7)
4. Vertebral bodies C7-T1 (SN: C8)
5. Vertebral bodies T1-T2 (SN: T1)

For delineation purposes, identification of vertebral bodies and nerve roots from C4 to T2 are recommended.

According to Brouwer and Hall [10, 13], the use of a 5 mm diameter tool is recommended to contour the BP. Anterior and middle scalene muscles could be contoured from C5 to insertion onto the first rib, as guidance for BP segmentation. The BP should be contoured from the foramina to the space between the anterior and middle scalene muscles.

On slices where there is no visible neural foramina, contour the space or soft tissue between the anterior and middle scalene muscles. The scalene muscles will end at the level of the subclavian neurovascular bundle.

Contour the BP as the posterior aspect of the neurovascular bundle until the axial level below clavicular head. If the BP is wrapped around the vascular bundle on the inferior slices, contour the brachial plexus divisions, cords, and terminal nerves by including the vascular structure into the axilla.

The first and second ribs would aid as the medial limit of the BP at subclavian space [8]. The BP contouring terminates at the medial limit of the second rib. The BP should be delineated inferiorly and laterally, to one or two CT slices below the clavicular head. Figures 13.2, 13.3, 13.4, and 13.5 show critical areas of the brachial plexus, for full view of the course of the

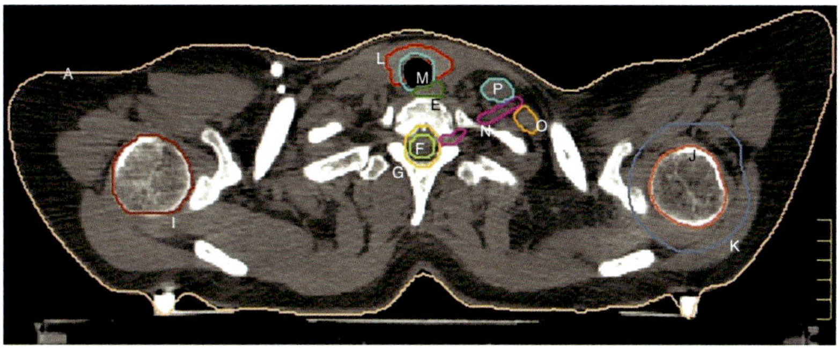

Fig. 13.2–13.5 *A* BODY, *B* Lungs, *E* Esophagus, *F* SpinalCord, *G* SpinalCord_PRV3, *I* Humerus_R, *J* Humerus_L, *K* Humerus_L_PRV10, *L* Thyroid, *M* Trachea, *N* BrachialPlex_L, *O* Scalene_M, *P* Scalene_A

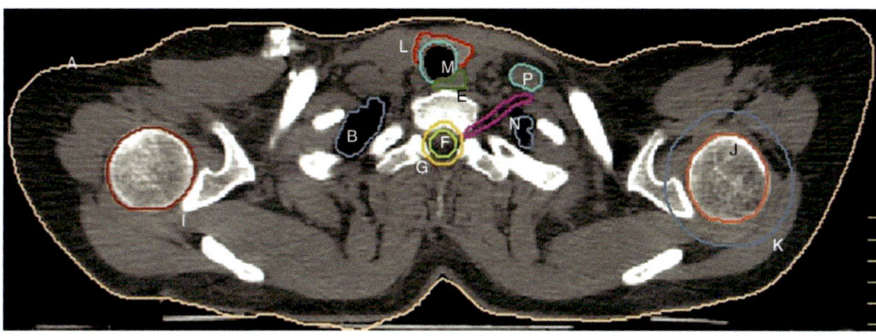

Fig. 13.3

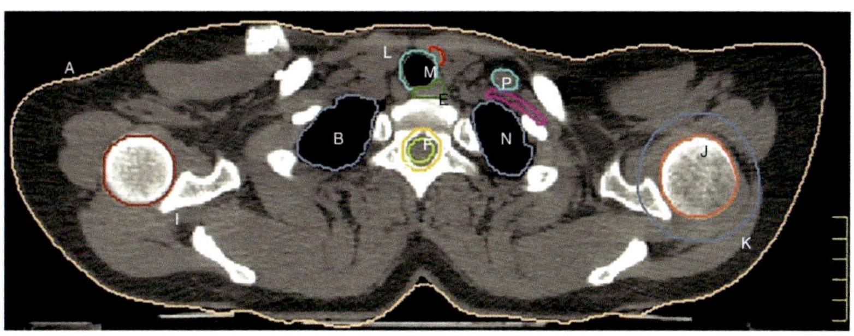

Fig. 13.4

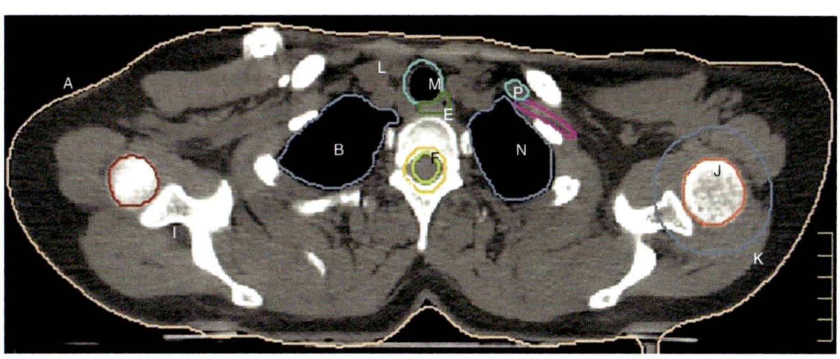

Fig. 13.5

brachial plexus, please view the electronic supplementary material.

13.5 Summary

Definition of volumes of interest has become one of the weakest links in contemporary Radiation Oncology. The contouring methods and treatment approaches have changed dramatically during the past decades, with the wide spread of technological advances and scientific network around the globe.

The quantitative analysis of normal tissues effects demanded for the improvement on organs and anatomical structures categorisation and standardisation, which became a priority of several working groups from RT community. The manual delineation of the Organs at Risk turns out to be an extensive time-consuming process, which could be eased with auto-segmentation tools available in most TPS and virtual simulator systems, nevertheless, human visual inspection remains the last checkpoint for contouring validation.

Unintended over- and/or under-contouring could lead to an unpredicted normal tissue complications with poor outcomes and patients QoL. Delineation skills and rationale are crucial for personalised RT, as it can contribute for better clinical care and promote evidence-based medicine.

In breast cancer RT, several guidance documents have been published towards standardisation and terminology of volumes of interest. Hereby, a compilation of the most relevant OARs were described and contoured, to guide and empower professionals for strengthening this crucial RT link.

References

1. Bentzen SM, Constine LS, Deasy JO, et al. Quantitative analyses of normal tissue effects in the clinic (QUANTEC): an introduction to the scientific issues. Int J Radiat Oncol Biol Phys. 2010;76(3):3–9. https://doi.org/10.1016/j.ijrobp.2009.09.040.
2. Standardizing nomenclatures in radiation oncology. The report of AAPM Task Group 263. 2018.
3. Mir R, Kelly SM, Xiao Y, et al. Organ at risk delineation for radiation therapy clinical trials: global harmonization group consensus guidelines. Radiother Oncol. 2020;150:30–9. https://doi.org/10.1016/j.radonc.2020.05.038.
4. Kaidar-Person O, Kostich M, Zagar TM, et al. Helical tomotherapy for bilateral breast cancer: clinical experience. Breast. 2016;28:79–83. https://doi.org/10.1016/j.breast.2016.05.004.
5. Feng M, Moran JM, Koelling T, et al. Development and validation of a heart atlas to study cardiac exposure to radiation following treatment for breast cancer. Int J Radiat Oncol Biol Phys. 2011;79(1):10–8. https://doi.org/10.1016/j.ijrobp.2009.10.058.
6. Milo ML, Offersen BV, Bechmann T, et al. Delineation of whole heart and substructures in thoracic radiation therapy: national guidelines and contouring atlas by the Danish Multidisciplinary Cancer Groups. Radiother Oncol. 2020;150:121–7. https://doi.org/10.1016/j.radonc.2020.06.015.
7. Duane F, Aznar MC, Barlett F, et al. A cardiac contouring atlas for radiotherapy. Radiother Oncol. 2017; 122:416–22. https://doi.org/10.1016/j.radonc.2017.01.008.
8. Kong FM, Ritter T, Quint D, et al. Consideration of dose limits for organs at risk of thoracic radiotherapy: atlas for lung, proximal bronchial tree, esophagus, spinal cord, ribs, and brachial plexus. Int J Radiat Oncol Biol Phys. 2011;81(5):1442–67. https://doi.org/10.1016/j.ijrobp.2010.07.1977.
9. Rancati T, Schwarz M, Allen AM. Radiation dose-volume effects in the larynx and pharynx. Int J Radiat Oncol Biol Phys. 2010;76(3):64–9. https://doi.org/10.1016/j.ijrobp.2009.03.079.
10. Brouwer C, Steenbakkers R, Bourhis J, et al. CT-based delineation of organs at risk in the head and neck region: DAHANCA, EORTC, GORTEC, HKNPCSG, NCIC CTG, NCRI, NRG Oncology and TROG consensus guidelines. Radiother Oncol. 2015;117:83–90. https://doi.org/10.1016/j.radonc.2015.07.041.
11. Nielsen MH, Berg M, Pedersen N, et al. Delineation of target volumes and organs at risk in adjuvant radiotherapy of early breast cancer: national guidelines and contouring atlas by the Danish Breast Cancer Cooperative Group. Acta Oncol. 2013;52(4):703–10. https://doi.org/10.3109/0284186X.2013.765064.
12. Offersen BV, Boersma LJ, Kirkove C, et al. ESTRO consensus guideline on target volume delineation for elective radiation therapy of early stage breast cancer. Radiother Oncol. 2015;114:3–10. https://doi.org/10.1016/j.radonc.2014.11.030.
13. Hall W, Guiou M, Lee NY, et al. Development and validation of a standardized method for contouring the brachial plexus: preliminary dosimetric analysis among patients treated with IMRT for head-and-neck cancer. Int J Radiat Oncol Biol Phys. 2008;72:1362–7. https://doi.org/10.1016/j.ijrobp.2008.03.004.

Breast Cancer Radiobiology: The Basics

14

Navita Somaiah and John R. Yarnold

14.1 Background

Good entry points to discussing the clinical radiobiology of hypofractionation are offered by the Ontario (1993–1996) and START-B (1998–2002) trials described by Brunt and Whelan elsewhere in this book [1–3]. The Canadian trial adopted 2.66 Gy fractions introduced by Ralston Paterson at The Christie Hospital, UK, in response to resource shortages in the 1940s. Paterson's 15-fraction schedule delivered 40 Gy in 3 weeks, and it co-existed in the UK for decades with 50 Gy in 25 fractions for postoperative local-regional radiation therapy after primary surgery [4].

The Ontario trial chose to test 16 fractions of 2.66 Gy as the number predicted by the LQ model to be equivalent to the control regimen of 50 Gy in 25 fractions in terms of late normal tissue changes (NTE), specifically breast cosmesis, assuming $\alpha/\beta = 3$ Gy. As with every application of the LQ model, it assumed complete repair of sublethal damage between fractions, no repopulation of target cells over the course of therapy and no redistribution in cell cycle phase in order to restrict the adjustment to the effect of fraction size. The relatively low value of 3 Gy reflects the relatively high sensitivity of late reacting normal tissues to changes in fraction size above conventional 2 Gy [5, 6]. The trial reported near-identical breast cosmesis and local tumour control in control and test regimens, the inference being consistent with breast cancer responding to the increased fraction size to a comparable degree as the dose-limiting normal tissues of the breast. The α/β estimate reflects the reduction in total dose from 50 Gy to 42.56 Gy needed to match the late NTE of the 25- and 16-fraction schedules, the 7.5 Gy difference offering a vivid indicator of fraction size sensitivity in action.

Based on $\alpha/\beta = 3$ Gy and the same assumptions relating to the LQ model described above, the Manchester schedule of 40 Gy in 15 fractions over 3 weeks schedule is equivalent to 46 Gy in 23 fractions of 2 Gy, so the hazard ratio of 0.8 ((0.67–0.96) 0.015) for 10-year physician-assessed breast shrinkage in test (15-fraction) compared to control (25-fraction) regimens in the START-B trial was expected [7]. The 15-fraction schedule was also non-inferior in terms of local control (HR 0.77, 95% CI 0.51–1.16; $p = 0.21$). This outcome is consistent with high fraction size sensitivity, but the 2-week difference in treatment time, in the Ontario and START-B trials, made it

N. Somaiah (✉)
Translational Breast Radiobiology, Institute of Cancer Research, The Royal Marsden NHS Foundation Trust, Sutton, UK
e-mail: Navita.somaiah@icr.ac.uk

J. R. Yarnold
Division of Radiotherapy and Imaging, The Institute of Cancer Research, The Royal Marsden NHS Foundation Trust, Sutton, UK
e-mail: John.Yarnold@icr.ac.uk

© The Author(s), under exclusive license to Springer Nature Switzerland AG 2022
O. Kaidar-Person et al. (eds.), *Breast Cancer Radiation Therapy*,
https://doi.org/10.1007/978-3-030-91170-6_14

impossible to rule out an effect of time on tumour control.

Why is the 2-week treatment time difference raised here? After all, low mean mitotic and labelling indices are characteristic of primary breast cancer, and accelerated repopulation during radiation therapy was not considered clinically relevant [8, 9]. This is likely true, but in START-B trial the 10-year HR for local control in the test compared to the control group was 0.77 (95% CI 0.51-1.16; $p = 0.21$), not statistically significant but describing the 1.4% lower rate of local recurrence observed after 40 Gy in 15 fractions compared to the 50 Gy control schedule (3.8 vs 5.2%) [7]. Assuming $\alpha/\beta = 3$ Gy for tumour control and no effect of time, 40 Gy in 15 fractions is equivalent to 46 Gy in 23 fractions, a lower dose intensity than the control schedule and expected to be 1% inferior in terms of local control. We have already mentioned that this is likely a chance effect, but in a discussion of clinical radiobiology it is reasonable to ask what the effect would be if the HR = 0.8 for local control after 40 Gy is real. In laryngeal carcinomas, at least 0.5 Gy/day can be 'wasted' compensating for accelerated repopulation from the fourth week of treatment onwards [10]. There was no hint of a superiority after 16 fractions in the Ontario trial, but in a post hoc, hypothesis-generating, test of time in START-B, Haviland estimated 0.6 Gy/day 'wasted dose' during weeks 4 and 5 of the 5-week regimen attributable to repopulation [11]. Radiation therapy is delivered to residual disease several weeks or months after primary surgery depending on adjuvant systemic therapies, so it is plausible to consider the possibility of cancer in a phase of accelerated repopulation from the start of treatment. The important point is not to argue whether or not a time effect for local control exists, we just don't know, but to point out that if it exists, it will attribute the time effect to enhanced fraction size sensitivity (reduce the α/β estimate) unless its impact is independently quantified and taken out of the basic LQ model and added as a separate term [11].

In terms of time-dependent effects, which do not all relate to repopulation, this is where the START-P (1986–1998) and START-A trials (1999–2002) [3, 7, 12–14] contribute, first by controlling for treatment time in all test and control groups (5 weeks) and second, by incorporating 2 dose levels of 13-fraction test regimens (5 fractions per fortnight) to ensure that the iso-effective regimens for late adverse effects and local tumour control can be estimated, if necessary by interpolation between test dose levels. By controlling for time-related effects and estimating iso-effects for both late normal tissue effects and tumour control, these trials generated unconfounded direct estimates of fraction size sensitivity. A direct α/β estimate for local tumour control was based on a 10-year total of 349 local tumour relapse events in 3646 women [7]. The 8.4 Gy reduction from 50 Gy to 41.6 Gy needed to match the anti-tumour effect of 3.2 Gy fractions with 25 fractions of 2.0 Gy generated an α/β estimate of 3.5 Gy (95% CI 1.2–5.7) unconfounded by time, and entirely consistent with prior predictions of relatively high sensitivity to fraction size. These set of trials offer the strongest evidence of breast cancers responding to increase in fraction size despite a significant drop in total dose, whilst avoiding any confounding effect of treatment time.

Is there anything to learn from the FAST-Forward trial apart from clinical indications that 26 Gy in 5 fractions over 1 week offers a safe and effective standard for patients prescribed postoperative local radiation therapy for early breast cancer? This pragmatic trial compared 2 test dose levels of a 5-fraction schedule delivered in 1 week with 40 Gy in 15 fractions over 3 weeks. Applying an α/β of 2.8 Gy for late NTE based on the combined estimates of α/β for late adverse effects in START-P/-A and FAST, the trial protocol predicted 27 Gy in 5 fractions of 5.4 Gy to be iso-effective with the 40 Gy schedule. As emphasised earlier, an application of original LQ model assumes complete sublethal damage repair between fractions, no redistribution in the cell cycle phase and no target cell repopulation. The lower test dose of 26 Gy in 5 fractions of 5.2 Gy was included in FAST-Forward, first to generate dose response data for late adverse effects, thereby ensuring that an iso-effective 5-fraction schedule could be determined, and second, to offer a safety margin if the assumptions described above (in relation to treatment time) were not met in practice. As it turned out, the observed iso-effect for NTE at 5 years was closer to 26 Gy than 27 Gy, suggesting a α/β value below 3 Gy. Estimates varied across multiple outcome measures based on clinician, patient and photographic assessments of late normal tissue effects, but are consistent with an α/β point estimate close to 2 Gy. This α/β value implies that 26 Gy in 5 fractions results in normal tissue effects comparable to 47 Gy given in 2 Gy equivalents.

How is this lower-than-expected α/β estimate for late normal tissue effects explained? The 95% confidence intervals of α/β point estimates for normal tissue endpoints in the FAST-Forward trial, whether scored by clinicians, patients or from photographs, all fall within the confidence intervals of α/β estimates for all late normal tissue effects reported in the FAST and START-P/-A trials. Statistically speaking the likeliest explanation is that different α/β estimates are internally consistent with each other. If the α/β estimate is truly closer to 2 Gy than 3 Gy, the likeliest mechanism is incomplete repair between 4 of the 5 fractions if treatment starts on a Monday or between 3 fractions if treatment is interrupted by a week-end. This represents a time effect to the extent that it would be less or absent if 5 fractions were given over 3 weeks, leaving more time to complete residual sublethal damage after fractions of 5.2 and 5.4 Gy. Robust quantitative data generated in human skin are consistent with a time effect for telangiectasia despite the complete absence of mitotic figures in capillary endothelium on serial skin biopsies during both conventional and hypofractionated radiation therapy post-mastectomy [15]. The absence of mitotic figures excluded endothelial repopulation, and the effect was considered to represent a very slow component of repair decaying with a $T_{1/2}$ of roughly 40 days, a phenomenon consistent with the experimental literature in animal systems [5]. In this context, the FAST trial (2004–2007), which served as a pilot trial for FAST-Forward, controlled for a potential time effect damage by testing 5 fractions of 5.7 Gy or 6.0 Gy once-weekly against 50 Gy in 5 weeks [16]. The α/β point estimate for any moderate or marked normal tissue effect was 2.5 Gy (CI), a point estimate 'halfway' between 3 Gy and 2 Gy. Differences in point estimates are likely chance effects, but in the context of a radiobiology discussion, a role for incomplete repair between daily fractions in FAST-Forward remains plausible.

There is one more mechanism that might explain or contribute to a reduction in α/β value for late NTE as fraction size increases. This relates to the milder acute skin reactions, especially moist desquamation, seen after 5-fraction regimens. Early reacting normal tissues are relatively insensitive to fraction size, leaving the reduction in total dose contributing disproportionately to reducing acute skin reactions. In FAST-Forward, the erythema was milder and of much shorter duration after 26 Gy and 27 Gy in 5 fractions compared to 40 Gy in 15 fractions [17]. Severe moist desquamation (α/β = 10+) in the inframammary fold or post-mastectomy chest wall can cause direct, so-called consequential, late normal tissue damage that shares the same high α/β as the causative early reaction and that can 'artificially' increase the α/β estimate of late normal tissue effects recorded in trials.

Does FAST-Forward tell us anything new or unexpected about anti-tumour effects of hypofractionation? Applying the $\alpha/\beta = 3.5$ for tumour estimated by START-P and START-A, which controlled for potential time effects, 26 Gy in 5 fractions is expected to be equivalent to 41 Gy in 2 Gy fractions in terms of tumour control. The difference between this equivalent total dose and the corresponding 45 Gy total dose equivalent to 40 Gy in 15 fractions assuming $\alpha/\beta = 3.5$ would be too small to detect at such high levels of local tumour control without many more thousands of patients. It is possible to ask if 26 Gy in 5 fractions would be expected to have any anti-tumour effect at all without a strong time effect contributing in addition. The adjusted α/β estimate derived from FAST-Forward was 3.7 Gy (95% CI 0.4–6.9), which despite very wide CI, does not suggest a significant time effect. The best one can say is that given the 5-year local control rate of 2.1% (95% CI 1.4–3.1) after 40 Gy in 15 fractions, the rate without any radiation therapy would be expected to be about 6% at 5 years and 10% at 10 years according to systematic overviews of radiation therapy effects. The non-inferior 5-year local relapse rate reported after 26 Gy in 5 fractions in FAST-Forward is therefore hardly consistent with an absence of effect.

After diving relatively deep into discussion based on randomised clinical trials, it is worth finishing by returning to the era of Ralston Paterson in mid-twentieth century. The first published estimate of α/β for breast cancer was mentioned in a single sentence of Discussion in a manuscript applying the LQ model to clinical data on hyper-fractionation by Bruce Douglas, a Canadian radiation biologist working at the Gray Laboratories in the early 1980s [18]. He estimated α/β to be 3.8 Gy based on a 1951 publication by Lionel Cohen from Johannesburg, South Africa [19]. Cohen had developed a precursor to the Ellis formula and used it to analyse treatment outcomes of his own patients and of previously published world literature totalling >1000 patients, deriving an exponent for $N = 2.4$, consistent with high fractionation sensitivity of clinical breast cancer, albeit without controlling for differences in time. The START-P trial opened in 1986 in response to Douglas' publication. Despite significant strides made with clinical trials, the cell and molecular basis of fraction size sensitivity is still relatively poorly understood. Recent evidence points to a strong influence of DNA double strand break repair pathways and cell cycle checkpoints [8, 9, 20–22]. Efforts to understand the basic biology of fractionation will no doubt complement future clinical applications of hypofractionation.

14.2 Summary

Over the years, protracted radiation therapy schedules spanning several weeks have been stepwise replaced by shorter, more convenient schedules. Radiobiological knowledge was used to prepare prospective clinical trials, which confirmed applicability of shorter schedules and, on its turn, provided further information to enhance our understanding of radiobiology of breast cancer and normal tissues.

References

1. Whelan T, MacKenzie R, Julian J, Levine M, Shelley W, Grimard L, et al. Randomized trial of breast irradiation schedules after lumpectomy for women with lymph node-negative breast cancer. J Natl Cancer Inst. 2002;94(15):1143–50.
2. Whelan TJ, Pignol JP, Levine MN, Julian JA, Mackenzie R, Parpia S, et al. Long-term results of hypofractionated radiation therapy for breast cancer. N Engl J Med. 2010;362(6):513–20.
3. Bentzen SM, Agrawal RK, Aird EG, Barrett JM, Barrett-Lee PJ, Bliss JM, et al. The UK Standardisation of Breast Radiotherapy (START) trial B of radiotherapy hypofractionation for treatment of early breast cancer: a randomised trial. Lancet. 2008;371(9618):1098–107.
4. Priestman TJ, Bullimore JA, Godden TP, Deutsch GP. The Royal College of Radiologists' fractionation survey. Clin Oncol. 1989;1(1):39–46.
5. Thames HD Jr, Withers HR, Peters LJ, Fletcher GH. Changes in early and late radiation responses with altered dose fractionation: implications for dose-survival relationships. Int J Radiat Oncol Biol Phys. 1982;8(2):219–26.
6. Withers HR, Peters LJ, Thames HD, Fletcher GH. Hyperfractionation. Int J Radiat Oncol Biol Phys. 1982;8(10):1807–9.
7. Haviland JS, Owen JR, Dewar JA, Agrawal RK, Barrett J, Barrett-Lee PJ, et al. The UK Standardisation of Breast Radiotherapy (START) trials of radiotherapy hypofractionation for treatment of early breast cancer: 10-year follow-up results of two randomised controlled trials. Lancet Oncol. 2013;14(11):1086–94.
8. Somaiah N, Yarnold J, Daley F, Pearson A, Gothard L, Rothkamm K, et al. The relationship between homologous recombination repair and the sensitivity of human epidermis to the size of daily doses over a 5-week course of breast radiotherapy. Clin Cancer Res. 2012;18(19):5479–88.
9. Somaiah N, Rothkamm K, Yarnold J. Where do we look for markers of radiotherapy fraction size sensitivity? Clin Oncol. 2015;27(10):570–8.
10. Withers HR, Taylor JM, Maciejewski B. The hazard of accelerated tumor clonogen repopulation during radiotherapy. Acta Oncol. 1988;27(2):131–46.
11. Haviland JS, Bentzen SM, Bliss JM, Yarnold JR. Prolongation of overall treatment time as a cause of treatment failure in early breast cancer: an analysis of the UK START (standardisation of breast radiotherapy) trials of radiotherapy fractionation. Radiother Oncol. 2016;121(3):420–3.

12. Yarnold J, Ashton A, Bliss J, Homewood J, Harper C, Hanson J, et al. Fractionation sensitivity and dose response of late adverse effects in the breast after radiotherapy for early breast cancer: long-term results of a randomised trial. Radiother Oncol. 2005;75(1):9–17.
13. Owen JR, Ashton A, Bliss JM, Homewood J, Harper C, Hanson J, et al. Effect of radiotherapy fraction size on tumour control in patients with early-stage breast cancer after local tumour excision: long-term results of a randomised trial. Lancet Oncol. 2006;7(6):467–71.
14. Bentzen SM, Agrawal RK, Aird EG, Barrett JM, Barrett-Lee PJ, Bliss JM, et al. The UK standardisation of breast radiotherapy (START) trial A of radiotherapy hypofractionation for treatment of early breast cancer: a randomised trial. Lancet Oncol. 2008;9(4):331–41.
15. Turesson I, Thames HD. Repair capacity and kinetics of human skin during fractionated radiotherapy: erythema, desquamation, and telangiectasia after 3 and 5 year's follow-up. Radiother Oncol. 1989;15(2):169–88.
16. Brunt AM, Haviland JS, Sydenham M, Agrawal RK, Algurafi H, Alhasso A, et al. Ten-year results of FAST: a randomized controlled trial of 5-fraction whole-breast radiotherapy for early breast cancer. J Clin Oncol. 2020;2020:1902750.
17. Brunt AM, Wheatley D, Yarnold J, Somaiah N, Kelly S, Harnett A, et al. Acute skin toxicity associated with a 1-week schedule of whole breast radiotherapy compared with a standard 3-week regimen delivered in the UK FAST-Forward Trial. Radiother Oncol. 2016;120(1):114–8.
18. Douglas BG, Castro JR. Novel fractionation schemes and high linear energy transfer. Prog Exp Tumor Res. 1984;28:152–65.
19. Cohen L. Radiotherapy in breast cancer I. The dose-time relationship theoretical considerations. Br J Radiol. 1952;25(300):636–42.
20. Somaiah N, Yarnold J, Lagerqvist A, Rothkamm K, Helleday T. Homologous recombination mediates cellular resistance and fraction size sensitivity to radiation therapy. Radiother Oncol. 2013;108(1):155–61.
21. Anbalagan S, Ström C, Downs JA, Jeggo PA, McBay D, Wilkins AC, Boyle S, Rothkamm K, Yarnold JR, Somaiah N. TP53 modulates radiotherapy fraction size sensitivity in normal and malignant cells. Sci Rep. 2021.
22. Eke I, Zong D, Aryankalayil MJ, Sandfort V, Bylicky MA, Rath BH, et al. 53BP1/RIF1 signaling promotes cell survival after multifractionated radiotherapy. Nucleic Acids Res. 2020;48(3):1314–26.

Dose Fractionation

15

Adrian Murray Brunt and Timothy Whelan

15.1 Background

In 2020 postoperative conventional fractionation for breast cancer (BCS, mastectomy with/without RNI) is considered to be 15 or 16 fractions delivering a dose of 40–42.5 Gy over 3 weeks. This is now being challenged by hypofractionation in 5 fractions over a week to the intact breast or chest wall. The previous standard of 50 Gy in 25 fractions of 2 Gy over 5 weeks was first tested in a randomised trial against the linear quadratic model by the START-pilot study [1] in the mid-1980s. This was backed up by START trial A [2], which was also a 3-arm study allowing radiobiological analysis and interpolation for an equivalent regimen.

15.2 Key Information for Clinical Practice

Two landmark trials commenced in the 1990s, the Ontario Clinical Oncology Group (OCOG) trial in Canada [3] and START trial B in the UK [4], comparing 42.5 Gy in 16 fractions and 40 Gy in 15 fractions respectively over 3 weeks with 50 Gy in 25 fractions over 5 weeks. These trials showed similar rates of local recurrence and normal tissue effects at 5 and 10 years for hypofractionation compared to historical conventional fractionation. The three START trials and the OCOG trial slowly led to 15/16/fractions over about 3 weeks becoming international standard practice [5]. The recent Danish-led HYPO trial also supports 40 Gy in 15 fractions over 3 weeks as a standard [6]. The main hypofractionation trials are the subject of Tables 15.1, 15.2, and 15.3. Table 15.1 gives the patient and tumour features of the patients.

15.2.1 Local Recurrence

The OCOG [7] and START [8] trials published long-term results showing that 15/16 fractions over 3 weeks is both safe and effective. The 10-year local recurrence rates are shown in Table 15.2. In an unplanned meta-analysis of 5861 patients in the START-pilot, -A and -B trials, Haviland et al. [8] reported no concerns with hypofractionation for local recurrence in any subgroups. This included age, nodal status, tumour grade, or use of chemotherapy. A central pathological review of the OCOG trial [9] showed that tumour grade and molecular subtype did not predict a response to hypofractionated RT.

A. M. Brunt (✉)
David Weatherall Building, School of Medicine, University of Keele, Keele, Staffordshire, UK
e-mail: m.brunt@keele.ac.uk

T. Whelan
Department of Oncology, McMaster University and the Juravinski Cancer Centre, Hamilton, ON, Canada
e-mail: twhelan@hhsc.ca

© The Author(s), under exclusive license to Springer Nature Switzerland AG 2022

O. Kaidar-Person et al. (eds.), *Breast Cancer Radiation Therapy*,
https://doi.org/10.1007/978-3-030-91170-6_15

Table 15.1 Demographic, clinical and treatment characteristics in 6 trials of hypofractionation for early breast cancer

	OCOG	START B	DBCG HYPO	Beijing	FAST	FAST forward[a]
Recruitment years	1993–1996	1999–2001	2009–2014	2008–2016	2004–2007	2011–2014
Median follow-up (years)	12.0	9.9	7.3	4.9	9.9	6.0
Control (Gy/fx/weeks)	50/25/5	50/25/5	50/25/5	50/25/5	50/25/5	40/15/3
1st test arm (Gy/fx/weeks)	42.5/16/3	40/15/3	40/15/3	43.5/15/3	30/5/5	27/5/1
2nd test arm (Gy/fx/weeks)	n/a	n/a	n/a	n/a	28.5/5/5	26/5/1
Total patients	1234	2215	1854	810	915	4096
Age (years)	Not reported	57.4 mean	59 median	49 median	62.9 mean	61 median
Age under 50 years	305	457	199	Over 50%	0	604
Mastectomy	0	177	0	810	0	264
Node positive	0	504	183[b]	810	0	756
T2/T3	240/0	795[c]	292/0	Not known	163/0	1211/76
Grade 3	233	509	303	232	98	1153
DCIS only	0	0	246	0	0	0
Chemotherapy	136	491	682	810	0	1174
Boost	0	868	430	0	0	1011
Regional radiotherapy	0	161	0	810	0	0

The figures are number of patients unless stated otherwise

[a] FAST-forward has a regional nodal radiotherapy sub-study that is yet to report

[b] DBCG HYPO trial node positive are micrometastasis only

[c] 220 patients greater than 3 cm, T3 allowed but numbers unknown

15.2.2 Normal Tissue Effects

Table 15.3 gives aspects of normal tissue effects from the trials with an attempt where possible to show similar aspects for comparison. START-B identified breast shrinkage, telangiectasia and oedema as significantly less in the 40 Gy/15 fractions arm with no significant differences for all other normal tissue effects [2, 8]. Both the OCOG and START-B trials saw a worsening of normal tissue effects with time, as expected, but no change in the relative comparison of the two arms. The HYPO trial reported that hypofractionation (40 Gy/15 fractions) is appropriate for all subgroups with regard to morbidity including those receiving chemotherapy, trastuzumab or letrozole. They also reported that large breast size and smoking increased breast induration (induration was the primary endpoint at 3 years) significantly but at no time did 40 Gy/15 fractions produce a worse outcome than 50 Gy/25 fractions. None of the three trials identified a subgroup for whom hypofractionation produced a worse outcome.

An important observation from these trials and others [10–13] is that acute toxicity of RT, e.g. skin erythema, desquamation and fatigue, was less with hypofractionation compared to conventional treatment. This is consistent with the radiobiological principle that acute reacting tissues are more sensitive to a reduction in total dose and less sensitive to an increase in fraction size [14].

In addition to an improvement in convenience and a reduction in resources required, hypofractionation provides important benefits with respect to acute and in some instances late toxicity that can improve patient quality of life.

15.2.3 Boost Fractionation

Conventional fractionation boost irradiation was used in: the START-B trial (43% of BCS, 10 Gy in 5 fractions); the HYPO trial (20%, 10 Gy in 5

Table 15.2 Local recurrence in 6 trials of hypofractionation for early breast cancer

Trial	Trial arm (Gy/fx)	5-year local relapse (95% CI)	10-year local relapse (95% CI)
OCOG[a]	50/25	3.2%	6.7%
	42.5/16	2.8%	6.2%
START-B	50/25	3.3% (2.4–4.6)	5.2% (3.9–6.9)
	40/15	1.9% (1.2–3.0)	3.8% (2.7–5.2)
DBCG HYPO[b]	50/25	n/a	3.3% (2.0–5.0)[c]
	40/15	n/a	3.0% (1.9–4.5)[c]
Beijing[d]	50/25	8.1% (5.4–10.6)	n/a
	43.5/15	8.3% (5.8–10.7)	n/a
FAST[e]	50/25	0.7% (0.2–2.8)	0.7% (0.2–2.8)
	30/5	1.0% (0.3–3.2)	1.4% (0.5–3.8)
	28.5/5	0.4% (0.05–2.6)	1.7% (0.6–4.4)
FAST forward	40/15	2.1% (1.4–3.1)	n/a
	27/5	1.7% (1.2–2.6)	n/a
	26/5	1.4% (0.9–2.2)	n/a

n/a not available

[a] The absolute difference at 5 years was 0.4% (95% CI, −1.5 to 2.4). At 10 years the absolute difference, 0.5% (95% CI, −2.5 to 3.5)

[b] Median follow-up 7.3 years. Absolute number of locoregional recurrences as first event in patients who had invasive carcinoma. 33 patients (2.1%) experienced a locoregional recurrence as first event, 19 patients in the 50-Gy group and 14 patients in the 40-Gy group (hazard ratio 0.75; 95% CI, 0.37 to 1.49; $P = 0.41$). DCIS, 14 patients (7.7%) experienced a locoregional recurrence 6 patients in the 50-Gy group and 8 in the 40-Gy group (hazard ratio 1.40; 95% CI, 0.49–4.05; $P = 0.53$)

[c] Loco-regional relapse reported. Median FU 7.26 years, results projected at 9 years

[d] Loco-regional relapse reported. 6 patients in each arm had chest wall recurrence

[e] Ipsilateral breast events were reported for 11/915 (1.2%) patients (50 Gy: 3; 30 Gy: 4; 28.5 Gy: 4)

fractions and 3%, 16 Gy in 8 fractions); and the FAST-Forward trial (26% of BCS, 20%, 10 Gy in 5 fractions and 6%, 16 Gy in 8 fractions). Shaitelman et al. [15] report 3-year cosmesis of 50 Gy/25 fractions with a boost of 10–14 Gy/5–7 fractions vs 42.6 Gy/16 fractions with a boost of 10–12.5 Gy/4–5 fractions. Adverse patient-reported outcome at 3 years, the primary outcome, was 8.2% in the hypofractionated group and 13.6% in the conventional, hypofractionated therefore non-inferior, $p = 0.002$. Any of the boost fractionations used in the trials can be used in practice. Since these trials, boost irradiation using hypofractionation of 10–12 Gy in 4 fractions or 12.5–13.7 Gy in 5 fractions also has been commonly used in Canada, the United Kingdom and other countries.

15.3 Special Considerations

15.3.1 Ductal Carcinoma In Situ (DCIS)

In the original hypofractionation trials patients with DCIS alone were not included. In the HYPO trial, 246 patients (13% of total) with DCIS only were included and no difference in local control was observed between hypofractionated or conventional fractionation. The Breast International Group and the Trans Tasmanian Radiation Oncology Group trial (BIG 3-07/TROG 07.01) double randomised patients with moderate to higher risk DCIS to boost radiation or no boost radiation ($n = 1608$) and, optionally, to hypofractionation of 42.5 Gy in 16 fractions or conventional fractionation of 50 Gy in 25 fractions ($n = 777$) [16]. The 5-year free from local recurrence rates were 93% in no boost group and 97% in the boost group (HR = 0.47, 95% CI = 0.31–0.72, $p < 0.001$). No differences were observed in local recurrence rates between patients randomised to hypofractionation or conventional fractionation (94% vs 94%, $P = 0.84$) supporting the use of hypofractionation for DCIS alone following BCS.

15.3.2 Post-mastectomy and Lymphatic RT

Only START, of the original hypofractionation trials, included patients following mastectomy or BCS with node positive disease that received

Table 15.3 Normal tissue adverse effects in 6 trials of hypofractionation for early breast cancer

Trial	Trial arm (Gy/fx)	Normal tissue effect being measured	Normal tissue effect at 5 years (%)	Normal tissue effect at 10 years (%)	Normal tissue effect being measured	Normal tissue effect at 5 years (%)	Normal tissue effect at 10 years (%)
OCOG	50/25	EORTC excellent/good global cosmetic rating[a]	79.2	71.3	RTOG-EORTC subcutaneous tissue grade 2/3[b]	6.1	10.4
	42.5/16		77.9	69.8		4.7	11.9
START-B[c]	50/25	Breast shrinkage	15.8	31.2	Breast induration moderate/marked (tumour bed)	12.1	17.4
	40/15		11.4	26.2		9.6	14.3
DBCG HYPO[d]	50/25	Favourable overall cosmetic outcome	75	n/a	Induration	12	n/a
	40/15		80	n/a		9	n/a
Beijing[e]	50/25	Late skin toxicity	22	n/a	Lymphoedema	21	n/a
	43.5/15		21	n/a		20	n/a
FAST	50/25	Any moderate/marked normal tissue effect[f]	7.5	9.1	Breast shrinkage moderate/marked[g]	6.3	7.6
	30/5		18.0	18.4		12.8	13.8
	28.5/5		9.9	14.6		7.5	13.9
FAST-Forward	40/15	Any moderate/marked normal tissue effect[h]	9.9	n/a	Breast shrinkage moderate/marked[i]	5.5	n/a
	27/5		15.4	n/a		8.2	n/a
	26/5		11.9	n/a		6.8	n/a

[a] At 5 years absolute difference 1.3% (95% CI −4.2% to 6.7%). At 10 years absolute difference 1.5% (95% CI −6.9% to 9.8%)

[b] The absolute difference at 5 years of grade 0 vs grade 1/2/3 favoured 42.5/16 and was −5.4% (95% CI −11.9 to 0.9%), and at 10 years the absolute difference was −2.8% (95% CI −11.7 to 6.5%)

[c] Breast shrinkage and induration were the most common late normal tissue effects at 10 years in START-B. Moderate or marked breast shrinkage significantly lower with 40 Gy than with 50 Gy (hazard ratio 0.80; 95%CI 0.67–0.96, $p = 0.015$) but not significantly lower for induration (hazard ratio 0.81; 95%CI 0.64–1.03, $p = 0.084$)

[d] Cosmesis hazard ratio 1.35 (95% CI 1.05–1.73) $p = 0.018$. Induration hazard ratio at 3 years primary endpoint, at 5 years 0.75 (95% CI 0.53–1.05) $p = 0.092$

[e] Report at a median of 58.5 months for grade 1–3

[f] 5-year prevalence of any moderate/marked breast NTE was estimated to be 10% higher (95% CI, 5% to 16%) for 30 Gy versus 50 Gy ($P < 0.001$), with no statistically significant difference between 28.5 Gy and 50 Gy 2% higher (95% CI, −2% to 7%; $P = 0.349$). At 10 years compared with 50 Gy were 9% (95% CI, 1–18%: $P = 0.032$) for 30 Gy and 5% (95% CI, 22–113%; $P = 0.184$) for 28.5 Gy

[g] At 5 years, risk ratios for moderate/marked breast shrinkage versus 50 Gy were 2.03 (95% CI, 1.15–3.58; $P = 0.017$) for 30 Gy and 1.20 (95% CI, 0.63–2.27; $P = 0.604$) for 28.5 Gy. No significant differences at 10 years

[h] At 5 years, any moderate or marked clinician-assessed normal tissue effects in the breast or chest wall showed a significant difference between 40 Gy and 27 Gy ($p = 0.0003$) but not between 40 Gy and 26 Gy ($p = 0.17$)

[i] Breast shrinkage was the most prevalent moderate or marked effect at 5 years and with a pre-specified cut-off of $p = 0.005$ for multiple testing, was not significant between 40 Gy and 27 Gy ($p = 0.0022$) nor between 40 Gy and 26 Gy ($p = 0.25$)

RNI. In the START-pilot, -A and -B trials 864/5861 (14.7%) of patients received RNI. Haviland et al. [17] reported late normal tissue effects observed in these patients. These studies occurred over an 18-year period (1986–2002) and patients were treated with a variety of surgical procedures, RT approaches (axillary RT and/or supraclavicular RT) and systemic therapies. Patient- and physician-assessed arm or hand swelling, and shoulder stiffness were similar for the hypofractionation regimens compared to conventional fractionation (50 Gy in 25 fractions). This data is limited by the different treatments received and the variability per trial in risk factors (which are well balanced between arms in each trial), but it does suggest that RNI with currently accepted hypofractionation schedules is not associated with increased morbidity.

Wang et al. [11] reported the results of a single institutional trial of post-mastectomy radiation therapy from the National Cancer Center in Beijing. In this trial, 810 women with primary tumours T3 to T4 or at least 4 positive axillary nodes were randomised to 43.5 Gy in 15 fractions of 2.9 Gy over 3 weeks or 50 Gy in 25 fractions to the chest wall, supraclavicular and level 3 axillary nodal regions. At 4.9-year median follow-up the risk of locoregional recurrence was similar between treatment arms and no significant increase in late effects such as lymphoedema, shoulder dysfunction or pneumonitis were observed. No cases of brachial plexopathy or rib fractures were reported. This data is limited by the lack of 3D planning used in the trial, but it is consistent with the findings from the START trials.

Overall, the data support chest wall and/or lymphatic radiation with commonly used hypofractionation schedules of 40–42.5 Gy in 15–16 fractions. A number of ongoing trials are formally evaluating this prospectively.

Brachial plexopathy is an uncommon complication following locoregional RT for breast cancer. Only one case was reported in the hypofractionation trials. A patient treated with 41.6 Gy in 13 fractions over 5 weeks (EQD_{2Gy} of 54 Gy assuming an α/β ratio of 2 Gy) in the START-A trial developed mild symptoms and signs of brachial plexopathy 2 years following treatment to the breast and supraclavicular fossa [17].

15.3.3 Breast Reconstruction

No patients with breast reconstruction following mastectomy were included in the original hypofractionation trials. Given the observation of similar or less late normal tissue effects in these trials, hypofractionation would be unlikely to result in any worse outcomes following breast reconstruction. A retrospective review of 267 patients following mastectomy with immediate breast reconstruction and 82 patients following breast conserving surgery with oncoplastic surgery treated with conventional fractionation (n = 126, 1.8–2 Gy) or hypofractionation (n = 223, 2.4–2.7 Gy per fraction) was reported from Korea [18]. No significant difference in major breast-related complications (requiring re-operation or re-hospitalisation) was observed between RT fractionations. In the United Kingdom and other European countries such as the Netherlands, patients with breast reconstruction are routinely treated with hypofractionation. A number of ongoing trials including Alliance 221505 (ClinicalsTrial.gov, NCT03414970) and the Dana-Farber trial (ClinicalsTrial.gov, NCT03422003) are currently evaluating the use of hypofractionation compared to conventional fractionation in patients with immediate or delayed reconstruction.

15.4 New Approaches

UK investigators have explored 5-fraction hypofractionation. The FAST trial randomised 915 women with node negative breast cancer after breast conserving surgery to 50 Gy in 25 fractions or two hypofractionated regimens of 30/28.5 Gy in 5 fractions of 6/5.7 Gy once weekly over 5 weeks [19]. At 5 years effects on photographic change in breast appearance were similar for 28.5 Gy but worse for 30 Gy compared to 50 Gy. Also for any moderate/marked physician-assessed breast adverse effect no differences were detected between 28.5 Gy and 50 Gy but significantly more were observed for 30 Gy compared to 50 Gy at 10 years (Table 15.3). Rates of local recurrence at 10 years were low (1.3%) and similar between arms. This information was used to provide an unadjusted α/β estimate for the normal tissue effects of 2.5–2.7 Gy, which was used to design the larger FAST-Forward trial. This trial evaluated 27 Gy in 5 fractions of 5.4 Gy or 26 Gy in 5 fractions of 5.2 Gy, both given daily over 1 week compared to the standard 40 Gy in 15 fractions in 3 weeks in 4096 women with node negative or positive breast cancer after breast conserving surgery or mastectomy [20]. At a median follow-up of 6 years, both 5 fraction regimens were shown to be non-inferior in terms of local recurrence compared to 40 Gy in 15 fractions. Late normal tissue effects as assessed by clinicians, patients and photographs were similar for 26 Gy but worse for 27 Gy compared to 40 Gy at 5 years. Based on the previous experience of the earlier hypofractionation trials suggesting that the relative effects of treatment did not appear to change over time [21] the UK adopted 26 Gy in 5 fractions as the new standard for chest wall, whole breast and partial breast RT at a consensus meeting in October 2020. Other countries are following this approach though some may wish to wait for longer term results or data from confirmatory trials before adopting the 5-fraction regimen.

15.5 Summary

Hypofractionation provides important benefits including an improvement in convenience, a reduction in resources required and a decrease in acute and in some instances late toxicity that can improve the quality of life of patients receiving breast or chest wall radiation therapy. In the early 2000s two landmark trials, the OCOG trial and the START-B trial, established that hypofractionation of 40–42.5 Gy in 15–16 fractions over 3 weeks in comparison to the historical conventional fractionation of 50 Gy in 25 fractions over 5 weeks resulted in similar rates of local recurrence and normal tissue effects leading to a new standard. Further trials have confirmed these findings and suggest that hypofractionation can be applied to patients in all subgroups, including with DCIS only or those requiring lymphatic irradiation. In 2020, the FAST-Forward trial was published demonstrating that 26 Gy in 5 fractions over 1 week was non-inferior to 40 Gy in 15 fractions in 3 weeks in terms of local recurrence at 5 years. Late effects were also similar between the fractionation schedules. The UK has adopted 26 Gy in 5 fractions as a new standard for breast or chest wall radiation therapy and some other countries are following this approach.

References

1. Owen JR, Ashton A, Bliss JM, Homewood J, Harper C, Hanson J, et al. Effect of radiotherapy fraction size on tumour control in patients with early-stage breast cancer after local tumour excision: long-term results of a randomised trial. Lancet Oncol. 2006;7:467–71. https://doi.org/10.1016/S1470-2045(06)70699-4.
2. Bentzen SM, Agrawal RK, Aird EG, Barrett JM, Barrett-Lee PJ, Bliss JM, et al. The UK standardisation of breast radiotherapy (START) trial A of radiotherapy hypofractionation for treatment of early breast cancer: a randomised trial. Lancet Oncol. 2008;9:331–41. https://doi.org/10.1016/S1470-2045(08)70077-9.
3. Whelan T, MacKenzie R, Julian J, Levine M, Shelley W, Grimard L, et al. Randomized trial of breast irradiation schedules after lumpectomy for women with lymph node negative breast cancer. J Natl Cancer Inst. 2002;94:1143–50. https://doi.org/10.1093/jnci/94.15.1143.
4. Bentzen SM, Agrawal RK, Aird EG, Barrett JM, Barrett-Lee PJ, Bentzen SM, et al. The UK standardisation of breast radiotherapy (START) trial B of radiotherapy hypofractionation for treatment of early breast cancer: a randomised trial. Lancet. 2008;371:1098–107. https://doi.org/10.1016/S0140-6736(08)60348-7.
5. Smith BD, Bellon JR, Blitzblau R, Freedman G, Haffty B, Hahn C, et al. Radiation therapy for the whole breast: executive summary of an American Society for Radiation Oncology (ASTRO) evidence-based guideline. Pract Radiat Oncol. 2018;8:145–52. https://doi.org/10.1016/j.prro.2018.01.012.
6. Offersen BV, Alsner J, Nielsen HM, Jakobsen EH, Nielsen MH, Krause M, et al. Hypofractionated versus standard fractionated radiotherapy in patients with early breast cancer or ductal carcinoma in situ in a randomized phase III trial: The DBCG HYPO trial. J Clin Oncol. 2020;38:3615–25. https://doi.org/10.1200/JCO.20.01363.
7. Whelan TJ, Pignol JP, Levine MN, Julian JA, MacKenzie R, Parpia S, et al. Long-term results of hypofractionated radiation therapy for breast cancer. N Engl J Med. 2010;362:513–20. https://doi.org/10.1056/NEJMoa0906260.
8. Haviland JS, Owen JR, Dewar JA, Agrawal RK, Barrett J, Barrett-Lee PJ, et al. The UK standardisation of breast radiotherapy (START) trials of radiotherapy hypofractionation for treatment of early breast cancer: 10-year follow-up results of two randomised

controlled trials. Lancet Oncol. 2013;14:1086–94. https://doi.org/10.1016/S1470-2045(13)70386-3.
9. Bane AL, Whelan TJ, Pond GR, Parpia S, Gohla G, Fyles AW, et al. Tumor factors predictive of response to hypofractionated radiotherapy in a randomized trial following breast conserving therapy. Ann Oncol. 2014;25:992–8. https://doi.org/10.1093/annonc/mdu090.
10. Arsenault J, Parpia S, Goldberg M, Rakovitch E, Reiter H, Doherty M, Lukka H, Sussman J, Wright J, Julian J, Whelan TJ. Acute toxicity and quality of life of hypofractionated radiotherapy for breast cancer. Int J Radiat Oncol Biol Phys. 2020;107:943–8. https://doi.org/10.1016/j.ijrobp.2020.03.049.
11. Wang S-L, Fang H, Hu C, Song Y-W, Wang W-H, Hu C, et al. Hypofractionated versus conventional fractioned postmastectomy radiotherapy for patients with high-risk breast cancer: a randomized, non-inferiority, open-label, phase 3 trial. Lancet Oncol. 2019;20:352–60. https://doi.org/10.1016/S1470-2045(18)30813-1.
12. Shaitelman SF, Schlembach PJ, Arzu I, et al. Acute and short-term toxic effects of conventionally fractionated vs hypofractionated whole-breast irradiation: a randomized clinical trial. JAMA Oncol. 2015;1:931–41. https://doi.org/10.1001/jamaoncol.2015.2666.
13. Brunt AM, Wheatley D, Yarnold J, Somaiah N, Kelly S, Harnett A, et al. Acute skin toxicity associated with a 1-week schedule of whole breast radiotherapy compared with a standard 3-week regimen delivered in the UK FAST-Forward trial. Radiother Oncol. 2016;120:114–8. https://doi.org/10.1016/j.radonc.2016.02.027.
14. Fowler JF. The linear-quadradic formula and progress in fractionated radiotherapy. Br J Radiol. 1989;62:679–94. https://doi.org/10.1259/0007-1285-62-740-679.
15. Shaitelman SF, Lei X, Thompson A, Schlembach P, Bloom ES, Arzu IY, et al. Three-year outcomes with hypofractionated versus conventionally fractionated whole-breast irradiation: results of a randomized, noninferiority clinical trial. J Clin Oncol. 2018;36:3495–503.
16. Chua B, Kunkler I, Gruber G, Olivotto IA, Whelan T, Link E, Westenberg H. A randomized phase III study of radiation doses and fractionation schedules in non-low risk ductal carcinoma in situ (DCIS) of the breast (BIG 3-07/TROG 07.01). Presented at the San Antonio Breast Cancer Symposium, San Antonio, Texas; December 9, 2020.
17. Haviland JS, Mannino M, Griffin C, Porta N, Sydenham M, Bliss JM, Yarnold JR. Late normal tissue effects in the arm and shoulder following lymphatic radiotherapy: results from the UK START (standardisation of breast radiotherapy) trials. Radiother Oncol. 2018;126:155–62. https://doi.org/10.1016/j.radonc.2017.10.033.
18. Kim D-Y, Park E, Heo CY, Jin US, Kim EK, Han W, Shin KH, Kim IA. Hypofractionated versus conventional fractionated radiotherapy for breast cancer in patients with reconstructed breast: toxicity analysis. Breast. 2021;55:37–44. https://doi.org/10.1016/j.breast.2020.11.020.
19. Brunt AM, Haviland JS, Sydenham M, Agrawal RK, Algurafi H, Alhasso A, et al. Ten-year results of FAST: a randomized controlled trial of 5-fraction whole-breast radiotherapy for early breast cancer. J Clin Oncol. 2020;38:3261–72. https://doi.org/10.1200/JCO.19.02750.
20. Brunt AM, Haviland JS, Wheatley DA, Sydenham MA, Alhasso A, Bloomfield DJ, et al. Hypofractionated breast radiotherapy for 1 week versus 3 weeks (FAST-Forward): 5-year efficacy and late normal tissue effects results from a multicentre, non-inferiority, randomised, phase 3 trial. Lancet. 2020;395:1613–26. https://doi.org/10.1016/S0140-6736(20)30932-6.
21. Yarnold J, Bentzen SM, Coles C, Haviland J. Hypofractionated whole breast radiotherapy for women with early breast cancer: myths and realities. Int J Radiat Oncol Biol Phys. 2011;79:1–9. https://doi.org/10.1016/j.ijrobp.2010.08.035.

Part IV

Radiation Therapy Preparation

Available Infrastructure

16

Orit Kaidar-Person, Maoz Ben-Ayun, Philip Poortmans, and Icro Meattini

16.1 Background

16.1.1 Available Infrastructure

Breast cancer patients often have several treatment options including surgery, systemic therapy and RT (e.g. volumes, fractionation) and need to be evaluated by a multidisciplinary team before final treatment recommendations are made, as each decision might influence other treatments. Treatment recommendations should take into consideration patient-related factors (e.g. age and comorbidities), disease-related factors (e.g. pathology features and stage), concomitant medications, and the patient's own preferences and circumstances as they will influence compliance. Radiation therapy, being an integral part of the treatment of most non-metastatic breast cancer patients and contributing to the management in the metastatic setting (e.g. pain and other symptoms relief, palliation for skin involvement, ablative treatment in oligometastatic patients), requires a broad understanding by the entire breast cancer team. Indications for RT for breast cancer patients should be managed serving the purpose of the treatment and not the other way around (e.g. doubtful appropriateness of using innovative techniques in the absence of demonstrated clinical benefits).

Technological advances were implemented over time into the RT system and improved at several crucial points for successful RT treatments. These include patient set-up imaging and adaptation before and during treatment, immobilisation, target volume definition and contouring, improved treatment plans by advanced TPS and various forms of respiratory control during treatment from vmDIBH to CPAP (discussed in Chap. 38). All this has contributed greatly to

O. Kaidar-Person (✉)
Radiation Oncology Unit, Sheba Medical Center, Ramat Gan, Israel

Sackler School of Medicine, Tel-Aviv University, Tel-Aviv, Israel

GROW-School for Oncology and Developmental Biology (Maastro), Maastricht University, Maastricht, The Netherlands
e-mail: Orit.kaidarperson@sheba.health.gov.il

M. Ben-Ayun
Radiation Department, Sheba Tel Hashomer, Ramat Gan, Israel
e-mail: maoz.Ben-Ayun@sheba.health.gov.il

P. Poortmans
Faculty of Medicine and Health Sciences, University of Antwerp, Antwerp, Belgium

Department of Radiation Oncology, Iridium Netwerk, Antwerp, Belgium
e-mail: philip.poortmans@gza.be

I. Meattini
Department of Experimental and Clinical Biomedical Sciences "M. Serio", University of Florence, Florence, Italy

Radiation Oncology Unit, Oncology Department, Azienda Ospedaliero-Universitaria Careggi, Florence, Italy
e-mail: icro.meattini@unifi.it

© The Author(s), under exclusive license to Springer Nature Switzerland AG 2022

O. Kaidar-Person et al. (eds.), *Breast Cancer Radiation Therapy*,
https://doi.org/10.1007/978-3-030-91170-6_16

more accurate treatment planning and delivery techniques to deliver therapeutic radiation doses more precisely to the target tissues while reducing the doses (and possible related subsequent risks) to the surrounding normal tissues, thereby improving the therapeutic ratio of RT.

16.1.2 Equipment, Personnel and Patient Load

Several groups and countries have published the needs for RT and defined minimum criteria for the infrastructure and staffing of a RT department, some specifically related for participation to clinical studies [1–5]. These requirements address various aspects of RT, including human resources mainly in relation to the workload [2], with recommendations for the number of full-time radiation oncologists, medical physicists, dosimetrist, and RTT per department related to the number of patients treated per year. Similarly, ranges (minimum–maximum) for each type of RT equipment (e.g. CT-simulator, Megavoltage Units) are defined as well. Fulfilment to these requirements will assure an appropriate workload for staffing (human resources) and infrastructure (equipment) that will allow for quality care without exhaustion. Indeed, overworked staff members may inevitably lead to human errors at all levels of the RT workflow, endangering safety and thereby compromising treatment outcomes. The number of patients and the complexity of the case mix dictate working hours and thereby define the number of machines and personnel needed. While staff should be allowed to work in shifts that will safeguard their performance, it should be kept in mind that the RT machines are limited in uptime as well. Table 16.1 summarised the EORTC-ROG recommended minimum requirements on infrastructure staffing and workload (in general, not specifically related to breast cancer care), and Fig. 16.1 shows the staffing and workload per discipline reported in the facility questionnaire database analyses [5].

The financial compensation for the staff should be sufficient in order not to drive them into doing extra-shifts for obtaining a proper income, jeopardising the effect of avoiding overworking of the team. Likewise, the RT equipment has a lifespan that depends on utilisation. It is likely that with increased workload, the equipment will wear out and require replacement sooner than would usually be expected.

It is important to realise that one of the major contributing factors for RT incidents is the introduction of new RT technologies and the increased level of computerisation in the department's workflow [6].

The perception that innovative techniques are flawless and reduce the workload of staff and machine should be considered as false. Many reported mistakes/incidents were at least partly attributed to insufficient understanding of the complexities involved in innovative technologies and the failure to fully understand its use in current practice, including properly balancing advantages and disadvantages in individual patient care, dose distributions and machines' limitations [7, 8]. Therefore, training of the RT teams is essential and we should avoid rushing in adopting new techniques before all preparations are carefully made.

As for breast cancer RT, we recommend that all members of the RT team will undergo specific

Table 16.1 EORTC-ROG recommended minimum requirements on infrastructure staffing and workload and their year of implementation

	1993	2008	2014
Maximum of patients per radiation oncologist	300	250–300	180–250 (maximum 300)
Maximum number of patients per medical physicist	500	500	500
Maximum number of patients per treatment unit	700	600	700

The table was adopted from Willmann et al. [5]

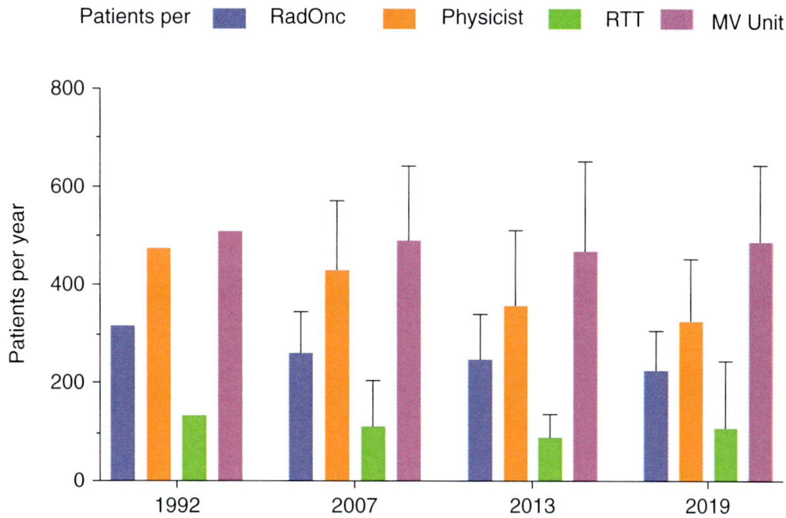

Fig. 16.1 Staffing and workload as reported in the EORTC-Facility Questionnaire database analyses. Years indicate the time of the respective analyses. Means of the parameters are depicted. Error bars denote one standard deviation. *RadOnc* radiation oncologist, *RTT* radiation therapist, *MV unit* treatment unit. The figure was adopted from Willmann et al. [5]

training which is available in various settings (e.g. ESTRO and ESO courses, national training courses). This training is required to acquire the necessary knowledge and skills for an optimal and efficient delivery of modern RT techniques to breast cancer patients.

16.1.3 Care Path-Workflow

Computerisation in the department workflow and electronical patient's files are the future. As part of the electronic files, it is recommended to create a care path-workflow to follow the status of the treatment plan. The care path-workflow should be designed according to the workflow of the department and allocate time for each speciality to perform their work properly. Some systems allow to create alerts to the team if the task is overdue. However, computerisation and electronical patient's files are not flawless. Therefore, proper QA measures for these processes, open feedback and communication between teams are crucial points for success. An example of patient's care path is displayed in Fig. 16.2.

16.1.4 Department's Learning Process

Documenting and learning of incidences and near-misses and adapting new preventing methods are essential. A quite environment without disturbances is essential for critical process, and the teams need to define a protocol for "time out" from all distractions to evaluate critical measures for treatment.

Highly trained personnel from all disciplines, combined with new innovative RT techniques, do not automatically assure treatment success, if all are not working as a team with free and constant communication. Therefore, routine time for team "huddle" for updates, strategising work, concerns, questions and more is essential and encourages open communication between teams (see quality assurance programmes in Chap. 6).

16.1.5 RT Equipment

Each component of RT equipment (simulation, mobilisation and treatment) should be considered, both individually and in combination, in the concept of serving the entire treatment chain. The vendors are part of the consideration and the concept of mono-vendor versus multi-vendor platforms should be fully understood in regard to advantages and disadvantages of each approach and compatibility with all relevant treatment indications, including supplementary equipment (i.e. breastboard, immobilisation devices, prone set-up) for patient positioning. The inter-exchangeability of patients between treatment machines in case of

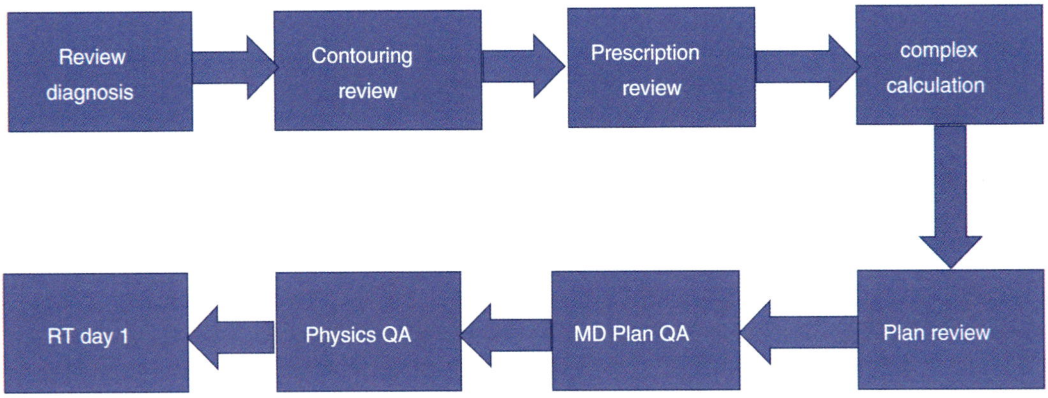

Fig. 16.2 Example for care path-workflow for treatment planning system. *MD* Radiation Oncologist, *QA* Quality assurence, *RT* Radiation therapy

Table 16.2 Key points for planning the infrastructure of breast RT unit

Equipment, personnel and patient load	• Follow global recommendation for the number of full-time radiation oncologists, physicists, dosimetrist and RTT per department per the estimated number of patients treated per year at your centre • Follow global recommendation for the number of each type of RT equipment (e.g. CT-simulator, megavoltage units) according to the estimated number of patients treated per year at your centre • Manage the working time to allow for the human resource and RT machine to fully recover for a workday • Take the time to fully study the new technologies, before putting them into service • Engage in specialised training for breast cancer
Scheduling	• 3–4 weeks following surgery to initiate RT should allow for adequate healing of the breast and axillary area • Allow to delay RT if additional workout is required to exclude the presence of residual disease, metastatic spread, need for chemotherapy or any new information that might change the therapeutic approach • The timing of last systemic therapy should be documented, especially in case of metastatic patients to avoid unwanted toxicity and RT should be scheduled accordingly • Prior to CT simulation, if the patient is still fertile, pregnancy must be ruled out, and the patient should be formally informed about the dangers in conception during RT • Schedule RT according to the radiation oncologist recommendation, at a date that will allow for volume delineation, planning and QA

scheduled or unforeseen downtime without (major) additional work for the team should be considered as an important prerequisite as downtimes are to be avoided. As it is known that for every day lost between 3 and 5 weeks of RT about 0.6 Gy/day is lost [9]. Multi-vendor platforms generally do not run smoothly in a synchronised way, increasing demands on technical and IT (Information Technology) departments, and on finances—also increasing the risks for downtime. Key points are presented in Table 16.2.

16.1.6 Scheduling Patients

Two important timing-related aspects for scheduling patients, to safeguard optimal disease control versus to reduce overload, might be in conflict in busy departments or exceptional circumstances such as a worldwide pandemic [10].

The optimal timing of RT after surgery has not been well defined, but there is a fair amount of data to guide us. Clinical trials that reported the benefit of post-operative RT BCS typically restricted the maximum interval between surgery and the start of RT to 6–8 weeks. While there is not much data about the minimal acceptable time from surgery to the beginning of external beam radiation, 3–4 weeks following surgery to initiate RT should allow for adequate healing of the breast and axillary area and, in the case of an ALND, for the patient to have regained adequate arm mobility to facilitate treatment planning. However, there is a fraction of patients in which RT can be/should be delayed: if additional work-out is required to exclude the presence of residual disease, metastatic spread or any new information that might change the therapeutic approach. However, more recent data support that for patients who are treated contemporary, starting RT shortly after BCS seems not to be associated with better long-term outcomes and that thereby this former quality indicator should be discarded, up to us in favour of maintaining an optimised overall treatment time depending on the fractionation scheduled used [11]. Therefore, especially for patients at low risk for recurrence or bearing metastatic disease, time intervals should not be taken too restrictively. Similarly, patients who completed adjuvant systemic therapy can be planned without time pressure, especially as they continue receiving targeted therapies (e.g. anti-HER2) or endocrine therapy. All this, however, should not be used as an excuse to postpone RT for breast cancer patients, even more because short intervals are a good indicator of a good flow of the overall process, which is a tremendously important quality indicator as such.

With new tumour genetic and molecular tests guiding the use of systemic therapies, we advise not to perform CT simulation until the decision about systemic therapy (mainly chemotherapy) has been clearly determined. Prior to scheduling CT simulation, one must exclude the possibility of pregnancy, document if the patient has a pacemaker and/or received previous irradiation (the three "P" of RT: pregnancy-pacemaker-previous RT). In case of a pacemaker, we recommend to consult with the cardiology team about the type and the model of the pacemaker and its function prior to RT, as some patients will need to be monitored at time of therapy. All are important to take into consideration when planning any oncological therapy. The type and timing of systemic therapy should be documented, especially in case of metastatic patients to avoid unwanted toxicity.

16.1.7 Technical Consideration in Booking Treatments

Booking and scheduling should be done based on the timeline recommended by the radiation oncologist according to the clinical case, and is recommended to be carried out by the secretary and RTT that have the full understanding of the time needed to plan treatment, perform appropriate QA, and allocate timeslot on the treatment unit needed with the specific treatment (e.g. with/without breath hold, patients that have difficulties in mobilisation or special needs). To take into consideration the time needed to prepare the treatment unit between patients, it is advised to have a system for the RTTs on the treatment units to reschedule the allocated timeslots in case needed and to alert the treating physician when a patient misses days from treatment. The system should allow the RTT to enter the scheduling system and to add additional fractions at the end and/or to plan bi-fractionations to respect the overall treatment time.

16.1.8 CT Simulation

The CT scan used for treatment planning should be equipped with appropriate positioning devices, identical to those at the treatment units. It is estimated that for at least 80% of the cases the same positioning/immobilisation device is sufficient (breastboard), but the team must be trained to allow individualisation for the few (~ maximal 20%) that will require it. Marking of positioning was traditionally done with tattoos, what should be reconsidered while the use of surface scanning (ideally combined with CBCT) should be planned (if not already in place) to replace all other position verification methods and obviating any marks on our patients, both permanent and temporary.

16.1.9 Treatment Planning and Fractionation

Nowadays, volume-based techniques in breast cancer based on delineated target volumes, and not any longer field-based RT, is the standard of care for breast cancer patients [12, 13]. However, target volume delineation and RT planning increases the workload on the RT team. While in some countries delineation is done by radiation oncologists, in others it is done by other staff members such as dosimetrists or RTT, and more recently automated contouring is being introduced and expected to decrease this workload again. Workload is also related to the number of RT sessions (fractions) which will mainly affect the RTTs and the machines and, to a lesser extent, also the radiation oncologists. Adoption of hypofractionation schedules that have the same clinical effect will reduce this workload, which will help to avoid that excessive workload makes it quite impossible for team members to actively supervise treatments, mentor and supervise new members, and address the patient needs at time of follow-up (for questions, acute and late side effects). Excessive workloads, especially in combination with a defective organisation, will impede the radiation oncologist from coming to the treatment machines and supervising treatments or interacting with the RTTs. Moreover, the motivation for clinical research is often frustrated by a lack of dedicated time for the staff members, which in the long run will not motivate new candidates with good academic records to join the team. Therefore, without an appropriate and dynamic workflow and manageable workload for all team members, there is a significant risk of shortages of staff members and downgrading of working conditions, leading to poor clinical performance and ultimately to the risk for "burnout" of staff members.

16.2 Summary

RT preparation is complex and composed of different aspects of treatment, but we should keep in mind that the breast cancer patients' journey is long and requires a number of diagnostic tests and procedures. However, no treatment like RT (mainly breast cancer) requires patients to daily expose in full conscience private/intimate body parts. Therefore, as part of our thrive for excellence, we advise that the staff get appropriate training addressing the psychological needs of the patients, understanding that patients are the owners of their bodies instead of considering the body just as an object to be treated. To cover the patients with a dedicated clothing/scarf at time of CT simulation or treatment can help them in maintaining control over their bodies and thereby indirectly their minds. Together with an appropriate infrastructure, carepath, pre-defined timelines, we assure holistic healthcare for our patients.

References

1. Atun R, Jaffray DA, Barton MB, et al. Expanding global access to radiotherapy. Lancet Oncol. 2015;16:1153–86.
2. Budiharto T, Musat E, Poortmans P, et al. Profile of European radiotherapy departments contributing to the EORTC Radiation Oncology Group (ROG) in the 21st century. Radiother Oncol. 2008;88:403–10.
3. Dunscombe P, Grau C, Defourny N, et al. Guidelines for equipment and staffing of radiotherapy facilities in the European countries: final results of the ESTRO-HERO survey. Radiother Oncol. 2014;112:165–77.
4. Borras JM, Lievens Y, Barton M, et al. How many new cancer patients in Europe will require radiotherapy by 2025? An ESTRO-HERO analysis. Radiother Oncol. 2016;119:5–11.
5. Willmann J, Poortmans P, Monti AF, et al. Development of staffing, workload and infrastructure in member departments of the European Organisation for Research and Treatment of Cancer (EORTC) radiation oncology group. Radiother Oncol. 2020;155:226–31.
6. Ortiz López P, Cosset JM, Dunscombe P, et al. ICRP publication 112. A report of preventing accidental exposures from new external beam radiation therapy technologies. Ann ICRP. 2009;39:1–86.

7. Ash D. Lessons from epinal. Clin Oncol. 2007;19:614–5.
8. Malicki J, Bly R, Bulot M, et al. Patient safety in external beam radiotherapy, results of the ACCIRAD project: current status of proactive risk assessment, reactive analysis of events, and reporting and learning systems in Europe. Radiother Oncol. 2017;123:29–36.
9. Haviland JS, Bentzen SM, Bliss JM, Yarnold JR. Prolongation of overall treatment time as a cause of treatment failure in early breast cancer: an analysis of the UK START (standardisation of breast radiotherapy) trials of radiotherapy fractionation. Radiother Oncol. 2016;121:420–3.
10. Coles CE, Aristei C, Bliss J, et al. International guidelines on radiation therapy for breast cancer during the COVID-19 pandemic. Clin Oncol. 2020;32:279–81.
11. van Maaren MC, Bretveld RW, Jobsen JJ, et al. The influence of timing of radiation therapy following breast-conserving surgery on 10-year disease-free survival. Br J Cancer. 2017;117:179–88.
12. Offersen BV, Boersma LJ, Kirkove C, Hol S, Aznar MC, Biete Sola A, Kirova YM, Pignol JP, Remouchamps V, Verhoeven K, Weltens C, Arenas M, Gabrys D, Kopek N, Krause M, Lundstedt D, Marinko T, Montero A, Yarnold J, Poortmans P. ESTRO consensus guideline on target volume delineation for elective radiation therapy of early stage breast cancer. Radiother Oncol. 2015;114(1):3–10.
13. Kaidar-Person O, Offersen BV, Boersma L, Meattini I, Dodwell D, Wyld L, Aznar M, Major T, Kuehn T, Strnad V, Palmu M, Hol S, Poortmans P. Tricks and tips for target volume definition and delineation in breast cancer: Lessons learned from ESTRO breast courses. Radiother Oncol. 2021;162:185–94.

Patient Positioning

17

Tamar Katzman

17.1 Positioning

The positioning of patients is one of the foundations of RT. Optimal positioning enhances patient's compliance and positioning reproducibility and enables the treatment volumes to be optimally targeted, while avoiding the OARs. Matters such as treatment technique, and patient specific issues (e.g. body habitus) must be considered prior to simulation, in order to ensure the best outcome.

Before positioning the patient, it is important to make sure the patient is feeling relaxed in her surroundings. Especially in patients affected by breast cancer, there may be body image issues which the patient is dealing with following surgery. Care, empathy, and privacy should be provided to the patient, with the RTT or nurse understanding that undressing for the simulation may not be a trivial matter for the patient.

Helping the patient feel comfortable is twofold beneficial:

1. Increases patient compliancy, helping the patient feel part of her treatment's team
2. Helps the patient relax, which decreases potential positioning variations during treatment

T. Katzman (✉)
Radiation Oncology, Sheba Medical Center, Ramat Gan, Israel
e-mail: Tamar.katzman@sheba.health.gov.il

The day of simulation, there is still some fear of the unknown—which can cause some physical tension in the patient's body. As the patient gets into the routine of treatment, naturally she progressively relaxes, which may cause a systematic error. A way to avoid this is to encourage the patient to relax and release all muscle tension when she lies down. This is true regardless of the position she is situated in.

Another important aspect of positioning is proper documentation, both in written/the electronic patient files and using drawings/pictures. Documentation errors are one of the major causes of incidences in RT [1]. To avoid errors, it is crucial to ensure that the position the patient is lying in during simulation is documented correctly and transferred to the rest of the team in a clear way.

In general, left-right symmetry should be aimed at to increase comfort and to decrease the risks of errors. The patient should be straightened from the suprasternal notch through the xiphoid process, and the symphysis pubis. If the axilla level 4 (formerly called supraclavicular) LN are being treated, the head could be turned to the contralateral side (i.e. if the left breast is treated, the head should be turned to the right). However, for elective LN RT, level 4 is behind the clavicle head and might be a bit superior to it (see Target volume definition and contouring section), so it is preferred to maintain symmetry and keep the head straight for all patients, resulting in an increased reproducibility and lower risks for

© The Author(s), under exclusive license to Springer Nature Switzerland AG 2022

O. Kaidar-Person et al. (eds.), *Breast Cancer Radiation Therapy*,
https://doi.org/10.1007/978-3-030-91170-6_17

errors. In advanced breast cancer cases, the level 4 might be cranial to the volumes of elective irradiation, then the head should be turned to the contralateral side. This will allow to avoid irradiation of the face.

If the patient is being treated in the prone position, the patient should be straightened through the vertebral bodies.

17.2 Standard Positioning

The most common practice for the positioning of breast cancer patients is supine on a breast board with both arms abducted, and the shoulders externally rotated. There are a number of commercially available breast boards, all of them CT-compatible and some MRI-compatible as well (Fig. 17.1). These generally share several design features, which are used to help achieve the goals of treatment. When utilised correctly, these features reduce set-up errors, and help to minimise the side effects of treatment.

These include:

1. The body of the breast boards are comprised from carbon fibre, which serves to minimise the attenuation of the treatment beam and does not produce artefacts during simulation procedures.
2. An angulation system, such that the torso and head of the patient is higher than the lower body. There is normally a choice of angles, and the optimal angle is decided upon at the time of simulation, based on the physical build of the patient, and the treatment technique.

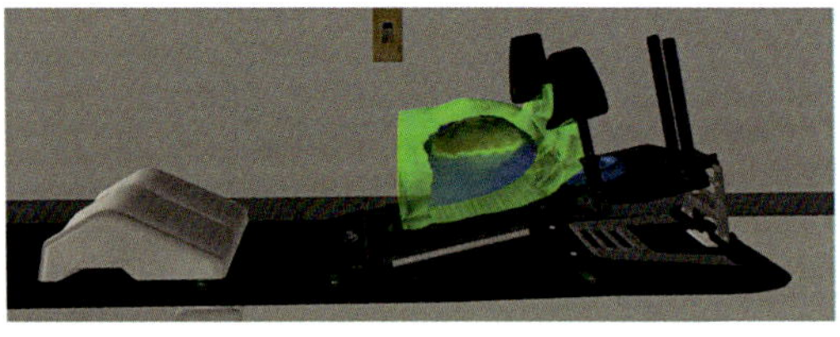

Fig. 17.1 Standardised supine breast board showing angulation, arm and wrist rests, and indexing. Note that sternum is horizontal. Picture courtesy of Vertual [2]. Available at: https://www.vertual.co.uk/. Accessed November 1, 2020

The reasons for the angulation system include: helping to reduce the amount of lung and heart in the vicinity of the target volumes and reducing skin folds both inframammary and between the breast and the axilla.

The optimal angle for planning purposes is such that the sternum is horizontal (parallel to the treatment couch) [3]. This angulation system should have an indexing solution on both sides. This indexation assists with straightening the patient, as well as positioning the patient. A reference mark/tattoo on the patient corresponds to a number on the index, and this indicates whether the patient is positioned on the breast board correctly. When using the angulation system, the RTTs need to be aware of the limitations of the set-up in the treatment room. For example, if the angle between the treatment couch and the breast board is very wide, there may be an issue of clearance between the gantry and the treatment couch for lateral oblique beams, for some arc positions and for IGRT.

Nowadays, many departments maintain a standard setting of the angle, most often between 7.5 and 12.5°. The advantages are that this completely avoids the risk of errors in angle settings and that a standard setting selected for a combination of a breast board with treatment machine can be chosen to avoid collisions in any of the 360° positions of the gantry.

3. Due to the angulation system patients may slide down the breast board. In order to combat that effect, a "stopper", most often a cushion made of foam, is placed caudal to the patients' bottom. The stopper is indexable and has several positions, which account for the varying heights of the patients. For example, a taller patient will require the stopper to be indexed further away from the angulated section of the breast board, than a shorter patient.
4. The head, arm, and wrist supports are adjustable. Once again, this allows the team to take into consideration the physical attributes of the patient, and position accordingly, keeping in mind the basic principles mentioned previously (comfort, reduction of side effects,

reproducibility, and reduction of dose to OAR). Also here, the use of fixed settings whenever possible decreases the risks of errors and avoids possible collisions with the gantry.

5. Ability to index the breast board to the treatment couch. This ensures that the breast board is straight, and stable. Furthermore, this helps with identifying a gross error in positioning in the treatment room. This is due to the fact that when indexing the breast board to the couch, the couch values in the treatment room should be reliable and within a certain tolerance. Values out of that tolerance could indicate a gross error in positioning.

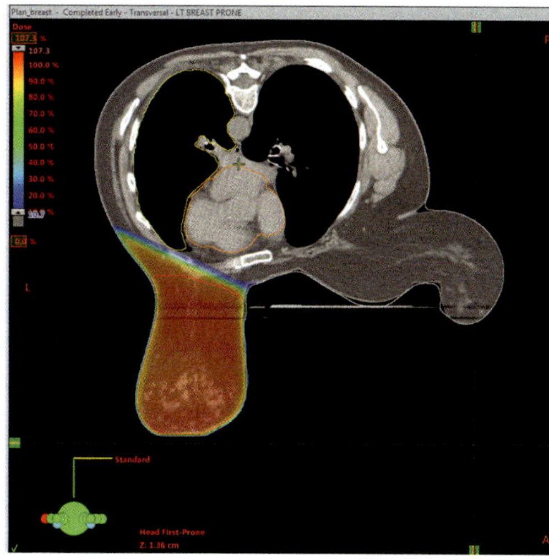

Fig. 17.2 Transversal view with dose colour wash showing a patient in the prone position. Picture courtesy of Dr. Yonina Tova & Sion Koren, Radiation Oncology, Ziv Medical Centre, Safed, Israel

17.3 Prone Positioning

Prone positioning of breast cancer patients has gained popularity over the last decade. An Australian study of breast radiation therapy showed that in 2014, 29% of centres surveyed offered prone breast radiation therapy, as opposed to only 5% a decade earlier [4]. However, a study of immobilisation techniques in the United Kingdom and Republic of Ireland showed that the use of prone positioning is not as popular as may have been expected [5].

Prone positioning is generally considered for large (pedunculated) breasted women who have an indication for breast-only RT. The main advantages of using this technique are dosimetric in nature. This position eliminates skin folds, and causes the breast shape to narrow, allowing for a more homogenous dose (Fig. 17.2) [6]. Additionally, for pedunculated breasts, prone positioning can reduce the dose to OARs such as lung and heart dose. However, in deeply seated tumours it might be challenging to sufficiently cover the target volumes. There are commercially available prone breast boards. Most are designed with a cutout where the treated breast hangs down (Fig. 17.3), and both arms are placed superolaterally to the head. The head rests on a cushion, and the patient is positioned so that the contralateral breast is out of the field (Fig. 17.4) [7]. These breast boards have some of the features of the supine breast board, including the ability to index, and some flexibility of hand and head position. A wedge pillow placed under the contralateral breast elevates the breast, allowing a wider range of gantry angles for treatment [8].

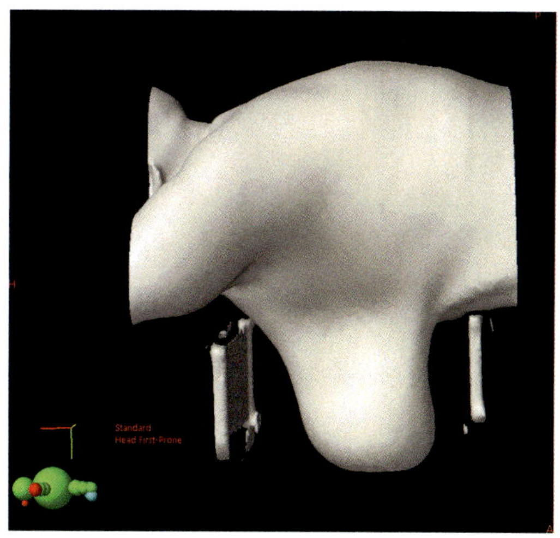

Fig. 17.3 View from the ipsilateral side of patient treated in the prone position. Note the breast hanging down. Picture courtesy of Dr. Yonina Tova & Sion Koren, Radiation Oncology, Ziv Medical Centre, Safed, Israel

One of the difficulties of treatment in the prone position is nodal irradiation [5], due to the position of the arms, and attenuation of the beam through the breast board. The crawl position

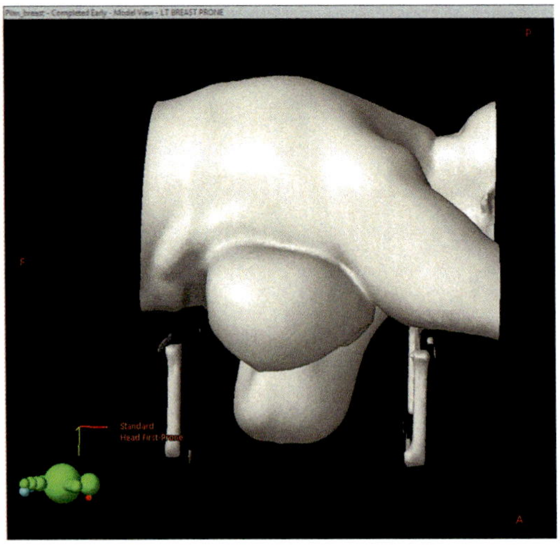

Fig. 17.4 View from the contralateral side of patient treated in the prone position. Note the untreated breast resting on the prone breast board, and the treated breast hanging down

(patient lies prone, with ipsilateral arm down) has been suggested to overcome this limitation [9].

17.4 Lateral Decubitus Positioning

An alternative positioning technique is the lateral decubitus position. This treatment technique has been successfully used for decades [10], although it is less common probably due to its highly artisanal approach. This position is useful for women with pedunculated breasts (Fig. 17.5).

In this position, the patient lies on her ipsilateral side. The ipsilateral breast rests on a specially designed platform, while the contralateral breast is moved in the dorsal direction. The patient's back is supported with a frame or firm pillow that is used for the purpose. The set-up marks are placed on the treated breast and the back of the patient. This set-up spares OAR and is tolerated well by patients. However, nodes cannot be treated using this set-up [11], and optimal reproducibility may be harder to achieve.

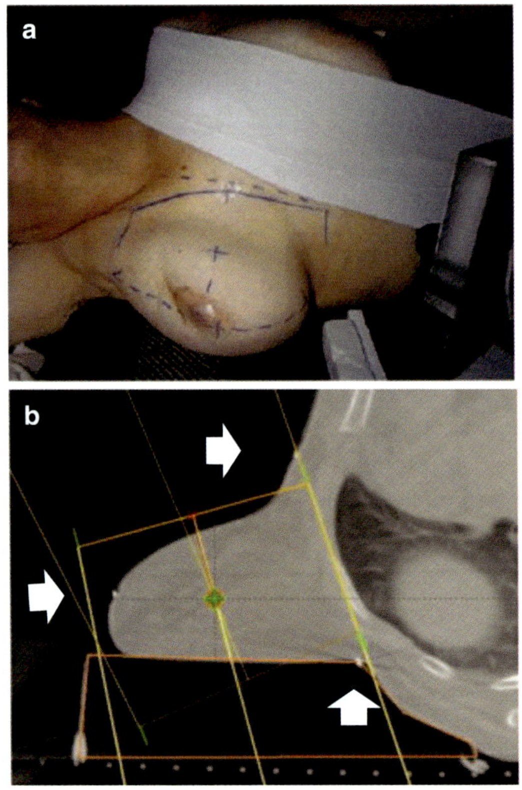

Fig. 17.5 Patient positioned in a lateral decubitus and immobilisation device, including a strap holding the contralateral breast (A) the breast lies on the flat part of the breast board. The edge of the angled side is marked by a metallic wire which is visible on CT scan (arrows). Taken with permission from Kirova et al. [11]

17.5 Challenges in Breast Positioning

The main challenges with breast positioning arise from two issues:

1. Patients who have difficulty raising their arms (often as a result of ALND, sometimes SLNB)
2. Patients with pendulous breasts

Some practical solutions for these challenges are outlined below.

1. Positioning of patients with difficulty raising their arms

There are instances when a patient is physically unable to raise their arms. Wherever possible, it is highly preferable to postpone the start of RT and not to force anything. Indeed, with the contemporary multidisciplinary approach, increasing the interval between surgery and initiation of radiation therapy is likely not negatively influencing outcomes [12]. During this time, lymphatic drainage therapy, physiotherapy and alike can greatly help the patient to regain arm functioning. If even then the mobility remains constrained, it is preferable for the ipsilateral arm of the affected breast to be abducted, thus avoiding radiation to the arm and symmetrical, thereby improving reproducibility. Adjusting the height, angle, and position of the arm and wrist rests can minimise the shoulder rotation. If that does not provide a satisfactory solution, and arm abduction cannot be achieved, a feasible solution is the use of a personalised positioning device such as an alpha cradle/vacuum bag [13, 14]. While these devices do provide a comparable level of reproducibility, they are time consuming to make, and therefore are not routinely used for breast positioning.

When using a personalised positioning cushion, the ipsilateral arm may be placed akimbo (arm bent at the elbow, with hand on hip) (Fig. 17.6), or by the patient's side. This will largely depend on the treatment technique at each centre and should be decided together with the radiation oncologist and treatment planning team. If using a 3DCRT technique, it may be optimised with the arm widely akimbo (smaller medial elbow angle, which translates to an increased distance from the elbow to the body), to allow a range of angles for planning in order to cover the PTVp (breast or chest wall). The arm by the side may be preferred for IMRT/VMAT planning.

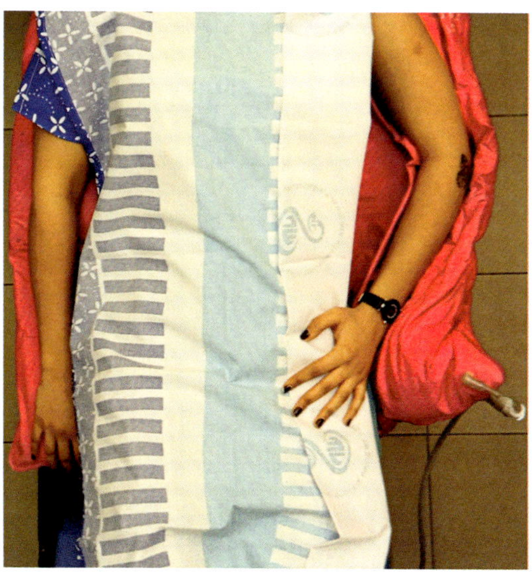

Fig. 17.6 Personal positioning device with arm akimbo. Picture courtesy of Sheba Medical Centre, Ramat Gan, Israel

If proton planning is implemented, the arm position is more flexible, as the treatment beam is en face [15], and may be an optimal solution in the case of limited arm mobility when available.

Depending on the planning method, the contralateral arm is often abducted (if possible), similar to the ipsilateral arm as it may facilitate some freedom with treatment planning. However, different institutions may have different protocols for the contralateral arm.

When creating a personalised positioning device for breast radiation therapy, it is useful to remember the protocols used when using a commercial immobilisation device, and to incorporate them as much as possible. The cushion should be formed in a wedge shape, or in conjunction with a breast board, to enable some angulation. A reference mark placed on the lateral sides of the personalised positioning device will mimic the indexation on the sides of the standard breast board, and the device should be indexed to the treatment couch.

Another option is to use the crawl prone positioning outlined above [9].

2. Patients with pendulous breasts

Patients with pendulous breasts provide both a challenge for reproducibility, and acute skin toxicity [16, 17]. Following, there is a brief outline of some methods used to overcome this issue (except prone and lateral positioning, discussed above).

Bras have been used in the prone position [18] to reduce set-up errors, and in the supine position mainly for women with pendulous breasts to reduce inframammary and lateral skin folds [18]. Commercial bras, or a patient's own bra (with the underwire removed) can be used. Whichever type is used, the bra needs to be marked up in a clear manner, so that it may be worn correctly for daily treatment. The bra is relatively easy to implement into use in a radiation therapy department, as it is used to enhance well-established techniques [19], with positioning being carried out as outlined previously. The use of a bra does not interfere with nodal irradiation if necessary. Diligence is required to check that a fold is not created between the axilla and the breast while reducing the inframammary fold. Also, the contralateral breast should be moved away from the midline so as not to interfere or limit anterior oblique beams (Fig. 17.7). One way to achieve this is to remove the cup of the bra from the contralateral breast, which allows the contralateral breast to fall naturally away from midline (Fig. 17.5).

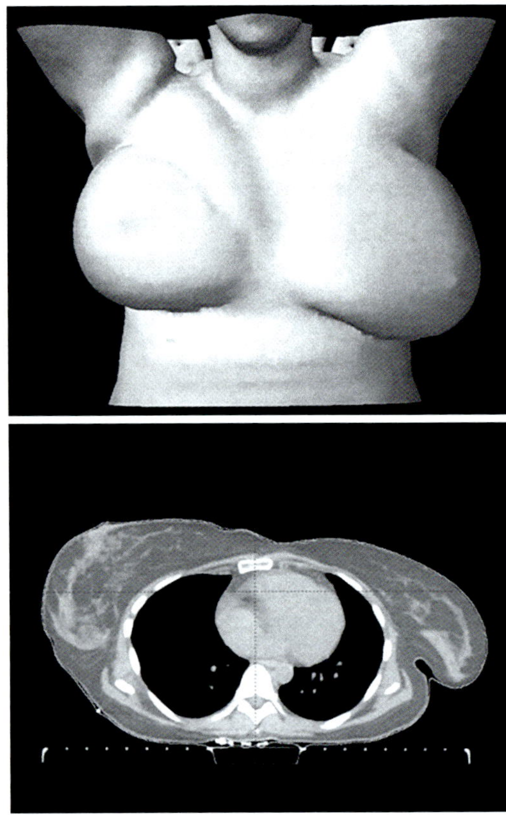

Fig. 17.7 Right breast treatment with bra. Top shows bird's eye view of patient. Note how the left breast falls away from the midline, unsupported by the bra. Bottom shows transverse view of CT. Picture courtesy of Sheba Medical Centre, Ramat Gan, Israel

Thermoplastic material can be used in a similar fashion to bras. This material, familiar e.g. from head and neck immobilisation, is warmed up either in a thermoplastic oven or warm water bath for a few minutes until it's flexible. It is then moulded to the patient's outline and attached to the sides of the breast board (Fig. 17.8) [20]. While this is a fairly rigid material, it is not clear whether the possible reduction of set-up errors outweighs the increased skin dose from this set-up [20, 21] (Fig. 17.9).

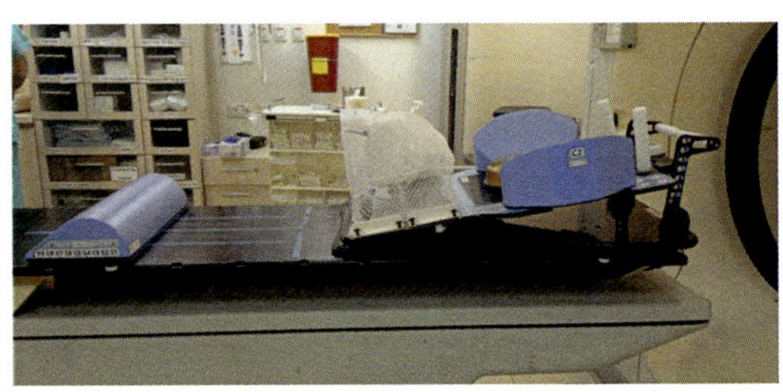

Fig. 17.8 Breast board with thermoplastic mask. Picture courtesy of Sheba Medical Centre, Ramat Gan, Israel

17.6 Summary

Treatment simulation procedure is one of the important steps in radiation planning. Optimal positioning enhances patient's compliance and positioning reproducibility and enables the treatment volumes to be ideally targeted, while avoiding the organs at risks. Patient positioning should be adjusted to allow correct RT planning and a safe delivery of treatment.

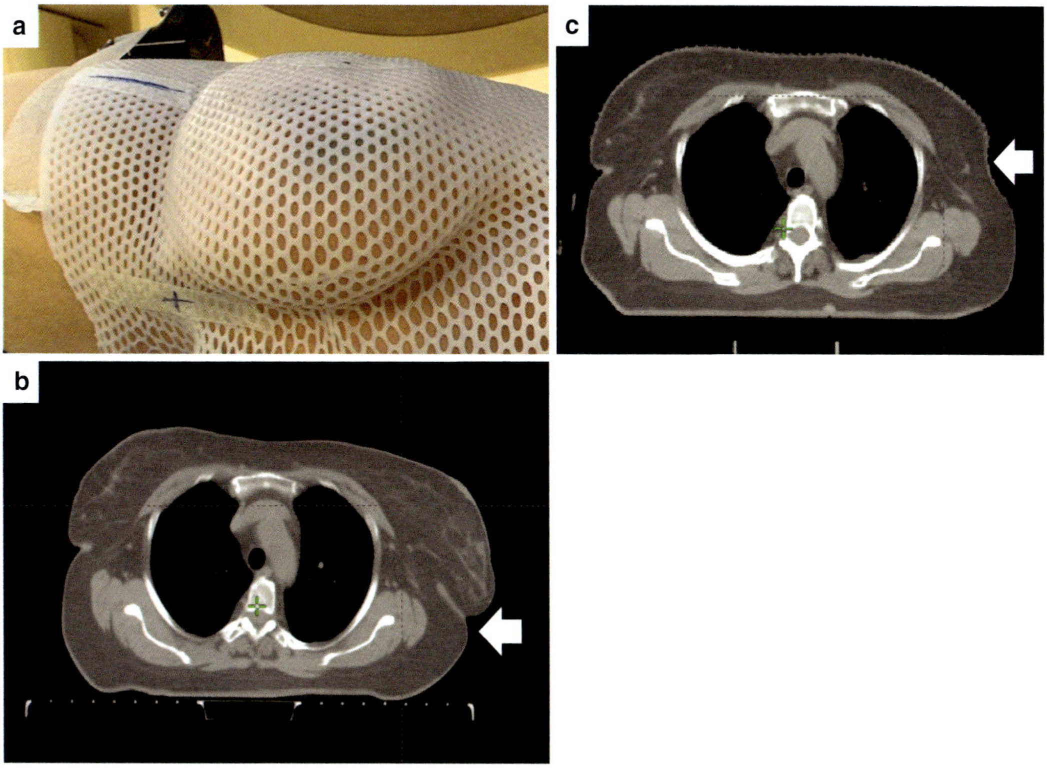

Fig. 17.9 Thermoplastic bra. (**a**) Thermoplastic bra used for planning and irradiation of the left breast of a patient with ptotic breast. (**b**) CT-simulation without the bra, arrow shows the lateral mammary fold a result of supine position. (**c**) CT-simulation with the thermoplastic bra, no lateral fold which aims to reduce potential toxicity and reproduce the position of the breast at time of treatment. Picture courtesy of Sheba Medical Centre, Ramat Gan, Israel

References

1. Yeung TK, Bortolotto K, Cosby S, Hoar M, Lederer E. Quality assurance in radiotherapy: evaluation of errors and incidents recorded over a 10 year period. Radiother Oncol. 2005;74(3):283–91. https://doi.org/10.1016/j.radonc.2004.12.003.
2. Vertual. 2020. Available at: https://www.vertual.co.uk/. Accessed November 1, 2020.
3. Thilmann C, Adamietz IA, Saran F, Mose S, Kostka A, Böttcher HD. The use of a standardized positioning support cushion during daily routine of breast irradiation. Int J Radiat Oncol Biol Phys. 1998;41(2):459–63.
4. Dundas KL, Pogson EM, Batumalai V, Boxer MM, Yap ML, Delaney GP, et al. Australian survey on current practices for breast radiotherapy. J Med Imaging Radiat Oncol. 2015;59(6):736–42.
5. Montgomery L, Flood T, Shepherd P. A service evaluation of the immobilisation techniques adopted for breast cancer patients with large and/or pendulous breasts, receiving external beam radiotherapy. J Radiother Pract. 2019;19:341–6.
6. Probst H, Bragg C, Dodwell D, Green D, Hart J. A systematic review of methods to immobilise breast tissue during adjuvant breast irradiation. Radiography. 2014;20(1):70–81.
7. Varga Z, Hideghéty K, Mező T, Nikolényi A, Thurzó L, Kahán Z. Individual positioning: a comparative study of adjuvant breast radiotherapy in the prone versus supine position. Int J Radiat Oncol Biol Phys. 2009;75(1):94–100.
8. Veldeman L, Speleers B, Bakker M, Jacobs F, Coghe M, De Gersem W, et al. Preliminary results on setup precision of prone-lateral patient positioning for whole breast irradiation. Int J Radiat Oncol Biol Phys. 2010;78(1):111–8.
9. Deseyne P, Speleers B, De Neve W, Boute B, Paelinck L, Van Hoof T, et al. Whole breast and regional nodal irradiation in prone versus supine position in left sided breast cancer. Radiat Oncol. 2017;12(1):89.
10. Fourquet A, Campana F, Rosenwald JC, Vilcoq JR. Breast irradiation in the lateral decubitus position: technique of the Institut Curie. Radiother Oncol. 1991;22(4):261–5.
11. Campana F, Kirova YM, Rosenwald JC, Dendale R, Vilcoq JR, Dreyfus H, Fourquet A. Breast radiother-

apy in the lateral decubitus position: a technique to prevent lung and heart irradiation. Int J Radiat Oncol Biol Phys. 2005;61(5):1348–54.
12. van Maaren MC, Bretveld RW, Jobsen JJ, Veenstra RK, Groothuis-Oudshoorn CG, Struikmans H, Maduro JH, Strobbe LJ, Poortmans PM, Siesling S. The influence of timing of radiation therapy following breast-conserving surgery on 10-year disease-free survival. Br J Cancer. 2017;117(2):179–88.
13. Graham P, Elomari F, Browne L. Armrest versus vacuum bag immobilization in the treatment of breast cancer by radiation therapy: a randomized comparison. Australas Radiol. 2000;44(2):193–7.
14. Nalder CA, Bidmead AM, Mubata CD, Tait D, Beardmore C. Influence of a vac-fix immobilization device on the accuracy of patient positioning during routine breast radiotherapy. Br J Radiol. 2001;74(879):249–54.
15. Depauw N, Batin E, Johnson A, MacDonald SM, Jimenez RB. Arms positioning in post-mastectomy proton radiation: feasibility and development of a new arms down contouring atlas. Phys Imaging Radiat Oncol. 2020;14:6–11. https://doi.org/10.1016/j.phro.2020.04.003.
16. Fernando I, Ford H, Powles T, Ashley S, Glees J, Torr M, et al. Factors affecting acute skin toxicity in patients having breast irradiation after conservative surgery: a prospective study of treatment practice at the Royal Marsden Hospital. Clin Oncol. 1996;8(4):226–33.
17. De Langhe S, Mulliez T, Veldeman L, Remouchamps V, van Greveling A, Gilsoul M, et al. Factors modifying the risk for developing acute skin toxicity after whole-breast intensity modulated radiotherapy. BMC Cancer. 2014;14(1):711.
18. Kawamura M, Maeda Y, Yamamoto K, Takamatsu S, Sato Y, Minami H, et al. Development of the breast immobilization system in prone setup: The effect of bra in prone position to improve the breast setup error. J Appl Clin Med Phys. 2017;18(4):155–60.
19. Arenas M, Hernández V, Farrús B, Müller K, Gascón M, Pardo A, et al. Do breast cups improve breast cancer dosimetry? A comparative study for patients with large or pendulous breasts. Acta Oncol. 2014;53(6):795–801.
20. Barrett-Lennard MJ, Thurstan SM. Comparing immobilisation methods for the tangential treatment of large pendulous breasts. Radiographer. 2008;55(2):7–13.
21. Zierhut D, Flentje M, Frank C, Oetzel D, Wannenmacher M. Conservative treatment of breast cancer: modified irradiation technique for women with large breasts. Radiother Oncol. 1994;31(3):256–61.

18 Simulation for Breast Cancer

Mirjam Mast and Filipe Cidade de Moura

18.1 Background

18.1.1 Simulation for Breast Cancer

For breast cancer irradiation preparation, a simulation process has to be performed. During this process the patient position will be determined. Furthermore, treatment simulation allows to locate the irradiation area (i.e. target volumes) and the critical organs (Organs At Risk, OARs) that need to be avoided or taken into consideration at the time of radiation treatment planning. A planning CT scan is commonly used for breast cancer irradiation simulation. For the RT workflow this is called CT simulation (i.e. this scan is not used for diagnostic purposes). The aim of the latter is to scan the patient in a reproducible position that will serve as treatment position, lying on RT-specific immobilisation devices (see Chap. 17). Different targets and indications require different positioning of the patient, to allow for a reproducible position and safe treatment. This chapter will focus on simulation for breast cancer, after BCS or mastectomy, with/without regional nodal irradiation.

M. Mast
Haaglanden Medical Center,
Leidschendam, The Netherlands
e-mail: m.mast@haaglandenmc.nl

F. Cidade de Moura (✉)
Escola Superior de Tecnologia de Saúde de Lisboa,
Instituto Politécnico de Lisboa, Lisboa, Portugal
e-mail: Filipe.moura@estesl.ipl.pt

18.2 Simulation Process

Usually, the patient is lying in the supine position on an inclined immobilisation device, preferably indexed to the treatment couch, with one or two arms raised [1, 2]. Depending on the target volumes that need to be irradiated, only local breast irradiation or more extensive irradiation including regional nodal areas, the head of the patient may be placed in a central position or turned to the contralateral side of the affected breast (see Chap. 17) [1, 2]. Nowadays, anatomically defined target volume definition guidelines have been introduced widely. This resulted in treatment volumes with more caudally located cranial borders, allowing a central position of the head irrespective of the target volumes to be included. The latter needs to be decided in the department according to the local medical protocols, taking into account that standardisation favours avoidance of errors. For patients with large pendulous breasts a prone or lateral decubitus position is a possibility [3].

There are different types of CT scanners from several manufacturers. Depending on the type of the CT simulator, the RTT needs to take precautions to avoid collision with the arms or the used immobilisation device. A specific option for RT

© The Author(s), under exclusive license to Springer Nature Switzerland AG 2022
O. Kaidar-Person et al. (eds.), *Breast Cancer Radiation Therapy*,
https://doi.org/10.1007/978-3-030-91170-6_18

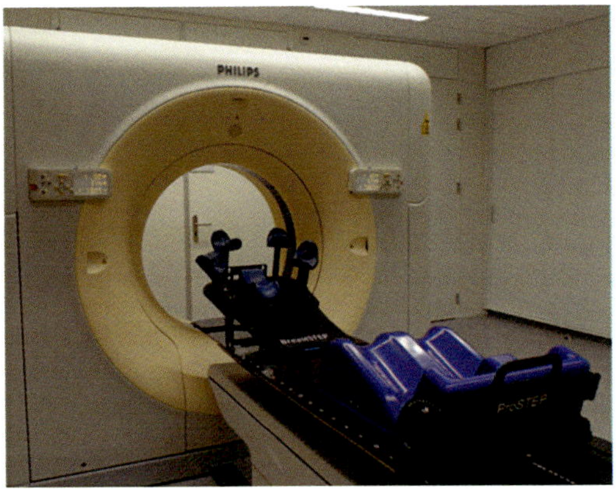

Fig. 18.1 Wide-bore RT CT scanner. Example of an inclined breast board immobilisation device (IT-V, Innsbruck). The use of the pelvic rest/stopper or knee/feet rest avoids the patient to slide down the immobilisation device

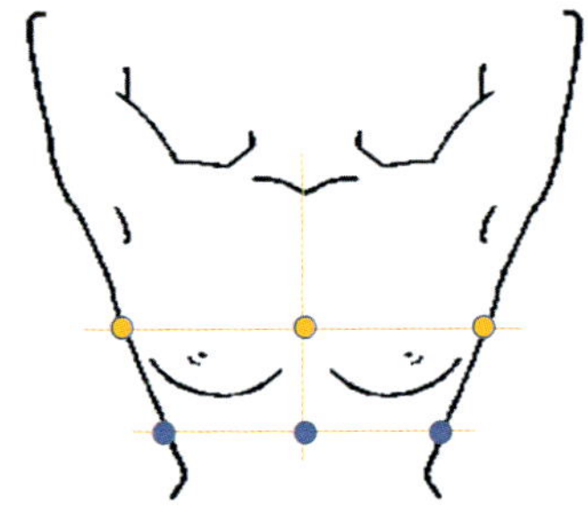

Fig. 18.2 An example of the position of the marks, this needs to be decided in the department. The reference point (0,0,0) is marked in blue. This might be a stable anatomical point to set the reference. The orange points could be helpful to outline the patient on the Linac

departments is a CT simulator with a large bore, providing the RTT more degrees of freedom in placing the patient on the RT immobilisation device on the CT simulation table and avoiding collisions with the patient (Fig. 18.1). To avoid the patient sliding down the inclined treatment couch, if the patient is positioned in supine position, additional devices can be added on the table to assist the patient to stay in the same position on the treatment table [4].

When the position of the patient is identified, the treatment planning reference point (or 0,0,0 point) is marked on the patient with a washable marker pen: one point at patient sagittal mid-line, two points at each side of the patient, all three halfway the chest since these are stable points. Cranial and/or caudal points can be added to improve patient alignment at sagittal level (Fig. 18.2). After that, artefact-free opaque markers are placed on this reference point, therefore the reference point will be visible during the treatment planning process.

The reference point is determined by using external fixed or mobile laser beams which are positioned in the CT simulator room, typically within a certain distance (i.e. 50 cm) to the CT isocentre, to allow for more working clearance. An accuracy of less than 2 mm between the imaging plane and the laser marking plane is a prerequisite for positioning the patient [5]. The reference point will be used on the linear accelerator to set-up the patient according to the position that was determined during the CT simulation, and will allow for manual/automatic movement to the planning isocentre. According to the protocols in the department several points can be placed. These points can be helpful to set-up the patient in the same position on the linear accelerator (Fig. 18.2).

Placing a radiopaque wire to mark the breast volume may be helpful at time of delineation. The wire, if done mindfully, may assist in identifying the borders of the CTV breast/chest wall. For example, the subcutaneous fold around the chest/breast from the breast itself, which is sometimes easier to identify on the patient (by appearance and palpation), especially in patients with small breasts and no infra-mammary fold. Thus, placing the wire correctly at the border of the glandular tissue as noted by palpation can be of assistance in identifying the inferior part of the breast in patients where the infra-mammary fold is not easily identified on CT simulation. The lumpectomy or mastectomy scar or other specific landmarks can be marked with a radiopaque wire as well, this is determined after consulting the radiation oncologist.

When all preparations are completed, using the external laser system to define the reference plane, the patient is moved into the CT simulator gantry. The distance from external lasers to the CT acquisition isocentre is fixed and set at the initial equipment/laser system installation.

During the acquisition phase, one or two scout views are made, depending on local standard operational procedures. On the scout views the RTT defines the field of view (FOV), to cover the entire body contour. The acquisition length would be enough to include all target volumes and OARs, plus a 5 cm margin to take into account the irradiation beams divergence and penumbra. Careful definition of the FOV and acquisition length must be performed, coupled with optimal pitch and slice thickness. For optimal reconstruction, the use of a helical CT scan is recommended with a pitch around 1:1, and a slice thickness of less than 5 mm, but preferably 3 mm. For breast cancer RT simulation, CT acquisition with intravenous contrast would not be necessary for defining the target volumes or OARs. Finally, the reference point and other points can be replaced by semi-permanent or permanent markers. Those markers need to be placed to guide the RTTs in positioning the patient on the linear accelerator. When a patient is lying in prone position, markers need to be placed on the patient's back and sides and another can be placed on the lateral aspect of the breast [3, 6]. More advanced technologies such as Surface Guided Radiation Therapy (SGRT) or adaptive linear accelerators provide meaningful changes on workflows in RT, with improvement of positioning and isocentre localisation, allowing for marker-less planning and treatment delivery. These techniques are described more extensively in the treatment delivery section.

The RTT is responsible for reporting the used immobilisation devices and if applicable other patient-specific positioning details. Colour photographs of the position of the patient can be of added value. The CT data is forwarded to the treatment planning system after the reconstruction of the images was completed. All this information is necessary for the next step in the RT workflow.

18.3 Positioning a Bolus at Time of Simulation

In some cases, a bolus is needed for PMRT or less often after BCS. We recommend that in such cases the bolus will be placed at time of CT simulation. By placing it at time of simulation it will provide information of how the bolus shapes to the body at the time of treatment planning, adjust for air gaps to reduce them as possible. A simulated bolus added in the treatment planning system will not reflect the true shape and size of the real bolus. Additionally, at time of CT simulation the team can adjust the bolus and cut/shape the bolus to areas that are at high risk and reduce the air gaps.

18.4 Deep Inspiration Breath-Hold (DIBH) Technique

When using a Deep Inspiration Breath-Hold (DIBH) technique in patients with left-sided breast cancer, or in some cases of right-sided irradiation, to reduce the dose to the heart and coronary arteries, lung, and liver (depending on patient's anatomy) a slightly adapted workflow needs to be used. As indicated in the positioning section, it is important to make sure the patient is feeling relaxed in her/his surroundings. If the patient is relaxed, it increases the chances to be more compliant with DIBH at time of simulation and treatment. Therefore, it would be recommended that RTTs first start with a clear explanation of the overall procedure that might include:

1. Demonstration of measuring/monitoring devices (optical surface detection (SGRT), spirometry)
2. Audio (e.g. intercom, earphones) and visual feedback (e.g. goggles, mirror, and screen)
3. Ensure a stable breathing cycle throughout the procedure
4. Breathing technique, with focus on upper chest (attention must be paid to avoid, arms and neck contraction, as well as back uplift)
5. Duration of deep inspiration breath-hold, preferably above minimum required time for full-length CT scan helical acquisition, typically between 15 and 30 s (optimal acquisition for reduction of temporal artefacts)

If the protocols in the department prescribe a free breathing and a DIBH scan, the same reference point is used. Furthermore, the position of the radiopaque wire needs to be checked in between these two CT scans.

18.5 Summary

For breast cancer irradiation, CT simulation is one of the important stages for treatment planning and delivery. The CT scan is used for delineation of the target volumes and the OAR, as well as for treatment planning dose calculation. After defining the position of the patient, the treatment planning reference point (0,0,0), and other essential markers, the CT scan will be performed. The reference points are used to position the patient on the Linac. The CT procedure can be performed in free breathing and breath-hold, both scans making use of the same reference point.

Advanced technologies such as optical surface devices and adaptive technologies would provide meaningful changes on workflows in RT, with improvement of positioning and isocentre localisation, allowing for marker-less planning and treatment delivery.

References

1. Xiang, et al. Which technique of positioning and immobilization is better for breast cancer patients in postmastectomy IMRT, single-pole or double-pole immobilization? J Appl Clin Med Phys. 2019;20:168–74. https://doi.org/10.1002/acm2.12506.
2. Goldsworthy, et al. Abducting both arms improves stability during breast radiotherapy: The Bi Arm study in radiotherapy. J Radiother Pract. 2011;10:250–9. https://doi.org/10.1017/S1460396910000452.
3. Huppert, et al. The role of a prone setup in breast radiation therapy. Front Oncol. 2011;31:1–8. https://doi.org/10.3389/fonc.2011.00031.
4. Jain, et al. Inter-fraction motion and dosimetric consequences during breast intensity-modulated radiotherapy (IMRT). Radiother Oncol. 2009;90:93–8. https://doi.org/10.1016/j.radonc.2008.10.010.
5. Mutic, et al. Quality assurance for computed-tomography simulators and the computed-tomography-simulation process: report of the AAPM Radiation Therapy Committee Task Group No. 66. Med Phys. 2003;30:2762–92.
6. Mitchell, et al. Interfraction and intrafraction setup variability for prone breast radiation therapy. Int J Radiat Oncol Biol Phys. 2010;76:1571–7. https://doi.org/10.1016/j.ijrobp.2009.07.1683.

Target Volume Definition and Contouring

19

Lise Bech Jellesmark Thorsen and Birgitte Vrou Offersen

19.1 Background

During recent years, RT planning for breast cancer has gone through major technological developments. In the 2D-era, the size and shape of treatment fields were determined using bony landmarks, and shielding of OARs was carried out based on planar projected images with limited detail on soft tissue [1]. With the introduction of 3DCRT, treatment techniques have been gradually refined from large, commonly tangential fields, over field-in-field planning to even more advanced approaches including modulated RT [2]. Even particle therapy has been introduced in highly selected patients with unfavourable anatomy or severe comorbidities [3]. Some techniques come with trade-offs between better target coverage at the cost of larger low-dose baths to OARs, whereas respiratory gated treatment offers a means of reducing incidental irradiation to heart and lungs while preserving target coverage [2, 4]. Common to all these advances is the increased ability to treat small target volumes to a high and homogeneously distributed dose with a steep dose gradient to adjacent OARs. The downside to this is that if the target delineation is of poor quality, we are able to miss the target with great accuracy: with improved precision, correct and consistent target volumes delineation becomes of utmost importance. Two major consensus guidelines on target volume delineation in early breast cancer are widely used. Both were developed with the purposes of improving consistency and reducing inter-observer variation. The RTOG guidelines were made available in 2009 (www.nrgoncology.org). They were based on the use of bony and muscular landmarks to include tissues that would have been treated with traditional treatment field design [5]. The concept of the ESTRO guidelines was a bit different, defining nodal targets based on lympho-vascular anatomy and including only the areas with high probability of containing lymph nodes [6, 7]. Apart from the philosophy behind, the main differences between the two guidelines concern the cranial boundary of the supraclavicular CTV, which is more generous in the RTOG definition, and the size of the IMN target volume, which is larger using the ESTRO guideline [8]. In mapping studies of loco-regional recurrences, both guidelines have very low rates of geographic miss when applied on patients with subclinical disease. In patients with locally advanced breast cancer, observed rates of geographic miss are higher, and more individualised approaches in contouring are encouraged [8]. Recommendations for more individualised target volume delineation are provided in the ESTRO consensus guideline [6, 7]. The following sections on target delinea-

L. B. J. Thorsen · B. V. Offersen (✉)
Department of Experimental Clinical Oncology, Aarhus University Hospital, Aarhus, Denmark
e-mail: liseb@oncology.au.dk; bvo@oncology.au.dk; Birgitte.Offersen@auh.rm.dk

© The Author(s), under exclusive license to Springer Nature Switzerland AG 2022

O. Kaidar-Person et al. (eds.), *Breast Cancer Radiation Therapy*,
https://doi.org/10.1007/978-3-030-91170-6_19

tion adhere to the ESTRO consensus guideline. We also recommend reading the complimentary chapters of breast and lymph node anatomy and lymph node volumes, the latter discuss the indications for RNI and which lymph node levels to be irradiated.

19.2 General Practical Advice for Delineation

- Go through the patient's diagnostic workup, surgeon's notes and pathology descriptions before embarking on delineation.
- Use a protocol for patient positioning including strict guidelines for choice of breast board, arm positioning, use of tattoos or other markers to help daily positioning reproducibility, and ensuring reproducibility of respiratory gated technique.
- Choose a Hounsfield Unit interval with high soft-tissue contrast—delineation software often comes with pre-set levels.
- Check your volumes in the coronal and sagittal planes as you contour—a smooth volume from the outset will spare you many corrections in the end.
- Use a template ensuring strict nomenclature and choice of colours for the individual volumes, as this facilitates pattern recognition when approving the delineation, eases communication and subsequent data harvesting.

19.3 Delineation of CTVp_breast

Practical advice

- Consider the configuration of the breast: firm/flat/ptotic?
- Start your delineation at a level where you clearly see the limits of the breast, then move cranially/caudally.
- Always include the primary tumour bed inside the CTVp_breast.

The CTVp_breast should contain all glandular breast tissue (Fig. 19.1). The extent of the breast gland may be difficult to distinguish from the surrounding subcutaneous fat. The cranial limit of the volume in most patients corresponds to caudal of the sternoclavicular joint. This derives from treatment planning in the days before CT scans, where the field border (50% isodose) in most guidelines was located at the caudal border of the sternoclavicular joint, and local recurrences from those days rarely occurred at or cranial to the border. If the tumour bed is located very cranially, the CTVp_breast should include the tumour bed with at least 1 cm margin.

The medial border may extend as far as the lateral edge of the sternum (e.g. in young firm breasts), but is often located more laterally. However, the breast gland is always lateral to the medial mammary branches from the internal mammary vessels, which are often identifiable in one or more images (Fig. 19.1b). These vessels should be identified in every patient, because they often indicate a more lateral border than the sternal edge. Note that a flaccid breast tends to flatten and droop in the lateral direction with placement of the patient in treatment position. This means that the lateral extent of the CTVp_breast depends on breast configuration and size. In some patients, the lateral border of the breast is clearly visible (e.g. a young firm breast). If not, find the lateral thoracic vessels; these mark the furthest possible lateral extension of the breast gland.

Pay attention that in the lateral direction the breast glandular tissue does not extend to the dorsal muscles, and in general it should be possible in the far majority of patients to reach a treatment plan where the dorsal muscles are not included with dose.

Caudally, delineate as long as the breast is visible. The ventral border of the CTVp_breast is cropped to 5 mm below the skin surface, unless the tumour involved the skin, in which case the skin around the scar should be included and a bolus applied. In depth, the dorsal border of the CTVp_breast extends to the surface of the pectoralis major muscle where present, otherwise to the ventral border of the ribs and intercostal muscles. Note that sometimes subcutaneous fat from the abdominal wall pushes the breast forward,

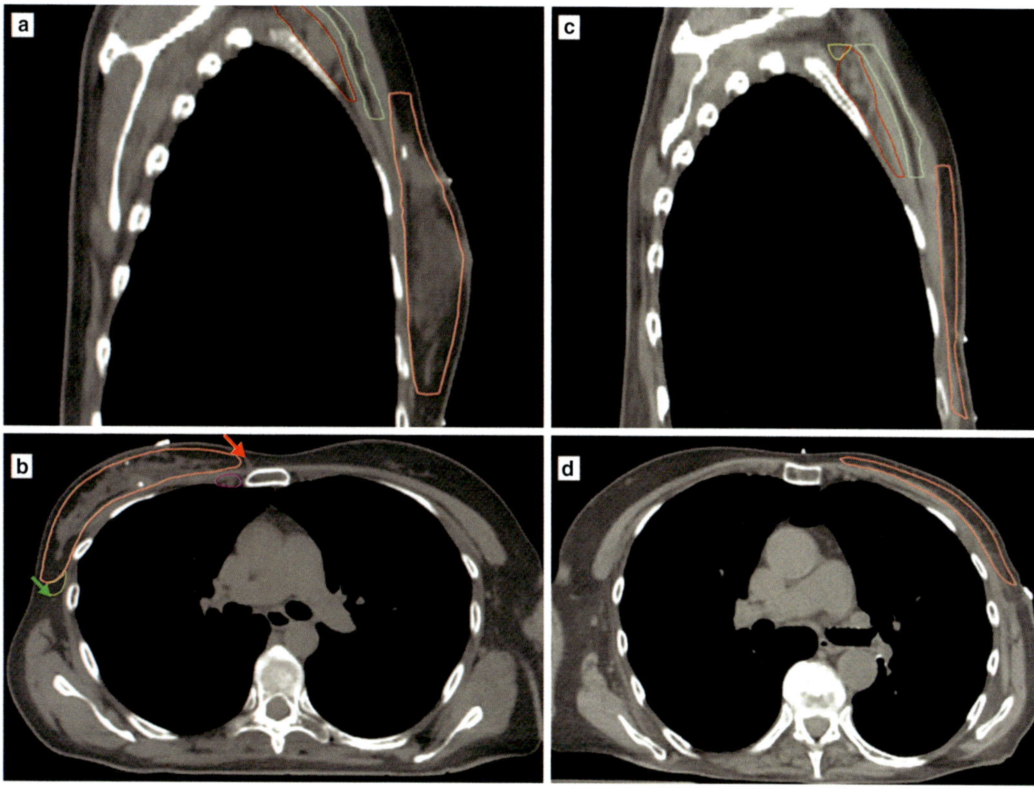

Fig. 19.1 (**a**) CTVp_breast (pink) in the sagittal view. Cranially, part of the interpectoral (light green) and CTVn_L2 (red) are visible. (**b**) Axial view of CTVp_Breast (pink). The arrows point at medial mammary branches of the internal thoracic artery (red arrow) and the lateral thoracic artery (green arrow). Panel (**c**, **d**) Sagittal (**c**) and axial (**d**) views of CTVp_thoracic wall

pushing the caudal part of the CTVp_breast more ventrally. In obese patients the abdominal fat may be quite helpful in pushing the breast glandular tissue ventrally and thus away from the heart; this phenomenon is usually more visible in MR-images.

19.4 CTVp_thoracic Wall

Practical advice

- Consider the configuration of the opposite breast and place radio-opaque markers where the breast used to be and on the scar.

The CTVp_thoracic wall should be delineated using borders as defined for the CTVp_breast (Fig. 19.1). Do not extend the volume further due to uncertainty about the position of the former breast—the surgical procedure involves pulling adjacent skin and subcutaneous tissue in to close the defect, and thus reduces the size of the CTVp_thoracic wall. Delineate the tissue from the ventral surface of the pectoralis major and/or muscular/bony chest wall, and crop 5 mm from the skin. If the area is very thin, do not routinely include the pectoralis major or any deeper parts of the chest wall—unless, of course, invasion was demonstrated, i.e. T4a-c disease (tumour invasion/adherence to the pectoralis muscle, in the absence of invasion to the deep chest wall structures does not qualify as T4). Instead, place a 5 mm bolus on the area and include the skin in the delineation. Note that in some countries the skin around the scar is part of the target in selected patients (pT3-4 disease). Therefore, in these cases a bolus is applied in case of chest wall irradiation.

To note, the surgeon may have extended the scar outside the breast region for better cosmetic outcome, but for treatment planning the relevant part of the scar is inside the breast region, unless the tumour was located at the border of the breast gland. In such cases, the CTVp_chest wall target should include the tumour bed with at least 1 cm margin.

19.5 Delineation of Nodal Volumes

Practical advice

- The nodal volumes consist of axillary levels 1–3, the interpectoral nodes, the IMN and the level 4, previously named the supraclavicular nodes. With correct delineation, the volumes should end up being interconnected.
- The nodal volumes in the periclavicular area follow the large veins in the area with a margin of 5 mm, as this is where the lymph nodes are situated. For the CTVn_IMN volume, lymph nodes are located along both the veins and arteries, thus both are included with 5 mm margin.
- To avoid irradiation of the scapula-humeral joint, delineate the humeral head and add a 1 cm margin around it as a PRV.
- Note any markings (e.g. clips) left by the surgeon, and read the surgical remarks to understand the markings.
- Note that these guidelines do not apply to patients with locally advanced disease, in whom we recommend individualised target-determination as also discussed in the ESTRO target consensus guideline [6, 7].

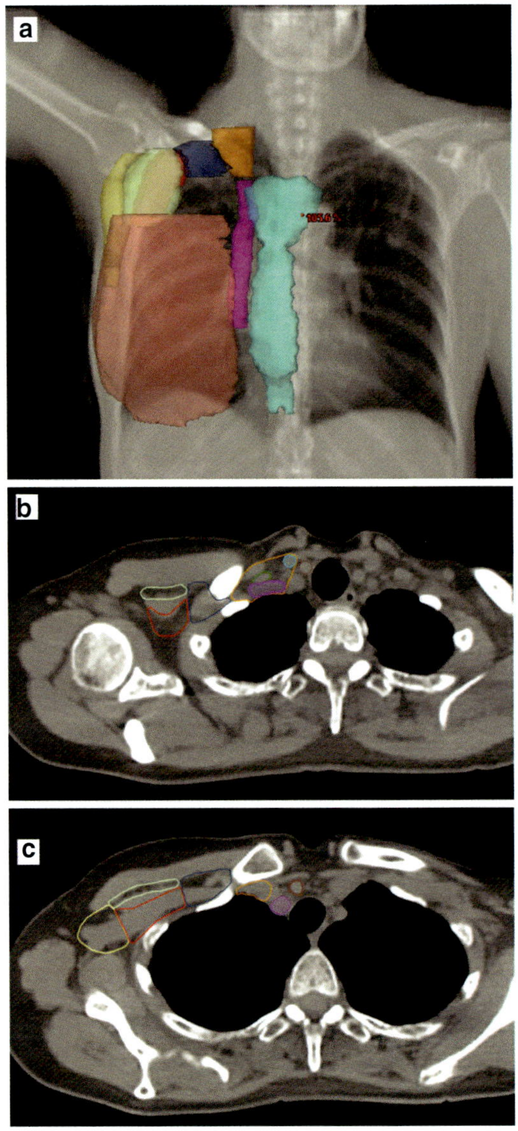

Fig. 19.2 (**a**) 3D view of the nodal volumes and CTVp_Breast. Panel (**b**, **c**) overviews of the interconnected lymph node volumes in the cranial (**b**) and more caudal (**c**) aspects. Pink: CTVp_Breast, orange: CTVn_L4, dark blue: CTVn_L3, red: CTVn_L2, light green: interpectoral muscles, magenta: CTVn_IMN, brown: carotid artery, green: scalenus anterior muscle, purple: subclavian artery, light blue: internal jugular vein, turquoise: sternum

19.6 Axillary Level 1: CTVn_L1

The axillary level 1 should include the axillary vein with a margin of 5 mm and all surgical scarring from ALND/SLNB (Fig. 19.2). In general, it is advisable to crop the volume to exclude the PRV from the scapula-humeral joint. Begin delineating at the slice 5 mm cranial to the axillary vein to compensate for partial volume effect. The medial border here matches the lateral border of the CTVn_L2 and the interpectoral nodes, while more caudally, the volume extends to the thoracic wall. In the ventral direction, the volume stops at the major and minor pectoral muscles. In the lateral direction, there is no clear anatomical boundary. Here, draw a line through the fatty tissue from the lateral edge of the major pectoral muscle to the ventro-lateral edge of the latissimus dorsi muscle. End the volume caudally at the level of costae 4–5, depending on extent of surgical scarring.

19.7 Axillary Level 2: CTVn_L2

The minor pectoral muscle defines this volume: Level 2 contains the volume dorsal to it, but extending in the dorsal direction to 5 mm dorsal to the axillary vein, limited by the ribs and intercostal muscles (Fig. 19.2). In the cranial direction, start delineating at one slice above the axillary artery. Move caudally dorsal to the minor pectoral muscle, extending the volume from its medial to its lateral edge. Stop at the caudal edge of the muscle. If you see scarring from axillary lymph node dissection at the caudal part of level 2, consider excluding it, as nodes have been surgically removed here.

19.8 The Interpectoral Lymph Nodes

This volume is the space between the major and the minor pectoral muscles (Fig. 19.2). Delineate the space with the same cranial/caudal/lateral/medial boundaries as CTVn_L2. At times, the space is largely imaginary, as the muscles lie very close to one another—in that case, delineate a thin strip of tissue ventral to the minor pectoral muscle.

19.9 Axillary Level 3: CTVn_L3

The axillary level 3, previously named the infraclavicular volume, lies medial to CTVn_L2 (Fig. 19.2). Medially, it contains the subclavian vein with a margin of 5 mm from the junction of the subclavian and jugular veins to laterally the medial edge of the minor pectoral muscle. Muscle and bone are excluded, meaning that the clavicle and the junction of the vessels become the medial limit, whereas the ventral border is the dorsal surface of the major pectoralis muscle. The dorsal border is 5 mm dorsal to the subclavian vein or the ribs/intercostal muscles, whichever comes first. The cranial limit is set at one CT-slice (usually 2–3 mm) cranial to the subclavian artery.

19.10 Axillary Level 4: CTVn_L4

The supraclavicular volume is different in patients with breast cancer, head and neck cancer and lymphoma, and therefore it is recommended to call it level 4 in a breast cancer patient. Cranially, the axillary level 4 includes the supraclavicular part of the subclavian vein with a margin of 5 mm (Fig. 19.2). In practice, this means that the volume begins one slice cranial to the subclavian arterial arch, which can be identified in the coronal view. Medially, the volume includes the internal jugular vein without a margin, excluding the internal carotid artery and the thyroid gland. Moving in the lateral direction, the ventral border of the volume is delineated dorsal to the sternocleidomastoid muscle, the sternothyroid muscle and the clavicle. The dorsal border is the pleura, and the caudal extension includes the tissue until 5 mm below the junction of the subclavian and the internal jugular vein. Laterally, the volume connects to the CTVn_L3 with the inclusion of the anterior scalene muscle, and caudally, it connects to the CTVn_IMN.

19.11 The IMN: CTVn_IMN

The IMN volume lies along the internal mammary vessels on the inner surface of the chest wall adjacent to the parietal pleura (Fig. 19.1b and 19.2a). The internal mammary arteries both originate from the subclavian arteries, whereas the internal mammary vein drains to the brachiocephalic venous trunk on the right, and to the subclavian vein on the left. Delineate the IMN volume around the vessels, adding a 5 mm margin around both the vein and artery, and crop for lung. As the veins end, taper the top of the volume around the arteries off to connect to the CTVn_L4. The caudal limit of CTVn_IMN is decided by tumour location. For most tumours, ICS 1–3 are included to the cranial part of the fourth rib, whereas for lower inner quadrant tumours, ICS 4 is also included, as lymphoscintigraphy studies have shown higher frequencies of IMN drainage to the lower ICS in this setting [9]. Use the sagittal view to determine the ICS.

19.12 Post-delineation

After completing delineation, inspect the overall result using the 3D view—by doing this systematically, you will gain pattern recognition skills and be able to identify important variations and mistakes (Fig. 19.2a). All volumes should be interconnected. An un-delineated upper medial part of the area between the IMN, CTVn_L3, CTVn_L2 and caudally the CTVp_breast/ CTVp_thoracic wall is acceptable.

19.13 Summary

In summary, the change to modern treatment planning with target-based rather than field-based techniques require correct and consistent target volume delineation. The best way to achieve this lies through practice in both the setting of mastectomy and BCS. We highly recommend interdisciplinary cooperation with surgeons and radiologists along with the use of recognised and updated guidelines in the field. The ESTRO consensus guidelines are currently being validated in two randomised trials on hypo- versus normo-fractionated loco-regional radiotherapy in patients with early breast cancer: the DBCG Skagen trial 1 (NCT02384733) and the HYPO-G01 (NCT03127995). The field of target volume delineation is in constant development and requires the dedicated and continuous attention of the clinician.

References

1. Thorsen LBJ, Thomsen MS, Overgaard M, Overgaard J, Offersen BV. Quality assurance of conventional non-CT-based internal mammary lymph node irradiation in a prospective Danish Breast Cancer Cooperative Group trial: the DBCG-IMN study. Acta Oncol. 2013;52:7.
2. Poortmans P, Aznar M, Bartelink H. Quality indicators for breast cancer: revisiting historical evidence in the context of technology changes. Semin Radiat Oncol. 2012;22(1):29–39.
3. Bradley JA, Mendenhall NP. Novel radiotherapy techniques for breast cancer. Annu Rev Med. 2018;69:277–88.
4. Hjelstuen MH, Mjaaland I, Vikstrom J, Dybvik KI. Radiation during deep inspiration allows loco-regional treatment of left breast and axillary-, supraclavicular- and internal mammary lymph nodes without compromising target coverage or dose restrictions to organs at risk. Acta Oncol. 2012;51(3):333–44.
5. Li XA, Tai A, Arthur DW, Buchholz TA, Macdonald S, Marks LB, et al. Variability of target and normal structure delineation for breast cancer radiotherapy: an RTOG multi-institutional and multiobserver study. Int J Radiat Oncol. 2009;73(3):944–51.
6. Offersen BV, Boersma LJ, Kirkove C, Hol S, Aznar MC, Biete Sola A, et al. ESTRO consensus guideline on target volume delineation for elective radiation therapy of early stage breast cancer. Radiother Oncol. 2015;114(1):3–10.
7. Offersen BV, Boersma LJ, Kirkove C, Hol S, Aznar MC, Sola AB, et al. ESTRO consensus guideline on target volume delineation for elective radiation therapy of early stage breast cancer, version 1.1. Radiother Oncol. 2016;118:205–8.
8. Loganadane G, Truong PT, Taghian AG, Tešanović D, Jiang M, Geara F, et al. Comparison of nodal target volume definition in breast cancer radiation therapy according to RTOG versus ESTRO atlases: a practical review from the transatlantic radiation oncology network (TRONE). Int J Radiat Oncol. 2020;107(3):437–48.
9. Estourgie SH, Nieweg OE, Olmos RA, Rutgers EJ, Kroon BB. Lymphatic drainage patterns from the breast. Ann Surg. 2004;239(2):232–7.

Target Volume Definition and Delineation Boost/PBI/SIB

20

Pierfrancesco Franco and Philip Poortmans

20.1 Background

Post-operative WBI is a standard of care for early-stage breast cancer patients after BCS [1, 2]. In node-negative early breast cancer patients, it reduces the rate of any breast cancer recurrence at 10 years from 31.0% to 15.6% and the 15-year breast cancer mortality rate from 20.5% to 17.2%, while the corresponding figures in node-positive early breast cancer patients are from 63.7% to 42.5% and from 51.3% to 42.8% [3]. An extra RT "boost" dose delivered to the primary tumour bed after BCS and WBI decreases local recurrence rates from 10.2% to 6.4% at 10 years and from 16.4% to 12.0% at 20 years [4]. As the relative reduction is similar among risk groups, the absolute reduction strongly depends on patient's and tumour's characteristics including patient's age, tumour biology and grade and resection margins [5]. Over the last 20 years, a significant decrease in loco-regional recurrence rates was seen following improvements in the multidisciplinary diagnostic approaches and therapeutic management, with only 1.8% loco-regional recurrence rates at 9 years seen in the "Young Boost Trial" (Fig. 20.1) [6, 7]. Moreover, the increased local control rate following a boost did not translate into a survival benefit and adverse cosmetic effects were noted, especially after high boost doses and large boosted volumes [4, 8, 9]. Therefore, boost delivery is advised to be restricted to patients having high-risk features for local relapse.

For low-risk patients, PBI was introduced to reduce treatment volumes and unintended dose to normal tissues, improve access and reduce costs. Originally, it was mainly aimed at reducing treatment duration but eligible patients can now be treated with a similar 5-day WBI fractionation schedule, wiping out this time benefit [10]. It can be delivered with EBRT, interstitial and intracavitary brachytherapy, and intra-operative electrons or low-energy photons, each of the techniques bearing their particular features [11]. In well-selected patients, local control rates are similar to those observed with WBI [12–15]. However, also for PBI, cosmetic outcomes depend strongly on dose-volume parameters and time interval between fractions for schedules delivering RT twice a day [16, 17].

Paradoxically, nowadays when breast imaging is more advanced, identifying the tumour bed is more challenging. It is mostly due to the fact that the old practice to place the boost field or volume over the location of the surgical scar visible upon inspection is completely outdated. This is mostly

P. Franco
Department of Translational Medicine, University of Eastern Piedmont, Novara, Italy
e-mail: pierfrancesco.franco@unito.it

P. Poortmans (✉)
Faculty of Medicine and Health Sciences, University of Antwerp, Antwerp, Belgium

Department of Radiation Oncology, Iridium Netwerk, Antwerp, Belgium
e-mail: philip.poortmans@gza.be

© The Author(s), under exclusive license to Springer Nature Switzerland AG 2022
O. Kaidar-Person et al. (eds.), *Breast Cancer Radiation Therapy*,
https://doi.org/10.1007/978-3-030-91170-6_20

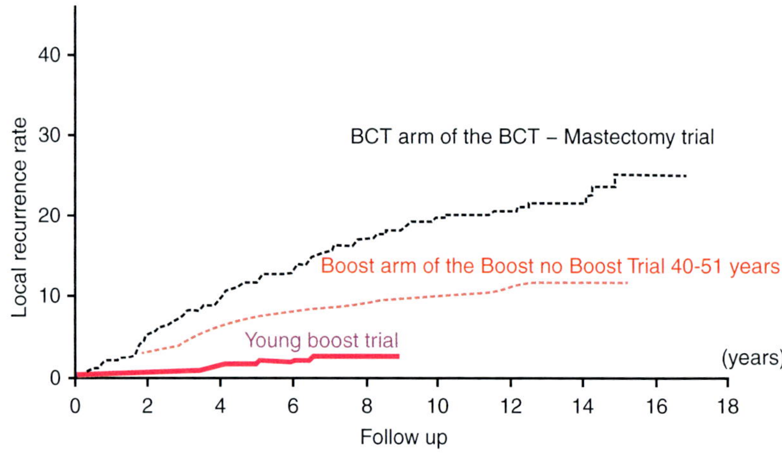

Fig. 20.1 Local breast recurrence rate in three consecutive trials on breast conserving therapy from 1980 till 2012. (Reproduced from [6])

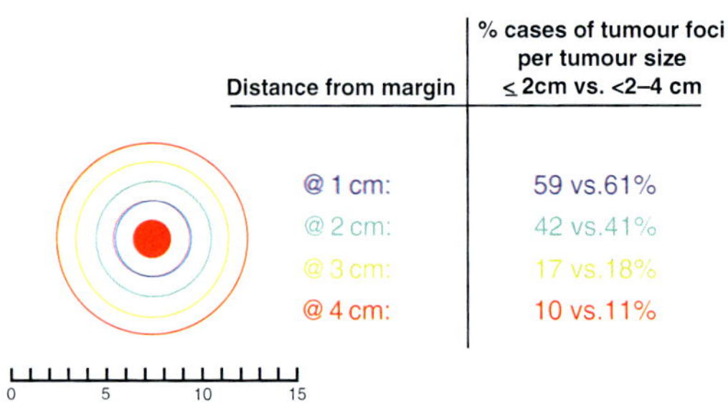

Fig. 20.2 The likelihood to observe residual tumour cells in the tissue surrounding of the primary tumour, up to 1 cm, 2 cm, 3 cm and 4 cm distance from the primary tumour, respectively, for tumour diameters up to 2 cm and tumour diameter between < 2 and 4 cm. (Based on [18])

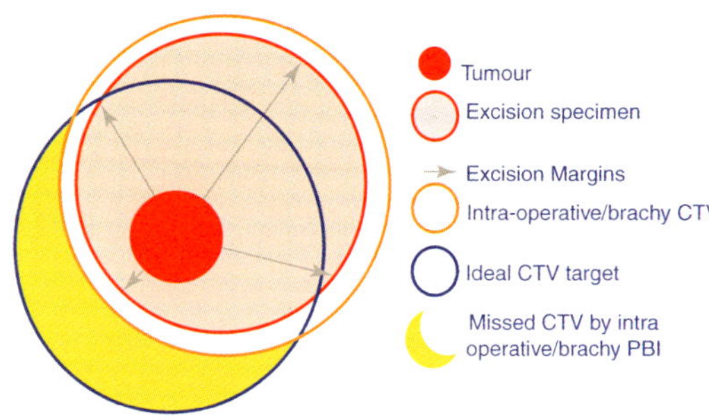

Fig. 20.3 Illustration highlighting the fact that breast tumours are most often eccentrically located within the lumpectomy specimen, with an anisotropic location of the CTV for boost/PBI that does not coincide with the surgical cavity. (Reproduced with permission from [19])

a result of the increased use of oncoplastic BCS techniques (see oncoplastic surgery section, Chap. 35), including remote positioning of the scar (e.g. at the edge of the areola) with/without relocation of breast tissue to different breast quadrants to reduce deformity and improve cosmesis. Even if applying anatomy-based treatment volume definition, pre- and post-operative imaging and all available clinical considerations, proper delineation of the target volume for boost and PBI is accompanied with many uncertainties. It is well known that with a conventional lumpectomy the amount of tissue removed around the primary tumour varies substantially (Fig. 20.2) [19], but with oncoplastic procedures, this may vary even more depending on the direction taken into account. Especially with closed cavity surgery it may be challenging to identify the surgical cavity, which is useful to help defining the primary tumour bed (but is not at all the same!). Pathology can describe reliably the microscopic tumour-free margins in all six spatial directions, enabling the correct estimation of the safety margin required. Both changing definition of surgical margins and increased use of primary systemic therapy (PST) influence the pathological examination that should reflect the estimated distribution of residual disease.

20.2 General Considerations

For both the boost (high-risk patients, after WBI) and PBI (low-risk patients, sole post-operative local treatment), the CTV is based on the distribution of tumour cells around the primary tumour which influences the pattern of local tumour relapse after BCS (Fig. 20.3) [4, 18, 20]. However, delineation of the target volume is subject to many uncertainties. It should be guided by a combination of preoperative imaging with post-operative findings including clinical examination, surgical scar, type of surgical procedure and visible post-operative effects including radio-opaque clips positioned within the excision cavity, all helping to define the original location of the primary tumour within the surgical cavity. The increased use of oncoplastic surgery, the refined specification in the pathology report, the more frequent use of primary systemic therapy, all underpin the importance of a thorough multidisciplinary collaboration to optimise target volume delineation. In any case, the surgical cavity or surgical bed most often poorly represents the CTV for boost/PBI (Fig. 20.2) [21]. Additionally, it is recommended to discuss with the surgeon the method for clipping the surgical bed, and to compare the clip location to the preoperative imaging of the primary tumour to assure the reliability of its location (e.g. migration of the clips, incorrect clipping on the pectoralis in attempt to reduce migration, unrelated to the primary location of the primary lesion within the tumour bed).

Several excellent guidelines describing CTV contouring for boost/PBI are available [22, 23]. However, they fail to be broadly adapted into daily clinical practice, where often the erroneous practice of considering the surgical cavity/bed as the target volume for the boost/PBI continues being advised [24]. The first attempts to set contouring guidelines after oncoplastic surgery, repositioning the CTV within the breast with volumes often separated both from each other and from the surgical scars, offer more insights into the thereto related challenges [25]. Optimal coordination and communication between surgeons, radiologists, pathologists and radiation oncologists is essential to ensure that the tumour bed and the margins around it are adequate to reliably define a correct CTV.

20.3 Definition of the Clinical Target Volume

20.3.1 The Primary Tumour Bed

The most appropriate approach is to first define the primary tumour bed, representing the area, within the breast, where the primary tumour was located preoperatively. Thereby, whereas the primary tumour bed should be located somewhere within the surgical cavity, in ideal circumstances it should be infinitely small and by no means include the entire surgical cavity.

As outlined in the guidelines published by the GEC-ESTRO Breast Cancer Working Group, the most appropriate delineation in clinical practice comprises the following steps: (a) the acquisition of a detailed knowledge of the surgical procedure on the primary tumour, including the preoperative imaging and detailed pathology report; (b) the correct localisation of the primary breast tumour before BCS and the transposition of this information onto the post-operative imaging; (c) the accurate calculation of the size of the safety margins from primary tumour bed to CTV, preferably in all directions (Fig. 20.4) [22].

20.3.2 The CTV

The CTV, by definition, constitutes the rim of tissue around the primary tumour bed. Therefore, it should be reconstructed from the latter as a starting point. As a minimum, the CTV can be constructed using isotropic expansion from the primary tumour bed by 1.5 cm or 2.0 cm, respectively for boost or PBI (Fig. 20.5).

Ideally, the surgical specimen should be orientated in space and tumour-free margins should be described by the pathologist in all six directions. If this can be correctly translated to the planning CT-scan, the volume of the CTV could be reduced by a factor of 1.9 [24]. If not given, the margin of 1.5/2.0 cm should be reduced by the minimal tumour-free margin (Fig. 20.6) [24, 26]. In case of wide tumour-free margins, exceeding 1.0 cm (1.5 cm for PBI), we advise to extend by 0.5 cm and not less, to accommodate for residual uncertainties. If the tumour-free margin exceeds the 1.5 cm in all directions, by definition, the entire CTV for the boost has been surgically removed and thereby the indication for a boost ceases.

The CTV boost/PBI should not extend outside of the CTV of the whole breast, limited deeply by the chest wall and the pectoral muscles and superficially by the skin. For this, we

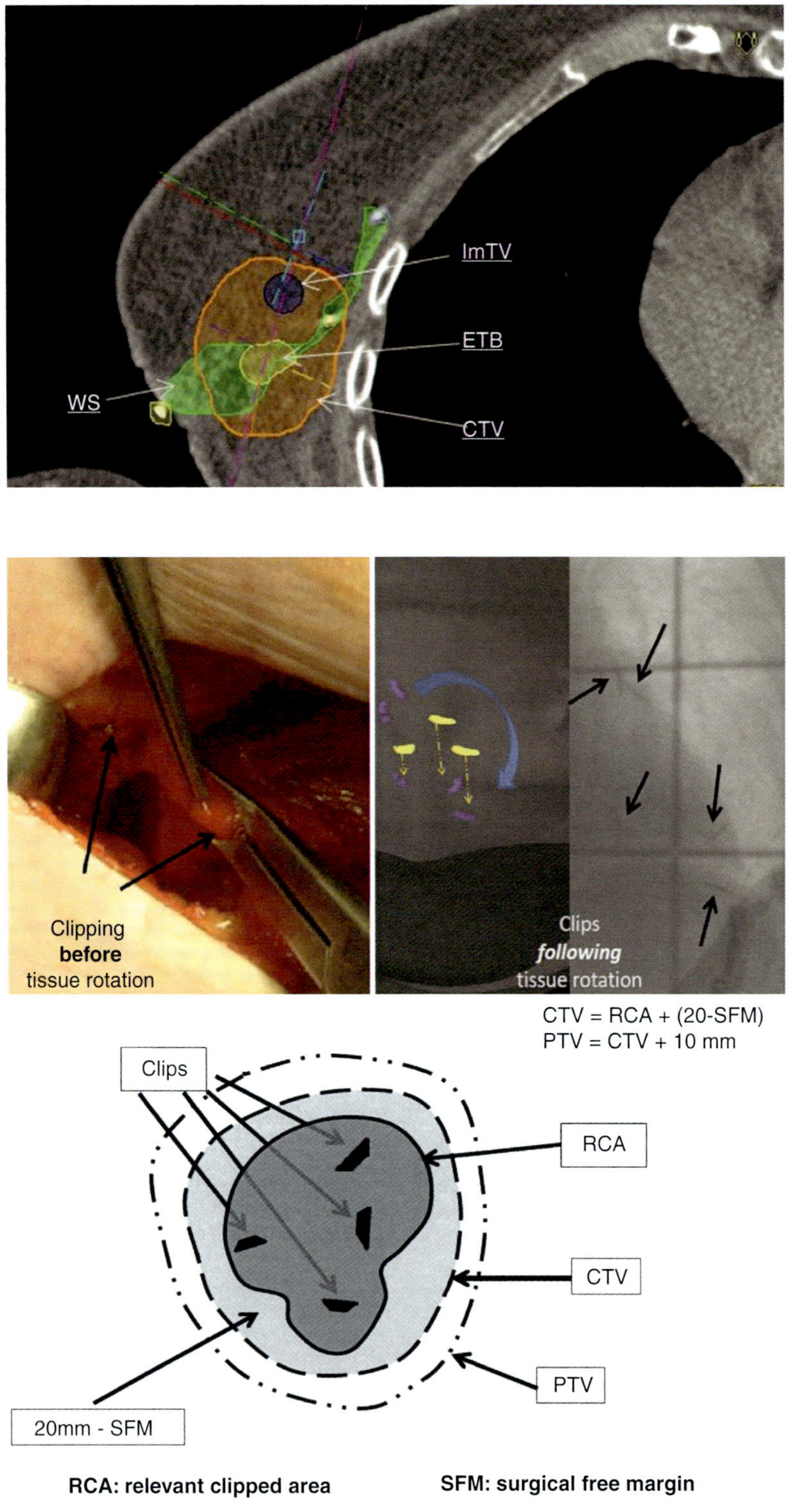

Fig. 20.4 GEC-ESTRO stepwise reconstruction of the CTV boost/PBI. *WS* whole surgical scar, *ImTV* Imaging related target volume, *ETB* estimated tumour bed, *CTV* clinical target volume. (Reproduced with permission from [22])

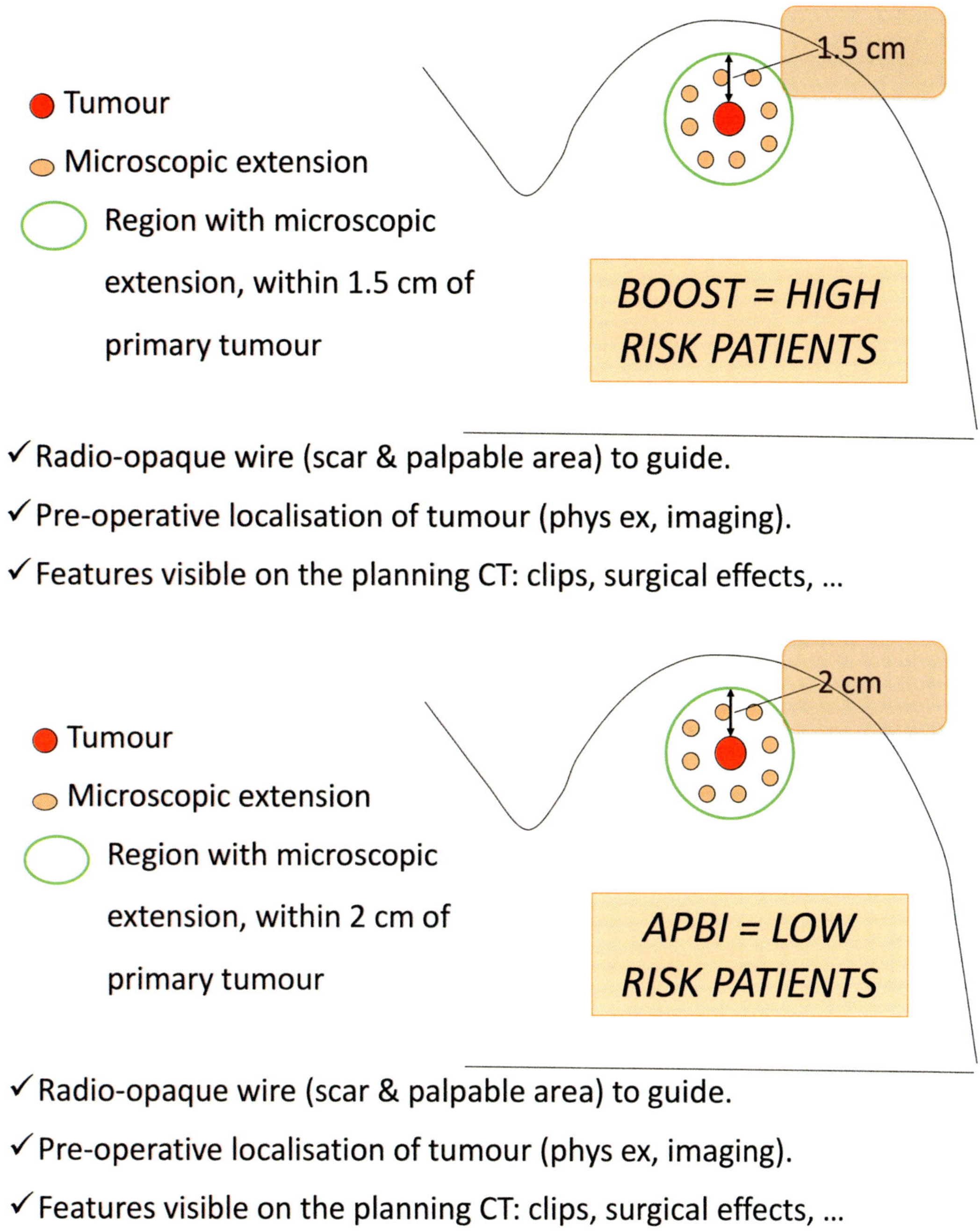

Fig. 20.5 Schematic representation of the definition of the CTV boost/PBI

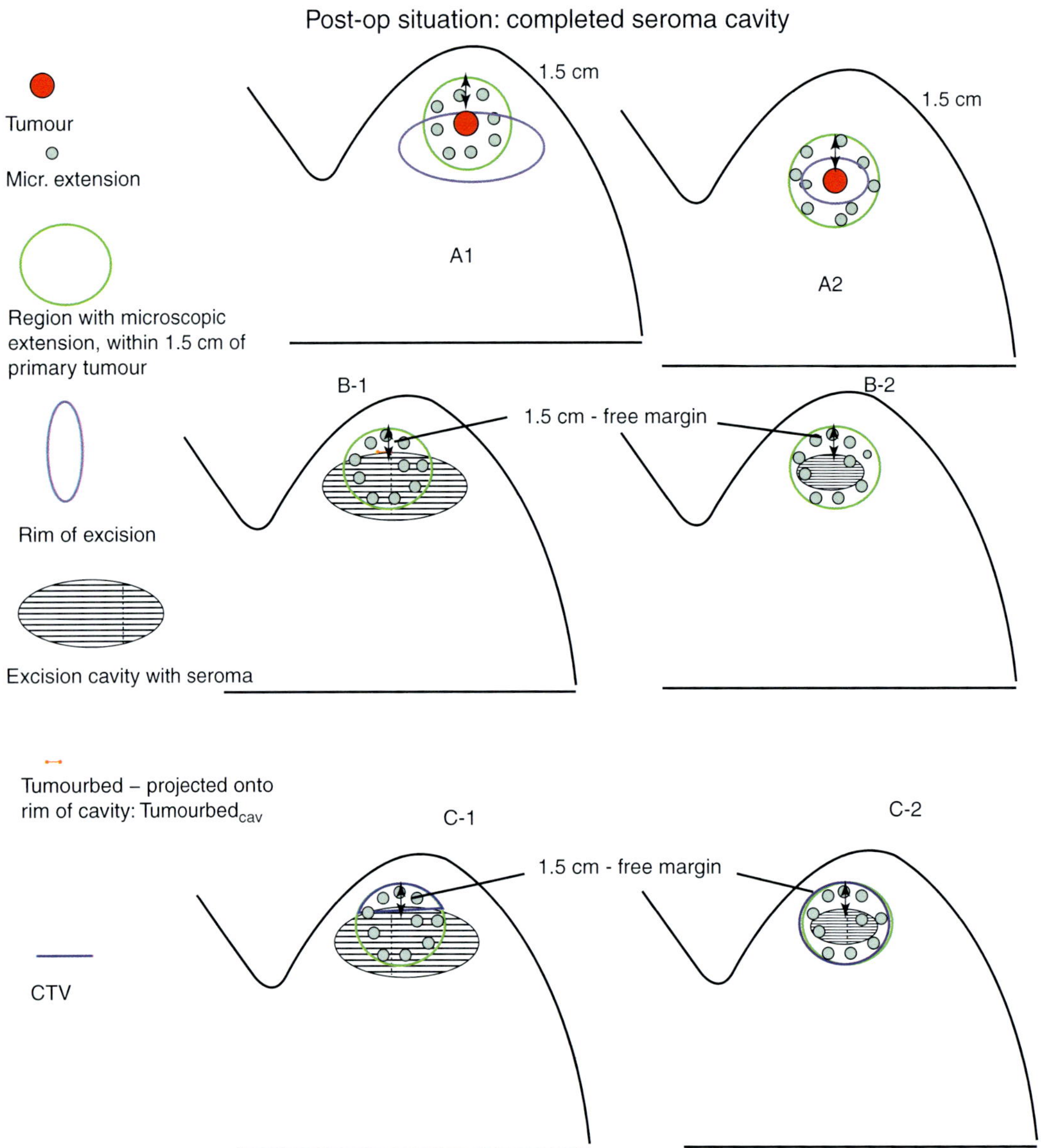

Fig. 20.6 Guideline used in the "Young Boost Trial" for generation of the CTV boost starting from the primary tumour bed (reproduced with permission from [24])

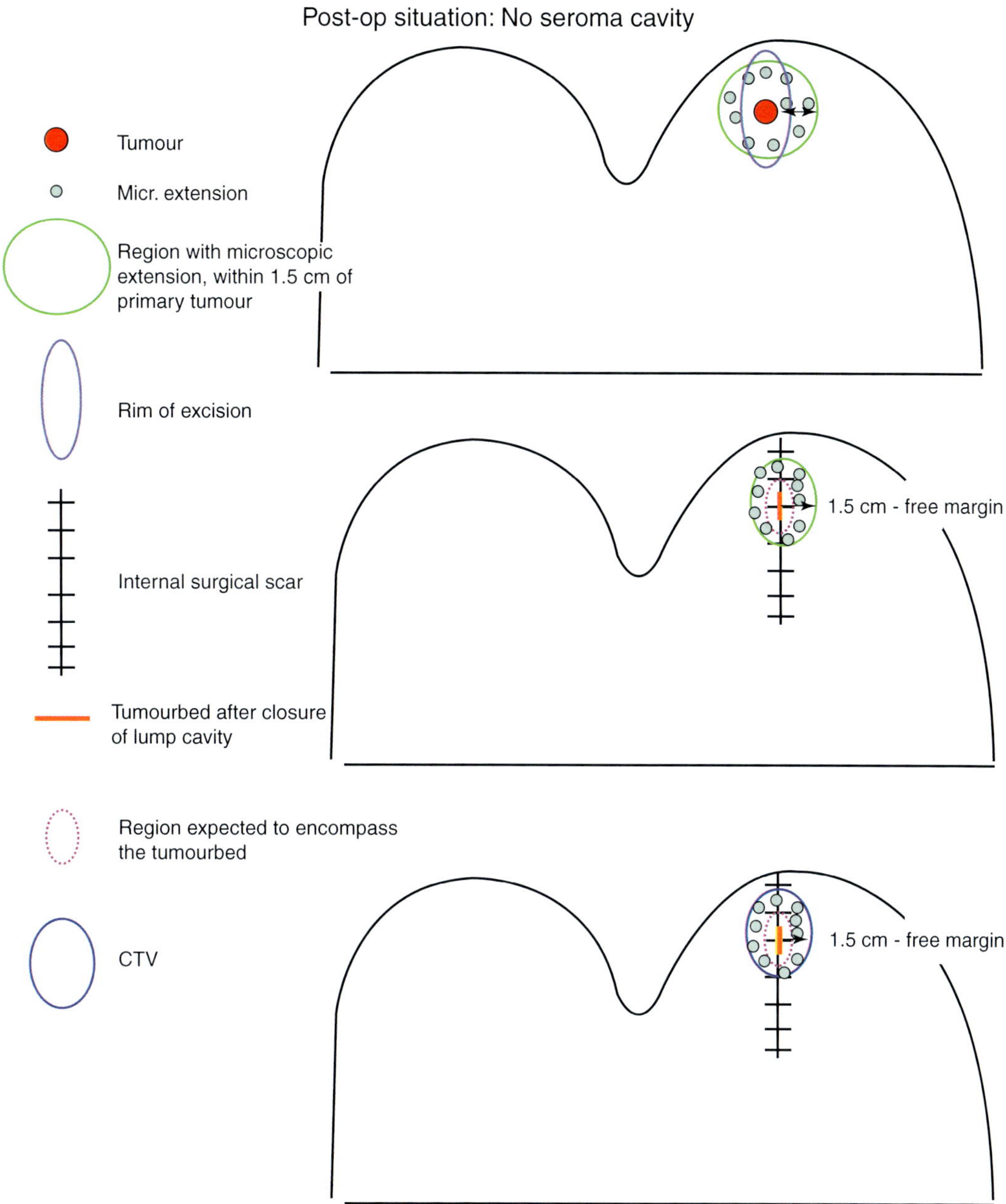

Fig. 20.6 (continued)

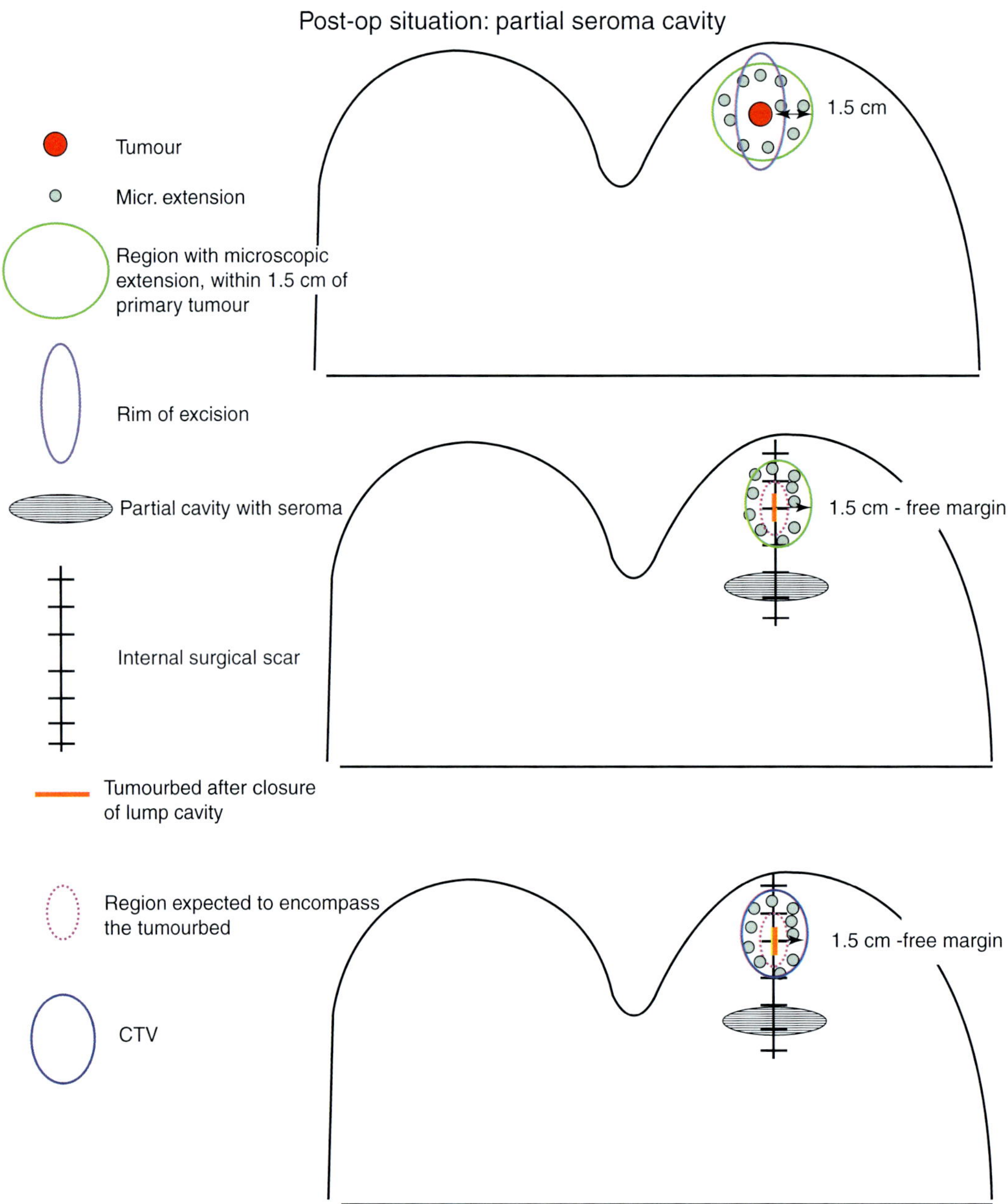

Fig. 20.6 (continued)

advise to first contour the CTV whole breast and thereafter to crop the CTV boost/PBI within the CTV breast using the treatment planning software delineation tool.

Important note: Most radiation oncologists contour directly the CTV boost, which is a conceptual error from both ICRU and anatomical perspectives. Experience also highlighted the fact that the introduction of the CT-scan for boost volume definition led to an increased irradiated volume, which is related to increased risks for fibrosis and adverse cosmetic effects [8, 27]. Therefore, when transitioning to correct 3-phased contouring (primary tumour bed–CTV boost/

PBI–PTV) do mind that target volumes don't get inappropriately increased.

20.3.3 Complicating Factors

In the case of open cavity surgery, fluid exudate enters the surgical cavity forming a seroma [28]. Whereas this seroma is by definition no part of the CTV, it will influence the delineation of the primary tumour bed and possibly also the expansion to the CTV (Fig. 20.5) [26].

While clinical findings, including the position of the scar and palpable surgical effects, preoperative imaging and the presence of surgical markers such as clips are all useful in defining the primary tumour bed, they may also be highly misleading. Especially the inappropriate use of clips and/or seroma is a point of concern, particularly when oncoplastic surgical techniques are used since they often lead to clip or seroma positions that are at wide distances from the CTV boost/PBI. Therefore, the following basic principles should be respected concerning the use of clips for delineation of the CTV:

- Breast surgeons should follow the GEC-ESTRO guidelines for the positioning of surgical clips [22]. They need to be fixed to the tumour bed during the surgical procedure before performing any breast tissue rotation. While in theory six clips should be used to represent the boundaries of resection in the six main directions, in clinical practice, at least four clips are recommended.
- Breast surgeons should participate in or at least observe the technical application of boost/PBI target volume delineations after various types of lumpectomy as part of their training in breast surgical oncology, as well as part of continuous medical education so they may understand the technical issues and the importance of bed marking.
- Radiation oncologists should participate in or observe various types of lumpectomy procedures (level 1 and 2 oncoplastic procedures) as part of their training in breast radiation oncology, as well as part of continuous medical education.

This would ensure optimal multidisciplinary collaboration and optimal targeted treatment in the modern era of breast conservation [29].

20.4 Special Considerations

Given the aformentioned considerations, which are subjected to multiple uncertainties, the CTV for boost/PBI should be rather considered as a a geometrical approximation than as an exact anatomical entity. The more extensive and precise the information, the smaller the additional margins required for handling uncertainties. As illustrated nicely using a peeled orange, the increase of a CTV measuring 5 cm in diameter by a margin around of merely 0.65 cm already doubles the volume from 60 to 120 cm^3 [30]. Therefore, multidisciplinary collaboration including mutual training should be mandated to improve both reliability and accuracy of delineation of the boost/PBI volumes.

Mathematics might help, using the formula to calculate the volume of a sphere ($4/3*pi*r^3$). This means that, for example, for a tumour measuring 2 cm in diameter, removed with a minimal tumour-free margin of 0.5 cm, the residual CTV amounts 29 cm^3 for a boost and 61 cm^3 for PBI. Whereas it is not feasible to use these values as an absolute target, it may help clinicians to have at least an estimation of the appropriateness of the size of the contoured CTV.

For PBI, the clear dose-volume relation for side effects, similar to that for the boost, urges to limit the size of the CTV PBI, generally advised to a maximum of 30% of the whole breast CTV [9, 16]. An example of other dose constraints for target and OARs to be respected during PBI can be found in Table 20.1. If this cannot be achieved, also for women with small-sized breasts, we strongly advice to use the fractionation schedule of the FAST-Forward trial, being 26 Gy in 5 consecutive fractions, to avoid increased risks of side effects as seen for example with 38.5 Gy in 10 fractions over 5 days [10]. In patients who are

Table 20.1 Dose prescriptions, dose objectives for target volumes and dose constraints for organs at risk used in the Florence APBI trial [15], the IRMA APBI trial (ClinicalTrials.gov Identifier: NCT01803958) and the IMPORT-HIGH boost trial (ClinicalTrials.gov Identifier: NCT00818051). In IMPORT-HIGH, all patients receive 40 Gy/15 fr/3 weeks on the whole breast with three different boost modalities

Target/OAR	Florence APBI trial	IRMA APBI trial	IMPORT HIGH trial (SIB)
Schedule	30 Gy/5 fractions/2 weeks	38.5 Gy/10 fractions b.i.d./1 week	Sequential boost up to 56 Gy/23 fr/4.6 weeks
			SIB up to 48 Gy/15 fr/3 weeks
			SIB up to 53 Gy/15 fr/3 weeks
PTV	V95% ($V_{28.5Gy}$) ≥ 95%	V90% ($V_{34.65Gy}$) ≥ 90%	PTV_{TB}: V95% (45.6 Gy or 50.4 Gy) > 95%
	D_{max} < 110% prescribed dose (33 Gy)	D_{max} < 120% prescribed dose (46.2 Gy)	PTV_{TB}: D_{mean} = 48 Gy or 53 Gy
			PTV_{TB}: V107% (51.4 Gy or 56.7 Gy) < 3%
Ipsilateral breast	V_{15Gy} < 50%	$V_{19.25Gy}$ < 60%	NR
		$V_{38.5Gy}$ < 100%	NR
Contralateral breast	D_{max} < 1 Gy	D_{max} < 1.16 Gy	D_{mean} < 0.5 Gy
Ispilateral lung	V_{10Gy} < 20%	$V_{11.6Gy}$ < 15%	V_{18Gy} < 15%
Contralateral lung	V_{5Gy} < 10%	NR	$V_{2.5Gy}$ < 15%
Heart	V_{3Gy} < 10%	$V_{1.9Gy}$ < 5% (left-sided breast cancer)	V_{13Gy} < 10%
		D_{max} < 1.9 Gy (right-sided breast cancer)	
Thyroid gland	NR	D_{max} < 1.9 Gy (right-sided breast cancer)	NR

treated twice daily, which we discourage, it is important to respect the time-gap between fractions to allow for normal tissue recovery.

For boost irradiation, careful attention should be paid in case of an excessively large CTV boost that the equilibrium between benefits and side effects should be respected, realising that the benefits are only considerably large for the patients at highest risks for local recurrences. If the boost volume cannot be reduced sufficiently, omission of the boost or lowering of the boost volume are both reasonable options.

In case of SIB, the same principles as for a sequential boost apply, except that planning can be done with smaller leaf settings around the PTV since electronic equilibrium is already obtained by WBI. Therefore, reducing the high-dose volume within the breast outside the boost volume (see treatment planning section, Chap. 25).

20.5 Final considerations

As indicated above, the old practice to simply place the boost field or volume over the location of the surgical scar is completely outdated. Boost volumes should be determinded according to pre- and post-operative imaging and multidisciplinary clinical considerations. For that, optimal and direct communication between specialists can aid in a correct definiton and delineation of the CTV for both boost and PBI.

References

1. Fisher B, Anderson S, Bryant J, et al. Twenty-year follow up of a randomized trial comparing total mastectomy, lumpectomy and lumpectomy plus irradiation for the treatment of invasive breast cancer. N Engl J Med. 2002;347:1233–41.

2. Veronesi U, Cascinelli N, Mariani L, et al. Twenty-year follow-up of a randomized study comparing breast-conserving surgery with radical mastectomy for early breast cancer. N Engl J Med. 2002;347:1227–32.
3. Early Breast Cancer Trialists' Collaborative Group (EBCTCG), Darby S, McGale P, Correa C, et al. Effects of radiotherapy after breast-conserving surgery on 10-year recurrence and 15-year breast cancer death: meta-analysis of individual patient data for 10,801 women in 17 randomised trials. Lancet. 2011;378:1707–16.
4. Bartelink H, Maingon P, Poortmans P, et al. Whole-breast irradiation with or without a boost for patients treated with breast-conserving surgery for early breast cancer: 20-year follow up of a randomised phase 3 trial. Lancet Oncol. 2015;16:47–56.
5. Vrieling C, van Werkhoven E, Maingon P, et al. Prognostic factors for local control in breast cancer after long-term follow-up in the EORTC boost vs no boost trial: a randomized clinical trial. JAMA Oncol. 2017;1(3):42–8.
6. Poortmans PMP, Arenas M, Livi L. Over-irradiation. Breast. 2017;31:295–302.
7. Kindts I, Laenen A, Peeters S, Janssen H, Depuydt T, Neven P, Van Limbergen E, Weltens C. Evaluation of a breast cancer nomogram to predict ipsilateral breast relapse after breast-conserving therapy. Radiother Oncol. 2016;119:45–51.
8. Brouwers PJAM, van Werkhoven E, Bartelink H, et al. Predictors for poor cosmetic outcome in patients with early stage breast cancer treated with breast conserving therapy: results of the Young boost trial. Radiother Oncol. 2018;128:434–41.
9. Borger JH, Kemperman H, Smitt HS, Hart A, van Dongen J, Lebesque J, Bartelink H. Dose and volume effects on fibrosis after breast conservation therapy. Int J Radiat Oncol Biol Phys. 1994;30:1073–81.
10. Murray Brunt A, Haviland JS, et al. Hypofractionated breast radiotherapy for 1 week versus 3 weeks (FAST-Forward): 5-year efficacy and late normal tissue effects results from a multicentre, non-inferiority, randomised, phase 3 trial. Lancet. 2020;23(395):1613–26.
11. Kaidar-Person O, Meattini I, Zippel D, Poortmans P. Apples and oranges: comparing partial breast irradiation techniques. Rep Pract Oncol Radiother. 2020;25:780–2.
12. Fastner G, Gaisberger C, Kaiser J, Scherer P, et al. ESTRO IORT Task Force/ACROP recommendations for intraoperative radiation therapy with electrons (IOERT) in breast cancer. Radiother Oncol. 2020;149:150–7.
13. Polgar C, Ott OJ, Hildebrandt G, et al. Late side-effects and cosmetic results of accelerated partial breast irradiation with interstitial brachytherapy versus whole-breast irradiation after breast-conserving surgery for low-risk invasive and in-situ carcinoma of the female breast: 5-year results of a randomised, controlled, phase 3 trial. Lancet Oncol. 2017;18:259–68.
14. Coles CE, Griffin CL, Kirby AM, et al. Partial-breast radiotherapy after breast conservation surgery for patients with early breast cancer (UK IMPORT LOW trial): 5-year results from a multicentre, randomised, controlled, phase 3, non-inferiority trial. Lancet. 2017;390:1048–60.
15. Meattini I, Marrazzo L, Saieva C, et al. Accelerated partial-breast irradiation compared with whole-breast irradiation for early breast cancer: long-term results of the randomized phase III APBI-IMRT-florence trial. J Clin Oncol. 2020;38:4175–83.
16. Olivotto IA, Whelan TJ, Parpia S, Kim DH, Berrang T, Truong PT, et al. Interim cosmetic and toxicity results from RAPID: a randomized trial of accelerated partial breast irradiation using three-dimensional conformal external beam radiation therapy. J Clin Oncol. 2013;31:4038–45.
17. Bentzen SM, Yarnold JR. Reports of unexpected late side effects of accelerated partial breast irradiation--radiobiological considerations. Int J Radiat Oncol Biol Phys. 2010;77:969–73.
18. Holland R, Veling SH, Mravunac M, Hendriks JH. Histologic multifocality of Tis, T1-T2 breast carcinomas. Implications for clinical trials of breast-conserving surgery. Cancer. 1985;56:979–80.
19. Bartelink H, Bourgier C, Elkhuizen P. Has partial breast irradiation by IORT or brachytherapy been prematurely introduced into the clinic? Radiother Oncol. 2012;104:139–42.
20. Mannino M, Yarnold J. Effect of breast-duct anatomy and wound-healing responses on local tumor recurrence after primary surgery for early breast cancer. Lancet Oncol. 2009;10:425–9.
21. van Mourik AM, Elkhuizen PH, Minkema D, et al. Multiinstitutional study on target volume delineation variation in breast radiotherapy in the presence of guidelines. Radiother Oncol. 2010;94:286–91.
22. Strnad V, Hannoun-Levi JM, Guinot JL, et al. Recommendations from GEC ESTRO Breast Cancer Working Group (I): target definition and target delineation for accelerated or boost Partial Breast Irradiation using multicatheter interstitial brachytherapy after breast conserving closed cavity surgery. Radiother Oncol. 2015;115:342–8.
23. Arthur DW, Winter KA, Kuerer HM, et al. Effectiveness of breast-conserving surgery and 3-dimensional conformal partial breast reirradiation for recurrence of breast cancer in the ipsilateral breast: the NRG oncology/RTOG 1014 phase 2 clinical trial. JAMA Oncol. 2019;21(6):75–82.
24. Boersma LJ, Janssen T, Elkhuizen PH, et al. Reducing interobserver variation of boost-CTV delineation in breast conserving radiation therapy using a pre-operative CT and delineation guidelines. Radiother Oncol. 2012;103:178–82.
25. Garreffa E, Hughes-Davies L, Russell S, et al. Definition of tumor bed boost in oncoplastic breast surgery: an understanding and approach. Clin Breast Cancer. 2020;20:e510–5.
26. Verhoeven K, Peeters S, Erven K, et al. Boost delineation in breast radiation therapy: isotropic versus anisotropic margin expansion. Pract Radiat Oncol. 2016;6:e243–8.

27. Al Uwini S, Antonini N, Poortmans PM, et al. The influence of the use of CT-planning on the irradiated boost volume in breast conserving treatment. Radiother Oncol. 2009;93:87–93.
28. Kirby AM, Coles CE, Yarnold JR. Target volume definition for external partial breast radiotherapy: clinical, pathological and technical studies informing current approaches. Radiother Oncol. 2010;94:255–63.
29. Aznar MC, Meattini I, Poortmans P, Steyerova P, Wyld L. To clip or not to clip. That is no question! Eur J Surg Oncol. 2017;43:1145–7.
30. Verellen D, De Ridder M, Linthout N, et al. Innovations in image-guided radiotherapy. Nat Rev Cancer. 2007;7:949–60.

21 Chest Wall Bolus

Jean-Philippe Pignol and Hannah M. Dahn

21.1 Background

In 2001 and 2017 the American Society of Clinical Oncology (ASCO) published guidelines for postmastectomy radiation therapy (PMRT) [1, 2]. Initially it recommended PMRT for patients with four or more positive nodes, when tumours invaded the chest wall or the skin, for "inflammatory" tumours, and tumours larger than 5 cm in diameter with metastatic nodes. In 2017 the indications were extended to include patients with 1–3 nodes positive with significant additional risk factors like lympho-vascular infiltration, aggressive biological subtype, or poor response to primary systemic treatment [2]. Additional studies suggested that PMRT may be recommended when only positive sentinel lymph nodes have been removed and no further axillary clearance is done, and for patients having persistent nodal disease after primary systemic treatment [3]. Regarding the PMRT technique, the ASCO panel of experts concluded: "*adequately treating the chest wall is mandatory*" [1]. However, the PMRT protocol details were not clarified, notably the dose/fractionation regimen, the need of a boost, or the use of a skin bolus. Also, there was no clear definition of what is included in the chest wall, notably if the dermis should be included in the clinical target volume (CTV). There is also no precision on the dose constraints on various chest wall volumes and more precisely for the skin.

J.-P. Pignol · H. M. Dahn (✉)
Dalhousie University, Halifax, NS, Canada
e-mail: Jean-Philippe.Pignol@nshealth.ca; Hannah.dahn@dal.ca

21.2 Rationale of Skin Bolus

A skin bolus is a piece of soft tissue equivalent material placed on the skin surface to reduce the "skin sparing" effect when megavoltage photons are used to treat the chest wall. The skin sparing effect is due to the dose build-up as electrons are put into motion towards the depth of the tissue. A dose maximum is reached at the electronic equilibrium point, when as many electrons are put into motion as are stopped after releasing all their energy. In shifting the position of the maximum towards the skin surface, the main justification of skin bolus is to ensure adequate dose distribution in the skin to reduce the risk of chest wall local recurrence [4].

Calculating the dose on the skin surface with standard treatment planning software is imprecise since those algorithms cannot handle well the dose absorbed before the build-up. Recently Monajemi [5] reported doses measured with optically stimulated luminescence dosimeters (OSLD) and tissue equivalent Gafchromic EBT3 films placed behind 3, 5, or 10 mm of Superflab on a breast phantom. Monajemi compared those values with those calculated using a treatment

© The Author(s), under exclusive license to Springer Nature Switzerland AG 2022
O. Kaidar-Person et al. (eds.), *Breast Cancer Radiation Therapy*,
https://doi.org/10.1007/978-3-030-91170-6_21

planning system (TPS) based on an analytical anisotropic algorithm (AAA) calculation engine [5]. There was a relatively good agreement between measured and calculated dose. Interestingly, for a pair of parallel-opposed tangential beams there was no major differences between 3 mm and 5 mm, or 10 mm of skin bolus, enabling to dose the skin to 102%, 103%, and 107%, respectively. This was in clear contrast with measurement performed without bolus with a skin surface dose measured only at 64%. Out of note, there were significant variations in the measurements and the calculation of the skin surface dose: 64% with EBT3 films, 62% with bare OSL, 77% with jacketed OSLD, and 68% with the TPS using voxel sizes of 2 mm. From this work, it appears that the dose calculation and measurement appear more stable after 2–3 mm, which is the thickness of the dermis [5].

21.3 Evidence for the Use of Bolus

There are several single centre retrospective series reporting on the absence of skin bolus benefit on the reduction of local recurrence [6–10]. A first series included 254 patients who were treated with PMRT at the St George Hospital in Sydney between 1993 and 2003 [6, 7]. A total of 143 patients received radiotherapy with a 1 cm thick bolus applied daily on the whole chest wall, 88 patients had an eight cm large parascar bolus applied daily, and 23 patients had no bolus. Multivariate analysis showed that the use of bolus was significantly associated with early cessation of treatment. The presence of lympho-vascular infiltration and incomplete radiotherapy were associated with a higher risk of chest wall recurrence. A second series included 106 locally advanced breast cancer patients receiving PMRT at the Allegheny General Hospital in Pittsburgh between 2005 and 2015 [8]. Half were treated with bolus and the other half without. The clinical and pathological characteristics were similar between groups. There were seven recurrences in total, four in the bolus group and three in the no-bolus group. There was more acute skin toxicity in the bolus arm, leading to more treatment interruption (37.7% versus 5.6%). Patients with treatment interruption were more likely to fail (17.4% versus 3.6%, $p = 0.03$). The third series was a retrospective review of 314 patients treated at the Kent Oncology Centre in the UK between 2005 and 2010 [9]. Turner reported no difference in local recurrence, 1% in 101 patients treated with bolus and 1.8% in 213 patients treated without bolus. There was also no difference in median time to relapse or in overall survival. However, there was significant difference in patient's characteristics between the two groups, notably more patients had close margin in the bolus group. Finally, in 2021 Nichol reported on 1887 patients treated with bolus (1569 patients) or without bolus (318 patients) between 2007 and 2011 in British Columbia [10]. The decision regarding omission of bolus was left to the treating radiation oncologist. It was omitted in 51% of the 550 patients having breast reconstruction and 4% of the patients without reconstruction. At 10 years there was a 1% difference in chest wall local recurrence, 0.9% versus 1.9%, depending on if a skin bolus was used or not. In this series there were significantly more patients with advanced nodal disease ($p < 0.001$), high grade ($p = 0.006$), and positive lympho-vascular infiltration ($p = 0.02$) in the bolus arm. Those are all factors associated with a higher risk of local recurrence [11].

These studies present the same methodological limitations: They are underpowered to test the equivalence of PMRT with or without bolus, the follow-up is limited, and being retrospective and non-randomised the bolus arm generally includes more aggressive cancer characteristics. It is also not possible from those studies to identify a subgroup, if any, that may benefit from a skin bolus.

21.4 Bolus Toxicity

If there is little evidence of a skin bolus benefit for PMRT, there are several studies showing that a skin bolus increases dramatically the occurrence of painful and severe acute skin toxicities [6–9, 12]. A prospective cohort evaluating acute side effect experienced by 257 patients treated in

Toronto was reported in 2015 [12]. A large proportion of patients had severe grade 3 toxicities measured with the NCI CTCAE scale, including 28.4% extensive (grade 3) moist desquamation and 22.2% severe (grade 3) pain impacting on the activity of daily life. The use of bolus was the most important independent risk factor for severe toxicity on univariate and multivariate analysis. When used daily, 41% of the patients had extensive moist desquamation and 32% severe pain. When used on alternate days the occurrence of toxicity was halved, with 22% experiencing extensive moist desquamation and 15% severe pain. Without bolus, only 4.2% of the patients had severe pain and none had moist desquamation.

If radiation acute skin toxicities generally resolve within 1–2 weeks [13], there is little data available regarding the frequency of long-term and permanent side effect of bolus. But three studies have demonstrated significant correlations between acute and permanent side effects [12, 14, 15]. So it is logical to assume that reducing PMRT acute skin toxicity could reduce permanent long-term toxicities. In 1991 Bentzen reported on 229 Danish patients receiving PMRT that those who had moist desquamation doubled the risk of developing severe telangiectasia, from 22% to 47%, which impacts the cosmetic outcome and the health-related quality of life [14]. In 2007, Lilla reported on 416 patients receiving adjuvant radiotherapy after breast-conserving surgery, a similar doubling of telangiectasia and fibrosis occured when severe acute skin reactions were present [15]. In 2016, the 10 years outcome of 241 patients included in a randomised clinical trial of adjuvant breast IMRT radiotherapy was reported [12, 16]. On univariate and multivariate analyses, the occurrence of pain during RT was significantly associated with persistence of chronic pain. Moist desquamation was significantly associated with late subcutaneous fibrosis and telangiectasia. It is unknown if the use of PMRT with skin bolus may worsen long-term toxicity compared to PMRT without bolus, but a precautionary principle would suggest omitting it whenever possible.

21.5 Variability in the Use of Bolus

Without clear consensus from societies and the absence of level 1 evidence, it is not surprising that the use of skin bolus would vary heavily between centres and countries. In 2007 the results of a global survey of 1035 radiation oncologists from around the world were reported [17]. They showed large differences in the clinical indication, frequency, and thickness of bolus. The respondents from the Americas used skin bolus for PMRT "*always*" in 82% of the responses, compared to 31% in Europe and 65% in Australasia. In Europe 20% of interviewees would never use bolus and 49% would use it depending on various factors. This proportion was larger in southern Europe with 52% of the radiation oncologists in Italy never using bolus, 20% in France, 14% in Germany, 12.5% in the UK, and 10% in Scandinavia and The Netherlands. Those findings were confirmed by two additional surveys published both in 2017 [18, 19]. For Australia and New Zealand, Nguyen reported that 91% of the radiation oncologists used skin bolus; however, they largely disagree on the optimal frequency, daily or alternate days [18]. Also, in the UK, Davis showed that 53.5% of radiation oncologists always use bolus after mastectomy without reconstruction, but only 17% used it when an immediate reconstruction is performed after mastectomy. The author concluded that this was illogical since there is no rationale why a breast reconstruction would change the skin target volume, especially when the prosthesis is placed behind the fascia pectoralis [19].

21.6 Unresolved Questions

The use of bolus is often the source of hot debates between specialists, as for many topics where evidence is lacking and where decisions are based on judgement call. There are several areas where additional knowledge and research would be helpful.

21.6.1 Target Volume and Dose

If PMRT has an impact on the local recurrence rate and survival by preventing the secondary spread of microscopic disease [20–23], it remains unclear where the microscopic disease remains. In 1986 Erwin Fisher reported the pathology finding of breast local recurrence for 1108 patients included in the NSABP-B06 study and treated with surgery alone [24]. Local recurrence was a rare event, but out of 110 cases the recurrence was found confined in the breast tissue, close to the surgical cavity, in 95% of the cases. In only 5% of cases the recurrence involved the skin or the nipple and this was highly associated with the presence of lympho-vascular infiltration. This suggests that unless there is an aggressive biology, with either skin involvement or the presence of diffuse lympho-vascular infiltration, the target volume should be limited to the lymphatic network at the bottom of the dermis, about 3 mm in depth. This is in contradiction with the International Commission on Radiological Protection (ICRP) that recommends including the dermis superficial layers of interest as well as the basal cell layer at about 70 μm [25].

The other question concerns the dose needed to sterilise microscopic cancer clusters in the lymphatics. Traditionally, in breast loco-regional adjuvant radiotherapy, a lower dose is delivered to the regional nodes compared to the breast and the seroma, especially if a boost is recommended. It is therefore possible that the 64% of surface dose would be enough [5].

21.6.2 Reconstruction and Cosmetic Complications of Skin Bolus

It is noticeable that in Nichol's retrospective study [10] half of the radiation oncologists worried about long-term bolus toxicity and its impact on breast reconstructions, so they did not use it in half of the patients, while the other half of radiation oncologists systematically used it [10]. Davis showed the same trend in the UK [19]. In 2016, Brooks reported a series of 560 retrospective patients who had breast reconstruction after mastectomy [26]. Ninety-seven patients (13%) also received RT. Radiation therapy doubled the risk of complication, from 27.6% to 58.8%, and double the rate of major complication from 21.8% to 45.4%. Major complications were defined as requiring additional surgery. In the non-irradiated group 7.1% required a permanent removal of the implant, while in the irradiated group 19.6% required such removal. On univariate and multivariate analyses, radiotherapy was the strongest risk factor of reconstruction complication (OR = 4.99, $p < 0.001$). The potential impact of radiation toxicity on the cosmetic outcome and reconstruction failure using skin bolus is unknown. There is unfortunately no data, and it is unknown if avoiding skin bolus to prevent moist desquamation and possibly long-term fibrosis may improve the rate of breast reconstruction success [27].

21.6.3 Absolute Benefit of Bolus

While there is no evidence for or against the use of a skin bolus, it may be possible to bracket the risk. There is a consensus that the modern risk of local relapse after PMRT is low, 3.5% without radiotherapy and 3% with [11]. This means that for the population of patients receiving PMRT the benefit of a bolus, increasing the dose to the first 3 mm from 63% to 85% or 90%, would be a fraction of 0.5% risk of local recurrence. Even without level 1 evidence it is hard to accept the dire skin side effect and pain for an unknown and likely very narrow benefit. The challenge is to define the ~5% of patients following the Fisher analysis that are at higher risk of true skin recurrence [24]. This might better be addressed by a consensus conference than a clinical trial [28, 29].

21.7 Summary

As indicated elsewhere in this book, ESTRO delineation guidelines for breast cancer published in 2015 and 2016, and later for immediate reconstruction in 2019, clearly state that if there is no evidence for skin involvement (T4), the skin is not considered as part of CTV_chest wall. This review suggests that in the absence of strong clinical evidence there is little justification for using a bolus outside of aggressive biology, namely extensive lympho-vascular infiltration and/or skin infiltration. Using bolus on alternate days halves the acute toxicity and a 3–5 mm tissue equivalent bolus might be enough.

References

1. Recht A, Edge SB, Solin LJ, et al. American Society of Clinical Oncology. Postmastectomy radiotherapy: guidelines of the American society of clinical oncology. J Clin Oncol. 2001;19:1539–69.
2. Recht A, Comen EA, Fine RE, et al. Postmastectomy radiotherapy: an American Society of Clinical Oncology, American Society for Radiation Oncology, and Society of Surgical Oncology focused guideline update. Ann Surg Oncol. 2017;24:38–51.
3. McBride A, Allen P, Woodward W, et al. Locoregional recurrence risk for patients with $T_{1,2}$ breast cancer with 1-3 positive lymph nodes treated with mastectomy and systemic treatment. Int J Radiat Oncol Biol Phys. 2014;89:392–8.
4. Andic F, Ors Y, Davutoglu R, et al. Evaluation of skin dose associated with different frequencies of bolus applications in post-mastectomy three-dimensional conformal radiotherapy. J Exper Clin Cancer Res. 2009;28:41.
5. Monajemi TT, Oliver PAK, Day A, et al. In search of a one plan solution for VMAT post-mastectomy chest wall irradiation. J Appl Clin Med Phys. 2020;21:216–23.
6. Cheng SH, Jian JJ, Chan KY, et al. The benefit and risk of postmastectomy radiation therapy in patients with high-risk breast cancer. Am J Clin Oncol. 1998;21:12–7.
7. Tieu MT, Graham P, Browne L, et al. The effect of adjuvant postmastectomy radiotherapy bolus technique on local recurrence. Int J Radiat Oncol Biol Phys. 2011;81:165–71.
8. Abel S, Renz P, Trombetta M, et al. Local failure and acute radiodermatological toxicity in patients undergoing radiation therapy with and without postmastectomy chest wall bolus: is bolus ever necessary? Pract Radiat Oncol. 2017;7:167–72.
9. Turner JY, Zeniou A, Williams A, et al. Technique and outcome of post-mastectomy adjuvant chest wall radiotherapy-the role of tissue-equivalent bolus in reducing risk of local recurrence. Br J Radiol. 2016;89:20160060.
10. Nichol A, Narinesingh D, Raman S, et al. The effect of bolus on local control for patients treated with mastectomy and radiotherapy. Int J Radiat Oncol Biol Phys. 2021;110:1360. https://doi.org/10.1016/j.ijrobp.2021.01.019.
11. Aalders KC, van Bommel AC, van Dalen T, et al. Contemporary risks of local and regional recurrence and contralateral breast cancer in patients treated for primary breast cancer. Eur J Cancer. 2016;63:118–26.
12. Pignol JP, Vu TT, Mitera G, et al. Occurrence of severe skin side effects and pain during post-mastectomy radiation therapy – a prospective cohort evaluation of patient and treatment factors. Int J Radiat Oncol Biol Phys. 2014;91:157–64.
13. Pignol JP, Olivotto I, Rakovitch E, et al. A multicenter randomized trial of breast intensity-modulated radiation therapy to reduce acute radiation dermatitis. J Clin Oncol. 2008;26:2085–92.
14. Bentzen SM, Overgaard M. Relationship between early and late normal-tissue injury after postmastectomy radiotherapy. Radiother Oncol. 1991;20:159–65.
15. Lilla C, Ambrosone CB, Kropp S, et al. Predictive factors of late normal tissue complications following radiotherapy for breast cancer. Breast Cancer Res Treat. 2007;106:143–50.
16. Pignol JP, Truong P, Rakovitch E, et al. Ten years results of the Canadian breast intensity modulated radiation therapy (IMRT) randomized controlled trial. Radiother Oncol. 2016;121(3):414–9.
17. Vu TTT, Pignol JP, Rakovitch E, et al. Variability in radiation oncologists' opinion on the indication of a bolus in post-mastectomy radiotherapy: an international survey. Clin Oncol. 2007;19:115–9.
18. Nguyen K, Mackenzie P, Allen A, et al. Breast interest group faculty of radiation oncology: Australian and New Zealand patterns of practice survey on breast radiotherapy. J Med Imaging Radiat Oncol. 2017;61:508–16.
19. Davis N, Jyothirmayi R. A nationwide survey of UK oncologists' views on the choice of radiotherapy regime for the reconstructed chest wall in breast cancer patients. Int J Breast Cancer. 2017;2017:6385432.
20. Hellman S. Stopping metastases at their source. N Engl J Med. 1997;337:996–7.
21. Ragaz J, Jackson SM, Le N, et al. Adjuvant radiotherapy and chemotherapy in node-positive premenopausal women with breast cancer. N Engl J Med. 1997;337:956–62.
22. Overgaard M, Hansen PS, Overgaard J, et al. Postoperative radiotherapy in high-risk premenopausal women with breast cancer who receive adjuvant chemotherapy. Danish Breast Cancer Cooperative Group 82b Trial. N Engl J Med. 1997;337:949–55.
23. Overgaard M, Jensen MB, Overgaard J, et al. Postoperative radiotherapy in high-risk postmenopausal breast-cancer patients given adjuvant tamoxifen: Danish Breast Cancer Cooperative Group DBCG 82c randomised trial. Lancet. 1999;353:1641–8.
24. Fisher ER, Sass R, Fisher B, et al. Pathologic findings from the National Surgical Adjuvant Breast Project (protocol 6). II. Relation of local breast recurrence to multicentricity. Cancer. 1986;57:1717–24.
25. International Commission on Radiological Protection. The Biological Basis for Dose Limitation in the Skin. ICRP Publication 59. Stockholm: ICRP; 1992.

26. Brooks S, Djohan R, Tendulkar R, et al. Risk factors for complications of radiation therapy on tissue expander breast reconstructions. Breast J. 2012;18:28–34.
27. Archambeau JO, Pezner R, Wasserman T. Pathophysiology of irradiated skin and breast. Int J Radiat Oncol Biol Phys. 1995;31:1171–85.
28. Kaidar-Person O, Dahn HM, Nichol AM, et al. A Delphi study and International Consensus Recommendations: The use of bolus in the setting of postmastectomy radiation therapy for early breast cancer. Radiotherapy and oncology : journal of the European Society for Therapeutic Radiology and Oncology. 2021;164:115–21.
29. Dahn HM, Boersma LJ, de Ruysscher D, et al. The use of bolus in postmastectomy radiation therapy for breast cancer: A systematic review. Crit Rev Oncol Hematol. 2021;163:103391.

Part V

Treatment Planning

Treatment Planning Including Dose Calculation

22

Henrik D. Nissen and Sandra Hol

22.1 Dose calculation

Dose calculation and validation for radiotherapy (RT) treatment planning is a wide and complex subject, and a detailed examination is well beyond the scope of the present work. Here we focus our discussion on a few points that are of particular interest for treatment planning for breast cancer patients, both for the individual plans and for comparing plans made with different treatment planning systems (TPS).

22.1.1 Past

Pencil beam (PB) algorithms are an older technique for dose calculation. They should no longer be used clinically for breast cancer patients, as they have significant deviations from measured dose in or near low density tissue like the lung. However, they have been used extensively until about 10 years ago and thus form a significant part of the calculated doses in clinical studies with long-term follow-up presented in the last decades and even up to today. For tangential treatment, PB overestimates dose to the lung inside the treatment field compared to modern algorithms, while doses outside the field are underestimated (Fig. 22.1). This has implications for the representation of the high dose region of the heart as well as the thoracic wall close to the lung, where calculated dose may be overestimated.

22.1.2 Present

Modern dose calculation algorithms (e.g. collapsed cone convolution type, AAA or Acuros XB) come close to measured data. There exist however still differences between the algorithms. Even when using measurements from the same linear accelerator to model the beam data, the resulting calculated dose distributions from a specific treatment plan with fixed monitor units (MU) (so keeping the actual physical dose delivered during treatment the same) may have mean or median doses vary in the order of 1–2% [1], and there are also relative differences in how dose is calculated in the lung and near the skin, as may be seen in Fig. 22.2. Variations may even be larger in smaller volumes, depending on how well beam data is modelled by the TPS and the details of the algorithm. This is especially relevant in low density tissue and on tissue-air/lung interfaces and should be kept in mind when comparing OAR doses between systems. Target doses will typically be normalised near the prescribed dose, so

H. D. Nissen (✉)
Department of Oncology, Vejle Hospital, Vejle, Denmark
e-mail: henrik.dahl.nissen@rsyd.dk

S. Hol
Instituut Verbeeten, Tilburg, The Netherlands
e-mail: hol.s@bvi.nl

© The Author(s), under exclusive license to Springer Nature Switzerland AG 2022
O. Kaidar-Person et al. (eds.), *Breast Cancer Radiation Therapy*,
https://doi.org/10.1007/978-3-030-91170-6_22

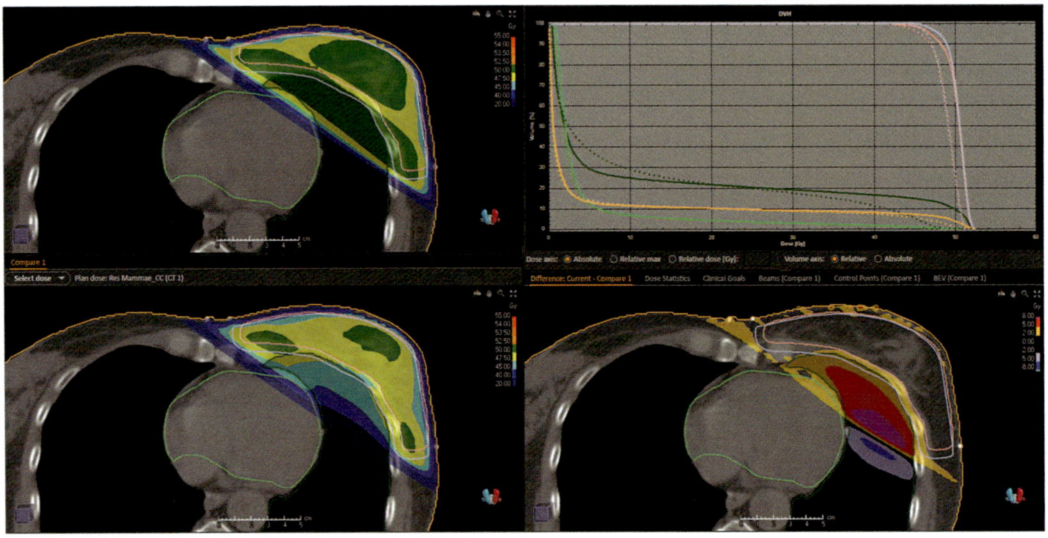

Fig. 22.1 Breast treatment plan calculated using a pencil beam algorithm (top-left) and a collapsed cone algorithm (bottom left). Both algorithms are from the Oncentra Masterplan TPS. Monitor units were kept fixed between recalculations, and both algorithms were optimised for clinical use on the same accelerator (i.e. the same physical dose would be delivered to the patient from both plans). The difference image (bottom-right) highlights the differences, and the DVH (top-right) shows the differences for the CTVp_breast (red), CTVn_IMN (blue), Lung (dark green), LAD (white), and Heart (light green)

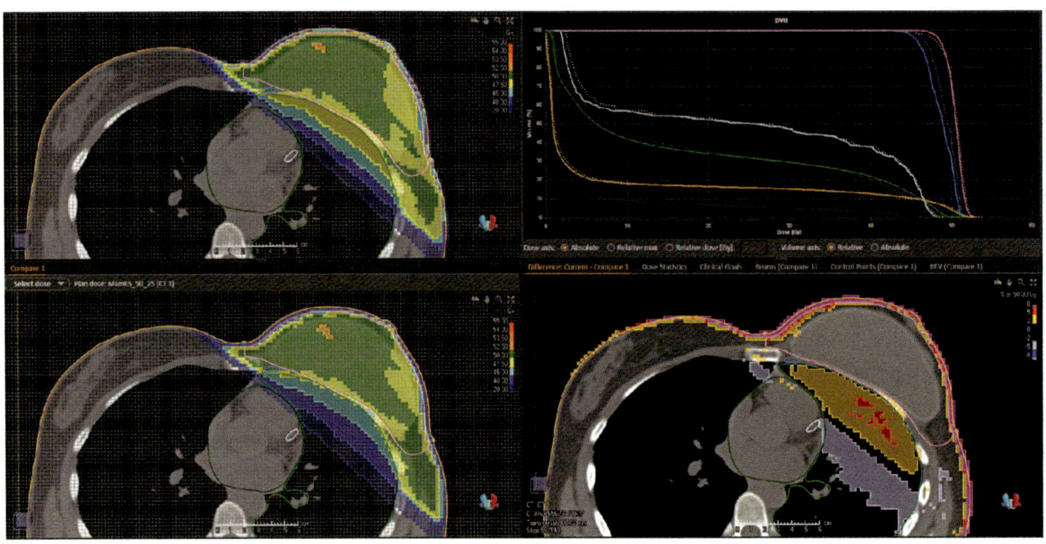

Fig. 22.2 Breast treatment plan calculated using two different implementations of a collapsed cone algorithm. Top-left is a collapsed cone algorithm using dose-to-water from RayStation (version 8.0.1, RaySearch Laboratories, Sweden) and bottom left is a collapsed cone algorithm using dose-to-medium from Oncentra Masterplan (version 4.3.0, Elekta, Sweden). The square grid shows the dose calculation grid, illustrating how variations in placement of the dose grid may affect especially skin dose. Doses are scaled to have the same average dose to CTVp_breast to better illustrate the relative differences in dose distribution in the lung and skin. The DVH (top-right) shows the differences for the CTVp_breast (red), CTVn_IMN (blue), Lung (light green), LAD (white), and Heart (dark green)

reported doses there will be similar, while in contrast the relative differences between lung dose may be clear for high dose regions, with lower doses being not strongly affected. Differences are also present in the dose build-up region near the skin (Fig. 22.2), with the difference between two collapsed cone algorithms being 10–20% in the first few mm in the present example, consistent with results from the literature [2, 3].

It is necessary to study the specific literature on a given TPS and dose calculation algorithm, to learn how a given system handles dose build-up compared to measurements. In the skin, dose calculation is very challenging due to the algorithms not fully handling the physics in this region as well as the finite voxel size leading to even more variations as the skin surface curves (Fig. 22.2). However, from about 4 mm below the skin surface, depending on the algorithm, the calculated doses with modern algorithms can be considered pretty accurate, with better precision near the skin with newer algorithms, especially Acuros XB and finer dose calculation grid [2, 4, 5]. Dose to the skin is often underestimated, so the calculated dose may be considered a lower limit for actual dose [3]. One study suggests that dose calculation accuracy near the skin can be increased by expanding body outline, to reduce the uncertainty related to boundary uncertainties [2]. However, for most patients the skin itself is not part of the CTV, so that should be cropped to underneath the skin while for dose (not volume) optimisation, even the PTV can be cropped to up to 5 mm underneath the skin. In case of involvement of the skin, where a high and well-documented dose is desired, bolus should be applied, both to create sufficient build-up and to shift the uncertainty of dose calculations out of the patient.

Out of field dose is a particular concern for breast cancer RT, as this relates to the risk of inducing heart disease or secondary cancers. In general, the TPS is not commissioned to calculate doses far outside the field border, and often dose is underestimated outside the field, with differences of up to 30% of local dose 3 cm outside the irradiated volume [6]. Mean doses are typically more reliable for OAR that are extending not too far from the irradiated volume, and where a significant part of the dose is delivered in smaller high dose volumes. For breast cancers, this means that mean heart dose is likely fairly reliable, but mean dose to contralateral breast and lung can be unreliable, even if dose to the parts closest to the treated breast is in-field and thus reliable. For a detailed discussion of out of field doses, the reader is referred to the AAPM task group 158 report [6].

22.1.3 (Near) Future

Monte Carlo dose calculation algorithms are considered the most exact method for dose calculations. These algorithms have been available for a long time and have shown excellent correlation with dosimetric measurements, but calculation times have been prohibitively long, making them unfit for routine clinical use. This is however changing, and Monte Carlo algorithms are already available in some commercial TPS. They have not seen extensive use in breast cancer patients yet, but in principle, they can perform more precise dose calculations not only in the breast and lung, but also in the surface region and outside the irradiated volumes.

22.2 3DCRT Tangential Treatment Planning

RT treatment planning for breast cancer has a long history, going back more than 50 years and current evidence for the benefits—and risks—of breast cancer RT, as described elsewhere in this book, are largely based on the tangential field technique. Since the turn of the millennium, CT-based conformal photon RT, generally using a similar tangential field set-up, has become the standard. In this section, we will focus on tangential fields for treating the breast, leaving loco-regional irradiation covering the axilla and supraclavicular regions and the internal mammary nodes to subsequent sections. We will also focus on patients in supine position as this is the most common, but general principles apply equally to patients in prone and lateral position. Alternative patient position is discussed in the chapter on patient positioning.

The main characteristic of the tangential technique is the use of opposed treatment fields, angled to include as much of the breast PTV as possible, while minimising the amount of lung and heart inside the field. The field borders inside the body are aligned as closely as possible to create a sharp penumbra of the beam and a strong dose fall-off gradient moving dorso-laterally away from the beam.

Before making treatment plans, it is necessary to have a set of dosimetric objectives for target volumes and constraints for OARs, defining what is considered a good treatment plan. These goals should be based on available evidence from relevant trials demonstrating tumour control for a given target coverage as well as studies examining NTCP and dose response for OAR. Organs at risk are discussed in Chap. 38 on techniques to reduce OAR dose and a review was recently published [7]. A common requirement for target coverage is at least 95% of the breast target volume should be covered by at least 95% of the prescribed dose. This is based on experience from both clinical practice and trials [8, 9]. For tumour bed boost the typical requirement is nearly full (98–100%) coverage with 95% of prescribed dose. For nodal targets the required dose is often a little lower at 85–90% of prescribed dose but the dose coverage should still be at least 95% of the target volume, but may depend on the balance between disease control and dose to OAR. In patients with advance nodal disease and high risk for residual subclinical nodal disease in the inoperable axilla levels, a high dose coverage is recommended. High dose volumes and dose inhomogeneity in the target volume are correlated to poorer cosmetic outcome after the treatment [10]. High dose volumes can be kept below 105–107% of prescribed dose in most cases, allowing up to 110% only in very small volumes. At this level of high dose volumes, radiation induced late effects in the breast can be kept at a low and acceptable rate [9, 11, 12].

Organs at risk dose constraints are available from many different sources, and there is significant heterogeneity in the constraints used in different publications. The main concerns regarding dose to OARs during treatment planning are dose to the heart (risk of cardiac events) [13], the lung (secondary cancers and RT-related pneumonitis) and, especially for younger patients, the contralateral breast (secondary cancers). For boost treatments dose to the brachial plexus should also be considered.

There are no known lower limits for these OAR, below which the dose can be considered safe, but local guidelines should be set based on what is considered an acceptable risk given the overall survival gains of RT for breast cancer. Such guidelines are available online from various societies, e.g. the Danish Breast Cancer Cooperative Group (DBCG) [14] or the American Society for Radiation Oncology (ASTRO) [8]. Guidelines should regularly be updated to take into account new knowledge of late effects and should be adapted if technical progress allows.

The first step to generating a good treatment plan lies in the definition of the target volume to be treated, the CTV. There are two main methods in use for defining the breast CTV. The older, derived from conventional-simulator based treatment set-up defines treatment fields based on anatomical fixed points like the mid-sternal and mid-axillary lines. Nowadays, anatomically based guidelines for target delineation like the ESTRO consensus guidelines [15] (see also Chap. 19 on Target volume definition and contouring) bring breast cancer RT planning to the level of most other tumour sites. For a recent comparison of delineation guidelines see sections about Target volume definition and contouring and section about Lymph node volumes (Chaps. 19 and 44) and the publication by Gee et al., [16]. From a treatment planning point of view, the choice of delineation guideline will affect the treatment plans from a fundamental point of view: the conventional set-up starts from the field that can afterwards be adjusted to some extent, while the anatomically based set-up starts from target volumes without predefining any field set-up, but differences between anatomically based guideline target definitions will also affect final field set-up. At the end, when using 3D-CRT, basically targets are defined slightly differently, which leads to slightly different placement of fields, which again will affect dose to organs at risk, especially the heart. From a dose reporting and quality assurance point of view, there is a clear advantage in selecting a guideline where targets are delineated, and delineation should be done before considering field placement, so the target volumes are based on intent-to-treat rather than ability-to-treat. For the individual patient this will not make a difference to the final treatment plan, which should always be optimised to achieve the best compromise between target coverage and OAR dose for the individual case, but for keeping track of changes in target coverage or OAR doses over time as techniques change, this is very important, as it allows quatifying the dose distribution including compromised target coverage due to OAR sparing modifications. This quantification is necessary, to be able to compare to, learn from and apply results from publications from other institutions on breast cancer treatment planning techniques. A corollary to this is that the quality of the delineations is important, and internal test cases should be delineated with intervals to maintain intra-institution consistency as well as consistency with guidelines, but even more importantly, the integrity of a delineation should be maintained. If a delineation is found to have errors when reviewed by other staff, it must of course be corrected, but this should be a fairly rare event among trained staff. However, if the delineation, the intended target, cannot be adequately covered with dose due to constraints on OAR doses, going back and reducing the original extent of the target delineation to achieve acceptable coverage should not be allowed, but rather it should simply be noted that optimal target coverage is not possible for the case, and the planning team should decide on how to compromise on target coverage or OAR dose to achieve the best result (or compromise) in the particular case.

Once the target is defined, a margin is added to the CTV. This is the PTV, which is a site-specific margin depending on fixation equipment and daily imaging technique to account for random and systematic errors in the positioning of the patient for daily treatment. This margin ensures the planned dose to the CTV is achieved even though the patient is not positioned perfectly every day. Typical PTV margins are 5–10 mm.

With the PTV defined, the medial border of the tangential fields for a typical patient anatomy is determined almost exclusively by two points: the medial and lateral part of the PTV closest to the thoracic wall. The field border then mostly determines low and medium (up to ~70% of prescribed dose) dose to the heart and lung for standard tangential treatment fields, allowing a first estimate of whether target coverage can be achieved while still observing the OAR dose constraints. The outer field border is usually expanded ~2–3 cm out from the PTV to include the air above the breast. This ensures a certain amount of robustness against anatomical changes of the patient outline due to, e.g. swelling of the breast or the appearance or disappearance of seroma in the breast.

Today CT-based, multi-field (often referred to as field-in-field (FiF) or forward planned IMRT) treatment plans should be considered the standard for tangential planning to achieve a homogeneous dose distribution. With the main fields defined by the PTV and scaled to deliver a dose close to the prescribed dose, the basic technique is to use wedged fields and/or subfields (manually adapted fields shielding part of the target, equivalent to segments in a step-and-shoot IMRT plan) to achieve a homogeneous dose distribution in the target. Depending on the shape and size of the target, the number of fields needed will increase to achieve better homogeneity and target coverage. While this is advantageous, it comes at the price of increased planning and treatment time.

Planning time may be reduced by using a hybrid technique, where about 80% of the prescribed dose is delivered with open fields and IMRT or VMAT is used to plan the remaining dose to ensure homogeneity, or by doing tangential VMAT or IMRT, where the field angles are limited to the angles also used for conformal tangential plans. When doing fully inverse optimised plans, they will often be more modulated than FiF plans, and it is necessary to consider how robust the specific technique will be to changes, e.g. swelling, affecting the body outline of the patient.

The dose should as a rule of thumb be delivered with the lowest beam energy available and preferably below ~10 MV to minimise neutron contamination, which occurs at higher beam energies. For large breast volumes the addition of higher energy beams might however have advantages, as they can significantly improve dose homogeneity.

Beyond the guidelines for indications, target volume definition and dose objectives, and OAR dose constraints, it is necessary to take into account patient-specific risk factors. The guidelines should be set up to handle most cases, but when all demands cannot be met or if there are special circumstances, these should be discussed within the planning team before or early in the treatment planning process. If guideline criteria cannot be met, there are standard strategies to explore initially: deep-inspiration breath hold is discussed in the section about techniques to reduce OAR dose. More advanced planning techniques like IMRT/VMAT or protons should be considered for their dose shaping abilities and, finally, compromising target coverage is a solution for some cases, depending on the location of the tumour bed and the tumour biology (see Chap. 24 about challenging anatomy and Chap. 39 about particle therapy). Aside from guideline deviations, these strategies should also be considered if there are specific risk factors, e.g. pre-existing heart or lung conditions—especially in conjunction with smoking [17], young age, or previous RT treatment in the area, which may necessitate increased demands on dose reduction to OAR.

For the particular case of a pacemaker or ICD in the field, it is often possible to have it moved to the contralateral side, but even then, special care should be taken to minimise neutron contamination (use low energy beams, <10 MV) and efforts should be made to minimise dose to the ICD or pacemaker, preferably keeping it below 2 Gy, although dose calculation from treatment planning systems are generally unreliable and underestimating dose far from the field edge [18].

Partial breast irradiation (PBI) is an evidence-based approach to reducing target volumes, which then results in reduced OAR dose [19]. The standard approach for treatment planning is the same tangential technique used for whole breast irradiation (WBI) just adapted to the smaller target volume. The net effect is that problems with OAR dose limits are exceedingly rare for these patients. The main considerations in planning these patients is the choice of beam angles, as the small target may allow for, e.g. almost anterior-posterior beams for a lateral target. While the atypical beam angle will minimise lung dose, it may also cause dose deposition in regions posteriorly to the target, that are not normally irradiated in standard breast cancer RT, and therefore there is limited experience with the risk of side effects. In such cases it may be a preferable solution to angle the beams more like a standard whole breast treatment plan, to keep the high dose volume inside the breast, even if the plan becomes less conformal, as here we have well established evidence for effect and no harm and let the OAR sparing be primarily from the reduced cranio-caudal extent. This should be discussed in the treatment planning team and noted in the department guidelines. A second, more complex approach strives for a more conformal dose around the PTV, for which non-coplanar beams, IMRT and VMAT can be used. The advantage of this approach is a decreased dose to the non-target breast tissue and a decreased volume that receives a significant dose, while the drawback is that lower dose volumes can be spread more in volumes that would receive no dose with the standard approach and where there is limited evidence for the long-term effects of low-dose irradiation. While the standard approach is safe and easy to apply for especially larger target volumes, the more complex approach could be preferable for smaller target volumes and when very intense dose prescriptions are used.

Boost planning can be divided into sequential boost and simultaneous integrated boost (SIB). Sequential boost planning is technically quite similar to PBI planning, especially the more advanced approach. Indeed, the above argument for keeping the high dose inside the breast is now reversed: where before the concern was giving a high dose to an area, which is not commonly irradiated to this dose, the concern in a boost is the cumulative effect of the combined effect of the primary treatment and the boost giving a worse cosmetic outcome [20]. Therefore, in the boost setting it is preferably to prioritise dose conformity around the boost target, to reduce the size of the high dose volume, even at the cost of irradiating from atypical angles. The same arguments apply for the SIB plans, but here the difference is often less pronounced, because dose gradients can be made sharper when the primary treatment and the boost are planned simultaneous. A special consideration when making SIB plans is whether to make the SIB as an add-on to the primary plan, by adding a few extra fields, or if the SIB is fully integrated in the plan, so any field may potentially contribute to the SIB dose. The advantage of the latter approach is that it will typically require fewer treatment fields in total, as there is no need to potentially remove hotspots from a region just to add a boost dose afterwards. The disadvantage comes into play, when a patient turns out to be difficult to position for the daily treatments, perhaps due to a large breast volume. In some exceptional cases, it can be difficult to find a position where both the whole breast and the boost volume are in an acceptable position for treatment. Here the first approach will allow a simple separation of the plan into a whole breast treatment and if necessary renewed imaging and repositioning to ensure optimal coverage of both the full breast and the boost volume.

22.3 Summary

Tangential treatment planning for breast cancer should be CT-based using multiple fields or fluency to ensure dose homogeneity. It is important to have consistently defined structures for planning and dose reporting to be able to track plan quality over time and be able to compare to data in the literature. Dose calculation with modern algorithms is generally reliable, but near-skin dose is still associated with significant uncertainties. Individual patients may have additional risk factors, which must be taken into account to make an optimal and individualised treatment plan.

References

1. Guebert A, Conroy L, Weppler S, et al. Clinical implementation of AXB from AAA for breast: plan quality and subvolume analysis. J Appl Clin Med Phys. 2018;19(3):243–50. https://doi.org/10.1002/acm2.12329.
2. Wang L, Cmelak AJ, Ding GX. A simple technique to improve calculated skin dose accuracy in a commercial treatment planning system. J Appl Clin Med Phys. 2018;19(2):191–7. https://doi.org/10.1002/acm2.12275.
3. Court LE, Tishler R, Xiang H, Allen AM, Makrigiorgos M, Chin L. Experimental evaluation of the accuracy of skin dose calculation for a commercial treatment planning system. J Appl Clin Med Phys. 2008;9(1):2792. https://doi.org/10.1120/jacmp.v9i1.2792.
4. Akino Y, Das IJ, Bartlett GK, Zhang H, Thompson E, Zook JE. Evaluation of superficial dosimetry between treatment planning system and measurement for several breast cancer treatment techniques. Med Phys. 2013;40(1):011714. https://doi.org/10.1118/1.4770285.
5. Hoffmann L, Alber M, Söhn M, Elstrøm UV. Validation of the Acuros XB dose calculation algorithm versus Monte Carlo for clinical treatment plans. Med Phys. 2018; https://doi.org/10.1002/mp.13053.
6. Kry SF, Bednarz B, Howell RM, et al. AAPM TG 158: measurement and calculation of doses outside the treated volume from external-beam radiation therapy. Med Phys. 2017;44(10):e391–429. https://doi.org/10.1002/mp.12462.
7. Wright JL. Toxicities of radiation treatment for breast cancer. New York, NY: Springer; 2019. ISBN 9783030116200.
8. Smith BD, Bellon JR, Blitzblau R, et al. Radiation therapy for the whole breast: executive summary of an American Society for Radiation Oncology (ASTRO) evidence-based guideline. Pract Radiat Oncol. 2018;8(3):145–52. https://doi.org/10.1016/j.prro.2018.01.012.
9. Thomsen MS, Berg M, Zimmermann S, Lutz CM, Makocki S, Jensen I, Hjelstuen MHB, Pensold S, Hasler MP, Jensen M-B, Offersen BV (2021) Dose constraints for whole breast radiation therapy based on the quality assessment of treatment plans in the randomised Danish breast cancer group (DBCG) HYPO trial. Clinical and Translational Radiation Oncology 28118–123 https://doi.org/10.1016/j.ctro.2021.03.009.
10. Mukesh MB, Barnett GC, Wilkinson JS, et al. Randomized controlled trial of intensity-modulated

radiotherapy for early breast cancer: 5-year results confirm superior overall cosmesis. J Clin Oncol. 2013;31(36):4488–95. https://doi.org/10.1200/JCO.2013.49.7842.
11. Offersen BV, Alsner J, Nielsen HM, et al. Hypofractionated versus standard fractionated radiotherapy in patients with early breast cancer or ductal carcinoma in situ in a randomized phase III trial: the DBCG HYPO trial. J Clin Oncol. 2020;38(31):3615–25. https://doi.org/10.1200/JCO.20.01363.
12. Coles CE, Griffin CL, Kirby AM, et al. Partial-breast radiotherapy after breast conservation surgery for patients with early breast cancer (UK IMPORT LOW trial): 5-year results from a multicentre, randomised, controlled, phase 3, non-inferiority trial. Lancet. 2017;390(10099):1048–60. https://doi.org/10.1016/S0140-6736(17)31145-5.
13. Laugaard Lorenzen E, Christian Rehammar J, Jensen MB, Ewertz M, Brink C. Radiation-induced risk of ischemic heart disease following breast cancer radiotherapy in Denmark, 1977-2005. Radiother Oncol. 2020;152:103–10. https://doi.org/10.1016/j.radonc.2020.08.007.
14. DBCG. National guideline for Radiotherapy; n.d.. https://www.dbcg.dk/.
15. Birgitte V, Offersen Liesbeth J, Boersma Carine, Kirkove Sandra, Hol Marianne C, Aznar Albert Biete, Sola Youlia M, Kirova Jean-Philippe, Pignol Vincent, Remouchamps Karolien, Verhoeven Caroline, Weltens Meritxell, Arenas Dorota, Gabrys Neil, Kopek Mechthild, Krause Dan, Lundstedt Tanja, Marinko Angel, Montero John, Yarnold Philip, Poortmans (2016) ESTRO consensus guideline on target volume delineation for elective radiation therapy of early stage breast cancer version 1.1. Radiother Oncol. 118(1):205–8. https://doi.org/10.1016/j.radonc.2015.12.027.
16. Gee HE, Moses L, Stuart K, et al. Contouring consensus guidelines in breast cancer radiotherapy: comparison and systematic review of patterns of failure. J Med Imaging Radiat Oncol. 2019;63(1):102–15. https://doi.org/10.1111/1754-9485.12804.
17. Taylor C, Correa C, Duane FK, et al. Estimating the risks of breast cancer radiotherapy: evidence from modern radiation doses to the lungs and heart and from previous randomized trials. J Clin Oncol. 2017;35(15):1641–9. https://doi.org/10.1200/JCO.2016.72.0722.
18. Miften M, Mihailidis D, Kry SF, et al. Management of radiotherapy patients with implanted cardiac pacemakers and defibrillators: a report of the AAPM TG-203[†]. Med Phys. 2019;46(12):e757–88. https://doi.org/10.1002/mp.13838. PMID: 31571229.
19. Haussmann J, Budach W, Corradini S, et al. No difference in overall survival and non-breast cancer deaths after partial breast radiotherapy compared to whole breast radiotherapy-a meta-analysis of randomized trials. Cancers (Basel). 2020;12(8):2309. https://doi.org/10.3390/cancers12082309.
20. Brouwers PJAM, van Werkhoven E, Bartelink H, et al. Predictors for poor cosmetic outcome in patients with early stage breast cancer treated with breast conserving therapy: results of the young boost trial. Radiother Oncol. 2018;128(3):434–41. https://doi.org/10.1016/j.radonc.2018.06.020.

23 Treatment Planning for Breast/Chest Wall and Regional Lymph Nodes Including the Internal Mammary Chain

Sandra Hol and Isabelle Mollaert

23.1 From 2D to Hybrid VMAT

Historically, two-dimensional (2D) radiation treatment preparation was based on setups using a conventional X-ray simulator. The field arrangement, the geometries, and positions were set during simulation based on fluoroscopy and planar radiographs. Treatment calculation was performed initially just at midline or in a single plane at the central axis of the breast, followed by several manually made slides and later on a couple of slides generated with a CT-extension mounted to the conventional simulator. The transition to three-dimensional (3D) imaging allowed full 3D dose calculation of whole breast irradiation. 3D conformal radiation therapy (3D-CRT) based on a tangential beam arrangement has been stepwise developed adding various methods, such as multileaf collimator (MLC) positioning, beam weight optimisation, different beam energies, and wedge pair combinations. With the introduction of 3D imaging and MLC it became apparent that, concerning collimator rotation, in many cases a trade-off was required between optimal orientation of the wedge and optimal direction of leaf motion, leading in many cases to the introduction of the so-called field-in-field techniques (some regard this as forward planning FiF IMRT) to generate homogenous dose distributions in all planes [1]. Intensity modulated radiation therapy (IMRT) represented the next level in the attempt to limit the dose variation in the target volume whilst reducing the dose to organs at risk as much as possible [2]. IMRT optimises the beam intensity using either step and shoot or dynamic sliding window techniques. More recently, volumetric-modulated arc therapy (VMAT) and hybrid VMAT, which is a combination of conventional tangential fields with VMAT, are being introduced to optimise dose homogeneity and healthy tissue sparing even further.

23.2 IMRT

IMRT is able to deliver a highly conformal dose to the target whilst maintaining a high degree of dose homogeneity. For most patients, reasonable dose coverage can be obtained with 6 MV photons only. However, with larger breast volumes mixed energy (6 and 10 MV) might be required for an improved coverage in depth whilst keeping the maximum dose as low as possible. Beam energies in excess of 10 MV should be avoided because of neutron generation and thereto-related radioprotection issues.

S. Hol (✉)
Instituut Verbeeten, Tilburg, The Netherlands
e-mail: Hol.s@bvi.nl

I. Mollaert
Iridium Cancer Network, Antwerp, Belgium
e-mail: Isabelle.mollaert@gza.be

© The Author(s), under exclusive license to Springer Nature Switzerland AG 2022
O. Kaidar-Person et al. (eds.), *Breast Cancer Radiation Therapy*,
https://doi.org/10.1007/978-3-030-91170-6_23

23.3 Gantry Angle

The choice of the gantry angle for the mediolateral (ML) and latero-medial (LM) tangential fields is the first and most important step following appropriate anatomy-based CTV contouring. An optimal gantry angle reduces the dose in the lungs, contralateral breast, and heart. By connecting a line from medial and lateral borders of the PTV_breast or chest wall and aligning the fields with this tangent line (Fig. 23.1a) will result in a good first estimation of the angles.

The overlap of the PTV with the lung, the heart, and the contralateral breast can be visualised by using the so-called beams eye view (BEV). The degree of overlap with the PTV can be reduced by adapting the beam angles (Fig. 23.1b, c). Care should be given also for the contralateral breast, especially in young patients.

23.4 MLC/Jaws/Collimator

When fitting the jaws (similarly for the MLC) around the PTV possible swelling of the breast during the radiation course should be taken into account (Fig. 23.2). Larger margins can be taken, for instance, in the lateral, caudal, and cranial direction. However, in the absence of an ALND and with ultrafractionation, these extra margins seem less required. We advise to collect IGRT-images to acquire estimations of required margins based on own experience in various clinical circumstances including variations in surgery and fractionation. In the medial direction the jaws are closely fitted to the PTV (e.g. 0.3 cm) with the leaves shielding the tissues outside of the PTV, including the contralateral breast and heart (Fig. 23.2b, red circle). Rotating the collimator can further improve the alignment with the breast.

23.5 Field-in-Field IMRT

Field-in-field IMRT is a step and shoot technique, where you divide your field into several subfields. Before adding subfields (Fig. 23.3a), the high isodose lines need to be evenly distributed over the PTV (Fig. 23.3b) and the condition of 95% of the prescription isodose line covering the PTV needs to be fulfilled (Fig. 23.3c). In the example, three subfields for each field are inserted into the plan (Fig. 23.3e). Small weights are inserted into the subfields and subtracted from the main fields. Variations of these weights with trial-and-error were used to create a homogeneous dose distribution (Fig. 23.3f). In the illustration of Fig. 23.3c, before inserting the subfields, the 105% isodose line should not cover the entire breast, to keep the maximum dose in the end result below 105% of the prescribed dose (Fig. 23.3d).

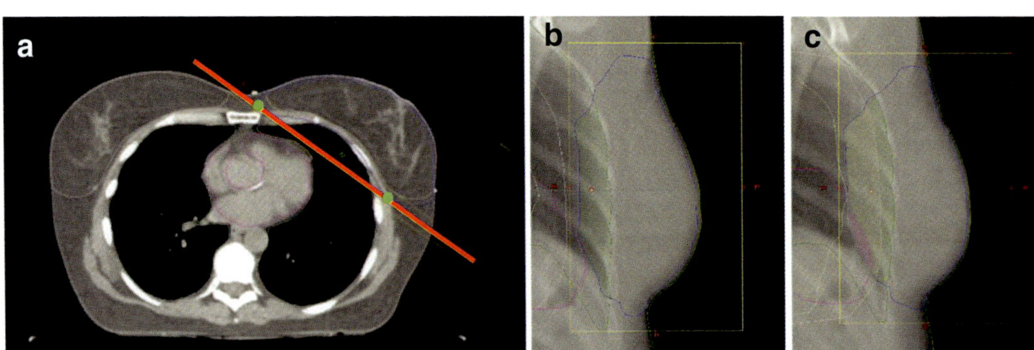

Fig. 23.1 Basic setup of tangential technique for breast/chest wall irradiation. (**a**) The tangential line (red line) connecting the medial and lateral PTV_breast borders (green dots) illustrate a good estimation for the angle of the tangential fields; (**b**) BEV visualising overlap with lung (light green), (**c**) FOV visualising overlap with heart (pink), lung (green), and contralateral breast (yellow)

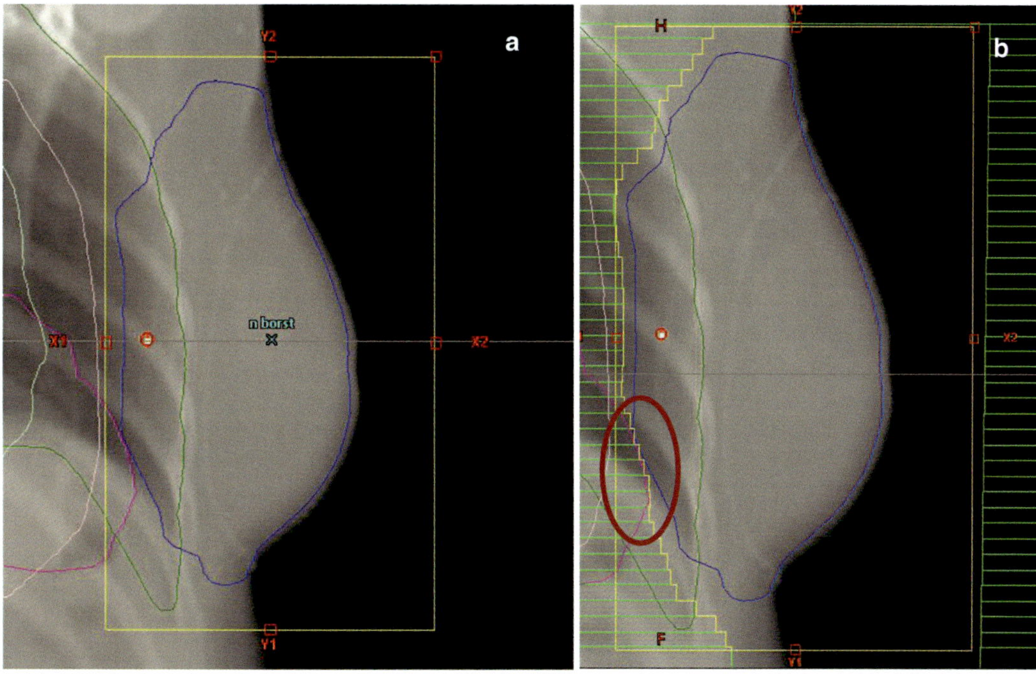

Fig. 23.2 Geometrically optimising tangential technique settings. (**a**) Jaws fit around the PTV (in blue) (BEV of ML field); (**b**) jaws and MLC fit around the PTV, where the leaves shield the heart if clinically acceptable (generally if primary tumour bed not close) (red circle) (BEV of ML field)

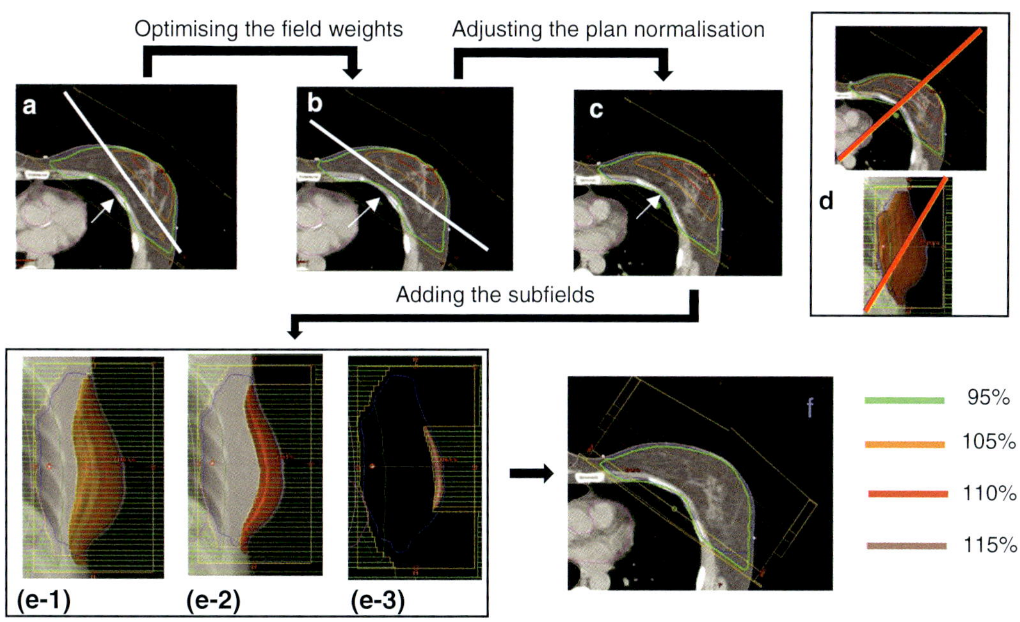

Fig. 23.3 Homogenising tangential technique dose distribution via Field-in-Field technique. (**a**) Starting with two tangential fields; (**b**) Even distribution of the high dose by optimising the field weights indicated by the white line; (**c**) covering of the PTV with the 95% isodose line by adjusting the normalisation indicated by the white arrow; (**d**) 105% of the prescription dose covering the PTV is not ideal to keep the maximum dose low; (**e**) The leaves are resp. covering the 105% (1-e-1), 110% (1-e-2), and 115% (1-e-3) of the prescription dose region for each subfield; (**f**) Final plan with optimised field weights

23.6 Dynamic MLC Sliding Window IMRT

With dynamic MLC sliding window there is a continuous leaf motion to create a fluence profile. Optimising the fluence map can be achieved following a forward planning method using the irregular surface compensator (ISC) [3] (Fig. 23.4a) with a fluence editor tool or inverse planning for IMRT. The irregular surface compensator calculates a fluence map based on the uneven body surface to obtain a homogeneous dose distribution at a certain depth (central plane inside the breast volume perpendicular to the beam incidence). In addition, the dose distribution for individual patients is modified with a fluence editor (Fig. 23.4b). In case of inverse planning, the dose constraints need to be specified before starting the optimisation algorithm. The optimiser will place the field border closely around the breast tissue. As a result, the fluence map outside the breast needs to be extended with the fluence editor tool in order to create robust plans taking into account breathing motion and possible breast swelling.

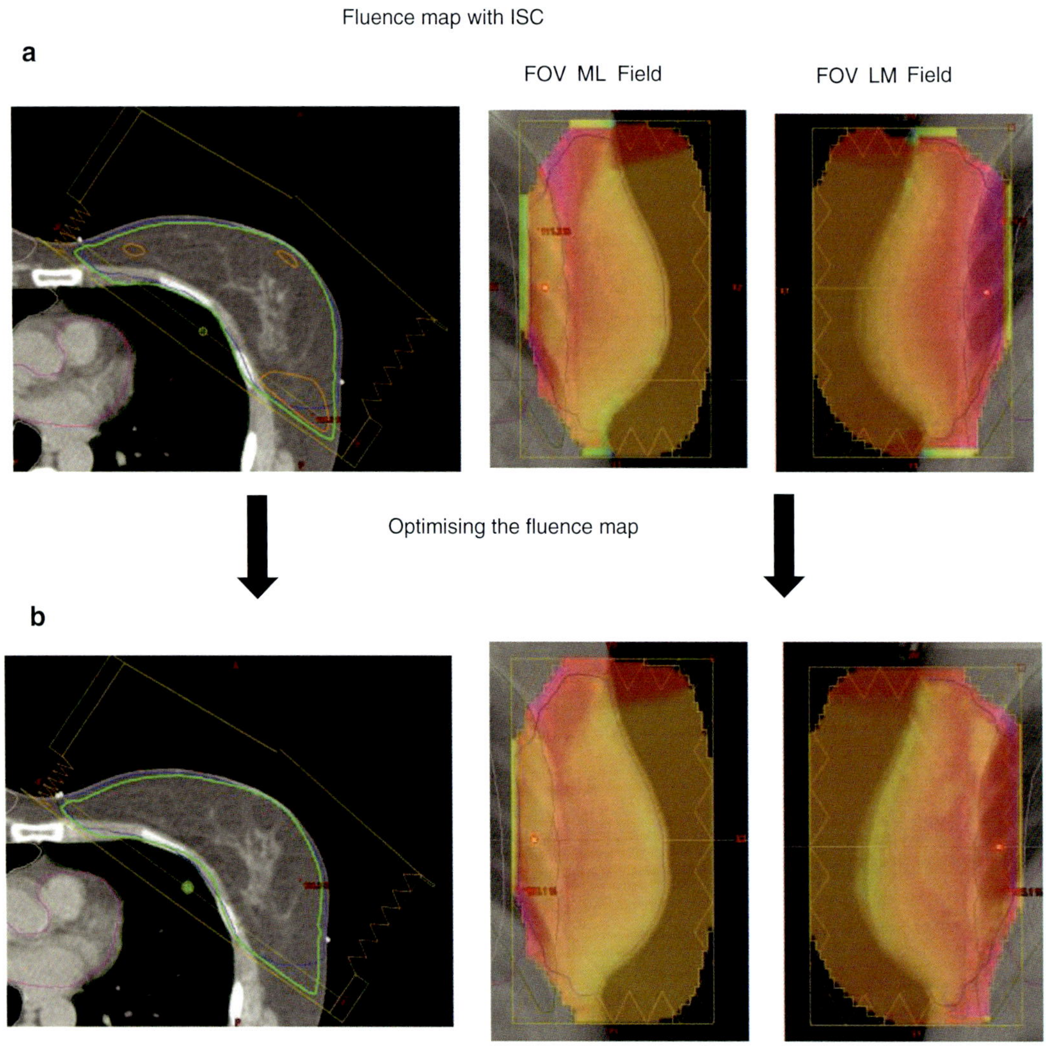

Fig. 23.4 Homogenising tangential technique dose distribution via IMRT. (**a**) Fluence map formed with irregular surface compensator (ISC) before optimisation, (**b**) fluence map after optimising using editor tool (FOV, field of view)

23.7 Treatment Planning Including the Lymph Node Areas

For axillary level 1–4 irradiation (Fig. 23.5a), the tangential fields to the breast/chest wall are combined with an adjacent field at an angle of about 345–350° (left anterior oblique (LAO)) or about 10–15° (right anterior oblique (RAO)), respectively, for a left or right breast. The isocentre is placed at the border of the adjacent fields. An opposing field of about 165–170° (right posterior oblique (RPO)) or about 190–195° (left posterior oblique (LPO)), generally with higher beam energy, can be added to improve coverage of the deeply located parts of the axillary lymph nodes regions. For nodal irradiation of only the base of the axilla (e.g. level 1–2 caudal from the axillary vessels), the tangential field setup for breast/chest wall can be extended on the cranial side. In case of nodal irradiation including the IMN, several approaches are possible, including the addition of an adjacent field parallel to the medial tangent field (Fig. 23.5b).

23.8 VMAT

In some cases, with very extensive and/or challenging anatomies and/or target volumes, volumetric-modulated arc therapy (VMAT) is a good alternative to the tangent fields-based 3DCRT or IMRT approach. Moreover, VMAT is gradually becoming the state-of-the-art technique at this moment due to its ease of use in the optimisation process as well as the efficiency of treat-

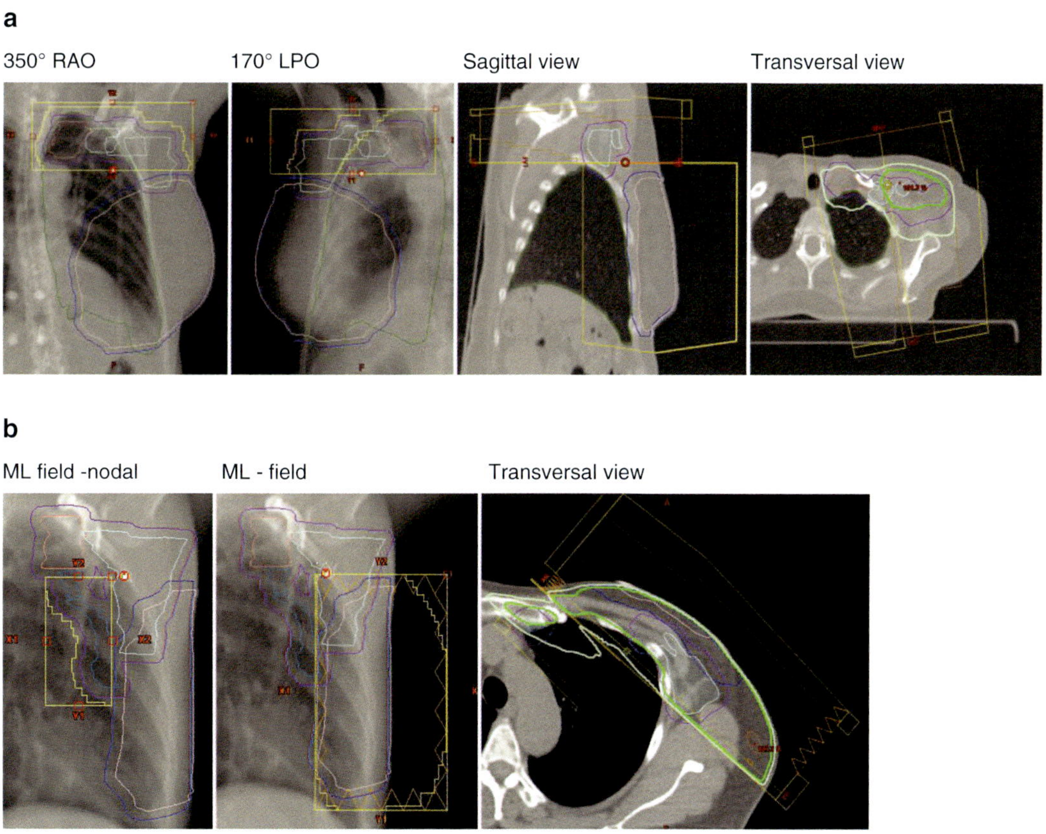

Fig. 23.5 Basic setup of tangential technique for breast/chest wall combined with regional lymph node irradiation. (**a**) Field setup for irradiation of the axillary lymph node levels 1–4, located superior to the left breast, using 350° RAO and 170° LPO fields; (**b**) Field setup for irradiation of the internal mammary lymph nodes, using tangent ML

ment delivery. In addition, the rotational character of the treatment renders it less prone to breathing motion and swelling issues during the course of treatment. Another reason for using VMAT could be when the heart dose is above 3.2 Gy with the other techniques including respiratory control or CPAP with or without respiratory control. In that case, treatment planning with VMAT might help to reduce the heart to below acceptable levels [4]. Two partial arcs are typically chosen with a start angle comparable to the angle of the ML field of the tangent setup and an ending-point angle in the range of 150–160° depending on the individual patient's anatomy. The collimator angle is set in a range of 10–20°, with complementary angles for the second arc. Due to the low dose bath inevitably adhered to rotational techniques, VMAT produces a slight increase in the low dose range of the dose in the heart and lungs compared to the static tangential fields [5]. As such, hybrid VMAT offers an interesting alternative in many situations. Using VMAT for breast RT, the DVH should be carefully evaluated including the low dose spectrum as it might result in a low dose bath, exposing a large volume of various organs to a low dose of radiation.

23.9 Hybrid VMAT

Hybrid VMAT is a combination of two tangential fields with VMAT that improves dose coverage and dose homogeneity within the target volumes compared to the tangent field setup combined with adjacent fields for nodal coverage. Hybrid techniques are mostly used for breast/chest wall including nodal irradiation. The isocentre is placed around the clavicle bone, depending on the combination of target volumes. First, a plan with open tangential fields is established (Fig. 23.6a). The jaw in cranial direction for the ML tangent field is set 0.5 cm superior to the isocentre and for LM fields 0.5 cm inferior to the isocentre. If pos-

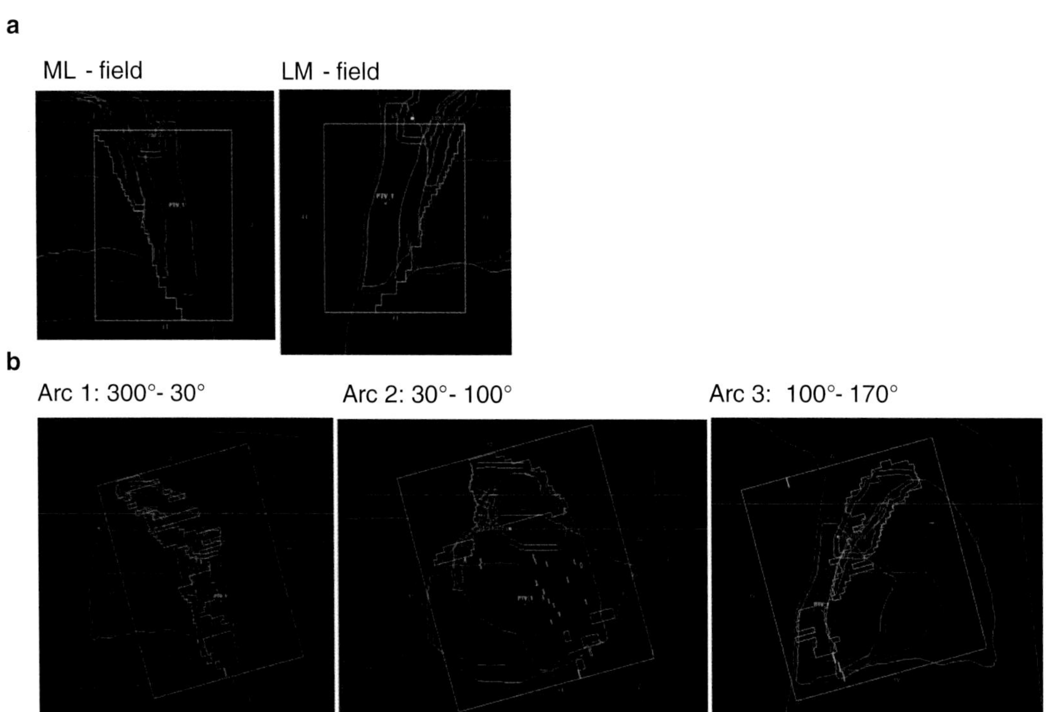

Fig. 23.6 Hybrid VMAT technique for breast/chest wall combined with regional lymph node irradiation. Hybrid VMAT with two tangent fields and three arcs: (**a**) beams eye view (BEV) of ML field and LM field; (**b**) BEV of three arcs, with gantry angles from 300° to 30° for arc 1, from 30° to 100° for arc 2 and from 100° to 170° for arc 3

sible, the axillary nodes and, if applicable, the IMN nodes on the same level as the breast are included in the tangential fields. The tangential field plan is used as a base plan for optimisation in the VMAT plan. The arcs make up 20% of the dose to the breast and 100% of the dose to the nodes above the clavicle. The VMAT plan (Fig. 23.6b) consists of three partial arcs rotating over 70°. The first arc starts at the same gantry angle as the ML field, the second and third arc starts, respectively, where the first or second ends. The arcs cover the entire target volume. There are two advantages of using three subarcs instead of one. First, the collimator angle can be changed per arc to keep the field width as small as possible. Second, it is a good beam setup for combining with voluntary moderate deep inspiration breath-hold (vmDIBH).

23.10 Summary

Over the last 3 decades, a gradual transition form 2D-radiation therapy over 3D-techniques and now motion-controlled and volumetric approaches has been made. While more advanced treatment techniques might be needed to obtain optimal dose homogeneity and low doses to OAR, especially for anatomically challenging cases, for most patients a straightforward less resource-demanding approach will suffice.

References

1. Morganti AG, Cilla S, de Gaetano A, et al. Forward planned intensity modulated radiotherapy (IMRT) for whole breast postoperative radiotherapy. Is it useful? When? J Appl Clin Med Phys. 2011;12:3451.
2. Hong L, Hunt M, Chui C, et al. Intensity-modulated tangential beam irradiation of the intact breast. Int J Radiat Oncol Biol Phys. 1999;44:1155–64.
3. Hideki F, Nao K, Hiroyuki H, Hiroshi K, Haruyuki F. Improvement of dose distribution with irregular surface compensator in whole breast radiotherapy. J Med Phys. 2013;38(3):115–9. https://doi.org/10.4103/0971-6203.116361.
4. Osman SOS, Hol S, Poortmans PM, Essers M. Volumetric modulated arc therapy and breath-hold in image-guided locoregional left-sided breast irradiation. Radiother Oncol. 2014;112:17–22. https://doi.org/10.1016/j.radonc.2014.04.00.
5. Tyran M, Mailleux H, Tallet A, Fau P, Gonzague L, Minsat M, et al. Volumetric-modulated arc therapy for left-sided breast cancer and all regional nodes improves target volumes coverage and reduces treatment time and doses to the heart and left coronary artery, compared with a field-in-field technique. J Radiat Res. 2015;56:927–37.

24 Treatment Planning for Challenging Anatomies

Sandra Hol, Orit Kaidar-Person, and Philip Poortmans

24.1 Background

The "Pareto principle", named after Vilfredo Federico Damaso Pareto who stated in 1906 that for many outcomes roughly 80% of consequences come from 20% of the causes, is often referred to as the "80/20 rule". For many medical applications, this means that for about 80% of the cases or indications a standard approach costing 20% of time and efforts will suffice, while for the remaining 20% individualised solutions are required, which are demanding up to 80% of the available resources. In case of RT, treatment planning procedures are set up for obtaining optimised dose distributions for the "average" patient. Whereas with individualisation of treatment planning a good compromise between dose objectives for the target volumes and dose constraints for the OARs can be obtained, some clinical cases demand creative and highly individualised approaches. Therefore, in most breast RT, a simple approach will do, and approximately 20% of the cases will be challenging to plan. In this section it is impossible to describe all imaginable challenging cases and indications. In some of them, compromises will have to be accepted, including balancing the coverage of target volumes against doses to OARs. However, for most challenges highly individualised and sometimes complex or even more challenging, out-of-the-box approaches may bring excellent clinically feasible solutions. The three cases that we present here just represent a few of them. However, the cases underline that with a combination of optimal usage of our technical infrastructure and tools with imagination and creativity, a lot is possible! The treatment plans are taken from real life cases and were aimed to fulfil the treating team's treatment objectives. Thereby, this short section is aimed to serve as a potential reference for RT planning teams in case of challenging cases.

S. Hol (✉)
Department of Radiation Oncology, Institute Verbeeten, Tilburg, The Netherlands
e-mail: hol.s@bvi.nl

O. Kaidar-Person
Radiation Oncology Unit, Sheba Medical Center, Ramat Gan, Israel

Sackler School of Medicine, Tel-Aviv University, Tel-Aviv, Israel

GROW-School for Oncology and Developmental Biology (Maastro), Maastricht University, Maastricht, The Netherlands
e-mail: Orit.KaidarPerson@sheba.health.gov.il

P. Poortmans
Faculty of Medicine and Health Sciences, University of Antwerp, Antwerp, Belgium

Department of Radiation Oncology, Iridium Netwerk, Antwerp, Belgium
e-mail: philip.poortmans@gza.be

24.1.1 Challenging Case 1: Pectus Excavatum

An 81-year-old female with an ILC of the left breast. Excellent KPS; no comorbidities. She

© The Author(s), under exclusive license to Springer Nature Switzerland AG 2022

O. Kaidar-Person et al. (eds.), *Breast Cancer Radiation Therapy*,
https://doi.org/10.1007/978-3-030-91170-6_24

underwent BCS with SLNB: stage pT1c N0 Mx, tumour grade 2, 1.1 cm, ER positive; PR negative; Her2 negative. Based on this, whole breast irradiation of 40 Gy in 15 fractions was prescribed.

The treatment planning CT-scan revealed a severe case of pectus excavatum, combined with an unfavourable position of the heart, not improving with respiratory control.

The treatment planning solution consisted of VMAT using 2 arcs from a gantry angle 300–150° and the other way around. Collimator angles were at 30° and 330° (Fig. 24.1).

The dose evaluation parameters were as follows (Table 24.1):

Conclusion: An excellent dose distribution to the target volumes could be combined with low doses to the OARs. The mean dose of 4.58 Gy to the contralateral breast is acceptable in view of the age >40 (and thereby low risk of breast cancer induction by RT).

24.1.2 Challenging Case 2: Including Sternal Bone Metastasis

A 48-year-old female presented with an IDC centrally in the left breast. Tumour stage was cT3 N1 M1 (solitary lesion at the level of the sternal bone), tumour grade 2. ER and PR were positive, Her2 negative. She received endocrine therapy with a good partial response on imaging. She did not undergo surgery because of stage IV. It was decided to give locoregional irradiation. Dose prescription was 44.66 Gy in 22 fractions (2.03 Gy per fraction) to the elective volumes (breast and all regional lymph nodes) and a high dose simultaneous integrated boost to 58.74 Gy in 22 fractions (2.67 Gy per fraction) to the primary tumour bed, the bone metastasis in the sternum and the visible lymph nodes in the axilla.

The treatment planning solution consisted of VMAT using 4 arcs and a number of "help volumes" to reduce the dose at the level of the tissue between the boost areas and in the lung, using both regular optimisation and biological optimisation objectives (Fig. 24.2).

The dose evaluation parameters were as follows (Tables 24.2 and 24.3):

Conclusion: An excellent dose distribution in several levels to the target volumes is combined with very acceptable doses to the organs at risk. The mean dose of 8.3 Gy to the contralateral breast is inevitable because of the high dose needed in the sternum which is right next to the contralateral breast.

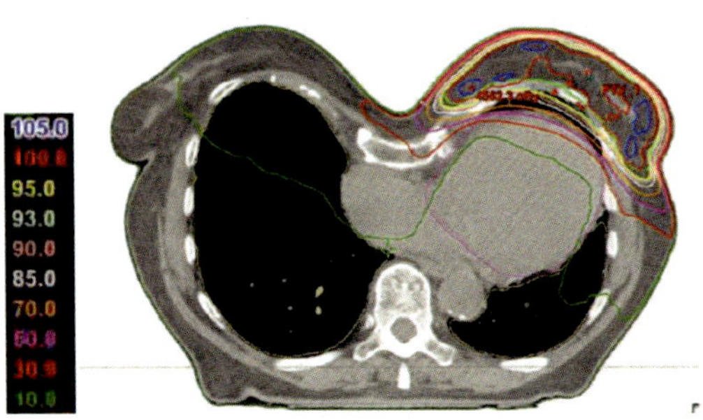

Fig. 24.1 Axial view of planning CT showing the dosimetric distribution (% isodose line of prescribed dose)

24.1.3 Challenging Case 3: Bilateral Locoregionally Advanced Breast Cancer with IMN Metastasis

A 74-year-old woman presented with bilateral breast cancer. A PET-CT scan showed uptake in both breast tumours, in right axillary and in right IMN lymph nodes, without pathological uptake elsewhere.

Table 24.1 The doses to OARs

Heart				Lungs				Contralateral breast	Spinal cord	PTV	CTV
MHD (cGy)	V20 (%)	V10 (%)	V5 (%)	MLD (cGy)	V30 (%)	V20 (%)	V5 (%)	Mean (cGy)	Dmax (cGy)	95% (%)	95% (%)
359	1.3	5	13.3	463	1.3	4.6	27.1	458	483	95.7	99.6

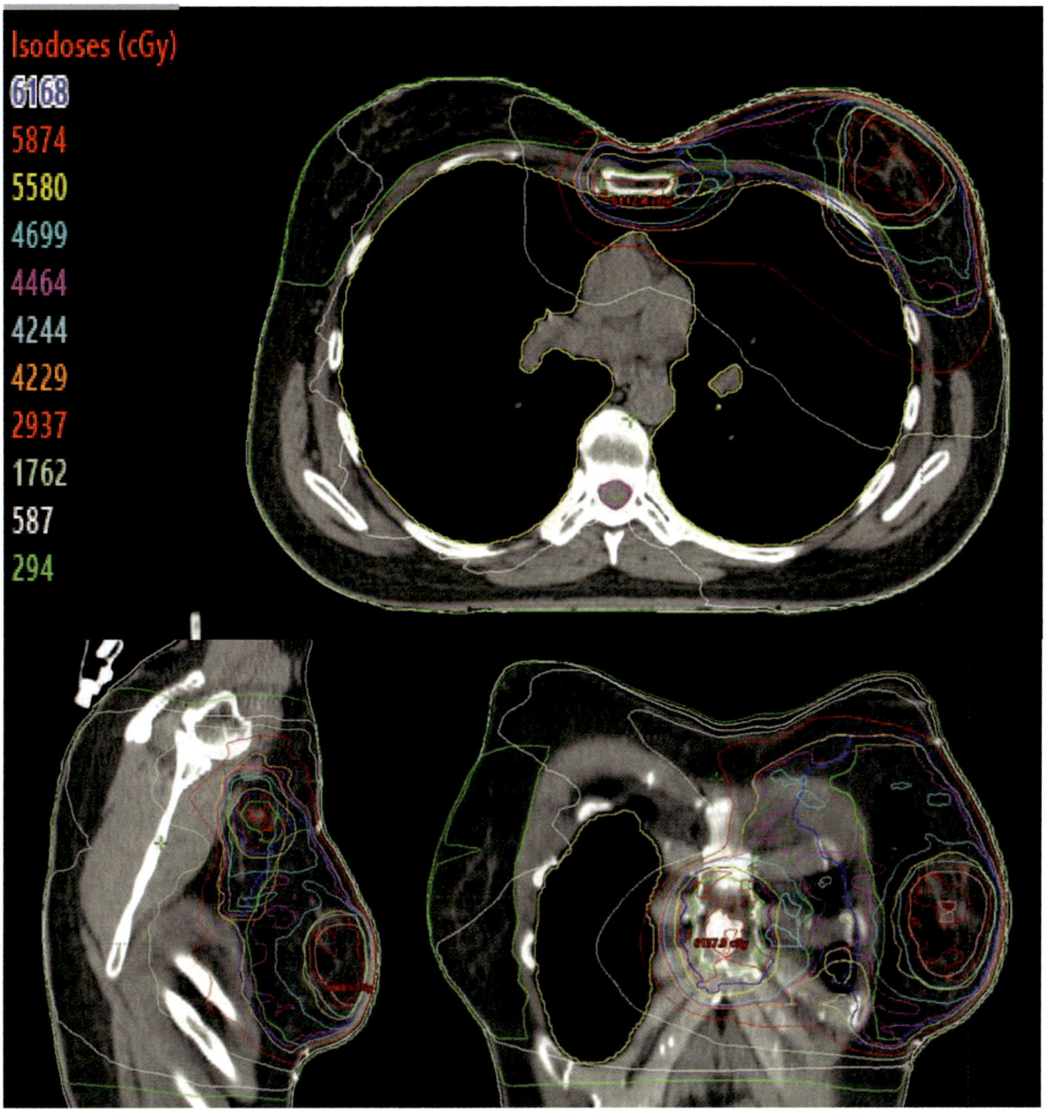

Fig. 24.2 Radiation planning CT showing the dosimetric distribution

Table 24.2 The doses to OARs

Heart				Lungs				Contralateral breast	Spinal cord
MHD (cGy)	V20 (%)	V10 (%)	V5 (%)	MLD (cGy)	V30 (%)	V20 (%)	V5 (%)	Mean (cGy)	Dmax (cGy)
528	3	12.3	33.1	1104	10.4	19.4	62.1	833	1879

Table 24.3 Clinical target volume versus planning target volume coverage

CTVbreast	**CTVIMN**	**CTVaxilla**	**CTVsupra**			
95% (%)	95% (%)	95% (%)	95% (%)			
99.5	100	100	100			
PTVbreast	**PTVIMN**	**PTVaxilla**	**PTVsupra**	**PTVbreastBoost**	**PTVaxBoost**	**PTVsternalboneBoost**
95% (%)	95% (%)	95% (%)	95% (%)	95% (%)	95% (%)	95% (%)
98.3	96.2	99.3	99.6	99.2	99.9	96.5

- Right-sided cT2 N1, treated with modified radical mastectomy. Pathological stage multifocal T2 N3: 3 IDC foci of 3.4 cm, 2.4 cm and 0.5 cm, respectively; all grade 2 with angioinvasion. ER and PR were positive; HER2 was negative. A total of 13 of the 16 axillary lymph nodes were pathologically involved, including extracapsular extension and invasion of the most cranially located node. Surgical margins were free of tumour.
- Left-sided cT2 N0, treated with simple mastectomy and SLNB. Pathological stage pT2 N1(sn): IDC of 2.5 cm; grade 1; tumour-free margins without angioinvasion. ER and PR were positive; HER2 was negative. The SLNB showed a macrometastasis with extracapsular extension. No ALND was done.

Postoperatively, she started with adjuvant endocrine therapy (aromatase inhibitor).

Dose prescription was 43.6 Gy in 20 fractions (2.18 Gy per fraction) to the elective volumes (bilateral chest wall; bilateral axillary levels 1–4 and right IMNs) and a simultaneous integrated boost to 53.4 Gy in 20 fractions (2.67 Gy per fraction) to the enlarged right IMNs.

The treatment planning solution consisted of VMAT using 2 isocentres with 2 arcs per isocentre. On the left side (isocentre 1) the arcs went from 300° to 170° and the other way around with collimator angles set to 10° and 350°. On the right side (isocentre 2) the arcs went from 60° to 200° and the other way around with collimator angles set to 10° and 350° (Fig. 24.3).

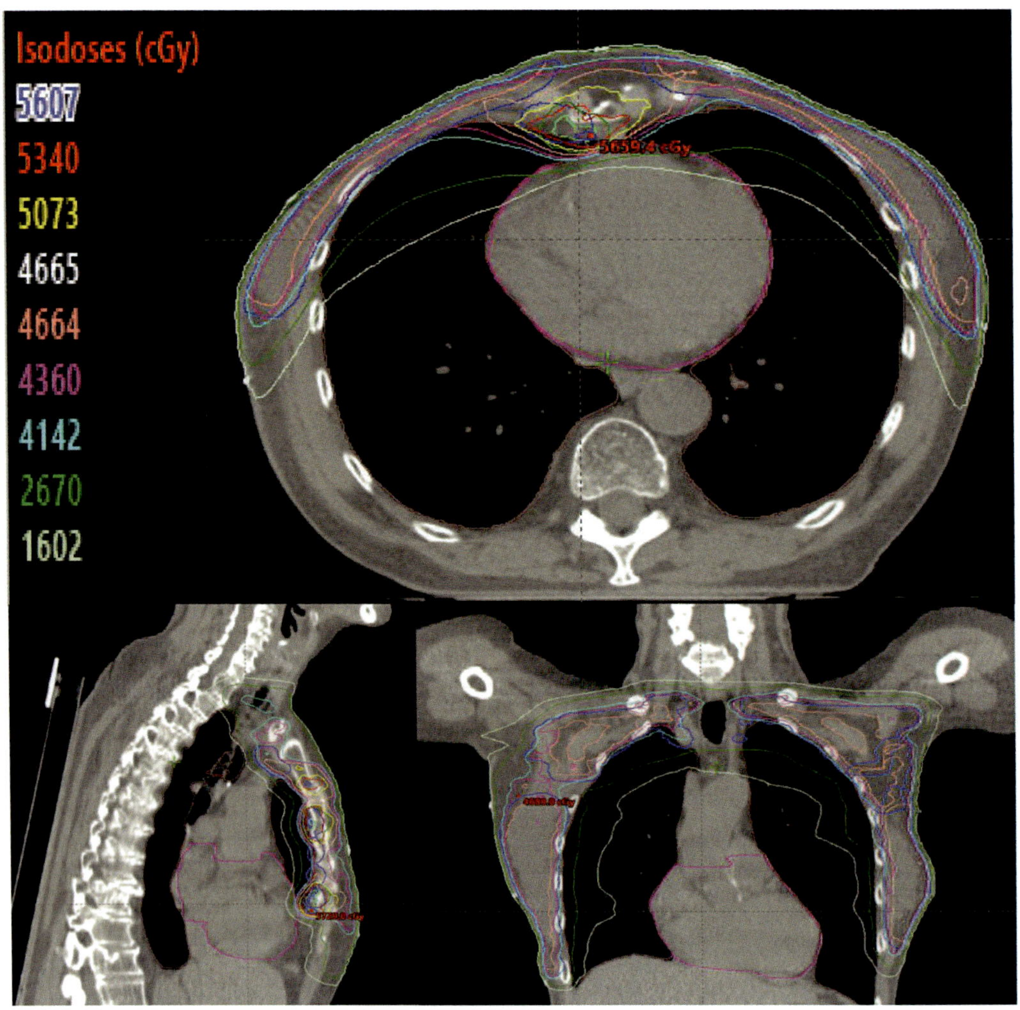

Fig. 24.3 Radiation planning CT showing the dosimetric distribution

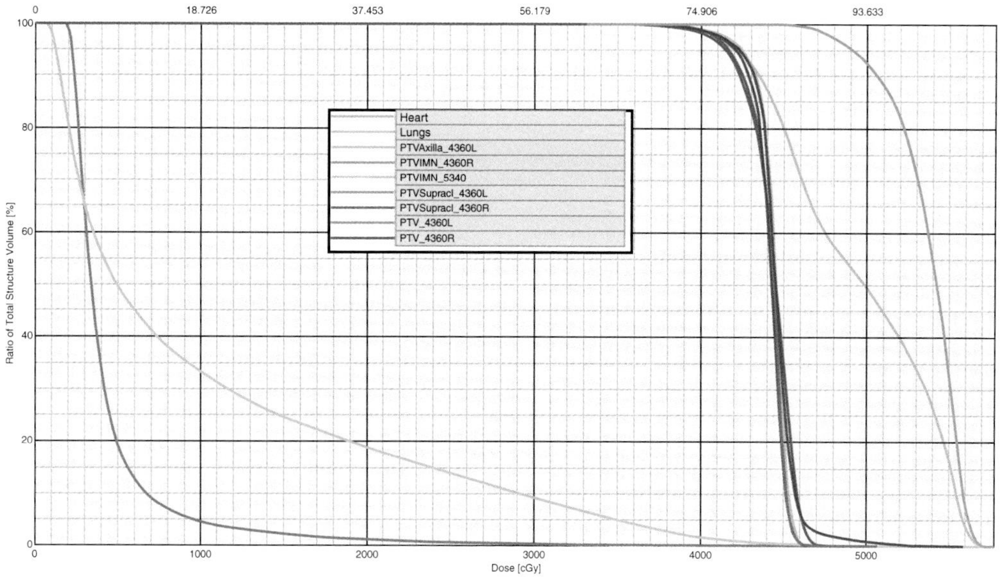

Graph 24.1 Dose volume histogram

Table 24.4 Doses to OARs

Heart				Lungs				Spinal cord
MHD (cGy)	V20 (%)	V10 (%)	V5 (%)	MLD (cGy)	V30 (%)	V20 (%)	V5 (%)	Dmax (cGy)
435	1.2	4.6	19.2	1023	9.2	18.9	49.6	1631

Table 24.5 Left side dose coverage

PTV chest wall	CTVchest wall	PTVaxilla	CTVaxilla
95% (%)	95% (%)	95% (%)	95% (%)
95.5	98.8	97.4	100

Table 24.6 Right side dose coverage

PTVChest wall	CTVChest wall	PTVaxilla	CTVaxilla	PTVIMN	CTVIMN	PTVIMNboost		CTVIMNboost
95% (%)	95% (%)	95% (%)	95% (%)	95% (%)	95% (%)	95% (%)	90% (%)	95% (%)
96.2	98.6	97.1	100	96.5	100	90	97.5	100

The dose evaluation parameters were as follows (Graph 24.1, Tables 24.4, 24.5, and 24.6):

Conclusion: An excellent dose coverage and homogeneity at two different dose levels to the target volumes are combined with doses below generally accepted constraints to the OARs.

24.2 Summary

The key to planning cases with challenging anatomies or challenging target volumes is to clearly define RT planning objectives. These include considering patient-related, disease-related, and treatment related factors. Patient-related factors such as age and comorbidities can dictate the dose constraints to various OARs: e.g. younger age will limit the dose allowed to the contralateral breast; chronic lung disease will limit the MLD and lung V_{5Gy}; and in a case of a patient with active heart disease, it is even more stringently advised to limit the cardiac doses to as low as possible but also avoid large doses to the coronary arteries. The disease control advantage by covering the IMNs should be weighed against the potential increase in cardiovascular dose. One should also take into consideration the different dose distribution and low dose spread that are linked to the different RT techniques such as tangential alignment versus volumetric IMRT (low dose bath, depending on the plan). Therefore, for different patients and cases the planning objective can be significantly different, and by working together and clearly defining the objectives of the treatment with a planning team, one can provide excellent planning, even for challenging cases.

25 Treatment Planning for Boost/SIB/PBI

Sandra Hol and Isabelle Mollaert

25.1 Background

An additional radiation dose (boost) to the primary tumour bed is indicated in case of high-risk breast cancer, while partial breast irradiation (PBI) can be used for low-risk breast cancer patients. For both indications, the clinical target volume is based on the distribution of tumour cells around the primary tumour which influences the pattern of local tumour relapse after breast conserving therapy. Optimal delineation of the tumour target volume is important for tumour control (in PBI and for boost) and for reducing the volume of breast tissue that is exposed to the higher boost doses. Subsequently, radiation planning and plan evaluation are important to reduce potential toxicity. Inappropriate field alignment can result in high doses within the breast that are outside the boost target volume or may result in increasing the low dose volume of the lung and/ or heart. This section discusses radiation treatment techniques for tumour bed irradiation, both boost and PBI.

S. Hol (✉)
Instituut Verbeeten, Tilburg, The Netherlands
e-mail: Hol.s@bvi.nl

I. Mollaert
Iridium Cancer Network, Antwerp, Belgium
e-mail: Isabelle.mollaert@gza.be

25.2 Tumour Bed Boost

A conventional sequential external beam boost to the primary tumour bed after whole breast radiation therapy can consist of two to three low energy beams using dynamic wedges or IMRT (Fig. 25.1a, b) or alternatively for a superficial PTV_boost, a direct electron field (Fig. 25.2). Replacing a low energy field with a higher energy field or adding supplementary fields can improve the dose homogeneity and the coverage of the PTV while decreasing the dose to the tissues outside of the PTV. Photon beam directions should preferably not be directed towards the heart or the contralateral breast. To reduce the dose in the lungs, the weight of the beams perpendicular to the breast may be limited. Often, simple beam setups lead to relatively higher doses to non-boost breast tissue, which is likely to contribute to adverse cosmetic outcomes. Therefore, also depending on the size of the breast, the position of the PTV_boost within the breast and individual anatomical particularities, the dose distribution can be optimised using dynamic wedges in craniocaudal direction, collimator rotation, and narrower MLC settings for perpendicularly oriented beams as well as non-coplanar beam arrangements.

An electron field is sometimes an attractive solution, for example, for small-sized breasts and for superficial tumours, especially located in the upper-inner quadrant. The energy is chosen

© The Author(s), under exclusive license to Springer Nature Switzerland AG 2022
O. Kaidar-Person et al. (eds.), *Breast Cancer Radiation Therapy*,
https://doi.org/10.1007/978-3-030-91170-6_25

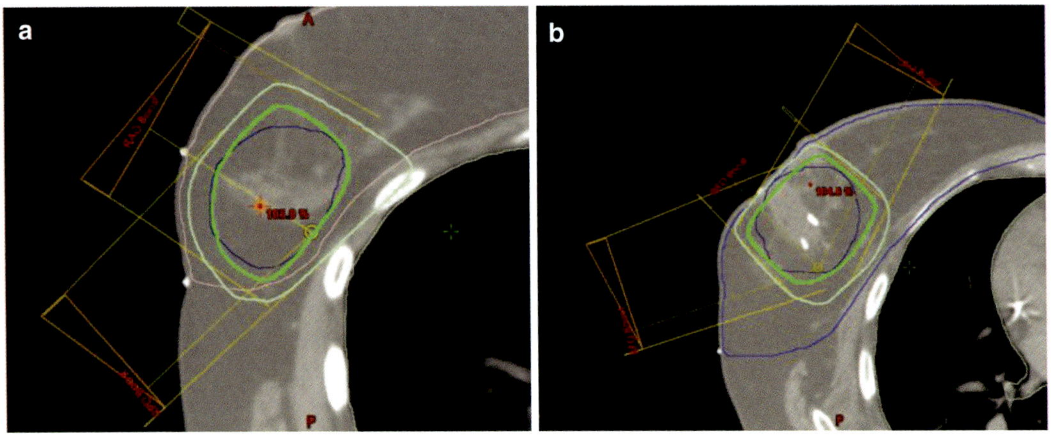

Fig. 25.1 (**a**) Boost located on the edge of the breast planned with two beams, (**b**) boost located in the middle of the breast planned with three beams. The 65% and 95% isodose lines are represented in light and dark green

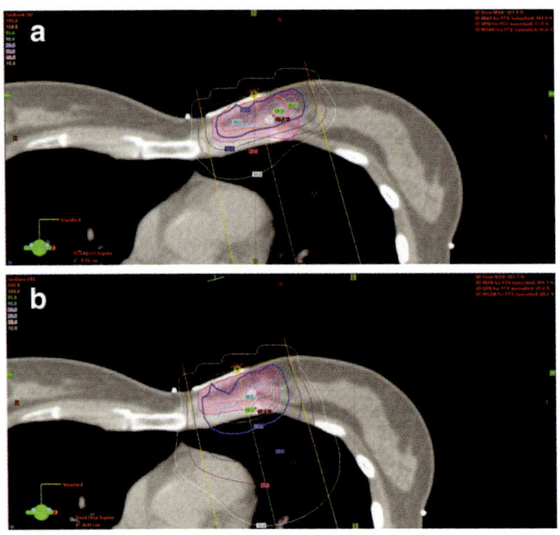

Fig. 25.2 Very medially located primary tumour in a young patient, for which a photon plan would have included part of the contralateral breast. A comparison was done between a 6 MeV and a 9 MeV electron plan. (**a**) Boost plan using 6 MeV electrons. The 80% isodose line misses a small part of the CTV_boost in depth, while in other directions covering the PTV_boost quite well. This plan was selected. (**b**) Boost plan using 9 MeV electrons with 0.5 cm bolus. The 80% isodose line covers the CTV_boost very generously in depth, while in other directions covering the PTV_boost quite well. This plan was, however, rejected as it extended into the ribs, with a lower-dose extension into the lungs and the heart

according to the deep end of the CTV alongside the beam axis, where CTV is equal to PTV. Due to the limited choice of energies, most often 6, 9, and 12 MeV, it can be a struggle to obtain a good balance between coverage, and limiting the dose behind the CTV, especially when this extends into the ribs and the lungs. On some occasions, adding a bolus of tissue equivalent material of, e.g. 0.5 cm can improve the dosimetric balance. However, this should not be combined with higher electron energies as this dramatically increases the skin dose, unless the skin is part of the CTV. Couch and gantry rotation are often applied to achieve the best beam setup, which can cause unforeseen collisions between the patient and the electron applicator. Therefore, attainable couch and gantry angles must be verified before actual treatment delivery.

25.3 Simultaneous Integrated Boost (SIB)

The planning of simultaneous integrated boost (SIB) starts with two tangential fields assigned to the PTV of the breast. The tangential fields are then combined with a beam setup for the boost as described above (25.2). However, as electronic equilibrium is already obtained by the tangential fields, the MLC's can be narrowly set, without any margin around the PTV_boost, leading to smaller volumes receiving higher doses compared to those obtained with sequential boost planning (Figs. 25.3 and 25.4). Moreover, during beam optimising, the dose to the PTV_breast can be optimised as well, taking into account the component delivered by the boost to the rest of the breast. In case of (hybrid) VMAT planning, no additional beams are added, as the boost area is included in the arcs, delivering 20% of the breast dose and, if indicated, the dose to the lymph node areas.

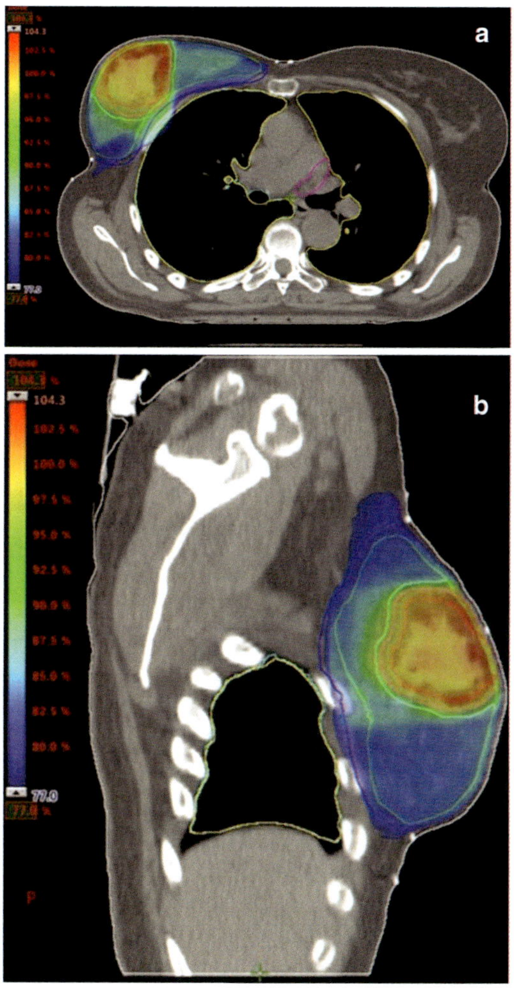

Fig. 25.3 (**a**) Axial view, (**b**) sagittal view. SIB-treatment planning for an upper-central tumour of the right breast. Treatment planning consists of inverse-planned IMRT (fixed beams) based on predefined objectives for CTV_Breast; PTV_Breast; CTV_Boost; PTV_Boost; lungs and heart. As can be appreciated, the dose distribution follows a 2-level pattern with a distinct separation of the elective whole breast and localised boost dose levels, as treatment planning for both takes into account the dose contribution from all fields/arcs

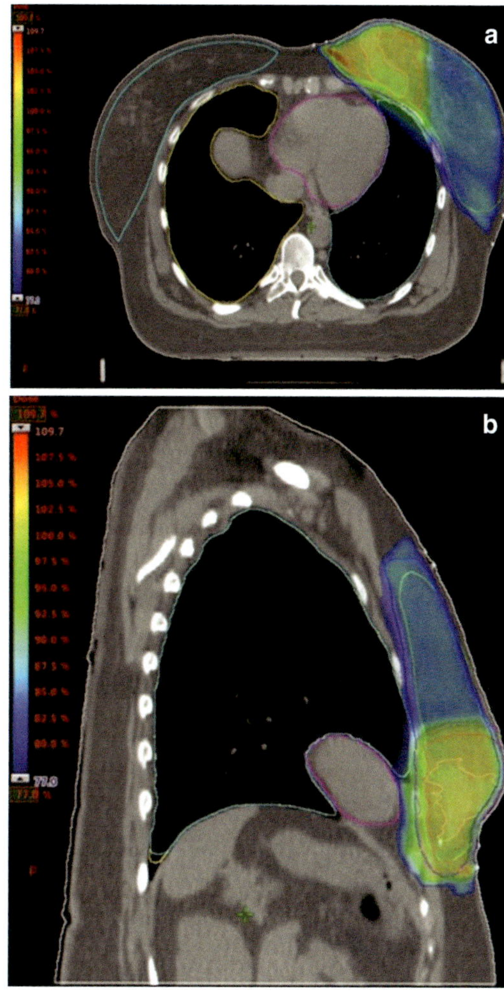

Fig. 25.4 (**a**) Axial view, (**b**) sagittal view. SIB-treatment planning for an inner-lower tumour of the left breast. Treatment planning consists of inverse-planned IMRT (fixed beams) based on predefined objectives for CTV_Breast; PTV_Breast; CTV_Boost; PTV_Boost; lungs and heart. As can be appreciated, the dose distribution follows a 2-level pattern with a distinct separation of the elective whole breast and localised boost dose levels, as treatment planning for both takes into account the dose contribution from all fields/arcs

25.4 Partial Breast Irradiation (PBI)

Treatment planning for partial breast irradiation (PBI) is similar to that of the planning of a sequential boost as described above (25.2). Alternatively, especially with fractionation schedules such as 26 Gy in 5 fractions in 1 week (5 consecutive days), a reduced-size breast plan can be used, where the two tangent fields are fitted around the PTV_PBI. Adjusting the angle of the tangent fields to the location of the tumour bed can further lower the dose to lung and heart (Fig. 25.5). Figure 25.6a, b is from the

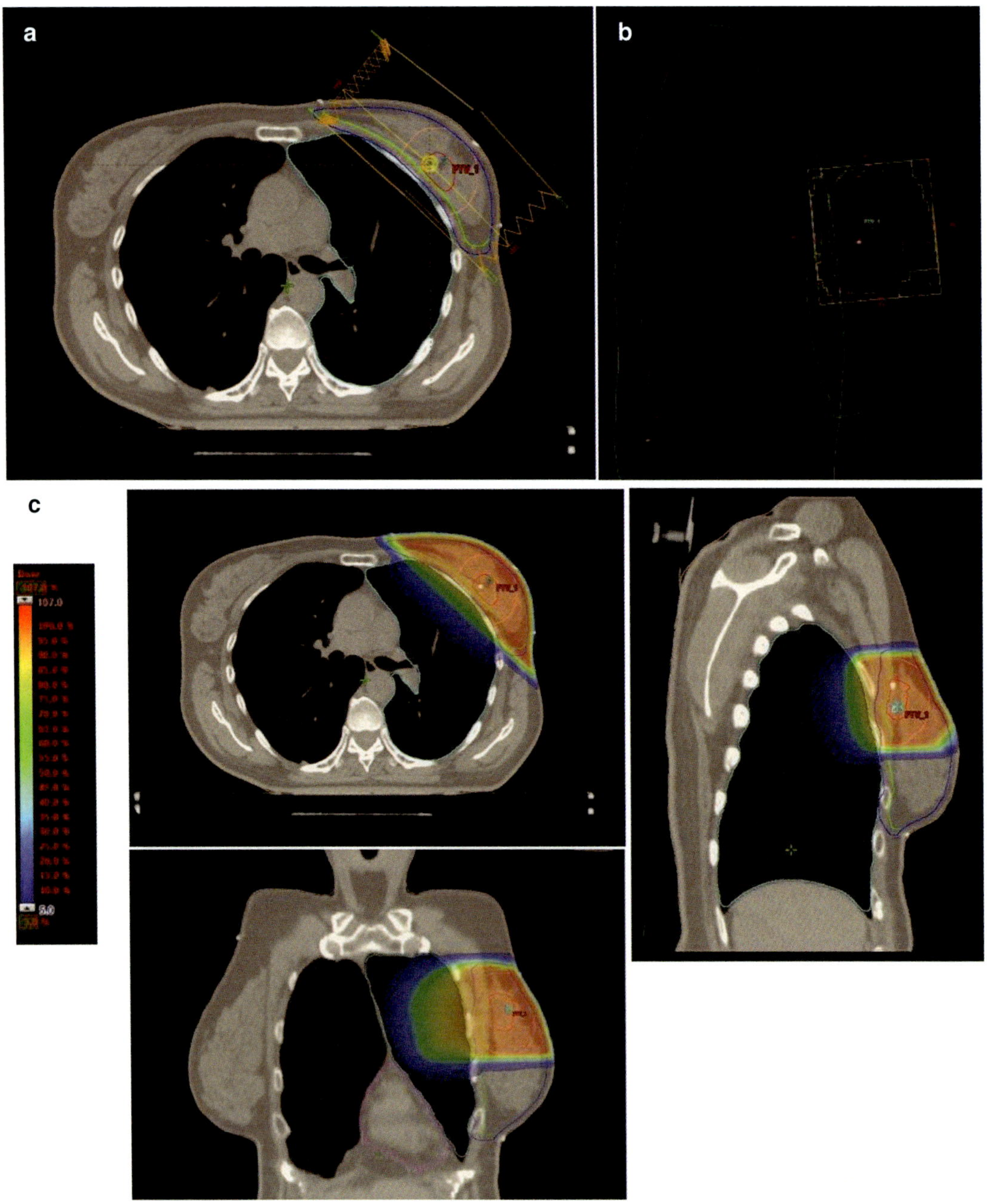

Fig. 25.5 (**a**) The angle of two tangent fields adjusted to the location of the tumour (**b**) BEV of the ML field (**c**) dose distribution of PBI for the transversal, sagittal and frontal plane

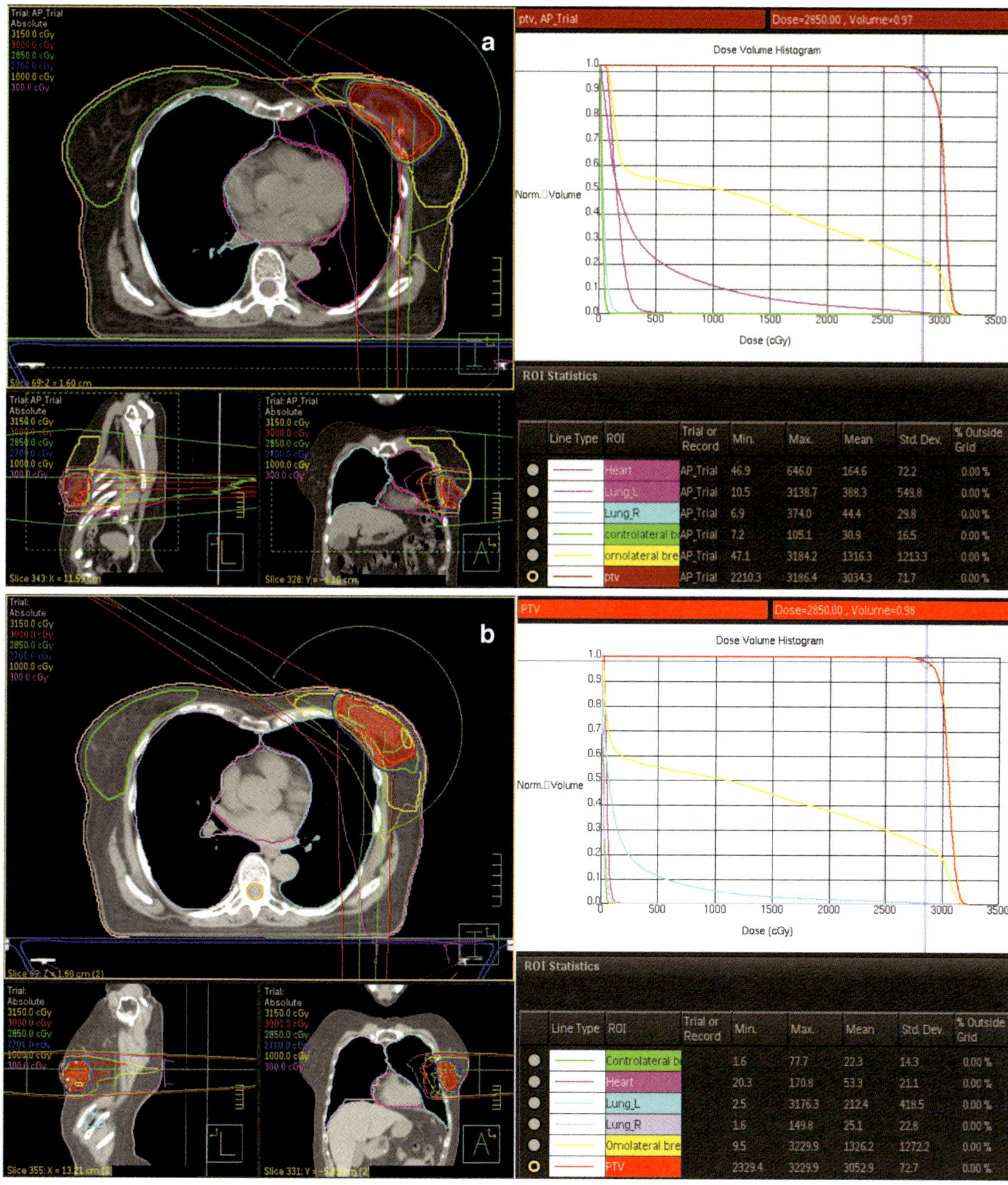

Fig. 25.6 Dose distributions and DVHs for an APBI VMAT treatment (30 Gy in 5 fractions) with a partial arc taken from the FLORENCE APBI trial [NCT02104895]. In (**a**) the treatment is planned on a free-breathing CT scan, while in (**b**) a DIBH CT is used. As can be observed by the DVH, mean heart dose, although quite limited for both treatments, is lowered from about 165 cGy using FB planning to 53 cGy when DIBH treatment is used

FLORENCE APBI trial [NCT02104895], 30 Gy in 5 daily fractions, given once every other day. The figures show dose distributions and DVHs planned with a partial arc using free-breathing and deep inspiration breath hold.

25.5 Summary

Following optimal delineation of the target volume for boost or PBI, radiation therapy planning should be performed meticulously. While for boost treatments, focus should lay on reducing dose to non-target breast tissue, for PBI adequate coverage carries the first priority. For both, doses to OAR, including the lungs and the heart, should be kept as low as possible.

26 Dosimetric Issues and the Transition from 3DCRT to IMRT/VMAT

Livia Marrazzo and Marianne Camille Aznar

26.1 Background

The target volume in breast RT can be largely heterogeneous depending on the stage, tumour biology, risk factors, nodal involvement, and the extent of surgery. More often it consists of the whole breast, but it can be reduced to the tumour bed (as in PBI) or it can extend to nodal regions (axillary levels I, II, III, and IV and/or IMN). Additionally, a dose boost on the tumour bed may be necessary. In postmastectomy patients, the target is the chest-wall (with nodal regions) but can also be very heterogeneous due to the eventual presence of prosthesis or tissue expander (see RT after breast reconstruction, Chap. 34).

This heterogeneity in target shape and extent, together with the anatomical differences among different patients, translates in a wide variety of RT techniques, each characterised by its own peculiarity and dosimetric issues. Generally, different target volumes may benefit from different irradiation techniques.

L. Marrazzo (✉)
Medical Physics Unit, Careggi University Hospital, Florence, Italy
e-mail: livia.marrazzo@unifi.it

M. C. Aznar
Manchester Cancer Research Center, University of Manchester, Manchester, UK
e-mail: marianne.aznar@manchester.ac.uk

26.2 The Transition from 3DCRT to IMRT/VMAT

3DCRT is considered conventional breast RT. Two (or more, with mixed energies and different wedge orientations) tangential fields with wedges are used to minimise dose to heart and ipsilateral lung. With this technique it can be challenging to achieve target homogeneity and conformity.

An improvement can be obtained by "modulated" tangential fields (generally called "field-in-field," FiF, when the optimisation method is forward planning and IMRT when inverse planning is used to obtain the modulation based on fluency), allowing a better dose homogeneity to target which translates into superior overall cosmesis and reduces the risk of skin telangiectasia [1] and the occurrence of moist desquamation [2] when compared with a standard wedged technique (Fig. 26.1).

Multiple fields [3] or helical [4] IMRT and VMAT [5] can improve target coverage, homogeneity, and dose conformity to the target, at the cost of an increase in low doses to contralateral organs (lung and breast) which may translate into an increased risk of secondary cancer [6]. Sparing of ipsilateral organs at risk can be equivalent to what is achievable with previous techniques or even be further improved.

In breast radiation therapy, VMAT, with today's technical implementations, is generally much simpler and faster to deliver compared to multiple fields

© The Author(s), under exclusive license to Springer Nature Switzerland AG 2022
O. Kaidar-Person et al. (eds.), *Breast Cancer Radiation Therapy*,
https://doi.org/10.1007/978-3-030-91170-6_26

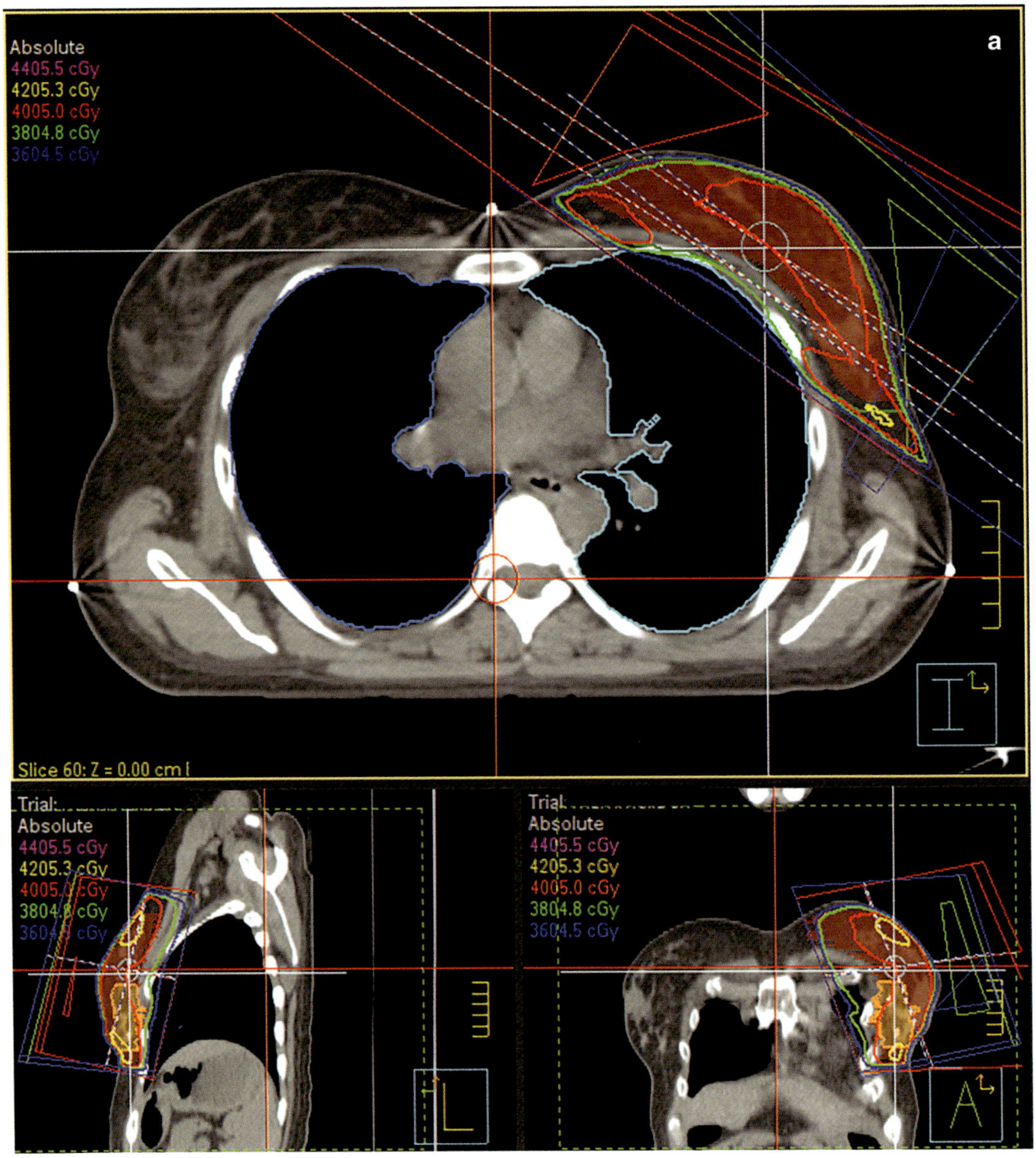

Fig. 26.1 Comparison of dose distribution: (**a**) 3DCRT plan with tangential 6 MV photon wedged beams (3 fields with multiple wedges orientations), (**b**) IMRT plan with two tangential 6 MV beams. The improvement in dose coverage and homogeneity is particularly evident in the sagittal and coronal view

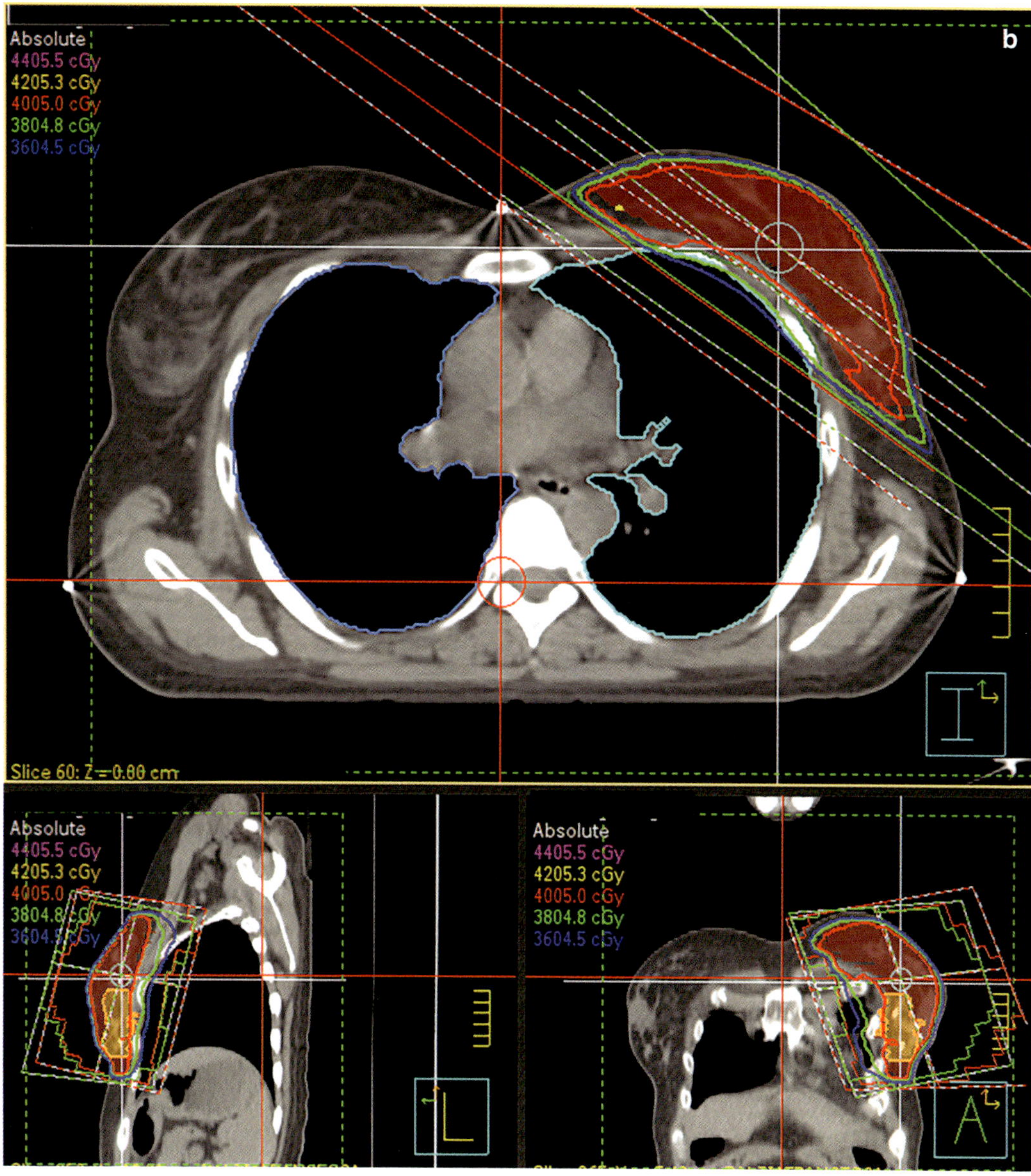

Fig. 26.1 (continued)

IMRT, while using much less monitor units as in the past [5]. VMAT is often delivered using partial arcs, in order to minimise the exposure of contralateral organs. Common beam configurations are presented in Fig. 26.2. Figure 26.2a shows a "bow-tie" approach, i.e. two opposing arcs covering around 60° of rotation, which is the closest to the tangential setup used in 3DCRT. Figure 26.2b shows a wider (180–220°) partial arc, allowing for more modulation, but also resulting in a larger "dose bath" compared to the "bow-tie" approach. "Bow-tie" arcs have been shown to increase the surface dose due

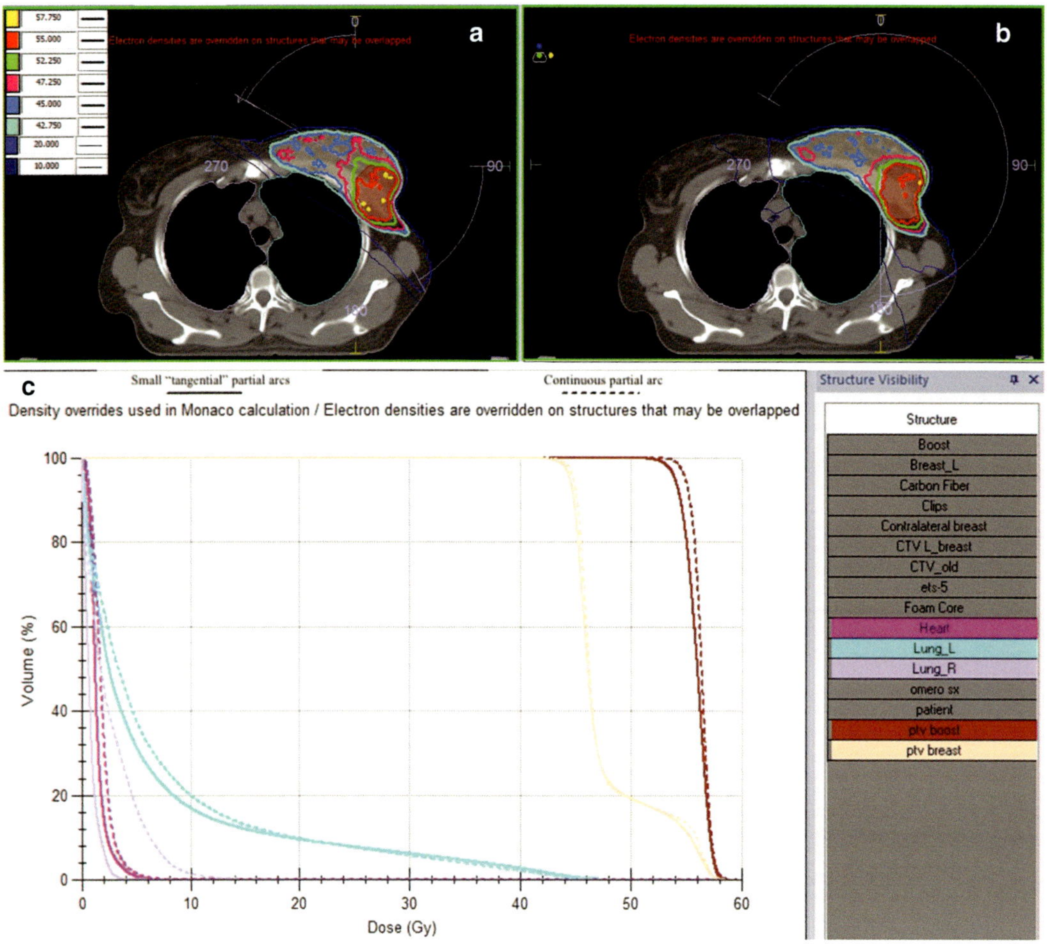

Fig. 26.2 Dose distribution for a VMAT left breast plan with simultaneous integrated boost 45/55 Gy in 20 fractions. (**a**) "bow-tie" arcs; (**b**) partial wider arc; (**c**) comparison between the DVH obtained with the two arc arrangements

to increased scattering compared to long partial arcs [7, 8]. The advantage of using wider arcs is the slightly better PTV coverage and sparing of ipsilateral OARs from high doses [9]. Instead, "bow-tie" arcs provide better sparing of contralateral breast and lung [7, 8, 10]. An example of DVH for these two arcs configurations is shown in Fig. 26.2c.

TomoDirect™ modality of TomoTherapy® has been also proposed as an option, although characterised by a lower conformity, with hotspots outside the PTV, which can be avoided by using more than two static angles [4].

The clinical settings in which these more complex techniques express their maximum potential are:

- in the case of nodal involvement, where 3DCRT would require multiple fields, complex geometries, fancy solutions (as the half-beam), and very long delivery times, often with suboptimal dose distributions;
- in challenging anatomical situations, where tangential beams cannot be used unless sacrificing target coverage or increasing doses to organs at risk;
- in bilateral breast treatments [11, 12], where contralateral breast is not an OAR and getting rid of the constraint on the contralateral breast allows an optimal sparing on lungs and heart. An example of dose distribution for a bilateral breast treatment with Helical TomoTherapy © is shown in Fig. 26.3.

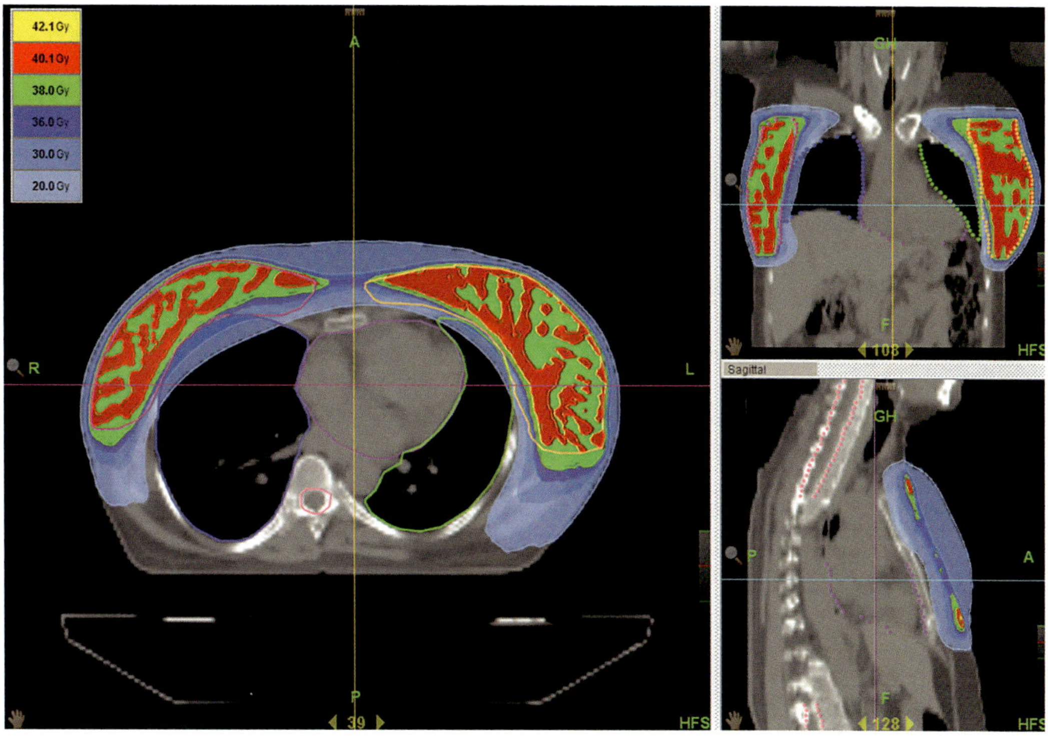

Fig. 26.3 Dose distribution for a bilateral breast treatment with helical tomotherapy

An additional advantage is the possibility of delivering a SIB (as shown in Fig. 26.2), thanks to the potentiality of modulating the dose distribution [13].

26.3 Dosimetric Issues

When moving from 3DCRT to more complex intensity modulated techniques, there are dosimetric issues arising that deserve some insights.

26.3.1 Robustness Towards Setup Errors and Deformations

One of the concerns is plan robustness towards setup errors and anatomical changes, with respect to which modulated dose distributions are likely to be more sensitive.

This might be particularly true in breast RT, where target is a non-rigid organ adjacent to the skin. Breast may expand or contract over the course of treatment (for instance, due to seroma), its position is affected by respiration and can be easily displaced or deformed by patient's setup errors [14, 15]. Tangential 3DCRT is, by essence, a robust technique: possible breast expansion is accounted for by "opening" the tangential fields into air, and breast contraction and setup errors will have a minimal impact on the dose distribution. In contrast, inverse-modulated techniques (IMRT/VMAT) are inherently less robust.

This is why some papers in the literature face with the evaluation of IMRT and VMAT plan robustness in breast RT, using either recalculation on daily CBCT, or deformable image registration (DIR) or simulation of patient displacement and/or breast swelling or shrinkage.

It is worth noting that the widespread use of advanced IGRT-procedures, including CBCT for daily online correction, allows to efficiently compensate for the effects of breast tissue deformations and swelling, as well as setup errors, thus allowing a safe use of VMAT/IMRT techniques. Moreover, variations are likely to be less important with the shorter fractionation schemes nowadays introduced in breast radiation therapy.

When comparing wedged 3DCRT, tangential IMRT, and multiple beams IMRT, dose distributions from the latter were shown to be more seriously affected by shape changes of the breast [14], while both patient and breast variations induced similar dose distribution deviations in 3DCRT and tangential IMRT plans, thus making tangential IMRT the preferred technique.

The dosimetric effect of soft tissue deformations and breast tissue swelling was shown to be similar for both VMAT and FiF plans if 3D image matching was used [16], thus suggesting that in VMAT treatments, a daily CBCT matching along with monitoring of the skin surface is recommended.

Though these considerations should not prevent the implementation of VMAT/IMRT techniques, it is sensible to deploy this check within the overall quality control/image verification process.

General reflections on plan robustness cannot predict the effect of large deformations, which should be evaluated in terms of their clinical relevance, and the potential need for replanning should be investigated [16].

Recently, robust optimisation tools, originally developed for proton beam therapy [17], have become available within commercial treatment planning systems, thus enabling to include setup uncertainties in plan optimisation [18, 19]. If such methods are applied to breast VMAT, the obtained plans result to be more robust than tangent 3DCRT plans to setup errors [18]. Additional robust optimisation strategies have been developed including organ motion [20]. The plan is optimised in the nominal (planning CT) scenario and over a number of simulated CTs generated by DIR based on user-defined organ motion. Organ motion-based robust optimisation VMAT is able to produce clinically acceptable organ-at-risk sparing plans for locoregional breast RT (including the IMN) that are robust to inter-fractional changes, therefore reducing the likelihood of replanning.

26.3.2 Interplay Effect

Despite the potential benefit provided by intensity modulated techniques, concerns have been raised regarding the breast motion resulting from patient breathing and which can affect the delivered dose distribution. In particular it could differ from the planned dose distribution due to the interplay between the breast motion and the MLC motion.

A common result of the studies investigating these aspects (both with simulations and in-phantom measurements) is that respiratory motion-induced dose variations are generally relatively insignificant [21].

It is worth noting that the potential impact of such effects is unique to the planning technique, the TPS used for segmentation, the extent of modulation, the characteristics of the delivery equipment and should be carefully investigated prior to the implementation of modulated techniques for breast radiation therapy.

Although interplay effects are likely of minor importance in modulated photon RT, DIBH might help further reduce their impact though a small amount of residual motion during each breath hold.

26.3.3 Skin Flash

In order to improve robustness of treatment delivery, a common practice in RT of superficial targets is to extend fluence outside the body to take into account breathing, possible anatomical changes and uncertainties in patient positioning. This procedure, commonly known as "skin flash" does not intend to treat the skin (which is not part of the CTV, except in specific cases where also a bolus should be applied), but aims to ensure proper target coverage in case of movements/swelling/deformations.

As mentioned previously, in tangential 3DCRT fields, the skin flash is manually performed when choosing the beam aperture.

In IMRT, the issue can be faced in several ways [3, 22, 23], such as using the skin flash tool when available (Eclipse™, Varian Medical Systems, Palo Alto, CA or Monaco, Elekta AB,

Stockholm, Sweden) or by properly opening the segments manually or through scripts after optimisation (Pinnacle[3], Philips Medical Systems, Fitchburg, WI). Not all the TPSs offer automatic solutions in case of VMAT, that not being based on a fixed field fluence delivery does not allow for an easy modification of control points aperture. While Monaco® TPS offers a skin flash option inside the VMAT plan optimiser, users of other TPSs had to work out alternative solutions. A pseudo skin flash strategy was proposed by Nicolini et al. [9], consisting in adding a 10 mm-thick soft tissue-equivalent virtual bolus out of the body contour (Fig. 26.3), then expanding the PTV of 10 mm of the body in the breast region and the PTV contours towards the external direction. Once the control points have been generated, a final dose calculation is performed after replacing the bolus density and the final dose distribution is eventually rescaled. The method was proved to be robust by several papers [9, 16, 24].

A method to select the optimal set of parameters to clinically implement the pseudo skin flash strategy was proposed by Lizondo et al. [25]. However, plan degradation is inevitable upon removal of the virtual bolus (Fig. 26.4) for final dose calculation and the further the target is expanded outside of the body in the virtual plan, the larger the plan degradation [20].

As already underlined in the session on robustness, with proper IGRT the movements/swellings/deformations can be efficiently detected and (at least partly) corrected and compensated for, thus reducing the need for skin flash. Also, when using VMAT, the varying direction of the incoming beams, inherently related to arc-based therapy, decreases the likelihood that movements/swellings/deformations significantly affect dose distributions and, thereby, reduces the utility of using a skin flash.

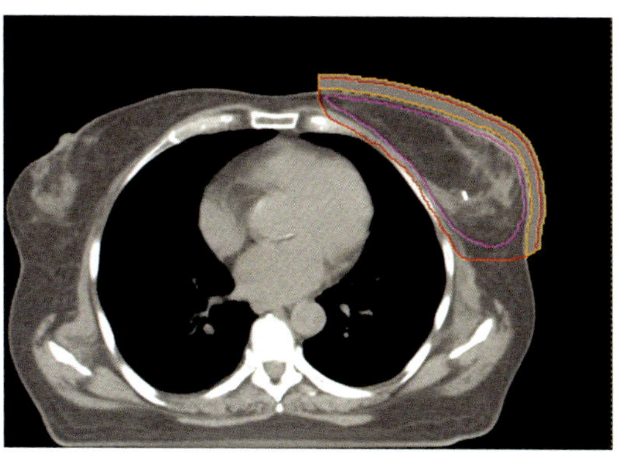

Fig. 26.4 Example of a virtual bolus for obtaining skin flash during VMAT planning

Figure 26.5 is an example of dose distribution degradation due to removal of the virtual bolus after optimisation.

Gas-filled temporary tissue expanders (not commonly used), containing both a substantial metallic component and a comparatively large volume of gas, are expected to produce increased dosimetric uncertainty in breast radiation therapy. This is due to the artefacts produced in CT images and also to the dose calculation uncertainties in the presence of high Z materials. If not properly handled (with appropriate density overrides) the dosimetric effects on dose distributions can be not negligible, and it is likely to be more important for intensity modulated techniques.

At the same time, inverse planning of modulated rotational RT treatments can produce modulated fluence distributions that compensate for the density heterogeneities in the implant [26]. This could arise some concerns on the robustness of these dose distributions.

26.4 Auto-Planning for Breast

In RT we are currently attending to the spread of automatic planning, which has the potential of improving plan quality and standardisation while reducing workload. Commercial TPSs have long allowed for planning templates or scripted solution, which can facilitate the work of the planner and offer some automation. However, automatic planning aims to offer a fully automated workflow (i.e. virtually no human interaction required to produce a plan). Since breast RT represents a large segment of RT treatments, generally 25–30% of a radiation oncology department, automation is likely to play an important role in this field and to have a large impact on workload and quality.

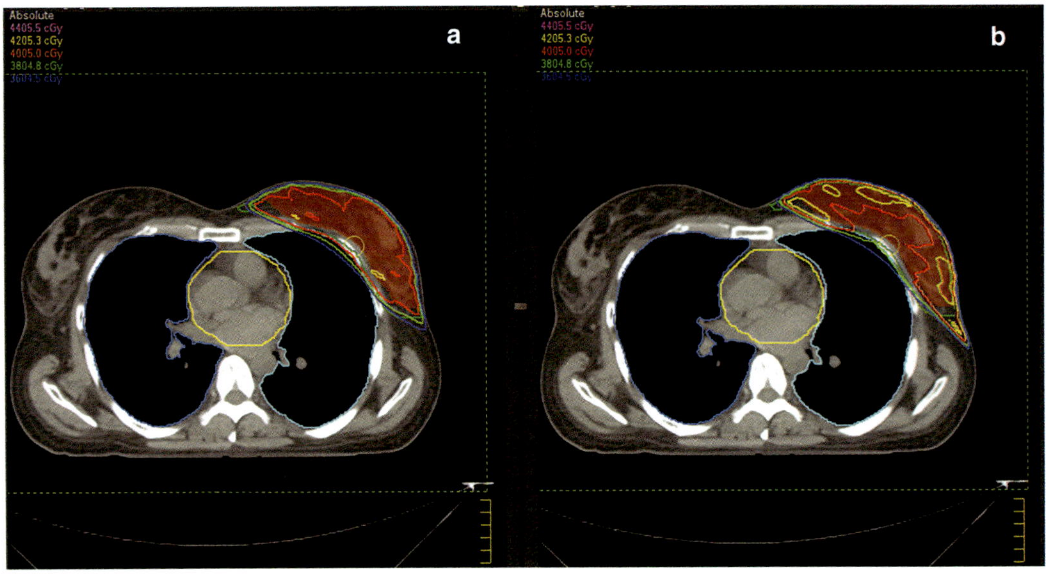

Fig. 26.5 Example of dose distribution degradation due to removal of the virtual bolus after optimisation: (**a**) dose distribution after first optimisation (virtual bolus in place); (**b**) dose distribution after virtual bolus removal and recalculation

In addition, automation in planning enables the bias-free comparison of different treatment techniques, since it allows to get rid of the dependence of plan quality on manual planning, thus enabling to finally answer to the question: which is the best technique for each breast cancer patient/patient group? Nowadays published papers on technique comparison are based on planning retrospective studies conducted with manual planning of few patients.

A further application would be patient selection, since the possibility of quickly producing plans for different techniques (e.g. the application of DIBH) and clinical scenarios would allow a posteriori (after planning) instead that an a priori selection of the best technique for each patient. The quick production of plans also has implications in adaptive radiation therapy, daily replanning, fast re-optimisation.

At last, the increase in standardisation plays a role in randomised clinical trials, since it reduces the level of variability in plan quality which may affect the clinical outcome.

Nowadays the available solutions for automated planning are [27]:

- Knowledge-based planning (atlas or model-based) as Eclipse™ Rapidplan™ (Varian)
- Template-based plan as Pinnacle^3 Auto-Planning (Philips)
- Multi-criteria optimisation as Erasmus-iCycle (Rotterdam) + Monaco® (Elekta) (a priori) and RayStation Plan Explorer (RaySearch Laboratories) (a posteriori)
- Several in-house systems based on script often focused on a single patient group or treatment technique.

Many applications of automated planning in breast RT make use of in-house scripts, alone [28, 29] or integrated in commercial systems [30, 31]. They are mainly on WBI [28, 30, 31] or WBI plus locoregional lymph nodes [29], make use of different irradiation technique, sometimes proposing a fully automated workflow from contouring to planning. A common result of these studies is that autoplans have, on average, more uniformity and consistency in plan parameters when compared with manual plans.

Pinnacle automated planning is applied to VMAT (A)PBI in [32], where automated planning was shown to be at least equivalent and overall superior to manual planning and to consistently reduce planning times. A commercial solution dedicated to breast is implemented in RayStation (RayAutoBreast). It is a fully automated treatment planning solution for tangential IMRT that performs segmentation of all relevant structures including the breast, placement of beams, setting IMRT optimisation parameters and objectives, dose calculation, and automated plan reporting, derived from the work of Princess Margaret Hospital [33, 34]. An application of automated plan for individualised selection of beam angles and treatment isocentre in tangential breast IMRT, based on graphic representations of mean doses to organs at risk in a large database of automatically generated IMRT plans, is presented in [35]. Except for Princess Margaret Hospital experience [34], no large studies on the application of fully automated planning to breast RT have been published up to now.

26.5 Summary

New RT techniques allow to individualise the RT volumes in breast cancer, as opposed to the volumes that were in the 2D era. Understanding of the target volumes, RT treatment objectives, and meticulous RT planning considering the anatomical differences among different patients are important steps for proper treatment. Breast cancer patients are treated with a curative intent, and the RT team should be familiar with each techniques peculiarity and dosimetric issues to assure an effective and safe treatment.

References

1. Mukesh MB, Barnett GC, Wilkinson JS, Moody AM, Wilson C, Dorling L, Hak CCW, Qian W, Twyman N, Burnet NG, Wishart GC, Coles CE. Randomized controlled trial of intensity-modulated radiotherapy for early breast cancer: 5-year results confirm superior overall cosmesis. J Clin Oncol. 2013;31(36):4488–95.
2. Pignol JP, Olivotto I, Rakovitch E, Gardner S, Sixel K, Beckham W, Vu TT, Truong P, Ackerman I, Paszat L. A multicenter randomized trial of breast intensity-modulated radiation therapy to reduce acute radiation dermatitis. J Clin Oncol. 2008;26(13):2085–92. https://doi.org/10.1200/JCO.2007.15.2488. PMID: 18285602.
3. Evans PM, Donovan EM, Partridge M, Childs PJ, Convery DJ, Eagle S, et al. The delivery of intensity modulated radiotherapy to the breast using multiple static fields. Radiother Oncol. 2000;57:79–89. https://doi.org/10.1016/s0167-8140(00)00263-2.
4. Reynders T, Tournel K, De Coninck P, Heymann S, Vinh-Hung V, Van Parijs H, Duchateau M, Linthout N, Gevaert T, Verellen D, Storme G. Dosimetric assessment of static and helical TomoTherapy in the clinical implementation of breast cancer treatments. Radiother Oncol. 2009;93(1):71–9. https://doi.org/10.1016/j.radonc.2009.07.005. PMID: 19682758.
5. Cozzi L, Lohr F, Fogliata A, Franceschini D, De Rose F, Filippi AR, et al. Critical appraisal of the role of volumetric modulated arc therapy in the radiation therapy management of breast cancer. Radiat Oncol. 2017;12:200. https://doi.org/10.1186/s13014-017-0935-4.
6. Abo-Madyan Y, Aziz MH, Aly MM, Schneider F, Sperk E, Clausen S, Giordano FA, Herskind C, Steil V, Wenz F, Glatting G. Second cancer risk after 3d-crt, imrt and vmat for breast cancer. Radiother Oncol. 2014;110:471–6.
7. Fogliata A, Seppälä J, Reggiori G, et al. Dosimetric trade-offs in breast treatment with VMAT technique. Br J Radiol. 2017;90:20160701.
8. Rossi M, Boman E, Kapanen M. Contralateral tissue sparing in VMAT radiotherapy of lymph node positive breast cancer. Med Dosim. 2019;44:117–21.
9. Nicolini G, Fogliata A, Clivio A, Vanetti E, Cozzi L. Planning strategies in volumetric modulated arc therapy for breast. Med Phys. 2011;38:4025–31. https://doi.org/10.1118/1.3598442.
10. Virén T, Heikkilä J, Myllyoja K, Koskela K, Lahtinen T, Seppälä J. Tangential volumetric modulated arc therapy technique for left-sided breast cancer radiotherapy. Radiat Oncol. 2015;10:79. https://doi.org/10.1186/s13014-015-0392-x.
11. Kim SJ, Lee MJ, Youn SM. Radiation therapy of synchronous bilateral breast carcinoma (SBBC) using multiple techniques. Med Dosim. 2018;43:55–68. https://doi.org/10.1016/j.meddos.2017.08.003.
12. Fiorentino A, Mazzola R, Naccarato S, Giaj-Levra N, Fersino S, Sicignano G, et al. Synchronous bilateral breast cancer irradiation: clinical and dosimetrical issues using volumetric modulated arc therapy and simultaneous integrated boost. Radiol Med. 2017;122:464–71. https://doi.org/10.1007/s11547-017-0741-y.
13. Nicolini G, Clivio A, Fogliata A, Vanetti E, Cozzi L. Simultaneous integrated boost radiotherapy for bilateral breast: a treatment planning and dosimetric comparison for volumetric modulated arc and fixed field intensity modulated therapy. Radiat Oncol. 2009;4:27. https://doi.org/10.1186/1748-717X-4-27.
14. van Mourik A, van Kranen S, den Hollander S, et al. Effects of setup errors and shape changes

on breast radiotherapy. Int J Radiat Oncol Biol Phys. 2011;79:1557–64. https://doi.org/10.1016/j.ijrobp.2010.07.032.
15. Topolnjak R, van Vliet-Vroegindeweij C, Sonke J-J, et al. Breast-conserving therapy: radiotherapy margins for breast tumor bed boost. Int J Radiat Oncol. 2008;72:941–8. https://doi.org/10.1016/j.ijrobp.2008.06.1924.
16. Rossi M, Boman E, Skyttä T, Haltamo M, Laaksomaa M, Kapanen M. Dosimetric effects of anatomical deformations and positioning errors in VMAT breast radiotherapy. J Appl Clin Med Phys. 2018;19(5):506–16. https://doi.org/10.1002/acm2.12409. PMID: 29978548; PMCID: PMC6123165.
17. Fredriksson A, Forsgren A, Hardemark B. Minimax optimization for handling range and setup uncertainties in proton therapy. Med Phys. 2011;38:1672–84.
18. Jensen C, Acosta Roa A. Robustness of VMAT and 3DCRT plans toward setup errors in radiation therapy of locally advanced left-sided breast cancer with DIBH. Phys Med. 2018;45:12–8.
19. Byrne M, Hu Y, Archibald-Heeren B. Evaluation of RayStation robust optimisation for superficial target coverage with setup variation in breast IMRT. Austr Phys Eng Sci Med. 2016;39:705–16.
20. Dunlop A, Colgan R, Kirby A, Ranger A, Blasiak-Wal I. Evaluation of organ motion-based robust optimisation for VMAT planning for breast and internal mammary chain radiotherapy. Clin Transl Radiat Oncol. 2019;16:60–6. https://doi.org/10.1016/j.ctro.2019.04.004. PMID: 31032432; PMCID: PMC6479013.
21. Liu Q, McDermott P, Burmeister J. Effect of respiratory motion on the delivery of breast radiotherapy using SMLC intensity modulation. Med Phys. 2007;34(1):347–51. https://doi.org/10.1118/1.2405323. PMID: 17278520.
22. Kestin LL, Sharpe MB, Frazier RC, Vicini FA, Yan D, Matter RC, et al. Intensity modulation to improve dose uniformity with tangential breast radiotherapy: initial clinical experience. Int J Radiat Oncol Biol Phys. 2000;48:1559–68. https://doi.org/10.1016/s0360-3016(00)01396-1.
23. Hong L, Hunt M, Chui C, Spirou S, Forster K, Lee H, et al. Intensity-modulated tangential beam irradiation of the intact breast. Int J Radiat Oncol Biol Phys. 1999;44:1155–64. https://doi.org/10.1016/S0360-3016(99)00132-7.
24. Tyran M, Tallet A, Resbeut M, Ferre M, Favrel V, Fau P, et al. Safety and benefit of using a virtual bolus during treatment planning for breast cancer treated with arc therapy. J Appl Clin Med Phys. 2018;19:463–72. https://doi.org/10.1002/acm2.12398.
25. Lizondo M, Latorre-Musoll A, Ribas M, Carrasco P, Espinosa N, Coral A, Jornet N. Pseudo skin flash on VMAT in breast radiotherapy: optimization of virtual bolus thickness and HU values. Phys Med. 2019;63:56–62. https://doi.org/10.1016/j.ejmp.2019.05.010.
26. Kairn T, Lathouras M, Grogan M, Green B, Sylvander SR, Crowe SB. Effects of gas-filled temporary breast tissue expanders on radiation dose from modulated rotational photon beams. Med Dosim. 2020;46:13. https://doi.org/10.1016/j.meddos.2020.06.003. PMID: 32660888.
27. Hussein M, Heijmen BJM, Verellen D, Nisbet A. Automation in intensity modulated radiotherapy treatment planning-a review of recent innovations. Br J Radiol. 2018;91(1092):20180270. https://doi.org/10.1259/bjr.2018027.
28. Lin TC, Lin CY, Li KC, Ji JH, Liang JA, Shiau AC, Liu LC, Wang TH. Automated hypofractionated IMRT treatment planning for early-stage breast cancer. Radiat Oncol. 2020;15(1):67. https://doi.org/10.1186/s13014-020-1468-9. PMID: 32178694; PMCID: PMC7077022.
29. van Duren-Koopman MJ, Tol JP, Dahele M, Bucko E, Meijnen P, Slotman BJ, Verbakel WF. Personalized automated treatment planning for breast plus locoregional lymph nodes using Hybrid RapidArc. Pract Radiat Oncol. 2018;8(5):332–41. https://doi.org/10.1016/j.prro.2018.03.008. PMID: 29907505.
30. Kisling K, Zhang L, Shaitelman SF, Anderson D, Thebe T, Yang J, Balter PA, Howell RM, Jhingran A, Schmeler K, Simonds H, du Toit M, Trauernicht C, Burger H, Botha K, Joubert N, Beadle BM, Court L. Automated treatment planning of postmastectomy radiotherapy. Med Phys. 2019;46(9):3767–75. https://doi.org/10.1002/mp.13586. PMID: 31077593; PMCID: PMC6739169.
31. Guo B, Shah C, Xia P. Automated planning of whole breast irradiation using hybrid IMRT improves efficiency and quality. J Appl Clin Med Phys. 2019;20(12):87–96. https://doi.org/10.1002/acm2.12767. PMID: 31743598; PMCID: PMC6909113.
32. Marrazzo L, Meattini I, Arilli C, Calusi S, Casati M, Talamonti C, Livi L, Pallotta S. Auto-planning for VMAT accelerated partial breast irradiation. Radiother Oncol. 2019;132:85–92. https://doi.org/10.1016/j.radonc.2018.11.006. PMID: 30825975.
33. Purdie TG, Dinniwell RE, Letourneau D, Hill C, Sharpe MB. Automated planning of tangential breast intensity-modulated radiotherapy using heuristic optimization. Int J Radiat Oncol Biol Phys. 2011;81(2):575–83. https://doi.org/10.1016/j.ijrobp.2010.11.016. PMID: 21237584.
34. Purdie TG, Dinniwell RE, Fyles A, Sharpe MB. Automation and intensity modulated radiation therapy for individualized high-quality tangent breast treatment plans. Int J Radiat Oncol Biol Phys. 2014;90(3):688–95. https://doi.org/10.1016/j.ijrobp.2014.06.056. PMID: 25160607.
35. Penninkhof J, Spadola S, Breedveld S, Baaijens M, Lanconelli N, Heijmen B. Individualized selection of beam angles and treatment isocenter in tangential breast intensity modulated radiation therapy. Int J Radiat Oncol Biol Phys. 2017;98(2):447–53. https://doi.org/10.1016/j.ijrobp.2017.02.008. PMID: 28463164.

Part VI

Radiation Therapy Delivery

27 Treatment Delivery

Dirk Verellen and Isabelle Mollaert

27.1 Background

Many factors influence the success of radiation therapy. Proper patient and disease evaluation, indication for radiation therapy, appropriate dose and fractionation are essential parts of the process, but defining the radiation volumes and assuring the precision and accuracy of radiation delivery are important factors for treatment success. Proper delivery of radiation will allow accurate target coverage and reduce the risk of toxicity. The current section will discuss radiation therapy delivery.

27.2 Treatment Verification Imaging

For treatment delivery, the patient can be aligned according to landmarks on the skin via a conventional laser-alignment system, which should reflect the patient's position during the CT-scan for simulation purposes. An alternative approach is positioning and monitoring of the patient set-up with an optical surface scanning system (i.e. SGRT), matching the real-time surface with the CT-based reference.

D. Verellen (✉) · I. Mollaert
Iridium Netwerk; Faculty of Medicine and Health Sciences, Antwerp University, Antwerp, Belgium
e-mail: Dirk.Verellen@gza.be; Isabelle.mollaert@gza.be

Different treatment confirmations can be used to verify the patient set-up and to ensure the precision and accuracy of treatment delivery. For tangential breast RT, a lateral and an anterior–posterior image (e.g. kV-kV or kV-MV imaging) are aligned with the corresponding digitally reconstructed radiographs (DRR), according to the ribs, sternum, chest wall, and vertebrae (Fig. 27.1). Based on the online image matching, couch corrections are performed if indicated. After the couch shifts, the tangential MV field image (electronic portal imaging (EPI)) is acquired to visualise the breast (Fig. 27.1: a.3/b.3). If the tangent field image exceeds the set-up tolerance, re-positioning or, in case of consistent and likely systematic deviations, re-simulation of the patient is required. Orthogonal imaging can be replaced by CBCT, which is especially useful in case of VMAT, to circumvent the final verification with a tangential MV field image.

27.3 Quality Assurance: In Vivo Dosimetry (IVD)

Traditionally, a diode or thermoluminescent dosimeter (TLD) was used for monitoring the dose delivered to a patient during treatment. The detector was placed on the patient's skin in the centre of the field where the dose gradient is small. The reading of the detector was com-

© The Author(s), under exclusive license to Springer Nature Switzerland AG 2022
O. Kaidar-Person et al. (eds.), *Breast Cancer Radiation Therapy*,
https://doi.org/10.1007/978-3-030-91170-6_27

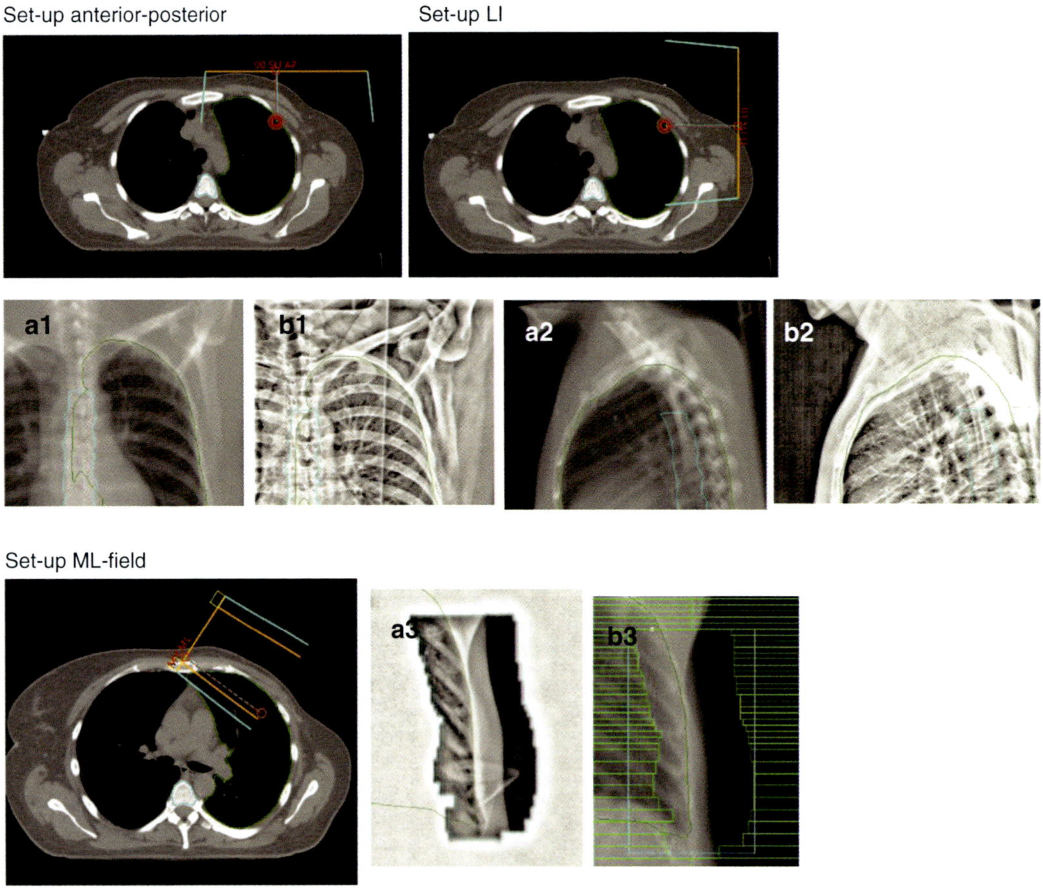

Fig. 27.1 Imaging verification with anterior–posterior kV image (a.1) and lateral kV image (a.2) with corresponding DRR (b.1/b.2) followed by an MV ML-field image (a.3) and ML-field DRR (b.3)

pared to the calculated dose delivered to a chosen checkpoint (AAPM report NO. 87 TG 62, 2005). However, this approach for IVD monitoring the breast had several drawbacks:

- Correct placement of the detector with respect to the beam axis is challenging on a breast.
- When using wedges, the placement with respect to the wedge angle is critical.
- In case of IMRT, this positioning became even more complicated.
- Point measurement at the patient's surface becomes useless in case of rotational delivery techniques and 3D reconstruction techniques are called for.
- Manual placement of detectors introduces additional set-up time.

In vivo dosimetry using electronic portal imaging device (EPID) can overcome the above indicated drawbacks [1]. The transit EPID images can be compared to the predicted dose or to a baseline (reference image from first treatment fraction) and evaluated with gamma analysis [2]. Compared with point measurements, more errors and deviations can be detected and translated to corrective actions. As an example, the shift in breast positioning as observed by analysing the delivered with the expected dose is illustrated in Fig. 27.2. On the left image, a shift of the thoracic wall is visualised with the in vivo software and on the right image the shift is confirmed by looking at the matching of the integrated images with the digitally reconstructed radiograph (DRR). In summary, novel

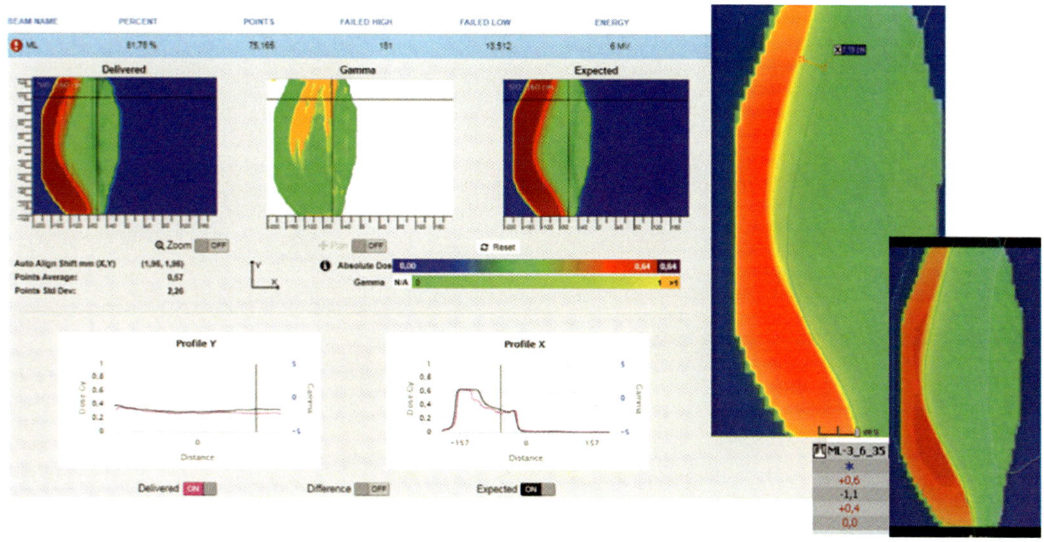

Fig. 27.2 Deviation in breast position. On the left, in vivo software results. On the right, offline review images where the integrated images could be matched with the digitally reconstructed radiograph (DRR) (Adapted with permission from [1])

technologies allowed us to treat and cure patients obtaining reduced adverse effects. However, all modern radiation therapy techniques are highly complex, thus increasing the potential for inaccuracy. This multi-step multidisciplinary framework is susceptible to errors that may occur due to several causes. Indeed, treatment verification imaging and QA in radiation therapy, integral part of the field of radiation oncology, gained increased interest in recent years and represent an essential part of treatment delivery.

27.4 Summary

Proper delivery of radiation will allow accurate target coverage and reduce the risk of toxicity. Therefore, the multidisciplinary RT team need to obtain accurate knowledge of the actual delivered dose distribution and the potential differences from the planned dose. This will ensure both target volumes coverage and reduce toxicity to OARs. Documentation, reporting, and understanding of pitfalls in RT delivery will strengthen knowledge and potentially improve patient's outcome.

References

1. Bossuyt E, Weytjens R, Nevens D, De Vos S, Verellen D. Evaluation of automated pre-treatment and transit in-vivo dosimetry in radiotherapy using empirically determined parameters. Phys Imaging Radiat Oncol. 2020;16:113–29.
2. Low DA, Dempsey JF. Evaluation of gamma dose distribution comparison method. Med Phys. 2003;30:2455–64.

Follow-Up During Treatment

28

Orit Kaidar-Person, Philip Poortmans, and Icro Meattini

28.1 Follow-Up During Treatment

Most guidelines do not address whether on-treatment-visits (OTV) should be scheduled in-advance or *on demand* in case of side effects or patient's preference. Ideally, OTV should be exclusively determined according to the potential side effects and their timing rather than stone-aged regulations, without adding potential workload to the team and redundant visits for the patients. Occurrence and severity of acute side effects during RT for breast cancer are mainly related to patient's anatomy, target volumes, doses, concomitant treatments, techniques, and individual radiosensitivity. Most of those factors translate into parameters that determine or can be derived from RT planning: dose homogeneity, skin dose and use of bolus, electron versus photon beams, total doses, and fractionation (all discussed in different sections of this book). In the past, patients systematically developed symptoms during treatment, especially due to protracted treatment regimens, field-based (instead of volume-based) RT techniques, and inhomogeneous dose delivery (see dosimetric issues and the transition from 3DCRT to IMRT/VMAT section).

Apart from skin reactions, mostly expressed in skin folds (inframammary and axillary) and in the upper-inner quadrants (more exposed to weather circumstances including the sun), symptoms related to 2DRT planning techniques also included oesophagitis in case of lymph nodal RT (IMN and peri-clavicular). Finally, the protracted period of daily RT delivery, especially combined with larger irradiated volumes, can also induce fatigue. Therefore, we used to have time-consuming weekly patients' OTV including psycho-social accompaniment.

Nowadays, with the combination of shorter treatment courses, conformal 3D-target volume-based RT, reduction of irradiated volumes and

O. Kaidar-Person (✉)
Radiation Oncology Unit, Sheba Medical Center, Ramat Gan, Israel

Sackler School of Medicine, Tel-Aviv University, Tel-Aviv, Israel

GROW-School for Oncology and Developmental Biology (Maastro), Maastricht University, Maastricht, The Netherlands
e-mail: Orit.KaidarPerson@sheba.health.gov.il

P. Poortmans
Faculty of Medicine and Health Sciences, University of Antwerp, Antwerp, Belgium

Department of Radiation Oncology Iridium Netwerk, Antwerp, Belgium
e-mail: philip.poortmans@gza.be

I. Meattini
Department of Experimental and Clinical Biomedical Sciences "M. Serio", University of Florence, Florence, Italy

Radiation Oncology Unit, Oncology Department, Azienda Ospedaliero-Universitaria Careggi, Florence, Italy
e-mail: icro.meattini@unifi.it

© The Author(s), under exclusive license to Springer Nature Switzerland AG 2022
O. Kaidar-Person et al. (eds.), *Breast Cancer Radiation Therapy*,
https://doi.org/10.1007/978-3-030-91170-6_28

doses, significantly less acute side effects are observed [1]. Moreover, currently patients are overall better informed and accompanied during their breast cancer treatment pathway, including for the RT component. Conversely, systemic therapies used preceding or concomitant with RT may increase acute toxicity (see "toxicity section" and "concomitant radiation and systemic therapy in the adjuvant and metastatic setting" sections). Therefore, while much less routine OTV is required compared to the past, its need should be ideally adopted case-by-case or using a pre-defined local protocol.

Indeed, high-level information and counselling on potential combination effects using ionising radiation and systemic therapies, one of the crucial background objectives of the radiation/clinical oncologist core curriculum [2], should be offered to the patient. The team should identify patients who might not be optimally informed (due to limited comprehension including disabilities, beliefs, age, linguistics). While every effort should be made to optimise full comprehension and informed consent, this is sometimes not fully achievable, which leads to higher levels of demands for close guidance through their treatment. Conversely, well-informed patients, who reviewed all possible available information on different media (e.g. flyers, video, social media, worldwide web) might be exposed to excessive out-of-the-context and even unreliable data and misinformation which eventually might cause stress and anxiety, likewise increasing the need for OTV. For patients with locally advanced breast cancer (e.g. inoperable patients, skin involvement), who have clinical evident disease, prescheduled OTV are encouraged, to record response to therapy. Factors that might indicate that patients will need scheduled OTV visits are listed in Table 28.1.

Some RT departments offer patients pre-RT sessions with a dedicated team (RTT, nurse) for guidance of care during RT to reduce the possibility of acute side effects, reduce pre-treatment anxiety, and improve treatment compliance. This can be organised as shared sessions for groups of patients or on individual basis, both potentially reducing OTV-related workload.

Table 28.1 Factors that might indicate that patients will need scheduled OTV

Factors to consider for scheduled OTV
• Extreme age (very young/older adults)
• Frail patients
• Comorbidities that might limit patient's compliance to RT or increase the risk of side effects
• Body habitus that is prone for toxicity:
– Large breast size
– Multiple skin folds, skin tags ("dogears")
– Challenging anatomy and proximity to OAR (e.g. oesophagus)
• Advance local disease, such as skin involvement
• RT-related:
– New RT fractionation/protocol/equipment
– Patients who are treated once a week (e.g. FAST protocol)
• Prone to difficulty in compliance with treatment position:
– Difficulties in upwards arm positioning
– Discomfort and pain
– Anxiety and stress
• Concomitant systemic therapy

It should be noted that with the increasing use of hypofractionation, and thereby shorter overall treatment courses, acute side effects may sometimes appear only (weeks) after completion of RT (mostly 3 weeks after initiation of treatment, or 2 weeks in case of preceding or concomitant systemic therapy). With the adoption of ultrafractionation for breast cancer (e.g. FAST FORWARD [3] or APBI-IMRT-Florence trial [4, 5] schedules with treatment delivery in 5 fractions over 1 week), or fractionations similar to the FAST protocol [6] (five fractions, once a week, over 5 treatment weeks) a remote contact with the patients 2–3 weeks after completion of RT could be advisable, when feasible: questionnaires (web-based or one of the electronic patient-reported outcome measures [PROM] tools); telephone; telemedicine, or even actual visits are all possible options. Due to the COVID-19 pandemic, the FAST FORWARD protocol was widely adopted [7, 8], even prior to full publication of the 5-year follow-up of the trial, and telemedicine has become an acceptable tool to evaluate toxicity while maintaining social distancing. Telemedicine allows for a triage to identify cases that may need actual visits for further care of toxicity [8]. The transition from the consept that "every patient must be seen every week" to "visits during RT are available on demand, when questions or side effects arise" takes time, as it requires a mindset change in the spirit of the patients and, often more difficult to obtain, of the health-care providers.

28.2 OTV Documentation

We advise that a different electronic-page format will be used for OTV, capturing information of the date of initial RT treatment, the number of fractions the patient received up to the date of evaluation out of the number of fractions given, and the total dose planned. This OTV page should record PROMs, which are designed to capture the common toxicities from radiation in a validated scale, including fatigue, pain, discomfort of the arm, and objective evaluation of the physician or nurse with validated toxicity grading (e.g. CTCAE). An example for OTV documentation is provided in Tables 28.2 and 28.3, which were modulated from the EORTC QoL BR23 and CTCAE. As these forms are helpful for OTV and after treatment follow-up, they can serve for reference in case a patient is coming for follow-up after RT is completed for evaluation of symptoms. Additionally, in the future, if department's RT protocols are modified this information can be used to compare side effects from treatment.

Table 28.2 Example for electronic OTV-form

Patient's reported outcomes				
During the past week:				
Please circle:				
1.1. Did you have any pain in your arm or shoulder?	Not at all	A little bit	Quite a bit	Very much
	1	2	3	4
1.2. Did you have a swollen arm or hand?	Not at all	A little bit	Quite a bit	Very much
	1	2	3	4
1.3. Was it difficult to raise your arm or to move it sideways?	Not at all	A little bit	Quite a bit	Very much
	1	2	3	4
1.4. Have you had any breast pain?	Not at all	A little bit	Quite a bit	Very much
	1	2	3	4
1.5. Have you had any breast swelling?	Not at all	A little bit	Quite a bit	Very much
	1	2	3	4
1.6. Have you had any increased breast sensitivity?	Not at all	A little bit	Quite a bit	Very much
	1	2	3	4
7. Have you had skin problems on the breast?	Not at all	A little bit	Quite a bit	Very much
(e.g. itchy, dry, flaky)?	1	2	3	4

Modulated from EORTC-Breast (QLQ-BR23) for the purpose of this section. Note that this format is not validated as a QoL measure, and an updated version, QLQ-BR45 is available

28.3 Summary

On-treatment-visits should be scheduled taking into consideration various factors including the needs of the patient, chances for side effects, and timing of side effects. However, OTV should be adjusted to the department workload and patients' need, as obligatory weekly OTV in many cases can overload both patients and treating teams. OTV should serve the patient to reduce potential side effects and possibly anxiety from therapy and to increase compliance.

Table 28.3 Example for physician of OTV

# Fraction:	**Cumulative dose to date (Gy):**
Plan total dose (Gy)/fractions:	
Comments* :	

* Special comments about target volumes, dose, and fractionation: example—nodal boost, bolus

Pain of skin	0 None	1 Mild	2 Moderate pain; limiting instrumental ADL	3 Severe pain; limiting self-care ADL	–	–
Fatigue	0 None	1 Fatigue relieved by rest	2 Fatigue not relieved by rest; limiting instrumental ADL	3 Fatigue not relieved by rest, limiting self-care ADL	–	–
Radiation dermatitis	0 None	1 Faint erythema or dry desquamation	2 Moderate to brisk erythema, mostly confined to skin folds and creases; moderate oedema	3 Confluent moist desquamation, other than skin folds and creases; bleeding induced by minor trauma or abrasion	4 Life-threatening consequences, skin necrosis, or ulceration of full thickness dermis; spontaneous bleeding from involved site; skin graft indicated	5 Death
Breast oedema	0 None	1 Asymptomatic breast enlargement	2 Symptomatic (e.g. pain or psychosocial impact)	3 Severe symptoms; intervention indicated; need to enlarge RT fields	–	–

Pain treatment : None/Tylenol/NSAID/Opioids/other_____________

Treatment used for dermatitis: calendula/hydrocortisone/Silver sulfadiazine/mepilex dressing/other_________

**Based on CTCAE v 4.0

References

1. Marta GN, Coles C, Kaidar-Person O, et al. The use of moderately hypofractionated post-operative radiation therapy for breast cancer in clinical practice: a critical review. Crit Rev Oncol Hematol. 2020;156:103090.
2. Benstead K, Lara PC, Eller Y, et al. Clinical oncology module for the ESTRO core curriculum. Radiother Oncol. 2020;156:19–22.
3. Murray Brunt A, Haviland JS, Wheatley DA, et al. Hypofractionated breast radiotherapy for 1 week versus 3 weeks (FAST-Forward): 5-year efficacy and late normal tissue effects results from a multicentre, non-inferiority, randomised, phase 3 trial. Lancet. 2020;395:1613–26.
4. Meattini I, Saieva C, Marrazzo L, et al. Accelerated partial breast irradiation using intensity-modulated radiotherapy technique compared to whole breast irradiation for patients aged 70 years or older: subgroup analysis from a randomized phase 3 trial. Breast Cancer Res Treat. 2015;153:539–47.
5. Meattini I, Marrazzo L, Saieva C, et al. Accelerated partial-breast irradiation compared with whole-breast irradiation for early breast cancer: long-term results of the randomized phase III APBI-IMRT-florence trial. J Clin Oncol. 2020;38:4175.
6. Group FT, Agrawal RK, Alhasso A, et al. First results of the randomised UK FAST Trial of radiotherapy hypofractionation for treatment of early breast cancer (CRUKE/04/015). Radiother Oncol. 2011;100:93–100.
7. Coles CE, Aristei C, Bliss J, et al. International guidelines on radiation therapy for breast cancer during the COVID-19 pandemic. Clin Oncol. 2020;32:279–81.
8. Machiels M, Weytjens R, Bauwens W, et al. Accelerated adaptation of ultrahypofractionated radiation therapy for breast cancer at the time of the COVID-19 pandemic. Clin Oncol (R Coll Radiol). 2020;33:e166.

Management of Acute Toxicity

29

Kim Cao and Ilanit Dromi Shahadi

29.1 Background

A consistent rate of patients affected by breast cancer treated with RT might develop acute skin toxicity. Though in most cases of mild intensity, breast RT side effects can significantly impact patients' health-related quality of life for a short period.

29.2 Key Information for Clinical Practice

29.2.1 Skin Toxicity

Acute radiation dermatitis is the most frequently observed side effect related to breast RT and affects up to 90% of patients (at different grades of toxicity), occurring within 2–4 weeks after the start of RT and until 1–2 week(s) after the end of treatment. The timing of skin toxicity is highly dependent on other factors such as systemic therapy. Radiation activates inflammatory pathways, affecting radiosensitive precursors of epidermal keratinocytes located in the stratum basale. Epidermis renewal by these stem cells is constant (3–4 weeks per cycle), resulting in delayed radiation induced effects, but is accelerated after preceding chemotherapy, thus these patients tend to develop skin toxicity earlier than those who were not treated with chemotherapy. Patients report symptoms such as discomfort, dryness or sweating, pruritus, and pain. On physical examination, there is mild erythema, and in a minority of cases moist desquamation. The most common identified risk factors for RT-related skin toxicity are: patient related factors such as breast size (related to RT planning, inframammary, and subcutis fold) [1, 2], smoking [3]; treatment-related factors: beam energy (inhomogeneous RT plan) [4], treatment technique [1, 5], the use of bolus as a tissue equivalent, and concomitant or previous systemic therapies.

An accurate assessment of radiation dermatitis according to RTOG or CTCAE scale (Table 29.1) is crucial and helps to determine symptomatic treatment. The use of quality of life PROMS (Patient-Reported Outcomes Measures) can also be useful to improve clinical practice. Homogeneous collection of these data from the beginning of treatment is important in order to have a baseline for patients and unbiased comparison over follow-up. Figures 29.1, 29.2, 29.3 and 29.4 show different presentations of acute skin reaction, occurring within 2 weeks from completion of RT course.

K. Cao (✉)
Institut Curie, Paris, France
e-mail: kim.cao@curie.fr

I. D. Shahadi
Sheba Medical Center, Ramat Gan, Israel
e-mail: Ilanit.Shahdi@sheba.health.gov.il

© The Author(s), under exclusive license to Springer Nature Switzerland AG 2022
O. Kaidar-Person et al. (eds.), *Breast Cancer Radiation Therapy*,
https://doi.org/10.1007/978-3-030-91170-6_29

Table 29.1 Toxicity scale

Grade	0	1	2	3	4
CTCAE V.5 [82]		Faint erythema or dry desquamation	Moderate to brisk erythema; patchy moist desquamation, mostly confined to skin folds and creases; moderate oedema	Moist desquamation in areas other than skin folds and creases; bleeding induced by minor trauma or abrasion	Skin necrosis or ulceration of full thickness dermis; spontaneous bleeding from involved site; skin graft indicated

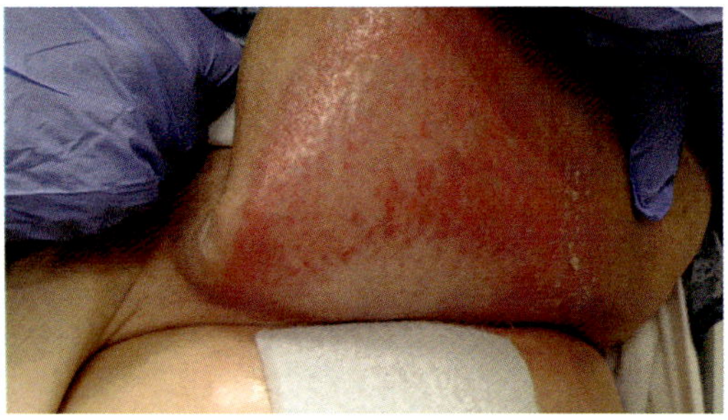

Fig. 29.1 Moist desquamation in the mammary fold of a patient with large ptotic breasts (grade 2)

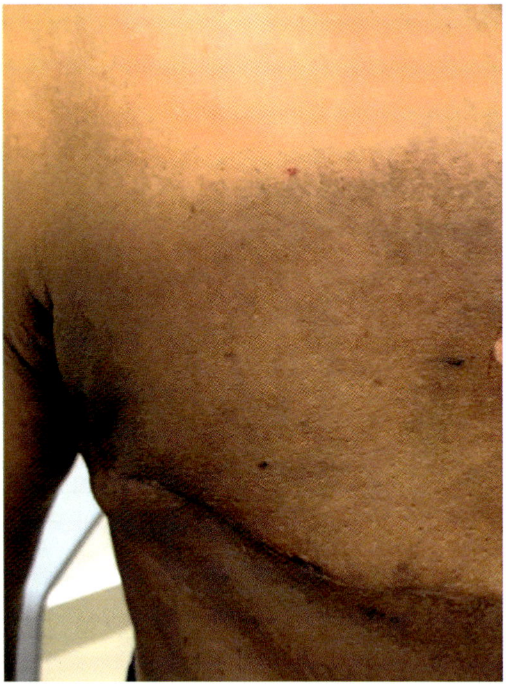

Fig. 29.2 Moderate erythema and early pigmentation of chest wall at the end of radiation course with bolus (grade 2)

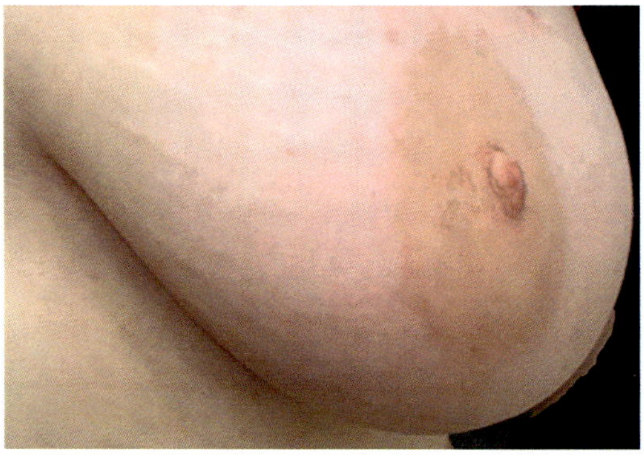

Fig. 29.3 Mild erythema of the breast skin (grade 1)

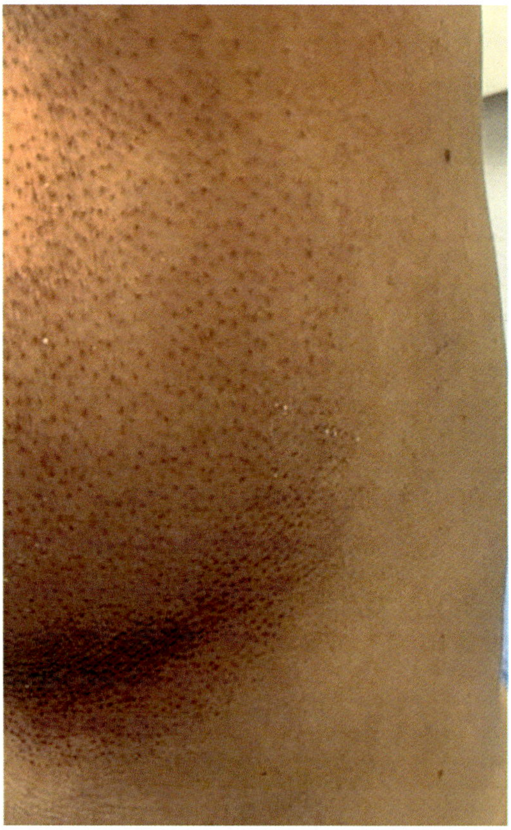

Fig. 29.4 Mild erythema of the breast skin with hyperpigmentation (grade 1)

29.2.1.1 Hygiene Counselling

Gentle skin washing with water, with or without mild soap is recommended during breast RT, supported by two randomised trials [6, 7]. The effect of deodorants on acute skin toxicity was assessed in two small randomised studies, and there is no evidence to avoid their use during the treatment period, including with axillary RT [8, 9]. Other practical tips and strict hygiene instructions, mainly based on expert clinical experience but not substantiated by evidence, are summarised in Table 29.2. Attention for patients who have ptotic breasts, as this area may be associated with fungal infection due to moist and poor hygiene, and this area is prone for RT-related acute side effects (Fig. 29.1).

29.2.1.2 Topical Corticosteroids

Corticosteroids have anti-inflammatory properties and a large number of trials have assessed their efficacy in the prevention and treatment of radiation dermatitis. The most studied is mometasone furoate [10–13]. In a recent study, this agent was compared with an emollient cream. A total of 124 patients underwent post-mastectomy RT with the use of daily bolus of 3–10 mm in all patients, of whom 66% were treated with 3DCRT (50 Gy in 25 fractions or 50.4 Gy in 28 fractions). There was a reduced incidence of moist desquamation in the group with mometasone compared with control group (43.8% vs. 66.7%, $p = 0.012$) [13]. However, these trials should be criticised for the total RT dose and fractionation and the use of bolus, all were proved by others to increase skin toxicity compared to moderate hypofractionation protocols and bolus omission. Mometasone efficacy was observed in a randomised trial including patients treated with hypofractionated breast RT (40 Gy in 15 fractions) ($n = 120$). In the mometasone group, mean RTOG scores were lower than in the control group treated with an emollient ($p = 0.046$), and there was a significant improvement in patients' quality of life according to the DLQI (Dermatology Quality of Life Index) [12]. In two smaller randomised studies, hydrocortisone cream and beclometasone spray, respectively, were shown to reduce the rate of grade 1–2 radiation dermatitis in breast cancer patients treated with conventional RT (1.8–2 Gy per fraction) [14, 15]. According to the MASCC (Multinational Association of Supportive Care in Cancer), topical steroids are the only recommended prophylactic treatment

Table 29.2 Treatment of breast cancer radiation dermatitis

Grade (CTCAE v5)	0	1	2	3	4
Timing[a]	–	Day 0–14	Day 10–28		
Treatments[a]	Patient education. Skincare measures: • Gentle daily washing with water with mild soap • Avoid skin irritation (e.g. avoid use of fragrance, avoid shaving the treated area or any other kind of hair removal; avoid scratching the treated area even in case of itchy skin; avoid exposure of the treated area to extreme temperatures) • Wear loose-fitting and sun-protective clothes (a cotton undershirt under a non-wire bra)	Consider hydrating lotions/creams	– Advise hydrating lotions/creams; consider bandages such as Mepilex®	Use hydrating lotions/creams; consider corticosteroid-containing cream or anti-infectants (silver sulfadiazine) – In case of documented infection: topical ± systemic antibiotics	Individualised care by a trained team is required: surgical treatment, skin graft.

[a]Revised from "Radiation therapy treatment effects", Bridget F. Koontz, 2017

for acute radiodermatitis [16]. However, the MASCC based these recommendations on studies that were conducted with small sample sizes. Although the results were in favour of the use of prophylactic topical steroids in reducing the acute effect of radiation dermatitis, we do not recommend for their routine use. By meticulous radiation planning, better dose homogeneity and the use of shorter radiation schemes (i.e. hypofractionation), and using a bolus only in patients who are at high risk for skin recurrence, the rates of acute dermatitis can be reduced. The MASCC report [16] did not address these factors within these trials, nor did the studies evaluated radiation quality assurance. Therefore, we do not recommend the use of prophylactic topical steroids (e.g. mometasone). Topical steroids can be considered in symptomatic patients, to reduce discomfort associated with itching. The treatment duration with topical steroids should be limited.

29.2.1.3 Topical Non-Steroidal Agents

Many randomised trials of small size have assessed the efficacy of topical skin care cream in order to alleviate radiation dermatitis effects, but except silver sulfadiazine, no one has shown clear clinical benefit. In a randomised study including breast cancer patients undergoing RT ($N = 102$), there was significantly less acute skin toxicity according to RTOG in the group treated with topical silver sulfadiazine versus the control group (skincare alone) ($p < 0.001$). Trolamine® have not shown efficacy in the preventive or curative setting [17, 18]. The RTOG 97–13 study compared Trolamine to best supportive care in women undergoing breast RT ($N = 172$). There was no difference for overall dermatitis between the two groups [17]. There is no demonstrated efficacy of acid hyaluronic cream [19, 20], calendula [21, 22], aloe vera gel [23], doxepin [24], and sucralfate cream [25].

29.2.1.4 Skin Dressings

Safetac-based films (Mepilex®, Mepitel®) are absorbent soft-silicone based dressings that provide a moist environment that promotes wound healing. In case of existing erythema, Mepilex film reduces the severity of skin reaction compared with aqueous cream in two controlled studies, but did not reduce the incidence of moist desquamation [26, 27]. In another monocentric randomised study, Mepitel® film was compared to aqueous cream in the prevention of radiation dermatitis for patients treated with non-hypofractionation breast RT ($N = 78$). Moist desquamation rate was lower in the Mepitel® group than in the control group (0% vs. 26%, $p < 0.001$). Of interest, there was no significant bolus effect [28]. There is no evidence of efficacy for the use of hydrophilic [29] or silver leaf nylon dressings in the preventive setting [30].

Treatments of breast cancer radiation dermatitis are summarised in Table 29.2.

29.2.2 Noncutaneous Acute Toxicity

29.2.2.1 Breast Swelling and Sensitivity

Patients can experience swelling of the breast or the chest wall, causing discomfort and pain, which persistent inflammation following surgery aggravated by RT. Risk factors include large breasts, a large seroma, extensive surgery with complete ALND [31, 32]. In a recent prospective study including women treated with breast conserving surgery followed by adjuvant breast RT ($N = 836$), 12% of patients reported breast oedema prior to the start of RT, 7.1% at 3 months, and 12.4% at 6 months [33]. These patients reported significantly higher levels of breast pain and a poorer QoL. Breast swelling is usually transient, typically resolving spontaneously within a few months after the end of treatment; if persisting, manual lymphatic drainage can be proposed.

29.2.2.2 Oesophagitis

Radiation oesophagitis is inflammation, oedema, erythema, and erosion of the mucosal surface of the oesophagus caused by radiation therapy to nearby or related structures. In case of breast cancer, it is mostly due to RT to regional nodes (medial supraclavicular area). Symptoms include throat pain and dysphagia, and the sensation that food is stuck [34, 35]. Most cases develop within

2–3 weeks post-initial treatment and 6 months for late development. Symptoms may be cumulative but are typically self-limiting, regressing 2–4 weeks after the completion of radiation treatment [34–39].

Studies of dosimetric factors which may influence the incidence and severity of oesophagitis in breast cancer patients receiving RT to the supraclavicular nodes concluded that >15% of RNI patients developed symptomatic oesophagitis. IMRT use was associated with higher rates of oesophagitis [40]. By limiting the mean dose to the irradiated oesophagus to <31 Gy during the planning process and ensuring that <1 cm of pharynx is included in the radiation field, oesophageal toxicity may be minimised [38, 41].

The most important measure to prevent this side effect is correct target volume delineation and RT planning. Early breast cancer needing elective nodal irraidation, who are planned according to ESTRO guidelines (2015, 2016), and if RT planning is done appropriately, patients are not expected to suffer from oesophagitis (see Chap. 19). In more advanced breast cases, with gross nodal disease (not elective nodal RT) in which the planned volumes are often more extensive, care should be given to reduce the dose to such OARs, without compromising coverage to high-risk volumes.

Treatment is supportive care with adequate hydration and nutrition intake. Dietary modifications are rarely necessary in breast cancer patients undergoing RT.

29.2.2.3 Arms Symptoms

The main treatment-related risk factors for breast cancer-related lymphoedema are axillary lymph node dissection (ALND) and regional lymph node radiation (RNI) [42–44]. RNI increases lymphoedema risk compared to breast/chest wall RT alone [44, 45]. Depending on RT planning, RNI may be associated with higher risk for late arm/shoulder morbidity [46].

Significant correlations ($p < 0.05$) were found between dose–volume histograms (DVHs), and arm stiffness, arm pain, use of arm and shoulder abduction difference, when arm/shoulder RT dose levels were approximately 15 Gy [47].

The START trials showed arm/shoulder pain in up to a third of the patients over 5 years after treatment, and around 20% of the patients complained about shoulder stiffness [48]. Several studies reported paraesthesia as a symptom after RT to the supraclavicular lymph nodes in breast cancer patients [49]. Two important mesures to reduce arm toxicity are: 1) not including the operated axilla in the irradiated volumes (see the EORTC 22922/10925 trial), unless there is residual disease, 2) Proper volume deliniation: The ESTRO guidelines (2015, 2016) for elective nodal delineation recommend adding a PRV to the humorous head, to reduce the unnecessary dose to the humeral head/arm and reduce the chances of arm/shoulder morbidity. Correct deliniation of the nodal volumes according to the ESTRO guidelines will also avoid the draining lymphatics from the arm and back, thus potentially reduce arm symptoms (lymphoedema and reduced mobility) (see Chap. 19).

In patients who suffer from arm/shoulder symptoms after treatment, physiotherapy is advised.

29.2.2.4 Fatigue

Radiation induced fatigue is described as a pervasive, subjective sense of tiredness persisting over time, interferes with activities of daily living, and is not relieved by adequate rest or sleep [50–53]. However, fatigue is mostly encountered in case of large RT volumes (e.g. Mantle fields), protracted RT schemes (e.g. 50 Gy in 25 fractions followed by a boost). For shorter RT schedules for early breast stage fatigue should be minimal. Fatigue at time of RT can be a result of systemic therapy, overall treatments, diagnosis of cancer and psychological/social distress. In general, RT may induce "early fatigue" (occurring during treatment or shortly after) and was described in up to 80% of patients [54–59]. Fatigue severity increases from the beginning to the middle of RT and remains elevated from the middle to the end of RT with a reduction in fatigue over weekends [54, 57]. Radiation induced fatigue decreases to pre-treatment levels within 4–8 weeks following the completion of the treatment [60]. However, the use of hypofractionated RT for breast cancer versus conventional fractionated RT was associated with less fatigue [61]. Acute RT side effects such as radiation dermatitis and prolonged RT (with sequential boost for example) were associated with fatigue at time of RT [62]. Radiation induced fatigue is frequently underestimated by medical and nursing staff, only about 50% of patients discuss it with a physician and in one-fourth of cases any intervention is proposed to the patient [63].

Different measures can be taken to reduce treatment-related fatigue. Aerobic exercise is the only intervention shown to consistently reduce radiation induced fatigue [50, 64–67]. The NCCN guidelines recommend a combination of endurance and resistance exercises to manage radiation induced fatigue [50, 68]. Most of these exercises are at least twice weekly and involve range of motion/flexibility, muscle strength, aerobic training, and mind/body fitness [50, 64]. Other interventions investigated include psychosocial interventions [69], cognitive-behavioural therapy [70], relaxation [54, 57–75], complementary and alternative therapies [76–78], Chinese medicine [79], energy conservation [80], and group psychotherapy [54, 81]. Patients should be reassured that fatigue could be a complication of the RT, not necessarily a symptom of cancer progression [54].

The NCCN Practice Guidelines in Oncology currently recommend five non-pharmacological interventions to manage fatigue related to cancer and/or cancer therapy (not specifically for RT-related fatigue), which include activity enhancement, psychosocial improvement, attention-restoring therapy, nutrition, and sleep. The NCCN guidelines recommend that after ruling out other causes of fatigue, the use of psychostimulants should be considered [50, 68]. However, this approach should be carefully applied, only after psychological evaluation, as most patients who are treated for early breast cancer have a curable disease. Disease progression should be rolled out if the fatigue is not improving and does not correlate with treatment burden (i.e. systemic therapy).

A few pharmacological agents have been found effective in the management of radiation-related fatigue. Correction of anaemia before or during the RT (mostly in metastatic/advance stage patients) [54, 71–73], treatment of other concomitant disturbances (dehydration, malnutrition, infections), and side effects of therapy may also help. Adjuvant therapies with antidepressants, tranquillisers, and analgesic agents have also been proposed in the literature [54, 55, 74]. Importantly, most of the breast cancer patients have a curable disease and current RT protocols for adjuvant RT are not associated with significant fatigue. We advocate to promote health-behaviour such activity enhancement, nutrition and sufficient sleep. Psychosocial distress should be identified and appropriate support should be offered.

29.3 Summary

Radiation dermatitis is the most frequent acute toxicity of breast RT. Hygiene instructions are recommended during the treatment. Swelling and sensitivity of the breast are usually transient side effects requiring no specific treatment and might be alleviated by cold compress. Patients with arm symptoms including arm stiffness due to RT and/or surgery should be reffered to physical therapy.

Fatigue is common during radiation therapy and shortly after it. Patients should be informed that RT-related fatigue is a transient side-affect and is not related to disease progression. Physical activity is encouraged during RT, and it is advised to rearrange activity-rest schedule in order to improve patient's ability to cope with the RT period.

References

1. Freedman GM, Li T, Nicolaou N, Chen Y, Ma CC-M, Anderson PR. Breast IMRT reduces time spent with acute dermatitis for women of all breast sizes during radiation. Int J Radiat Oncol Biol Phys. 2009;74(3):689–94.
2. Chen M-F, Chen W-C, Lai C-H, Hung C, Liu K-C, Cheng Y-H. Predictive factors of radiation-induced skin toxicity in breast cancer patients. BMC Cancer. 2010;10(1):508.

3. Sharp L, Johansson H, Hatschek T, Bergenmar M. Smoking as an independent risk factor for severe skin reactions due to adjuvant radiotherapy for breast cancer. Breast Edinb Scotl. 2013;22(5):634–8.
4. Pignol J-P, Vu TTT, Mitera G, Bosnic S, Verkooijen HM, Truong P. Prospective evaluation of severe skin toxicity and pain during postmastectomy radiation therapy. Int J Radiat Oncol Biol Phys. 2015;91(1):157–64.
5. Pignol J-P, Olivotto I, Rakovitch E, Gardner S, Sixel K, Beckham W, et al. A multicenter randomized trial of breast intensity-modulated radiation therapy to reduce acute radiation dermatitis. J Clin Oncol. 2008;26(13):2085–92.
6. Campbell IR, Illingworth MH. Can patients wash during radiotherapy to the breast or chest wall? A randomized controlled trial. Clin Oncol R Coll Radiol G B. 1992;4(2):78–82.
7. Roy I, Fortin A, Larochelle M. The impact of skin washing with water and soap during breast irradiation: a randomized study. Radiother Oncol. 2001;58(3):333–9.
8. Théberge V, Harel F, Dagnault A. Use of axillary deodorant and effect on acute skin toxicity during radiotherapy for breast cancer: a prospective randomized noninferiority trial. Int J Radiat Oncol Biol Phys. 2009;75(4):1048–52.
9. Lewis L, Carson S, Bydder S, Athifa M, Williams AM, Bremner A. Evaluating the effects of aluminum-containing and non-aluminum containing deodorants on axillary skin toxicity during radiation therapy for breast cancer: a 3-armed randomized controlled trial. Int J Radiat Oncol Biol Phys. 2014;90(4):765–71.
10. Boström A, Lindman H, Swartling C, Berne B, Bergh J. Potent corticosteroid cream (mometasone furoate) significantly reduces acute radiation dermatitis: results from a double-blind, randomized study. Radiother Oncol J Eur Soc Ther Radiol Oncol. 2001;59(3):257–65.
11. Miller RC, Schwartz DJ, Sloan JA, Griffin PC, Deming RL, Anders JC, et al. Mometasone furoate effect on acute skin toxicity in breast cancer patients receiving radiotherapy: a phase III double-blind, randomized trial from the north central cancer treatment group N06C4. Int J Radiat Oncol Biol Phys. 2011;79(5):1460–6.
12. Hindley A, Zain Z, Wood L, Whitehead A, Sanneh A, Barber D, et al. Mometasone furoate cream reduces acute radiation dermatitis in patients receiving breast radiation therapy: results of a randomized trial. Int J Radiat Oncol Biol Phys. 2014;90(4):748–55.
13. Ho AY, Olm-Shipman M, Zhang Z, Siu CT, Wilgucki M, Phung A, et al. A randomized trial of mometasone furoate 0.1% to reduce high-grade acute radiation dermatitis in breast cancer patients receiving postmastectomy radiation. Int J Radiat Oncol Biol Phys. 2018;101(2):325–33.
14. Shukla PN, Gairola M, Mohanti BK, Rath GK. Prophylactic beclomethasone spray to the skin during postoperative radiotherapy of carcinoma breast: a prospective randomized study. Indian J Cancer. 2006;43(4):180–4.
15. Meghrajani CF, Co HS, Arcillas JG, Maaño CC, Cupino NA. A randomized, double-blind trial on the use of 1% hydrocortisone cream for the prevention of acute radiation dermatitis. Expert Rev Clin Pharmacol. 2016;9(3):483–91.
16. Wong RKS, Bensadoun R-J, Boers-Doets CB, Bryce J, Chan A, Epstein JB, et al. Clinical practice guidelines for the prevention and treatment of acute and late radiation reactions from the MASCC skin toxicity study group. Support Care Cancer. 2013;21(10):2933–48.
17. Fisher J, Scott C, Stevens R, Marconi B, Champion L, Freedman GM, et al. Randomized phase III study comparing best supportive care to Biafine as a prophylactic agent for radiation-induced skin toxicity for women undergoing breast irradiation: radiation therapy oncology group (RTOG) 97–13. Int J Radiat Oncol Biol Phys. 2000;48(5):1307–10.
18. Szumacher E, Wighton A, Franssen E, Chow E, Tsao M, Ackerman I, et al. Phase II study assessing the effectiveness of Biafine cream as a prophylactic agent for radiation-induced acute skin toxicity to the breast in women undergoing radiotherapy with concomitant CMF chemotherapy. Int J Radiat Oncol Biol Phys. 2001;51(1):81–6.
19. Kirova YM, Fromantin I, De Rycke Y, Fourquet A, Morvan E, Padiglione S, et al. Can we decrease the skin reaction in breast cancer patients using hyaluronic acid during radiation therapy? Results of phase III randomised trial. Radiother Oncol. 2011;100(2): 205–9.
20. Pinnix C, Perkins GH, Strom EA, Tereffe W, Woodward W, Oh JL, et al. Topical hyaluronic acid vs. standard of care for the prevention of radiation dermatitis after adjuvant radiotherapy for breast cancer: single-blind randomized phase III clinical trial. Int J Radiat Oncol Biol Phys. 2012;83(4):1089–94.
21. Pommier P, Gomez F, Sunyach MP, D'Hombres A, Carrie C, Montbarbon X. Phase III randomized trial of *Calendula officinalis* compared with trolamine for the prevention of acute dermatitis during irradiation for breast cancer. J Clin Oncol. 2004;22(8):1447–53.
22. Sharp L, Finnilä K, Johansson H, Abrahamsson M, Hatschek T, Bergenmar M. No differences between calendula cream and aqueous cream in the prevention of acute radiation skin reactions—results from a randomised blinded trial. Eur J Oncol Nurs. 2013;17(4):429–35.
23. Heggie S, Bryant GP, Tripcony L, Keller J, Rose P, Glendenning M, et al. A phase III study on the efficacy of topical aloe vera gel on irradiated breast tissue. Cancer Nurs. 2002;25(6):442–51.
24. Shariati L, Amouheidari A, Naji Esfahani H, Abed A, Haghjooy Javanmard S, Laher I, et al. Protective effects of doxepin cream on radiation dermatitis in breast cancer: a single arm double-blind randomized clinical trial. Br J Clin Pharmacol. 2020;86:1875–81.
25. Wells M, Macmillan M, Raab G, MacBride S, Bell N, MacKinnon K, et al. Does aqueous or sucralfate

cream affect the severity of erythematous radiation skin reactions? A randomised controlled trial. Radiother Oncol J Eur Soc Ther Radiol Oncol. 2004;73(2):153–62.
26. Diggelmann KV, Zytkovicz AE, Tuaine JM, Bennett NC, Kelly LE, Herst PM. Mepilex Lite dressings for the management of radiation-induced erythema: a systematic inpatient controlled clinical trial. Br J Radiol. 2010;83(995):971–8.
27. Paterson D. Randomized intra-patient controlled trial of Mepilex Lite dressings versus aqueous cream in managing radiation-induced skin reactions postmastectomy. J Cancer Sci Ther. 2012;4(11):347–56. https://www.omicsonline.org/randomized-intra-patient-controlled-trial-of-mepilex-lite-dressings-versus-aqueous-cream-in-managing-radiation-induced-skin-reactions-postmastectomy-1948-5956.1000166.php?aid=8898. Accessed 8 Nov 2020.
28. Herst PM, Bennett NC, Sutherland AE, Peszynski RI, Paterson DB, Jasperse ML. Prophylactic use of Mepitel film prevents radiation-induced moist desquamation in an intra-patient randomised controlled clinical trial of 78 breast cancer patients. Radiother Oncol. 2014;110(1):137–43.
29. Bazire L, Fromantin I, Diallo A, de la Lande B, Pernin V, Dendale R, et al. Hydrosorb® versus control (water based spray) in the management of radio-induced skin toxicity: results of multicentre controlled randomized trial. Radiother Oncol. 2015;117(2):229–33.
30. Aquino-Parsons C, Lomas S, Smith K, Hayes J, Lew S, Bates AT, et al. Phase III study of silver leaf nylon dressing vs standard care for reduction of inframammary moist desquamation in patients undergoing adjuvant whole breast radiation therapy. J Med Imaging Radiat Sci. 2010;41(4):215–21.
31. Degnim AC, Miller J, Hoskin TL, Boughey JC, Loprinzi M, Thomsen K, et al. A prospective study of breast lymphedema: frequency, symptoms, and quality of life. Breast Cancer Res Treat. 2012;134(3):915–22.
32. Boughey JC, Hoskin TL, Cheville AL, Miller J, Loprinzi MD, Thomsen KM, et al. Risk factors associated with breast lymphedema. Ann Surg Oncol. 2014;21(4):1202–8.
33. Young-Afat DA, Gregorowitsch ML, van den Bongard DH, Burgmans I, van der Pol CC, Witkamp AJ, et al. Breast edema following breast-conserving surgery and radiotherapy: patient-reported prevalence, determinants, and effect on health-related quality of life. JNCI Cancer Spectr. 2019;3(2):pkz011. https://doi.org/10.1093/jncics/pkz011.
34. Nesheiwat Z, Akbar H, Kahloom A, Mahajan M. Radiation esophagitis. Treasure Island, FL: StatPearls; 2020.
35. Baker S, Fairchild A. Radiation-induced esophagitis in lung cancer. Lung Cancer Targets Ther. 2016;7:119–27. https://doi.org/10.2147/LCTT.S96443.
36. Murro D, Jakate S. Radiation esophagitis. Arch Pathol Lab Med. 2015;139:827–30. https://doi.org/10.5858/arpa.2014-0111-RS.
37. Coia LR, Myerson RJ, Tepper JE. Late effects of radiation therapy on the gastrointestinal tract. Int J Radiat Oncol Biol Phys. 1995;31(5):1213–36.
38. Trowers E, Thomas C, Silverstein FE. Chemical-and radiation-induced esophageal injury. Gastrointest Endosc Clin N Am. 1994;4(4):657–75.
39. Gong B, Jiang N, Yan G, Wang S, Deng C, Wei S, Zhao Y. Predictors for severe acute esophagitis in lung cancer patients treated with chemoradiotherapy: a systematic review. Curr Med Res Opin. 2016;32(10):1701–8.
40. Yaney A, Ayan AS, Pan X, Jhawar S, Healy E, Beyer S, Lindsey K, Kuhn K, Tedrick K, White JR, Bazan JG. Dosimetric parameters associated with radiation-induced esophagitis in breast cancer patients undergoing regional nodal irradiation. Radiother Oncol. 2020;155:167–73. https://doi.org/10.1016/j.radonc.2020.10.042.
41. West K, Schneider M, Wright C, Beldham-Collins R, Coburn N, Tiver K, Gebski V, Stuart KE. Radiation-induced oesophagitis in breast cancer: factors influencing onset and severity for patients receiving supraclavicular nodal irradiation. J Med Imaging Radiat Oncol. 2020;64(1):113–9. https://doi.org/10.1111/1754-9485.12943.
42. Tsai RJ, Dennis LK, Lynch CF, et al. The risk of developing arm lymphedema among breast cancer survivors: a meta-analysis of treatment factors. Ann Surg Oncol. 2009;16:1959–72. https://doi.org/10.1245/s10434-009-0452-2.
43. Shaitelman SF, Chiang YJ, Griffin KD, et al. Radiation therapy targets and the risk of breast cancer-related lymphedema: a systematic review and network meta-analysis. Breast Cancer Res Treat. 2017;162:201–15. https://doi.org/10.1007/s10549-016-4089-0.
44. Warren LE, Miller CL, Horick N, Skolny MN, Jammallo LS, Sadek BT, Shenouda MN, O'Toole JA, MacDonald SM, Specht MC, Taghian AG. The impact of radiation therapy on the risk of lymphedema after treatment for breast cancer: a prospective cohort study. Int J Radiat Oncol Biol Phys. 2014;88(3):565–71. https://doi.org/10.1016/j.ijrobp.2013.11.232.
45. Gillespie TC, Sayegh HE, Brunelle CL, et al. Breast cancer-related lymphedema: risk factors, precautionary measures, and treatments. Gland Surg. 2018;7:379–403. https://doi.org/10.21037/gs.2017.11.04.
46. Blomqvist L, Stark B, Engler N, Malm M. Evaluation of arm and shoulder mobility and strength after modified radical mastectomy and radiotherapy. Acta Oncol. 2004;43(3):280–3. https://doi.org/10.1080/02841860410026170.
47. Johansen S, Fosså K, Nesvold IL, Malinen E, Fosså SD. Arm and shoulder morbidity following surgery and radiotherapy for breast cancer. Acta Oncol. 2014;53(4):521–9. https://doi.org/10.3109/0284186X.2014.880512.
48. Hopwood R, Haviland JS, Sumo G, Mills J, Bliss JM, Yarnold JR, et al. Comparison of patient-reported breast, arm and shoulder symptoms and body image after

radiotherapy for early breast cancer: 5-year follow-up in the randomised standardisation of breast radiotherapy (START) trials. Lancet Oncol. 2010;11:231–40.
49. Lundstedt D, Gustafsson M, Steineck G, Alsadius D, Sundberg A, Wilderäng U, et al. Long-term symptoms after radiotherapy of supraclavicular lymph nodes in breast cancer patients. Radiother Oncol. 2012;103:155–60.
50. Hsiao C, Daly B, Saligan LN. The etiology and management of radiotherapy-induced fatigue. Expert Rev Qual Life Cancer Care. 2016;1(4):323–8.
51. Berger AM, Mooney K, Alvarez-Perez A, et al. Cancer-related fatigue, version 2.2015. Concisely and updated review on cancer-related fatigue from clinical practice guidelines in oncology. J Natl Compr Canc Netw. 2015;13(8):1012–39.
52. Bower JE. Cancer-related fatigue–mechanisms, risk factors, and treatments. Nat Rev Clin Oncol. 2014;11(10):597–609. https://doi.org/10.1038/nrclinonc.2014.127.
53. Piper BF, Cella D. Cancer-related fatigue: definitions and clinical subtypes. J Natl Compr Canc Netw. 2010;8(8):958–66.
54. Jereczek-Fossa BA, Marsiglia HR, Orecchia R. Radiotherapy related fatigue: how to assess and how to treat the symptom. A commentary. Tumori. 2001;87:147–51.
55. Hickok JT, Morrow GR, McDonald S, Bellg AJ. Frequency and correlates of fatigue in lung cancer patients receiving radiation therapy: implications for management. J Pain Symptom Manage. 1996;11:370–7.
56. Smets EM, Garssen B, Schuster-Uitterhoeve AL, de Haes JC. Fatigue in cancer patients. Br J Cancer. 1993;68:220–4.
57. Smets EM, Visser MR, Willems-Groot AF, Garssen B, Old-enburger F, van Tienhoven G, de Haes JC. Fatigue and radio-therapy: (A) experience in patients undergoing treatment. Br J Cancer. 1998;78:899–906.
58. Smets EM, Visser MR, Willems-Groot AF, Garssen B, Schuster-Uitterhoeve AL, de Haes JC. Fatigue and radio-therapy: (B) experience in patients 9 months following treatment. Br J Cancer. 1998;78:907–12.
59. Vogelzang NJ, Breitbart W, Cella D, Curt GA, Groopman JE, Horning SJ, Itri LM, Johnson DH, Scherr SL, Portenoy RK. Patient, caregiver, and oncologist perceptions of cancer-related fatigue: results of a tripart assessment survey. The fatigue coalition. Semin Hematol. 1997;34(suppl 2):4–12.
60. Dhruva A, Dodd M, Paul SM, Cooper BA, Lee K, West C, Aouizerat BE, Swift PS, Wara W, Miaskowski C. Trajectories of fatigue in patients with breast cancer before, during, and after radiation therapy. Cancer Nurs. 2010;33(3):201–12.
61. Kishan AU, Wang P-C, Sharif J, Kupelian PA, Steinberg ML, McCloskey SA. Clinical indicators of psychosocial distress predict for acute radiation-induced fatigue in patients receiving adjuvant radiation therapy for breast cancer: an analysis of patient-reported outcomes. Int J Radiat Oncol Biol Phys. 2016;95:946–55.
62. Nakamura N, Ito R, Takahashi O, Haga C, Shikama N, Akahane K, Ogita M, Mizuno N, Tamaki S, Sekiguchi K. Fatigue during breast radiation therapy and its predictive factors. Int J Radiat Oncol. 2013;87(2):S205.
63. Donovan KA, Jacobsen PB, Andrykowski MA, et al. Course of fatigue in women receiving chemotherapy and/or radiotherapy for early stage breast cancer. J Pain Symptom Manage. 2004;28:373–80.
64. Stubbe CE, Valero M. Complementary strategies for the management of radiation therapy side effects. J Adv Pract Oncol. 2013;4(4):219–31.
65. Mustian KM, Morrow GR, Carroll JK, et al. Integrative nonpharmacologic behavioral interventions for the management of cancer-related fatigue. Oncologist. 2007;12(Suppl 1):52–67. https://doi.org/10.1634/theoncologist.12-S1-52.
66. Mustian KM, Peppone L, Darling TV, Palesh O, Heckler CE, Morrow GR. A 4-week home-based aerobic and resistance exercise program during radiation therapy: a pilot randomized clinical trial. J Support Oncol. 2009;7:158–67.
67. Mock V, Pickett M, Ropka ME, Muscari Lin E, Stewart KJ, Rhodes VA, McDaniel R, Grimm PM, Krumm S, McCorkle R. Fatigue and quality of life outcomes of exercise during cancer treatment. Cancer Pract. 2001;9:119–27.
68. NCCN Clinical Practice Guidelines in Oncology. Current and comprehensive guideline for cancer-related fatigue including radiotherapy-induced fatigue. Cancer-related fatigue. J Natl Compr Canc Netw. 2016;1:1–56.
69. Rahmani S, Talepasand S. The effect of group mindfulness—based stress reduction program and conscious yoga on the fatigue severity and global and specific life quality in women with breast cancer. Med J Islam Repub Iran. 2015;29:175.
70. Armes J, Chalder T, Addington-Hall J, et al. A randomized controlled trial to evaluate the effectiveness of a brief, behaviorally oriented intervention for cancer-related fatigue. Cancer. 2007;110(6):1385–95. https://doi.org/10.1002/cncr.22923.
71. Dicato M, Duhem C, Berchem G, Ries F. Clinical benefit from erythropoietin. Curr Opin Oncol. 2000;12:297–302.
72. Lavey RS. Clinical trial experience using erythropoietin during radiation therapy. Strahlenther Onkol. 1998;174(suppl 4):24–30.
73. Spaeth D, Marchal C, Bataillard A, Blanc-Vincent MP. Updating 1999 of standards, options and recommendations (SOR) for the clinical use of erythropoietin in oncology Federation of the French Cancer Centres. Bull Cancer. 1999;86:631–9.
74. Okuyama T, Akechi T, Kugaya A, Okamura H, Imoto S, Nakano T, Mikami I, Hosaka T, Uchitomi Y. Factors correlated with fatigue in disease-free breast cancer patients: application of the cancer fatigue scale. Support Care Cancer. 2000;8:215–22.
75. Decker TW, Cline-Elsen J, Gallagher M. Relaxation therapy as an adjunct in radiation oncology. J Clin Psychol. 1992;48:388–93.

76. Bardy J, Finnegan-John J, Molassiotis A, et al. Providing acupuncture in a breast cancer and fatigue trial: the therapists' experience. Complement Ther Clin Pract. 2015;21(4):217–22. https://doi.org/10.1016/j.ctcp.2015.08.003.
77. Zick SM, Alrawi S, Merel G, et al. Relaxation acupressure reduces persistent cancer-related fatigue. Evid Based Complement Alternat Med. 2011;2011:142913. https://doi.org/10.1155/2011/142913.
78. Zick SM, Wyatt G, Murphy S, et al. Acupressure for persistent cancer-related fatigue in breast cancer survivors (AcuCrft): a study protocol for a randomized controlled trial. BMC Complement Altern Med. 2012;12:132. https://doi.org/10.1186/1472-6882-12-132.
79. Yang L, Li T-T, Chu Y-T, et al. Traditional Chinese medical comprehensive therapy for cancer-related fatigue. Chin J Integr Med. 2015;22(1):67–72. https://doi.org/10.1007/s11655-015-2105-6.
80. Barsevick AM, Dudley W, Beck S, et al. A randomized clinical trial of energy conservation for patients with cancer-related fatigue. Cancer. 2004;100(6):1302–10. https://doi.org/10.1002/cncr.20111.
81. Forester B, Kornfeld DS, Fleiss JL, Thompson S. Group psychotherapy during radiotherapy: effects on emotional and physical distress. Am J Psychiatry. 1993;150:1700–6.
82. Common Terminology Criteria for Adverse Events (CTCAE) Version 5. Published: November 27. US Department of Health and Human Services, National Institutes of Health, National Cancer Institute.

Part VII

After Completion of Radiation Therapy

30 Follow-up Guidelines, Evidence, and Recommendations

Merel Kimman, Marjan van Hezewijk, and Liesbeth J. Boersma

30.1 Background

30.1.1 Guidelines and Aims of Follow-up

After curative treatment for breast cancer, survivors will generally attend regular follow-up examinations. In most countries, guidelines prescribe follow-up visits every 3–4 months in the first 2–3 years, every 6–12 months up to 5, and annually thereafter [1, 2]. Routine blood tests, measurement of tumour markers, and/or surveillance imaging studies beyond mammography are not recommended in otherwise asymptomatic patients with no specific findings on clinical examination [1, 2]. The timing of the first mammography is no earlier than 6 months after surgery and definitive radiation therapy, and subsequent mammograms should be performed annually. The exact frequency, duration, and intensity (i.e. use of MRIs, bone scans, chest radiographs, liver ultrasounds, pelvic exams, computed tomography scans, etc.) differ per country and hospital and may depend on factors such as the age of the patient, tumour characteristics, or treatment modality. The guidelines do not specify who should perform the follow-up. Generally, alternations between medical specialties ensure that all types of therapy-related complications are adequately monitored. However, continuity of care by having a specialised health care professional acting as a patient navigator throughout follow-up is strongly recommended as well [2].

The aims of follow-up are to detect early local recurrences or contralateral breast cancer and to evaluate and treat therapy-related complications (such as menopausal symptoms, osteoporosis, and second cancers). For patients who received radiation therapy, monitoring and treatment of late toxicity is important, with a focus on cosmetic outcome, fibrosis, shoulder function, lymphoedema, pain, and cardiac and pulmonary toxicity. Importantly, follow-up also aims to provide psychological support and information and refer to specialised rehabilitation facilities and services, if needed. Depression and intense fatigue frequently occur in the months following the end of adjuvant chemotherapy and/or radiation therapy. In addition, there may be long-term survivorship issues involving work, family, and sexuality. Assessing and addressing these various quality of life issues

M. Kimman (✉)
Department of Clinical Epidemiology and Medical Technology Assessment, Care and Public Health Research Institute (CAPHRI), Maastricht University Medical Center, Maastricht, The Netherlands
e-mail: merel.kimman@mumc.nl

M. van Hezewijk
Radiotherapiegroep, Arnhem, The Netherlands
e-mail: m.vanhezewijk@radiotherapiegroep.nl

L. J. Boersma
Department of Radiation Oncology (Maastro), GROW-School for Oncology and Reproduction, Maastricht University Medical Center, Maastricht, The Netherlands
e-mail: liesbeth.boersma@maastro.nl

© The Author(s), under exclusive license to Springer Nature Switzerland AG 2022

O. Kaidar-Person et al. (eds.), *Breast Cancer Radiation Therapy*,
https://doi.org/10.1007/978-3-030-91170-6_30

is an important aspect of follow-up care. Specific survivorship programmes can enable patients to return to a normal life after breast cancer [3, 4]. Finally, follow-up care should encourage a healthy lifestyle, including regular exercise, a healthy diet, and cessation of smoking [5].

30.2 Key Information for Clinical Practice

30.2.1 The Evidence-Base for Follow-up Aimed to Detect Recurrences

Ten-year overall survival of breast cancer patients exceeds 70% in most European regions, with 89% survival for local and 62% for regional disease [6, 7]. Patients who develop a loco-regional recurrence have a higher risk of developing distant metastases and have worse survival compared to patients without recurrence [8]. There is no evidence, however, that routine or intensive follow-up aimed at early identification of recurrences improves prognosis [8, 9]. Most recurrences are detected on routine mammography or by women themselves in between scheduled follow-up visits. Therefore, alternative strategies for follow-up have been proposed, varying in frequency of visits, follow-up providers, and settings (e.g. telephone, e-consult) [9]. Since high-level evidence for any particular follow-up strategy is lacking there is opportunity for health professionals and patients to make a shared decision regarding the most suitable care for the individual patient [10]. A patient decision aid can help patients understand their own preferences and make informed choices. Use of such a decision aid appears promising in terms of positive effects on shared decision-making, choice evaluation, and costs [11]. Furthermore, a personal recurrence risk, based on patient, tumour, and treatment characteristics, could identify patients with low recurrence risk who might benefit from less frequent follow-up [12]. More frequent follow-up may be required for specific subgroups of patients, for example, those with familial breast cancer associated with BRCA mutations, patients with an advanced stage at initial diagnosis who are at higher risk of distant metastases, or those with a risk factor for the development of brain metastases (e.g. young age, pulmonary metastases, negative hormone receptor status, and HER2 amplification) [2, 6, 8, 13, 14].

30.2.2 The Evidence-Base for After Care to Deal with (Late) Treatment Effects and Distress

Optimising Quality of Life (QoL) by detection of side effects and distress, providing psychosocial support and information, and coaching to deal with fear of recurrence are crucial aims of follow-up. Yet, such QoL outcomes may be underestimated by clinicians and underreported by patients leading to suboptimal care [15, 16]. PROMs are increasingly being used in routine clinical care to more accurately characterise these outcomes. In The Netherlands, for example, the Distress Thermometer is used to detect distress in cancer patients and facilitate support for those patients who most need and want it [17, 18]. Furthermore, studies have shown that the systematic collection of QoL related PROMs can have a positive impact on symptom management, QoL, and patient–provider communication [19–22]. Effects are then most pronounced when results of the PROMs are fed back to the health care provider or patient and used to support care [20]. Specifically for radiation therapy, PROM data can be used to monitor toxicity >10 years after therapy and identify patients who need attention because of severe complaints. Moreover, patients are more willing to return a PROM than attend the clinic at this time. Hence, PROMs have the potential to reduce the number of visits to the radiation oncology clinic [23].

Finally, increasing evidence is emerging that points towards lifestyle factors having an effect on the prognosis of patients with breast cancer through impacting on the risk of recurrence or other health outcomes. For example, regular exercise provides functional and psychological benefits [4] and possibly reduces the risk of recurrence. A recent systematic review and meta-analysis of the impact of lifestyle on the risk of a second new primary cancer in the contralateral breast identified BMI is a modifiable risk factor for contralateral breast [24]. Nevertheless, most of the evidence is not sufficient to warrant a strong evidence-based recommendation.

30.3 Recommendations

After curative treatment for breast cancer, patients are generally followed clinically for at least 5 years after their treatment. An annual mammography and clinical examination remain the mainstay of follow-up, but high-level evidence for this is lacking. There is no evidence to perform more intensive follow-up, including scans. Yet, if evidence emerges that treatment of oligometastases prolonged survival, this may be reconsidered. On the basis of current evidence, we recommend:

- No more frequent or intensive follow-up than currently recommended in ESMO and ASCO guidelines (i.e. an annual mammography).
- The use of nomograms and PROMs to support personalised follow-up, identifying patients for whom less frequent follow-up would be safe and preferred, and those who need additional psychosocial support and coaching.
- To increase attention to the potential health benefits of a healthy lifestyle.
- Continuity of care by having a specialised health care professional, preferably a breast care nurse, as a patient navigator throughout follow-up.
- Implementation of PROMs to systematically monitor the quality of care.

References

1. Khatcheressian JL, et al. Breast cancer follow-up and management after primary treatment: American Society of Clinical Oncology clinical practice guideline update. J Clin Oncol. 2013;31(7):961–5.
2. Cardoso F, et al. Early breast cancer: ESMO clinical practice guidelines for diagnosis, treatment and follow-up†. Ann Oncol. 2019;30(8):1194–220.
3. Chlebowski RT, Aiello E, McTiernan A. Weight loss in breast cancer patient management. J Clin Oncol. 2002;20(4):1128–43.
4. Mustian KM, et al. Comparison of pharmaceutical, psychological, and exercise treatments for cancer-related fatigue: a meta-analysis. JAMA Oncol. 2017;3(7):961–8.
5. Runowicz CD, et al. American Cancer Society/American Society of Clinical Oncology breast cancer survivorship care guideline. CA Cancer J Clin. 2016;66(1):43–73.
6. Allemani C, et al. Predictions of survival up to 10 years after diagnosis for European women with breast cancer in 2000–2002. Int J Cancer. 2013;132(10):2404–12.
7. Pan H, et al. 20-year risks of breast-cancer recurrence after stopping endocrine therapy at 5 years. N Engl J Med. 2017;377(19):1836–46.
8. Geurts YM, et al. Patterns and predictors of first and subsequent recurrence in women with early breast cancer. Breast Cancer Res Treat. 2017;165(3):709–20.
9. Moschetti I, et al. Follow-up strategies for women treated for early breast cancer. Cochrane Database Syst Rev. 2016;2016(5):Cd001768.
10. Harnett A, et al. Diagnosis and treatment of early breast cancer, including locally advanced disease—summary of NICE guidance. BMJ. 2009;338:b438.
11. Klaassen LA, et al. A novel patient decision aid for aftercare in breast cancer patients: a promising tool to reduce costs by individualizing aftercare. Breast. 2018;41:144–50.
12. Witteveen A, et al. Personalisation of breast cancer follow-up: a time-dependent prognostic nomogram for the estimation of annual risk of locoregional recurrence in early breast cancer patients. Breast Cancer Res Treat. 2015;152(3):627–36.
13. Arvold ND, et al. Brain metastases after breast-conserving therapy and systemic therapy: incidence and characteristics by biologic subtype. Breast Cancer Res Treat. 2012;136(1):153–60.
14. Barnholtz-Sloan JS, et al. Incidence proportions of brain metastases in patients diagnosed (1973–2001) in the metropolitan Detroit cancer surveillance system. J Clin Oncol. 2004;22(14):2865–72.
15. Di Maio M, et al. Symptomatic toxicities experienced during anticancer treatment: agreement between patient and physician reporting in three randomized trials. J Clin Oncol. 2015;33(8):910–5.
16. Trotti A, et al. Patient-reported outcomes and the evolution of adverse event reporting in oncology. J Clin Oncol. 2007;25(32):5121–7.
17. Ploos van Amstel FK, et al. Distress screening remains important during follow-up after primary breast cancer treatment. Support Care Cancer. 2013;21(8):2107–15.
18. Tuinman MA, Gazendam-Donofrio SM, Hoekstra-Weebers JE. Screening and referral for psychosocial distress in oncologic practice. Cancer. 2008;113(4):870–8.

19. Kotronoulas G, et al. What is the value of the routine use of patient-reported outcome measures toward improvement of patient outcomes, processes of care, and health service outcomes in cancer care? A systematic review of controlled trials. J Clin Oncol. 2014;32(14):1480–501.
20. Graupner C, et al. Patient outcomes, patient experiences and process indicators associated with the routine use of patient-reported outcome measures (PROMs) in cancer care: a systematic review. Support Care Cancer. 2020;29(2):573–93.
21. van Egdom LSE, et al. Implementing patient-reported outcome measures in clinical breast cancer care: a systematic review. Value Health. 2019;22(10):1197–226.
22. Riis CL, et al. Are patient-reported outcomes useful in post-treatment follow-up care for women with early breast cancer? A scoping review. Patient Relat Outcome Meas. 2019;10:117–27.
23. Brouwers P, et al. Are PROMs sufficient to record late outcome of breast cancer patients treated with radiotherapy? A comparison between patient and clinician reported outcome through an outpatient clinic after 10 years of follow up. Radiother Oncol. 2018;126(1):163–9.
24. Akdeniz D, et al. The impact of lifestyle and reproductive factors on the risk of a second new primary cancer in the contralateral breast: a systematic review and meta-analysis. Cancer Causes Control. 2020;31(5):403–16.

Evaluation of Late Toxicity

31

Carlotta Becherini and Lorenzo Livi

31.1 Background

Clinicians constantly weigh anticipated benefits of RT against risks of treatment-associated toxicities. Early toxicity may lead to treatment discontinuation, which might negatively impact on outcomes. Late toxicity causes physical, emotional, and financial burden on patients, their families and caretakers. The development of increasingly complex multimodal, new techniques and multiagent treatment programmes creates further challenges. More quantitative measures of severity are lacking to evaluate radiation-induced late toxicity.

31.2 Relevant Information for Clinical Practice

First of all, it should be recognised that the vast majority of breast cancer patients that was treated with RT will develop no or only minor late side effects. Therefore, the value of routine follow-up for screening of side effects is very low, at the best. To avoid excessive medical visits, including all costs and other conveniences, a system for follow-up "on demand" seems to be preferable. For this, easy access for the patients needs to be organised. As a separate note, routinely scheduled follow-up visits can be of added value in the framework of clinical trials and research, in which case an adapted schedule that tappers-off over time might offer sufficient information without being an excess burden to the patients.

31.2.1 Skin Evaluation

Telangiectasia

- *Follow-up:*
  - Documentation in the preoperative/before RT is essential for comparison at the time of follow-up.
  - During the first examination, it is important to precisely describe the affected area (size, depth, morphological aspects, and colour) to assess the efficacy of treatment in the future.
- *Possible screening tools for signs and symptoms.*
  - Tissue compliance meter (TCM) measurements in the treated breast compared to the untreated breast [1].

C. Becherini (✉)
Department of Radiation Oncology, A.O.U. Careggi, University of Florence, Florence, Italy

L. Livi
Department of Radiation Oncology, A.O.U. Careggi, University of Florence, Florence, Italy

Department of Experimental and Clinical Biomedical Sciences "Mario Serio", University of Florence, Florence, Italy
e-mail: lorenzo.livi@unifi.it

© The Author(s), under exclusive license to Springer Nature Switzerland AG 2022

O. Kaidar-Person et al. (eds.), *Breast Cancer Radiation Therapy*,
https://doi.org/10.1007/978-3-030-91170-6_31

  - High-resolution ultrasonography (HRUS) is a noninvasive and easily repeatable technique that detects focal lesions from dermal and subdermal tissues quickly and accurately [2].
  - When the clinical presentation is unclear or suspicious, a biopsy and histopathological examination are obligatory.

Fibrosis/Chest Wall Pain

- *Follow-up:*
  - Documentation in the preoperative/before RT is essential for comparison at the time of follow-up.
- *Possible screening tools for signs and symptoms.*
  - Tissue compliance meter (TCM), for quantitative and objective recording of soft tissue consistency [1].
  - High-resolution ultrasonography (HRUS) could be useful but fibrosis could be hampered by pronounced oedema [3].
  - Differential diagnosis between RIF and malignancy can be confirmed by imaging [4].

Lymphatic evaluation

- *Follow-up:*
  - Preoperative measurement should be obtained [5] followed by regularly scheduled postoperative measurements for 3–5 years, only if lymph nodes were treated (surgery/elective nodal RT).
  - Postoperative regular visits depending on department/national protocols and grade of toxicity.
  - Increased vigilance for identifying subclinical or early-stage lymphoedema (relative volume changes of 5–10%) for best opportunity of early intervention and treatment.
- *Possible screening tools for signs and symptoms.*
  - Critical Preoperative Baseline Measurement.
  - Relative Volume Change (RVC) evaluation:

    $RVC = ([A2 \times U1]/[U2 \times A1]) - 1$ ($A2$, volume of the affected limb at given time point; $A1$, volume of the affected limb at baseline; $U1$, volume of the unaffected limb at baseline; $U2$, volume of the unaffected limb at given time point) [6].
  - Objective Screening Measures.

    Serial arm circumference measurements (compared to unaffected limb): Measure in at least six reproducible points (for instance, 10 cm above and 10 cm below the olecranon process) [7].

    Volumetric measurement via water displacement.

    Perometry (uses infrared light to estimate cross-sectional measurement, it also identifies subclinical lymphoedema) [8].

    Bioimpedance spectroscopy (may not detect early- or late-stage lymphoedema when tissues become fibrotic) [9].

    Lymphoscintigraphy.

Brachial Plexus evaluation

- Documentation in the preoperative/before RT is essential for comparison at the time of follow-up as some of the patients will have symptoms related to surgery and not plexopathy.
  - Possible screening tools from signs and symptoms.

    Magnetic Resonance Imaging (MRI).
    - MRI may be helpful in distinguishing neoplastic plexopathy from radiation-induced plexopathy.
    - Radiation plexopathy does not produce nerve enhancement, although an increase in T2 signal may be present [10].
  - Electromyography (EMG).
    - EMG may reveal fasciculations more pronounced than clinical symptoms but is otherwise of little diagnostic benefit [11].
    - Myokymia (localised quivering of muscles) is present in radiation plexopathy 60% of the time and less often in neoplastic plexopathy [12].

Lung evaluation

- *Follow-up:* during regular follow up visits.
- *Possible screening tools for signs and symptoms.*
  - Chest X-ray or chest CT when symptomatic.
    Most common pulmonary changes on CT include patchy, unilateral, or bilateral reticular markings, ground-glass opacities, inter/intra-lobular septal linear thickening, lung consolidation, and fibrosis [13]. Rarely, RT can be associated with bronchiolitis obliterans organising pneumonia (BOOP).
  - Unclear benefit of lung function tests (e.g. spirometry with lung diffusion capacity test) for determining the grade of radiation-induced pneumonitis (RIP).
  - Most patients exhibit normal levels of C-reactive protein (CRP) and diagnostic differentiation from bacterial pneumonia remains challenging [14]. Nevertheless, the performance of bronchial lavage sampling with subsequent cytology for differential diagnosis of RIP from infectious lung disease is currently under investigation [15].

Heart evaluation

- *Follow-up:*
  - Assessment of baseline risk of potential cardiotoxicity is crucial.
- *Possible screening tools for signs and symptoms.*
  - Three-dimensional echocardiography [16].
    Including left ventricular ejection fraction, global longitudinal strain, left ventricular diastolic function, left ventricular filling pressure, pulmonary pressure, and right ventricular function [17].
  - Cardiac magnetic resonance [18].
    Limitations in availability and cost.
    Myocardial tissue characterisation (including detection of myocardial oedema and fibrosis).
  - Cardiac computed tomography [19].
    Not routinely used (better in detecting coronary artery calcification).
  - Myocardial perfusion studies.
  - Troponin T and N-terminal pro brain natriuretic peptide [20, 21].

Quality of life evaluation

- *Follow-up:*
  - Preoperative and before RT, at regular follow up visits.
- *Possible screening tool for signs and symptoms.*
  - The quality of life can be evaluated with EORTC QLQ-C30 and EORTC QLQ-BR45 questionnaires.
  - BREAST-Q questionnaire [22] can be used to measure patient-reported satisfaction.
  - Disorder specific questionnaires.

Table 31.1 summarises evaluation of late toxicities. We recommend to review the section of "reporting" (Chap. 32) that covers toxicity scales used at clinic and "management of late toxicity" section (Chap. 33) that covers treatments of late toxicity.

31.3 Summary

Currently, a more analytic approach is growing around the evaluation of late toxicities. There is no evidence to perform more intensive follow-up for late toxicity. Pre-treatment evaluation can help to identify patients who are prone for late toxicity. Long periods of observation are required to adequately assess effects of RT alone or combined with surgical resection, cytotoxic drugs, and endocrine therapy. Early detection, appropriate evaluation, and early intervention could improve both patients' QoL and our knowledge of late toxicities.

Table 31.1 Evaluation of late toxicities: summary

Site	Side effect	Follow-up	Screening tools/diagnostic tools	Differential diagnosis
Skin/ subcutis	Telangiectasia	Preoperative Before radiation therapy 3 months after RT, regular visit for a minimum of 2 years	• Examination of skin and subcutaneous tissue (palpation and inspection) • TCM measurements • HRUS • MRI for suspicious presentation	Second cancers, angiosarcoma
	Fibrosis/chest wall pain			Second cancers, nephrogenic systemic fibrosis (NSF, also known as nephrogenic fibrosis dermopathy)
Lymphatics	Lymphoedema	Preoperative Postoperative regular visit every 6–12 months for a minimum of 2–3 years	• Clinical examination • Preoperative baseline measurement • RVC evaluation • Objective screening measures – Serial arm circumference measurements – Volumetric measurement via water displacement – Perometry – Bioimpedance spectroscopy – Lymphoscintigraphy	Evaluated for alternate causes of new swelling including tumour recurrence, infection, and thrombosis
Brachial plexus	Brachial plexopathy	3 months after RT, regular visit for a minimum of 3–5 years	• Clinical examination • MRI • EMG	Neoplastic plexopathy (more pain at presentation 98% vs. 10%; rapid progression; unusual myokymia)
Lung	Radiation-induced lung injuries	3 months after RT, regular visit for a minimum of 3–5 years	• CXR or chest CT when symptomatic • CRP • Bronchial lavage sampling • Lung function tests	Bacterial pneumonia, infectious lung disease, Bronchiolitis obliterans organising pneumonia (BOOP)
Heart	Cardiac damage	Before radiation therapy 3 months after RT, regular visit for a minimum of 5 years	• Clinical examination • 3D echocardiography • Cardiac magnetic resonance • Cardiac computed tomography • Myocardial perfusion studies • Troponin T and N-terminal pro–brain natriuretic peptide	RT-related coronary artery disease and conduction system disease same morphological features as non-RT related RT-related valvular disease: interruptions of elastic fibres without rheumatic endocarditis changes RT-related pericarditis: protein-rich exudates in the pericardial sac and fibrin in the mesothelial lining pericardial cavity

References

1. Wernicke AG, et al. Tissue compliance meter is a more reproducible method of measuring radiation-induced fibrosis than late effects of normal tissue-subjective objective management analytical in patients treated with intracavitary brachytherapy accelerated partial breast irradiation: results of a prospective trial. Breast J. 2013;19(3):250–8.
2. Giovagnorio F, et al. Color Doppler sonography of focal lesions of the skin and subcutaneous tissue. J Ultrasound Med. 1999;18:89–93.
3. Huang YP, et al. High-frequency ultrasound assessment of skin fibrosis: clinical results. Ultrasound Med Biol. 2007;8:1191–8.
4. Hoeller U, et al. Radiation-induced plexopathy and fibrosis. Strahlenther Onkol. 2004;180(10):650–4.
5. Stout Gergich NL, et al. Preoperative assessment enables the early diagnosis and successful treatment of lymphedema. Cancer. 2008;112:2809–19.
6. Ancukiewicz M, et al. Standardized method for quantification of developing lymphedema in patients treated for breast cancer. Int J Radiat Oncol Biol Phys. 2011;79:1436–43.
7. Tidhar D, et al. Measurement issues in anthropometric measures of limb volume change in persons at risk for and living with lymphedema: a reliability study. J Pers Med. 2015;5:341–53.
8. Brunelle C, et al. Establishing and sustaining a prospective screening program for breast cancer-related lymphedema at the Massachusetts General Hospital: lessons learned. J Pers Med. 2015;5(2):153–64.
9. Seward C, et al. A comprehensive review of bioimpedance spectroscopy as a diagnostic tool for the detection and measurement of breast cancer-related lymphedema. J Surg Oncol. 2016;114:537–42.
10. Wouter van Es H, et al. Radiation-induced brachial plexopathy: MR imaging. Skeletal Radiol. 1997;26(5):284–8.
11. Jaeckle KA. Neurologic manifestations of neoplastic and radiation-induced plexopathies. Semin Neurol. 2010;30(3):254–62.
12. Roth G, et al. Post-radiation brachial plexopathy. Persistent conduction block. Myokymic discharges and cramps. Rev Neurol (Paris). 1988;144(3):173–80.
13. Cleverley JR, et al. Drug-induced lung disease: high-resolution CT and histological findings. Clin Radiol. 2002;57(4):292–9.
14. Wang Z, et al. The role of procalcitonin in differential diagnosis between acute radiation pneumonitis and bacterial pneumonia in lung cancer patients receiving thoracic radiotherapy. Sci Rep. 2020;10:1–6.
15. Toma CL, et al. The bronchoalveolar lavage pattern in radiation pneumonitis secondary to radiotherapy for breast cancer. Maedica. 2010;5(4):250–7.
16. Jacob S, et al. Early detection and prediction of cardiotoxicity after radiation therapy for breast cancer: the BACCARAT prospective cohort study. Radiat Oncol. 2016;11:54.
17. Yu AF, et al. Assessment of early radiation-induced changes in left ventricular function by myocardial strain imaging after breast radiation therapy. J Am Soc Echocardiogr. 2019;32(4):521–8.
18. Karamitsos TD, et al. Myocardial tissue characterization and fibrosis by imaging. JACC Cardiovasc Imaging. 2020;13(5):1221–34.
19. Milgrom SA, et al. Coronary artery dose-volume parameters predict risk of calcification after radiation therapy. J Cardiovasc Imaging. 2019;27(4):268–79.
20. Skyttä T, et al. Troponin T-release associates with cardiac radiation doses during adjuvant left-sided breast cancer radiotherapy. Radiat Oncol. 2015;10:141.
21. D'Errico MP, et al. N-terminal pro-B-type natriuretic peptide plasma levels as a potential biomarker for cardiac damage after radiotherapy in patients with left-sided breast cancer. Int J Radiat Oncol Biol Phys. 2012;82(2):e239–46.
22. Pusic AL, et al. Development of a new patient-reported outcome measure for breast surgery: the BREAST-Q. Plast Reconstr Surg. 2009;124(2):345–53.

Reporting of Late Toxicity

32

Carlotta Becherini and Lorenzo Livi

32.1 Background

Quantification of toxicity is inherently more complex than quantification of efficacy, in part because the set of possible adverse events is virtually unlimited and in part because adverse events vary widely in severity from individual to individual even after the same therapeutic approach. Even when studies include toxicity data, the lack of standards for reporting and data analysis means that comparisons between studies are often not possible or lack credibility [1].

Nevertheless, in comparison with other areas of cancer research, the field of RT has been a front runner regarding awareness and reporting of late morbidity [2].

C. Becherini (✉)
Department of Radiation Oncology, A.O.U. Careggi, University of Florence, Florence, Italy

L. Livi
Department of Radiation Oncology, A.O.U. Careggi, University of Florence, Florence, Italy

Department of Experimental and Clinical Biomedical Sciences "Mario Serio", University of Florence, Florence, Italy
e-mail: lorenzo.livi@unifi.it

32.2 Key Information for Clinical Practice

32.2.1 Skin Late Toxicity

In a routine clinical practice, two scales are used to assess the grade of chronic radiation dermatitis. The toxicity criteria of the RTOG and the EORTC assess two aspects of chronic radiation dermatitis: skin and subcutaneous tissue [3]. More detailed assessment can be done through the CTCAE [4].

32.2.2 Lymphoedema

Several classification systems are also used to describe lymphoedema, including the Campisi staging system, and those of the American Physical Therapy Association and the NCI's CTCAE [4]. Recently, the Cancer-Related Lymphedema of the Upper Extremity (CLUE) tool was developed and validated to standardise clinical examinations for lymphoedema, providing a single score accounting for multiple constructs [5].

The most commonly used is the staging system of the International Society of Lymphology (ISL) [6]. The ISL combines two criteria to

© The Author(s), under exclusive license to Springer Nature Switzerland AG 2022
O. Kaidar-Person et al. (eds.), *Breast Cancer Radiation Therapy*,
https://doi.org/10.1007/978-3-030-91170-6_32

classify lymphoedema: the "softness" or "firmness" of the limb:

- Stage "0": subclinical or latent condition where swelling is not evident.
- Stage I: early accumulation of fluid relatively high in protein content (e.g. in comparison with "venous" oedema) which subsides with limb elevation. Pitting may occur.
- Stage II: changes in solid structures, limb elevation alone rarely reduces tissue swelling, and pitting is manifest. Later, the limb may not pit as excess subcutaneous fat and fibrosis develop.
- Stage III: encompasses lymphostatic elephantiasis where pitting can be absent and trophic skin changes such as acanthosis, alterations in skin character, and thickness, further deposition of fat and fibrosis.

Within each stage, a limited but nonetheless functional severity assessment has utilised simple excess volume differences assessed as minimal (>5 < 20% increase in limb volume), moderate (20–40% increase), or severe (>40% increase).

The lymphoedema quality-of-life study (LYMQOL) is a condition-specific, validated questionnaire used to assess the effectiveness of lymphoedema-related treatment plans [7].

32.2.3 Brachial Plexopathy

One of the most commonly used scores to grade brachial plexus neuropathy is the modified LENT-SOMA score [8]. Pain could be reported through the Neuropathic Pain Symptom Inventory (NPSI), which is a 12-item scale, with each item scored on a 10-point numerical rating scale. Scores range from 0 to 120 [9].

Weakness was assessed in radiation induced brachial plexopathy studies using the Medical Research Council scale [10, 11], which provides a semiquantitative estimation of muscle strength.

32.2.4 Lung

In clinical practice, RTOG criteria and the CTCAE are the ones most widely used [3, 4]. However, most patients will not show any clinical symptoms.

The severity of radiation induced lung fibrosis can be radiologically measured with the help of semiquantitative grading (1–5 points) using radiographic features [12]:

- Mild to moderate RILF: "scar-like" patterns as characterised by streaky opacities,
- Severe RILF: "mass-like" patterns as depicted by focal consolidation and/or ground glass opacification with air bronchograms and/or traction bronchiectasis.

32.2.5 Heart

Radiation induced cardiac disease holds a wide range of deleterious effects on the heart, ranging from preclinical findings to symptomatic clinical disease, including pericarditis, coronary artery disease (CAD), myocardial infarction, valvular heart disease, rhythm abnormalities, and non-ischemic myocardial and conduction system damages. The symptoms and signs of radiation induced cardiac toxicity are, for the most part, indistinguishable from those encountered in patients with heart disease due to other aetiologies. Therefore, clinical assessment is frequently done with the same staging system of non-RT related counterparts.

We recommend that the LENT-SOMA system [8] can be considered to describe cardiac effects, as it explicitly addresses clinical, radiological, and functional assessments of cardiac dysfunction.

32.2.6 Patient-Reported Outcome Measures

In 2017, the International Consortium for Health Outcomes Measurement has developed a standard set of value-based patient-reported outcome measures [13]. EORTC QLQ-C30 and -BR45 and the Body Image after Breast Cancer Questionnaire (BIBCQ) were frequently used as reliable cancer-related quality-of-life and body image-related questionnaires [13, 14], among several tools reported in literature (Table 32.1). Importantly, it is known that the toxicity burden faced by the patients may be greater than acknowledged by physicians [15].

Patient-reported outcome measures related to breast RT have been investigated and they include skin changes, breast shrinkage, breast hardness, and low aesthetic outcome, which negatively impact the psychosocial well-being [16]. Aesthetic outcomes can also be measured by patients themselves according to Harris et al. on a 4-category scale: excellent, good, fair, or poor [17], either with Body Image Scale [18] or in a more detailed way using self-assessment questionnaire such as used in a number of clinical trials.

Table 32.1 Summary of late toxicities assessment tools

Site	Disorder	Staging system	Patient-reported outcome measures
Skin[a]/subcutis/chest wall	Telangiectasias Fibrosis/chest wall pain	• NCI's CTCAE • RTOG • EORTC / LENT-SOMA	• Patient-reported outcome common terminology criteria of adverse events (PRO-CTCAE) • Harvard scale (Cosmesis) • Body image scale
Lymphatics	Lymphoedema	• Staging system of the International Society of Lymphology (ISL) • Campisi staging system • American Physical Therapy Association (APTA) • NCI's CTCAE	• The lymphoedema quality-of-life study (LYMQOL) • Lymphoedema life impact scale (LLIS) questionnaire • Upper limb lymphoedema (ULL)-27 • MOS—short form McGill pain questionnaire • World Health Organization International Classification of Functioning Disability and Health (WHO-ICF) • Medical outcome study—short form (SF-36)
Brachial plexus	Brachial plexopathy	• EORTC / LENT-SOMA	• Neuropathic pain symptom inventory (NPSI) • 36-item short form health survey and the patient global impression of change (PGIC) • Medical Research Council scale for weakness
Lung	Radiation induced lung injuries (RILI)	• NCI's CTCAE • RTOG • EORTC / LENT-SOMA	• EORTC QLQ-C30 • Lung module 13 (QLQ-LC13)
Heart	Cardiac damage	• EORTC / LENT-SOMA • Disease specific grading tools (e.g. American Heart Association, syntax score)	• EORTC QLQ-C30

[a]Late skin toxicity includes dryness, reduced skin elasticity, hyperpigmentation, depigmentation, etc

32.3 Summary

Early detection and evaluation, through the employment of univocal measures agreed by international societies, could improve both patients' QoL and knowledge of late toxicities themselves (summarised in Table 32.1). Given the variety of treatment modalities and the importance of evaluating the impact of treatment de-escalation, it is important to share decisions with patients. Thereby, data-driven patient education comparing patients reported outcome measures between treatment options can help to define treatment goals. Those goals can be any combination of oncological outcomes such as recurrences or survival, side effects, and quality-of-life.

References

1. Trotti A, et al. The need for adverse effects reporting standards in oncology clinical trials. J Clin Oncol. 2004;22:19–22.
2. Bentzen SM, et al. Quantitative analyses of normal tissue effects in the clinic (quantec): an introduction to the scientific issues. Int J Radiat Oncol Biol Phys. 2010;76:3–9.
3. Cox JD, et al. Toxicity criteria of the radiation therapy oncology group (RTOG) and the European Organization for Research and Treatment of cancer (EORTC). Int J Radiat Oncol Biol Phys. 1995;31(5):1341–6.
4. National Cancer Institute, National Institutes of Health, U.S. Department of Health and Human Services. Common Terminology Criteria for Adverse Events (CTCAE) Version 5.0. Published: November 27, 2017. Accessed 24 Oct 2020.
5. Spinelli B, et al. Intra- and interrater reliability and concurrent validity of a new tool for assessment of breast cancer-related lymphedema of the upper extremity. Arch Phys Med Rehabil. 2019;100:315–26.
6. Executive Committee of the International Society of Lymphology. The diagnosis and treatment of peripheral lymphedema: 2020 consensus document of the International Society of Lymphology. Lymphology. 2020;53(1):3–19.
7. Keeley V, et al. A quality of life measure for limb lymphoedema (LYMQOL). J Lymphoedea. 2010;5(1):26–37.
8. LENT-SOMA. LENT-SOMA scales for all anatomic sites. Int J Radiat Oncol Biol Phys. 1995;31(1049):1091.
9. Bouhassira D, et al. Development and validation of the neuropathic pain symptom inventory. Pain. 2004;108:248–57.
10. Delanian SE, et al. Randomized, placebo-controlled clinical trial combining pentoxifylline–tocopherol and clodronate in the treatment of radiation-induced plexopathy. Int J Radiat Oncol Biol Phys. 2020;107(1):154–62.
11. Medical Research Council. Aids to the examination of the peripheral nervous system, memorandum no. 45. London: HMSO; 1981.
12. Benveniste MF, et al. Recognizing radiation therapy-related complications in the chest. Radiographics. 2019;39:344–66.
13. Ong W, et al. A standard set of value-based patient-centered outcomes for breast cancer: the International Consortium for Health Outcomes Measurement (ICHOM) initiative. JAMA Oncol. 2017;3:677–85.
14. Kanatas A, et al. Patient-reported outcomes in breast oncology: a review of validated outcome instruments. Tumori. 2012;98:678–88.
15. Mukesh M, et al. The Cambridge breast intensity-modulated radiotherapy trial: comparison of clinician-versus patient-reported outcomes. Clin Oncol. 2016;28:354–64.
16. Al-Ghazal S, et al. Does cosmetic outcome from treatment of primary breast cancer influence psychosocial morbidity? Eur J Surg Oncol. 1999;25:571–3.
17. Harris J, et al. Analysis of cosmetic results following primary radiation therapy for stages I and II carcinoma of the breast. Int J Radiat Oncol Biol Phys. 1979;5:257–61.
18. Hopwood P, et al. A body image scale for use with cancer patients. Eur J Cancer. 2001;37(2):189–97.

33 Management of Late Toxicity

Carlotta Becherini and Lorenzo Livi

33.1 Background

Late toxicity refers to a group of side effects that occur months and years after radiation therapy treatment, which is characterised by many different symptoms or conditions of variable severity occurring over time. Figures 33.1, 33.2, 33.3, 33.4, 33.5 and 33.6 are pictures of different types of late toxicity. Most patients will present with mild changes including de/hyperpigmentation (Figs. 33.1 and 33.2).

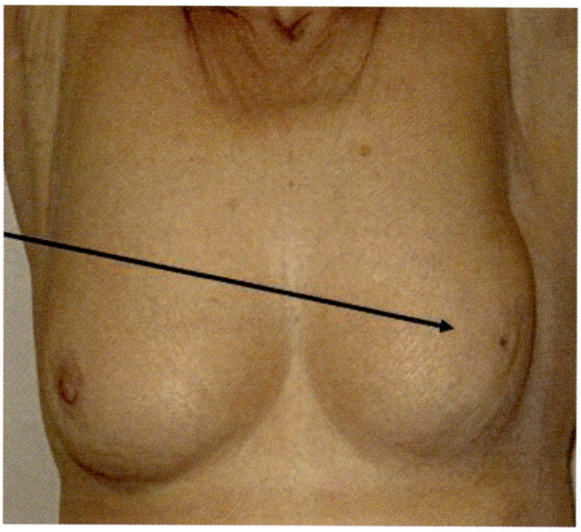

Fig. 33.1 A patient with mild late effects: no difference in colour between the breasts. Nipple/areola lighter on treated side compared to untreated side

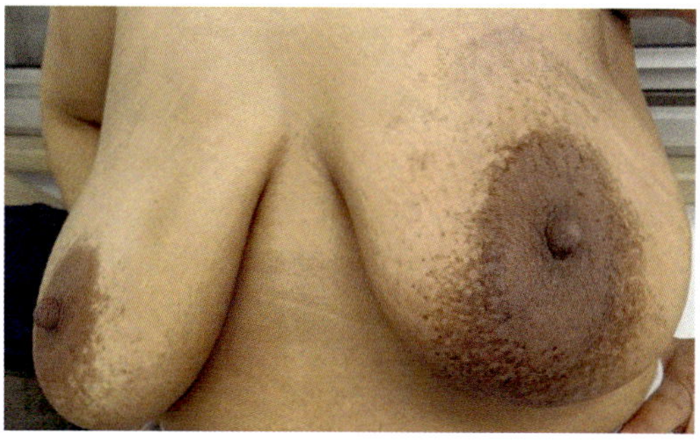

Fig. 33.2 A patient with late effects with pigmentation of breast skin, especially in the area of nipple/areola

33.2 Key Information for Clinical Practice

33.2.1 Telangiectasias (Fig. 33.3)

- *Symptoms:* Dilatation of the capillaries causing them to appear as small red or purple clusters, often spidery in appearance, on the skins.
- *Timing:* 2–6+ months.

C. Becherini (✉)
Department of Radiation Oncology, A.O.U. Careggi, University of Florence, Florence, Italy

L. Livi
Department of Radiation Oncology, A.O.U. Careggi, University of Florence, Florence, Italy

Department of Experimental and Clinical Biomedical Sciences "Mario Serio", University of Florence, Florence, Italy
e-mail: lorenzo.livi@unifi.it

© The Author(s), under exclusive license to Springer Nature Switzerland AG 2022
O. Kaidar-Person et al. (eds.), *Breast Cancer Radiation Therapy*,
https://doi.org/10.1007/978-3-030-91170-6_33

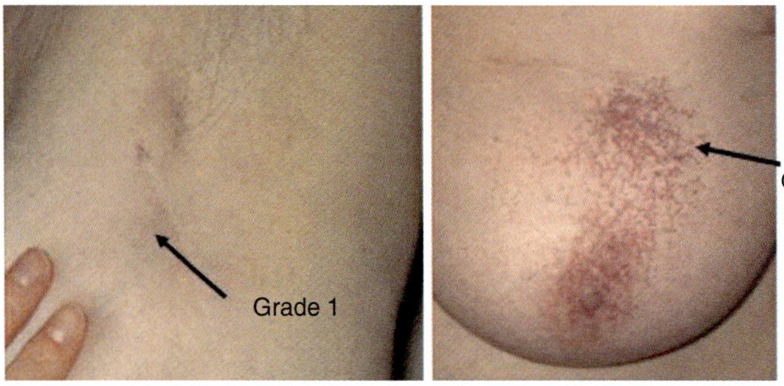

Fig. 33.3 Telangiectasia. Small dilated vessels grading: 0 = none, 1 = <1/cm^2, 2 = 1–4/cm^2, 3 = >4/cm^2

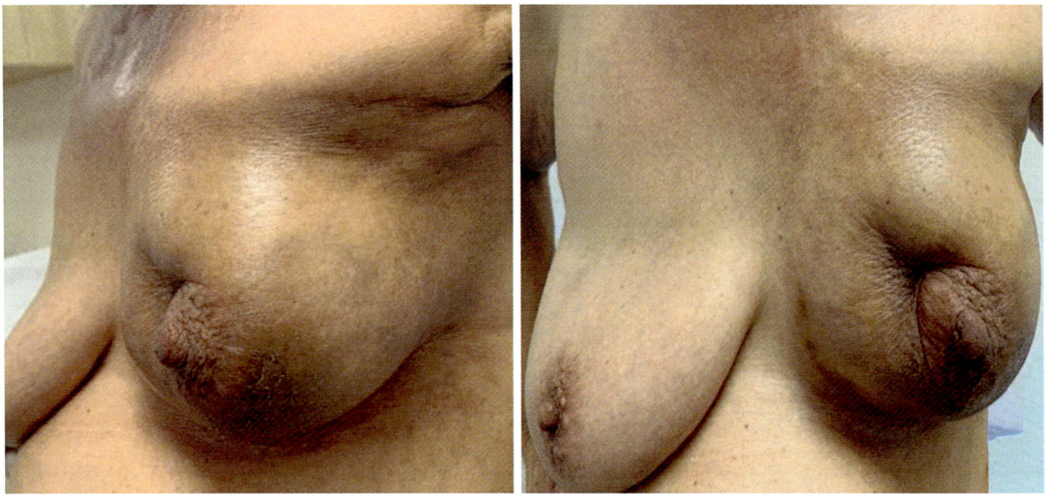

Fig. 33.4 Morphea-like fibrosis, stiffness of the breast and deformation, 1 year after completion of whole breast irradiation and boost

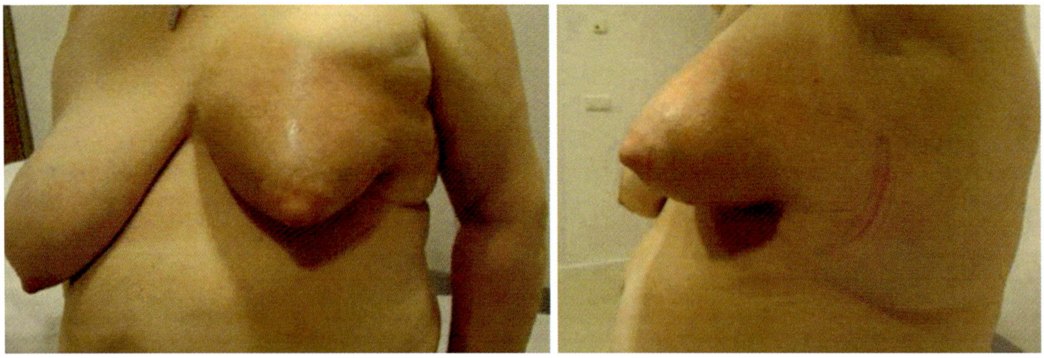

Fig. 33.5 Morphea-like fibrosis, stiffness of the breast and deformation, 1 year after completion of whole breast irradiation and boost

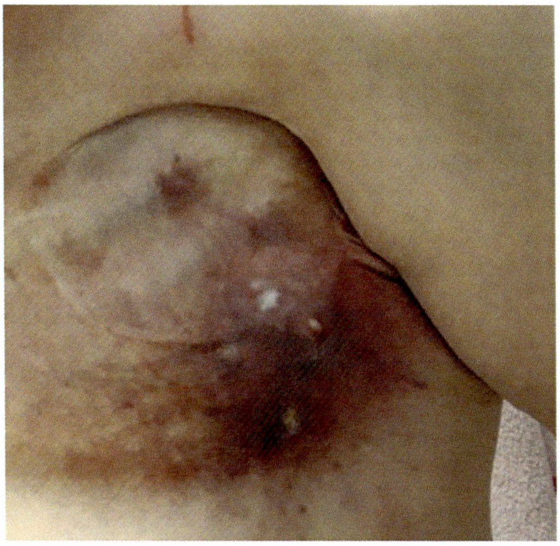

Fig. 33.6 Fibrosis, chest wall necrosis (proven histologically), 30 years after halsted mastectomy and chest wall RT

- *Prevention:*
  - The local control benefit of a breast boost should be weighed against the potential long-term complication, such as telangiectasias [1, 2].
  - Bolus should be applied in limited cases (see bolus section, Chap. 21).
  - Use of high-energy electron beams (>10 MeV) is associated with increased telangiectasias rates compared to lower energy electrons or photons [3].
  - Field-in Field planning (i.e. forward planned IMRT) leading to dose homogeneity showed to decrease telangiectasias compared to standard RT [4, 5].
- *Management:*
  - Long pulsed dye laser treatment [6].
  - Treatment of post-irradiation morphea (rare late complication) includes topical and intralesional corticosteroids, phototherapy, and systemic immunosuppressive agents in various combinations [7].

33.2.2 Fibrosis/Chest Wall Pain

- *Symptoms:* Pain, breast shrinkage and firmness, cutaneous induration, contraction, ulceration, delayed wound healing, arm oedema, decreased shoulder range of motion.
- *Timing:* 4–12+ months.
- *Prevention:*
  - Utilisation of a breast boost should be weighed against the potential long-term complication [1, 2].
  - Bolus should be applied in limited cases (see bolus section, Chap. 21).
  - Use of high-energy electron beams (>10 MeV) is associated with increased fibrosis rates compared to lower energy electrons or photons [3].
  - Minimise the breast volume receiving over 107% of the prescribed dose. If this is not achievable with 3D technique, consider using IMRT.
  - Counsel risk associated with reconstructive options.
  - Consider prophylactic oral pentoxifylline (PTX) 400 mg two or three times a day and oral vitamin E (400–1000 IU) daily for at least 6 months in patients at high risk for radiation fibrosis (i.e. severe acute dermatitis, breast oedema, planning to undergo reconstruction) [8–10].

    Patients should not take PTX while on blood thinners.

    If patients develop nausea while taking PTX, the dose may be reduced to 200 mg twice a day.

    PTX and vitamin E should be discontinued 1 week before any planned invasive procedure.
- *Management:*
  - *Anti-inflammatories.*

    Ibuprofen 400 mg two to three times a day.

    Naproxen 250–500 mg a day.

- *Neuropathic pain.*
  Duloxetine 60 mg once a day.
  Gabapentin 300–1200 mg three times a day.
  Pregabalin 75–150 mg twice a day.
- Oral PTX (400 mg two or three times a day) and oral vitamin E (400–1000 UI daily) for at least 6 months to avoid rebound fibrosis [11].
- Oral PTX-vitamin E-clodronate (PENTOCLO protocol). This protocol can be considered if pain is associated with osteoradionecrosis of ribs/costo-chondral joint. PENTOCLO protocol: 800 mg PTX, 1000 IU vitamin E, and 1600 mg clodronate 5 days per week alternating with 20 mg prednisone and 1000 mg ciprofloxacin 2 days per week [12].
- Conflicting evidence to support hyperbaric oxygen therapy. It can be used only for patients with no evidence of recurrence/cancer.

The risk for radiation-induced fibrosis and telangiectasia after brachytherapy alone seems to depend on the skin dose delivered [13]. Proton therapy did not increase the risk for radiation fibrosis compared with APBI with photons [14], although higher skin toxicity was observed.

In case of mastectomy and reconstruction, some advice that tissue expanders should be maximally expanded prior to RT and not further expanded after RT owing to RT-induced oedema and tightening of the skin around the expander [15].

33.2.3 Lymphoedema

- *Symptoms:* Abnormal swelling that can develop in the arm, hand, breast, or torso; increase heaviness and/or pain, and increases the risk of delayed wound healing and cellulitis.
- *Timing:* 6+ months.
  - Early onset (<12 months postoperatively): associated with axillary lymph node dissection.
  - Late onset (>12 months): associated with regional lymph node radiotherapy and axillary lymph node dissection.
- *Prevention:* appropriate reduction of axillary surgery and nodal irradiation volumes based on disease characteristics (see Chap. 19).
  - In clinically node-negative patients, the rates of breast cancer related lymphoedema were significantly reduced with the use of sentinel node dissection over complete axillary lymph node dissection (5% vs. 20%) [16].
  - In patients with up to 2 positive nodes after sentinel node dissection, axillary radiation is associated with a lower incidence of lymphoedema compared to axillary nodal dissection (23% vs. 11%) [17].
  - Increased risk to develop lymphoedema adding a supraclavicular field (9.9%), posterior axillary boost (14.7%), and internal mammary boost (8.3%) [18].
  - Surgery for Lymphoedema Prevention:
    Axillary reverse mapping (ARM) [19].
    Lymphatic Microsurgical Preventative Healing Approach (LYMPHA) [20].
- *Recommended prophylaxis.*
  - Maintain ideal body weight.
  - Aggressively manage localised infections to prevent cellulitis.
  - Range of motion and weight-bearing exercise.
  - Physiotherapy.
- *Management:* The treatment is mostly a conservative multimodal approach, which aims to improve patient comfort and reduce limb volume [21]. Treatment options in order of increasing symptom toxicity:
  - Exercise [22].
  - Limb elevation (3.1% reduction in arm volume) [23].
  - Compression garments (32% vs. 15.8% reduction at 24 weeks, compared to elastic hosiery alone) [24].

- Minimise the risk of infection [25].
- Manual lymphatic drainage (more effective for patients under the age of 60 years and an intervention time of 1 month) [26].
- Complete decongestive therapy.
- Intermittent pneumatic compression [27].
- For severe lymphoedema, surgical intervention may be considered (lymphatic bypass procedures, vascularized lymph node transfer, etc.) [28].

There is no compelling evidence to suggest that compression garments especially need to be worn during air travel [25]. Hyperbaric oxygen is not certainly effective; the data about this are conflicting, and it is not recommended in case of active malignancy [29].

Evidence supporting avoidance of blood pressure measurements on the affected arm is conflicting. In the absence of level I evidence, the National Lymphedema Network recommends avoidance of excessive constriction on the affected arm, if possible [21].

33.2.4 Brachial Plexopathy

- *Symptoms:*
  - Numbness, paresthesia, dysesthesia, pain, and/or motor weakness in the hand/arm/shoulder.
  - Progression of symptoms is gradual in about two-third of cases and the patients may initially present with paresthesia and pain and later progress to have motor weakness in the affected upper limb.
- *Timing:* 8–12+ months (median 1.5 years).
- *Prevention:*
  - Decrease total dose and dose per fraction [30].
  - Avoid irradiating large volumes of the brachial plexus ($V_{40Gy} \geq 13.5$ cm^3) [31].
  - Reduce maximum dose to the brachial plexus of <55 Gy [31].
- *Management:* Treatment options in order of increasing symptom toxicity.
  - Symptomatic treatment and supportive care.

    Neuropathic pain: Gabapentin 300–1200 mg three times a day or pregabalin 75–150 mg twice a day.

    Paraesthesia: Benzodiazepines (such as diazepam 2–10 mg three to four times a day).

    Weakness: Physical therapy.
  - No evidence to support hyperbaric oxygen [32].
  - Nerve transfer (minimal evidence to support) [33].
  - Dorsal column stimulators, transdermal electrical nerve stimulation, neurolysis with omentoplasty could be helpful in managing radiation plexopathy [34].

33.2.5 Lung

- *Symptoms:*
  - *Pneumonitis:* Cough, shortness of breath, increased oxygen requirements, pleuritic chest pain, and/or pyrexia. If treated, typically resolves.
  - *Fibrosis:* Dyspnoea. It is an irreversible effect which can result in reduced lung capacity.
- *Timing:*
  - *Pneumonitis:* 4 weeks to 12 months.
  - *Fibrosis*: 6–12+ months.
- *Prevention:*
  - When treating comprehensive nodal RT, keep ipsilateral lung $V_{20Gy} < 35\%$, if possible [35].
  - When treating standard tangents, keep ipsilateral lung $V_{20Gy} < 20\%$, if possible [35].
  - When treating hypofractionated dose scheme (mostly 40 Gy in 15 fractions), keep ipsilateral lung $V_{30} < 10\%$ [36].
  - When treating supraclavicular nodes and internal mammary nodes, consider deep inspiration breath-hold to decrease lung volume inside the irradiated field [37].
  - When planning vIMRT, consider also the low dose lung volumes (V_{5Gy}) and dose to both lungs.

- *Management:*
  - *Asymptomatic or with mild symptoms:*
    Supportive care (e.g. antitussives therapy).
  - Avoid glucocorticoid treatment unless symptoms become bothersome or pulmonary function declines by more than 10%.
  - *Severe symptoms and evidence of respiratory impairment:*
    Oral glucocorticoid therapy (e.g. Prednisone 60 mg per day for 2 weeks following dose reduction by 10 mg per 1–2 weeks) [38].
    If the patient is stable or improved, the prednisone dose is gradually tapered to 0.5–0.75 mg/kg per day for the ensuing 4–6 weeks. Thereafter, it is gradually tapered to zero after 3–6 months if the patient remains stable.

33.2.6 Heart

- *Symptoms:* Angina, syncope, dyspnoea, sick sinus syndrome, pleuritic chest pain, non-anginal chest pain fever.
- *Timing:* 5–30 years.
  - During treatment (weeks) or after treatment up to 10 years: Pericardial disease.
  - 6 months to 20 years: Conduction system disease
  - 4–11 years: Asymptomatic Valvular disease
  - 5–20 years: Coronary artery disease
  - 10 years: Symptomatic myocardial injury
  - >16 years: Symptomatic valvular disease
- *Prevention:*
  - Ensure that dose to the hearth is as low as possible.
  - In left-sided breast cancers, or right-sided breast cancers involving irradiation of the internal mammary nodal chain, consider deep inspiration breath-hold, respiratory gating, CPAP (see sections on Techniques to reduce OAR dose, Chap. 38) [37].
  - Encourage lifestyle modifications (smoking cessation, diabetes control, weight loss, dietary modifications, and exercise) to minimise cardiac risk [39].
- *Management:* Treatment options in order of recommended use.
  - Refer to a cardiologist if heart failure or coronary artery disease is suspected.

33.3 Recommendations

The right knowledge and management of late toxicity could reduce patients' discomfort, allowing the physician to introduce prevention's strategy whenever it could be possible (Table 33.1).

33.4 Summary

RT increases the risk for late toxicity, but the absolute rates for late pulmonary and cardiac disease were reported to be low at 15-years follow up [40]. Meticulous volume-based RT planning, dose homogeneity, moderate hypofractionation, and limiting skin dose are associated with reduced acute toxicity and potentially reduce the rates of late toxicity. Lifestyle changes are for patient well-being and can reduce potential late effects and improve QoL. Measures such as avoiding sun direct exposure, smoking cessation, healthy nutrition, physical activity are strongly advised. Other interventions, as indicated in Table 33.1 can be considered in case of late toxicity.

Table 33.1 Late toxicities management summary

Site	Side effect	Timing	Mild	Moderate/severe	Prevention
Skin	Dryness Decrease elasticity	0-years	Mild pH-neutral or non-alkaline soaps Rich moisturises	Consider PTX and vitamin E	Limit use of high energy (>10 MeV electron beams) Limit the use of bolus Limit skin dose Homogenous RT plan Avoid sun exposure, limiting the amount of time spent in direct sunlight, and use sunscreen, high ultraviolet protective factor clothing
Skin	Telangiectasia/ pigmentation changes	2-years	Observation	Laser therapy	Limit use of high energy (>10 MeV electron beams) Limit the use of bolus Avoid sun exposure, limiting the amount of time spent in direct sunlight, and use sunscreen, high ultraviolet protective factor clothing
Skin	Morphea	3 years		Topical and intralesional corticosteroids, phototherapy, and systemic immunosuppressive agents	Limit use of high energy (>10 MeV electron beams) Limit the use of bolus Limit skin dose Homogenous RT plan
	Chronic ulceration and necrosis	2-years		Special dressings (e.g. silver or adsorbent dressing) If severe, require surgical management (from simple removal to advanced reconstructions, skin flaps or artificial skin) In case of NED, consider hyperbaric chamber	Limit use of high energy (>10 MeV electron beams) Limit the use of bolus Limit skin dose Homogenous RT plan

(continued)

Table 33.1 (continued)

Site	Side effect	Timing	Mild	Moderate/severe	Prevention
	Fibrosis/chest wall pain	4-years	Anti-inflammatories • Ibuprofen 400 mg two to three times a day • Naproxen 250–500 mg twice a day Neuropathic pain • Duloxetine 60 mg once a day • Gabapentin 300–1200 mg three times a day • Pregabalin 75–150 mg twice a day	Oral pentoxifylline and vitamin E for at least 6 months Pentoxifylline (400 mg two or three times a day) Vitamin E (400–1000 UI daily) PENTOCLO protocol: 800 mg PTX, 1000 IU vitamin E, and 1600 mg clodronate 5 days per week alternating with 20 mg prednisone and 1000 mg ciprofloxacin 2 days per week In case of NED, consider hyperbaric chamber	Limit use of high energy (>10 MeV electron beams) Limit the use of bolus PTX and vitamin E
Lymphatics	Lymphoedema	6–12 months (surgery) 18–24 months (axillary surgery + regional node RT) 36–48 months (sentinel + regional node RT)	Physical therapy, avoid trauma to involved arm • Stage I: Simple lymphatic drainage + compression garments • Stage II: Intensive physiotherapy (complete decongestive therapy) • Stage III: Intensive physiotherapy +/− intermittent pneumatic compression (IPC)	Lymphatic bypass procedures Vascularized lymph node transfer	De-escalation of axillary surgery: prefer sentinel node biopsy if applicable & correct delineation of target volumes (Chap. 19) General measures for self-care (e.g. monitoring, skincare, weight reduction, exercise) Limb elevation Properly fitted compression garments
Brachial plexus	Brachial plexopathy	8–12 months	Neuropathic pain • Gabapentin or pregabalin Paresthesia • Benzodiazepines (i.e. diazepam 2–10 mg three or four times a day) Physical therapy	Dorsal column stimulators, transdermal electrical nerve stimulation, neurolysis	Limit the dose, rarely an issue with elective doses but mind when a boost is required Delineate the brachial plexus to avoid hot spots at that region Careful planning in case of nodal boost
Lung	Radiation-induced lung injuries	Pneumonitis: 4 weeks to 12 months Fibrosis: 6–12+ months	Asymptomatic/mild symptoms: supportive care (e.g. antitussive therapy)	Severe symptoms (pulmonary function declines >10%): Oral glucocorticoid therapy (e.g. prednisone 0.75–1 mg/kg, per day)	Comprehensive breast/chest wall and nodal RT: Keep ipsilateral lung $V_{20Gy} < 35\%$ Breast/chest wall only: Keep ipsilateral lung $V_{20Gy} < 20\%$ Mind V_{5Gy}, especially for vIMRT
Heart	Cardiac damage	5–10 years	Referral to cardiology	Referral to cardiology	Minimise mean dose to heart Lifestyle risk-reduction (diet, exercise, tobacco avoidance)

NED no evidence of disease, i.e. malignancy, *PTX* pentoxifylline, *vIMRT* volumetric intensity modulated radiation therapy, *RT* radiation therapy

References

1. Bartelink H, European Organisation for Research and Treatment of Cancer Radiation Oncology and Breast Cancer Groups, et al. Whole-breast irradiation with or without a boost for patients treated with breast-conserving surgery for early breast cancer: 20-year follow-up of a randomised phase 3 trial. Lancet Oncol. 2015;16(1):47–56.
2. Torres MA, et al. Postmastectomy and regional nodal radiation for breast cancer. J Clin Oncol. 2020;38(20):2299–309.
3. Huang EY, et al. Predictive factors for skin telangiectasia following post-mastectomy electron beam irradiation. Br J Radiol. 2002;75(893):444–7.
4. Barnett GC, et al. The Cambridge breast intensity-modulated radiotherapy trial: patient- and treatment-related factors that influence late toxicity. Clin Oncol. 2011;23(10):662–73.
5. Barnett GC, et al. Randomized controlled trial of forward-planned intensity modulated radiotherapy for early breast cancer: interim results at 2 years. Int J Radiat Oncol Biol Phys. 2012;82(2):715–23.
6. Rossi AM, et al. Radiation-induced breast telangiectasias treated with the pulsed dye laser. J Clin Aesthet Dermatol. 2014;7(12):34–7.
7. Fruchter R, et al. Characteristics and treatment of postirradiation morphea: a retrospective multicenter analysis. J Am Acad Dermatol. 2017;76(1):19–21.
8. Jacobson G, et al. Randomized trial of pentoxifylline and vitamin E vs standard follow up after breast irradiation to prevent breast fibrosis, evaluated by tissue compliance meter. Int J Radiat Oncol Biol Phys. 2013;85(3):604–8.
9. Magnusson M, et al. Pentoxifylline and vitamin E treatment for prevention of radiation-induced side-effects in women with breast cancer: a phase two, double-blind, placebo-controlled randomised clinical trial (Ptx-5). Eur J Cancer. 2009;45(14):2488–95.
10. Delanian S, et al. Striking regression of chronic radiotherapy damage in a clinical trial of combined pentoxifylline and tocopherol. J Clin Oncol. 1999;17(10):3283–90.
11. Delanian S, et al. Kinetics of response to long-term treatment combining pentoxifylline and tocopherol in patients with superficial radiation-induced fibrosis. J Clin Oncol. 2005;23(34):8570–9.
12. Delanian S, Chatel C, Porcher R, Depondt J, Lefaix JL. Complete restoration of refractory mandibular osteoradionecrosis by prolonged treatment with a pentoxifylline-tocopherol-clodronate combination (PENTOCLO): a phase II trial. Int J Radiat Oncol Biol Phys. 2011;80(3):832–9.
13. Rabinovitch R, et al. RTOG 95–17, a phase II trial to evaluate brachytherapy as the sole method of radiation therapy for Stage I and II breast carcinoma—year-5 toxicity and cosmesis. Brachytherapy. 2014;13(1):17–22.
14. Galland-Girodet S, et al. Long-term cosmetic outcomes and toxicities of proton beam therapy compared with photon-based 3-dimensional conformal APBI: a phase 1 trial. Int J Radiat Oncol Biol Phys. 2014;90(3):493–500.
15. Schechter SW, et al. Immediate breast reconstruction can impact postmastectomy irradiation. Am J Clin Oncol. 2005;28(5):485–94.
16. DiSipio T, et al. Incidence of unilateral arm lymphoedema after breast cancer: a systematic review and meta-analysis. Lancet Oncol. 2013;14(6):500–15.
17. Donker M, et al. Radiotherapy or surgery of the axilla after a positive sentinel node in breast cancer (EORTC 10981-22023 AMAROS): a randomised, multicentre, open-label, phase 3 non-inferiority trial. Lancet Oncol. 2014;15(12):1303–10.
18. Shah C, et al. Factors associated with the development of breast cancer-related lymphedema after whole-breast irradiation. Int J Radiat Oncol Biol Phys. 2012;83(4):1095–100.
19. Ahmed M, et al. Systematic review of axillary reverse mapping in breast cancer. Br J Surg. 2016;103:170–8.
20. Feldman S, et al. Single institution experience with lymphatic microsurgical preventive healing approach (LYMPHA) for the primary prevention of lymphedema. Ann Surg Oncol. 2015;22:3296–301.
21. Executive Committee of the International Society of Lymphology. The diagnosis and treatment of peripheral lymphedema: 2020 consensus document of the International Society of Lymphology. Lymphology. 2020;53(1):3–19.
22. McNeely ML, et al. Conservative and dietary interventions for cancer-related lymphedema: a systematic review and meta-analysis. Cancer. 2011;117(6):1136–48.
23. Swedborg I, et al. Lymphoedema post-mastectomy: is elevation alone an effective treatment? Scand J Rehabil Med. 1993;25(2):79–82.
24. Badger CM, et al. A randomized, controlled, parallel-group clinical trial comparing multilayer bandaging followed by hosiery versus hosiery alone in the treatment of patients with lymphedema of the limb. Cancer. 2000;88(12):2832–7.
25. Asdourian MS, et al. Precautions for breast cancer-related lymphoedema: risk from air travel, ipsilateral arm blood pressure measurements, skin puncture, extreme temperatures, and cellulitis. Lancet Oncol. 2016;17(9):e392–405.
26. Liang M, et al. Manual lymphatic drainage for lymphedema in patients after breast cancer surgery: a systematic review and meta-analysis of randomized controlled trials. Medicine (Baltimore). 2020;99(49):e23192.
27. Shao Y, et al. Intermittent pneumatic compression pump for breast cancer-related lymphedema: a systematic review and meta-analysis of randomized controlled trials. Oncol Res Treat. 2014;37(4):170–4.

28. Granzow JW. Lymphedema surgery: the current state of the art. Clin Exp Metastasis. 2018;35:553–8.
29. Gothard L, et al. Randomised phase II trial of hyperbaric oxygen therapy in patients with chronic arm lymphoedema after radiotherapy for cancer. Radiother Oncol. 2010;97(1):101–7.
30. Guenzi M, et al. Hypofractionated irradiation of infra-supraclavicular lymph nodes after axillary dissection in patients with breast cancer post-conservative surgery: impact on late toxicity. Radiat Oncol. 2015;20(10):177.
31. Lundstedt D, et al. Radiation therapy to the plexus brachialis in breast cancer patients: analysis of paresthesia in relation to dose and volume. Int J Radiat Oncol Biol Phys. 2015;92(2):277–83.
32. Pritchard J, et al. Double-blind randomized phase II study of hyperbaric oxygen in patients with radiation-induced brachial plexopathy. Radiother Oncol. 2001;58(3):279–86.
33. Tung TH, et al. Nerve transfer for elbow flexion in radiation-induced brachial plexopathy: a case report. Hand. 2009;4(2):123–8.
34. Warade AC, et al. Radiation-induced brachial plexus neuropathy: a review. Neurol India. 2019;67(7):S47–52.
35. Blom Goldman U, et al. Radiation pneumonitis and pulmonary function with lung dose-volume constraints in breast cancer irradiation. J Radiother Pract. 2014;13(2):211–7.
36. Lee BM, et al. Hypofractionated radiotherapy dose scheme and application of new techniques are associated to a lower incidence of radiation pneumonitis in breast cancer patients. Front Oncol. 2020;11(10):124.
37. Nissen HD, et al. Improved heart, lung and target dose with deep inspiration breath hold in a large clinical series of breast cancer patients. Radiother Oncol. 2013;106(1):28–32.
38. Murofushi KN, et al. Radiation-induced bronchiolitis obliterans organizing pneumonia (BOOP) syndrome in breast cancer patients is associated with age. Radiat Oncol. 2015;26(10):103.
39. Darby SC, et al. Risk of ischemic heart disease in women after radiotherapy for breast cancer. N Engl J Med. 2013;368(11):987–98.
40. Poortmans PM, Struikmans H, De Brouwer P, Weltens C, Fortpied C, Kirkove C, Budach V, Peignaux-Casasnovas K, van der Leij F, Vonk E, Valli M, van-Tienhoven G, Weidner N, Noel G, Guckenberger M, Koiter E, vanLimbergen E, Engelen A, Fourquet A, Bartelink H; EORTC Radiation Oncology and Breast Cancer Groups. Side Effects 15 Years After Lymph Node Irradiation in Breast Cancer: Randomized EORTC Trial 22922/10925. J Natl Cancer Inst. 2021;113(10):1360–8.

Part VIII

Specific Technical Topics

34 Postmastectomy Irradiation in the Setting of Implant-Based Breast Reconstruction

Orit Kaidar-Person and Alice Ho

34.1 Background

Postmastectomy radiation therapy is indicated for patients who are at high risk of local and regional recurrence. These mostly include patients with nodal burden and/or high-risk features of the primary tumour. Breast reconstruction is increasingly performed in breast cancer patients receiving mastectomy, aiming to increase health-related QoL by restoring the breast shape [1]. PMRT in the setting of breast reconstruction is challenging, as surgical techniques evolved in the aim of improving aesthetic outcomes, while PMRT is associated with increased risk for reconstruction complications and can compromise aesthetic results. Additionally, the shape of the reconstructed breast may be challenging for proper PMRT planning [2].

Current PMRT techniques used in the setting of immediate breast reconstruction (IBR), regardless of the reconstruction type, are similar to postoperative RT in the case of BCT rather than volume-based adapting to the type of mastectomy and reconstruction procedure, targeting only areas of residual breast tissue and areas that are at risk of recurrence (see ASTRO and ESTRO guidelines comparison) [3–5]. The use of target volume-based RT planning may reduce the dose to OARs and other non-target tissues and thereby RT-related toxicity, without compromising target coverage. In 2019, ESTRO published consensus guidelines for PMRT irradiation for early-stage breast cancer in the setting of immediate implant-based reconstruction. The work on consensus guidelines in case of autologous-based reconstruction is still ongoing; however, ESTRO published together with the EUBREAST a narrative review of the management of patients who underwent autologous-based IBR and are planned for PMRT [6, 7]. The target volumes recommended by ESTRO are based on literature research and expert consensus and were mainly based on anatomy, including lymphatic drainages within the gland and the subcutaneous and deep plexus, location of residual breast tissue after mastectomy, patterns of recurrence, and previous ESTRO guidelines for chest wall and regional nodes irradiation [8–10]. Key considerations are based on the observation that most of the local recurrences after mastectomy, regardless of the surgical procedure, occur at the subcutaneous tissue and residual breast tissue, followed by the skin (together, between 75 and 100% in reported literature) [11, 12]. In case of

O. Kaidar-Person (✉)
Radiation Oncology Unit, Sheba Medical Center, Ramat Gan, Israel

Sackler School of Medicine, Tel-Aviv University, Tel-Aviv, Israel

GROW-School for Oncology and Developmental Biology (Maastro), Maastricht University, Maastricht, The Netherlands
e-mail: Orit.KaidarPerson@Sheba.health.gov.il

A. Ho
Department of Radiation Oncology, Harvard Medical School, Massachusetts General Hospital, Boston, MA, USA
e-mail: alice.ho@mgh.harvard.edu

© The Author(s), under exclusive license to Springer Nature Switzerland AG 2022

O. Kaidar-Person et al. (eds.), *Breast Cancer Radiation Therapy*,
https://doi.org/10.1007/978-3-030-91170-6_34

autologous-based reconstruction, recurrences were described at the autologous flap margins near the native breast skin-envelop (i.e. near the native chest wall skin that was not removed at the time of mastectomy) [13–15].

Chest wall recurrences invading into the pectoral muscle are less frequent than recurrences at the subcutaneous/skin level and may be a result of a tumour bed adjacent to or invading the muscle, or inter-pectoral lymph node recurrence [16, 17]. Areas that are at potential risk for residual subclinical disease include the nipple–areola complex (NAC) for early invasive cancer that includes extralesional DCIS (especially low-grade DCIS) which often presents as skip lesions, leaving the base of the nipple free of DCIS, but might have skip lesion in the ducts in the actual unresected nipple core [18], cases of central tumours, and patients with advanced lymph node status (N2 and N3 stage). These were found to have a higher positive nipple margin rate in case of NSM, thus this should be taken into consideration when discussing the type of procedure and at time of PMRT planning [19].

Another point of consideration when assessing patterns of local recurrence after mastectomy and cosmesis following reconstruction and RT is the variability in flap thickness between institutions and individual surgeons. Although flap thickness can be prospectively assessed, it is hypothesised that thin flaps may lead to increase capsular contracture and suboptimal cosmesis, particularly when postoperative RT is delivered. The use of prepectoral implants may minimise this complication, as fibrosis of the stretched muscle overlying the implant is thought to be an aetiology for capsular contracture [20–22]. This hypothesis, while attractive, requires data from uniformly planned studies with large numbers of patients in whom pre- versus postpectoral implants followed by RT are evaluated for reconstruction failure and cosmesis. Moreover, the oncological safety of these procedures should be evaluated in all breast cancer patients who are undergoing these procedures, regardless of PMRT.

Adaptation to of the PMRT volumes based on ESTRO's recommendations necessitates a comprehensive understanding of not only the patients breast's anatomy and regional lymphatics drainage patterns (which guide the most common indications for PMRT), tumour location within the intact breast prior to the procedure, disease stage (e.g. certain fractures were found to be associated with increased risk of NAC involvement as described above), but also the surgical procedure of the mastectomy and IBR. All are essential in guiding delineation of the clinical target volume of the chest wall (CTVp_chest wall) and lymphatic drainage (CTVn) [6, 7].

In cases that information is missing, or patients with more advanced disease, treatment volumes should be as historically done, covering all areas that are at high risk of recurrence, including the chest wall and lymphatic drainage as indicated without excluding the transplanted/implanted tissue/material.

34.2 Presurgical Considerations

The decision of the type of mastectomy and reconstruction should be discussed at a preoperative multidisciplinary meeting and includes appropriate assessment of the potential need for PMRT. The indications for PMRT are according to the risk of recurrence, but there is no consensus if the amount of residual breast tissue should be an indication for PMRT for patients who are otherwise not candidates for PMRT based on disease related risk [4].

34.3 PMRT

Per ESTRO guidelines, the skin is not part of the CTVp in early breast cancer patients; however, the subcutaneous lymphatic plexus (which is assumed to be the initial course of lymphatic drainage of the breast gland) is part of the CTVp as is any residual breast glandular tissue. During a total mastectomy/simple mastectomy/modified radical mastectomy, part of the skin is removed and the remaining skin is pulled together and sutured, reducing the surface size of the subcutaneous to be included within the CTVp_chest wall compared to a CTVp_breast (Fig. 34.1). This entails that, in contrast to older handbook, the area of the CTVp_chest wall should be significantly smaller compared to the surface occupied by the removed breast.

In contrast, IBR is mostly performed with skin-sparing (with removal of nipple–areolar complex) or nipple sparing (with preservation of skin and nipple–areolar complex) mastectomy. As more native breast skin is preserved, there remain more residual draining lymphatics and potentially residual breast glandular tissue [23]. The location of the residual glandular tissue after mastectomy varies in individual patients and depending on surgical procedure performed (with/without skin or nipple sparing), surgical technique, and surgeon expertise [4, 22]. Common locations of residual glandular tissue are upper outer quadrant and NAC (in case of NSM) [4, 23]. Surgeons may have a tendency to leave more residual breast glandular tissue in case of NSM/SSM and IBR, to facilitate reconstruction, reduce potential complications, and better aesthetic outcome [24, 25]. Notably, approximately 5–10% of the glandular tissue is retained after more traditional surgeries (i.e. not NSM/SSM) such as total mastectomy or modified radical mastectomy [23].

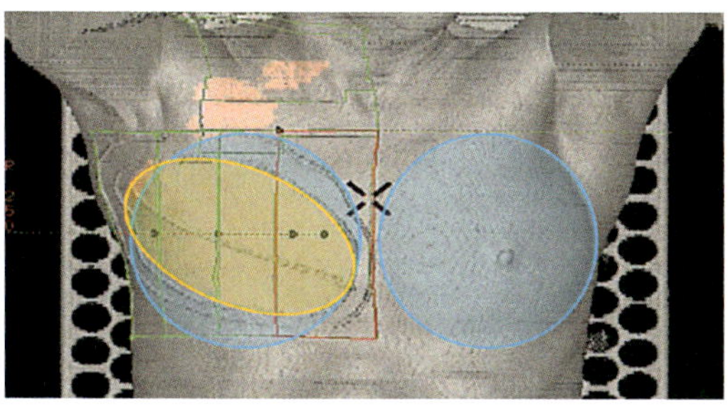

Fig. 34.1 This patient underwent an MRM including ALND. The blue shapes or the left breast projected to the right chest wall. The orange shape is the CTVp_chest wall. The difference is surface between the two is equivalent to the amount of skin that has been excised

Therefore, awareness for the possibility of residual breast tissue should be raised, and in some cases also potential residual tumour cells (especially tumour deposits within the subcutaneous of the native skin breast) [26].

At the time of patient simulation, we recommend that the borders of native breast skin be determined in conjunction with the surgeon and marked before planning CT scanning. Especially as in some cases IBR is performed with a myocutaneous flap. In these cases, autologous flap skin and subcutaneous are not part of the CTVp. The CT simulation scans and other postoperative imaging (if done) should also be reviewed for residual tissue that is not evident on physical examination. The markings should be documented in the notes used for RT planning.

Per ESTRO recommendations, the CTVp_chest wall is the volume anterior to the major pectoral muscle (Fig. 34.2a, b). The pectoralis is not considered part of the CTVp and should only be included in case of muscle invasion, and even

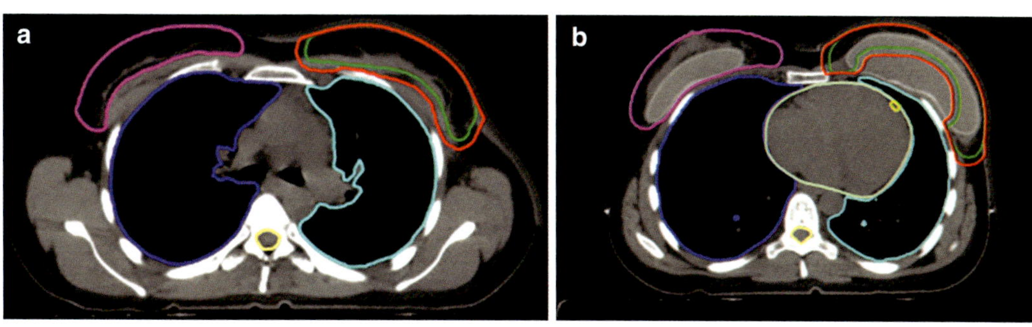

Fig. 34.2 Figure 34.2a, b are showing delineation according to ESTRO's guidelines in the setting of subpectoralis implant-based IBR. (**a**) Showing the superior part of the chest wall. Green is the CTV, Red is the PTV, Pink contralateral breast. (**b**) At the level of the heart (light blue) and left anterior descending artery (yellow). Green is the CTV, Red is the PTV, Pink contralateral breast. The figures are taken from ESTRO-FALCON website, used for educational purposes

in that case most often only partially [8]. Since the pectoral muscle is often not well developed in females and not as obvious on CT simulation or after surgical intervention, knowing the location of the implant should guide delineation (pre/post-pectoral muscle) [12, 27]. In general, the implant (tissue expander or permanent implant) may be positioned pre- or below the major pectoral muscle. In both cases, additional materials, e.g. de-epithelialized dermal flap, synthetic mesh, or a bio-mesh of animal or human tissues (acellular dermal matrix, ADM) are often used to provide complete coverage of the implant. In case of post-pectoral implant, it is usually sutured to the inferior part of the pectoral muscle to achieve a "pocket" to hold the implant. In case of a pre-pectoral implant this is secured in position with a mesh/ADM covering the largest part of the superficial surface of the implant, and the CTVp includes all the volume that encompasses the implant up the pectoral muscle [28, 29].

Per ESTRO recommendation for CTVp_chest wall cranio-caudal borders should be defined by careful clinical examination at the time of CT simulation, taking into account the position of the contralateral breast. The medial and lateral borders should be recommendations for chest wall delineation, according to potential residual glandular tissue and anatomy [8, 9].

For proper planning, it is recommended that certain volumes will be delineated. These include: the implant/autologous flap, the transplanted tissues (skin, fat, muscle). Other OARs that should be delineated for treatment planning purposes include heart, lungs, thyroid and, in case of axillary lymph node irradiation with a local boost, the brachial plexus.

Regardless of the procedure, the transplanted tissues (skin, fat, autologous muscle) and synthetic materials (implant, tissue expander, ADM) are not part of the CTVp. While limiting the dose to these volumes is expected to reduce IBR with PMRT-related side effects, there are not recommendations to spare these volumes, yet [30]. In general, an objective to limit the dose at 50–70% at non-target volumes is feasible and could already significantly reduce side effects.

34.4 Fractionation Regimens in the Setting of Breast Reconstruction

Practice patterns vary widely in terms of fractionation for breast cancer patients with implant reconstructions. In the USA and Israel, the most commonly used fraction sizes to the reconstructed chest wall and regional lymph nodes are 1.8–2 Gy to a total dose of 50–50.4 Gy. In some European countries, including the UK, Belgium, and the Netherlands, hypofractionation regimens (e.g. 40 Gy delivered in 15 fractions over 3 weeks) are more commonly employed based on long-term data from the START A/B and the Ontario Clinical Oncology Group trial trials showing reduced toxicity of hypofractionation schemes compared to the historical conventional fractionation (total dose of 50–50.4 Gy) [31, 32], which was assumed to result in reduced toxicity in case of IBR similar to BCT or chest wall (see section on dose and fractionation). In the USA, randomised controlled trials such as FABREC (NCT03422003) and RTCharm (NCT03414970) are comparing historical conventional fractionation vs. hypofractionated regimens in breast cancer patients with immediate reconstructions, with primary endpoints based on patient-reported outcome measures. These studies will provide important data on whether or not hypofractionated radiation may improve quality of life as well as reconstruction outcomes. The 2021 St. Gallen panel and the ESTRO-ACROP guidelines (2022) endorsed modrate hypofractionation also in the setting of PMRT and IBR, and regional node irradiation [33, 34].

34.5 Bolus

Bolus is commonly used for PMRT chest wall irradiation (without reconstruction). It is a tissue equivalent material placed on the skin that is representing the anterior border of the target volume and is used during the PMRT to increase the dose to the chest wall skin and subcutaneous to reduce the risk local recurrences (see section about the chest wall bolus, Chap. 21) [35]. Bolus use and protocols (thickness and schedule) vary significantly between institution [36–39].

As bolus was found to be the most important independent risk factor for severe skin toxicity in case of PMRT, due to the increased skin surface volume receiving higher radiation dose [35] and the lack of evidence-based recommendations on if/when to use bolus case of SSM/NSM, its use highly varies between institutions. In some institutions, bolus is routinely used in any IBR (because the skin and subcutaneous are preserved and considered high-risk target volumes) to allow full coverage of these volumes (within the 95% isodose line). Per ESTRO recommendations, based on dosimetric evaluation by the DBCG, due to the shape of the reconstructed breast which resembles the shape of the native breast, using tangential field-in-field planning, only the lateral side of the reconstructed breast tends to have the skin-sparing effect compared to other regions of the breast mound. Therefore, until further data become available, the routine use of a bolus in case of IBR is not recommended by ESTRO consensus guidelines and should be considered on an individual basis if there is a concern for a high-risk area that is not getting full coverage [40].

34.6 PMRT Boost

The use of the boost in case of mastectomy was common to provide an additional radiation dose to the chest wall scar with the aim to reduce local recurrences as a result of tumour cell seeding and the area that the native chest wall skin is approximated [41]. A retrospective study by Massachusetts General Hospital [41] evaluated whether to deliver a chest wall boost to the mastectomy scar or chest wall was independently associated with reconstruction complications in the setting of breast reconstruction. The cohort included patients who had delayed reconstruction procedures. The study showed that radiation boost was significantly associated with infection, skin necrosis, and implant exposure. For implant reconstruction patients, boost was independently associated with higher risks of implant failure. Most importantly, the addition of the boost was not associated with improving local tumour control, even in high-risk subgroups [41]. Therefore, we do not recommend routine use of boost in case of IBR, and if clinically indicated, it should be used with great caution to limit the risk of complications.

34.7 Timing of Reconstructions Relative to PMRT

Reconstructions can be immediate, delayed, or a hybrid of the two approaches, called delayed–immediate (Fig. 34.3). Immediate reconstructions are performed at the time of the mastectomy, whereas delayed reconstructions are usually performed 6–12 months after the completion of mastectomy and adjuvant therapy. Practical and aesthetic considerations must be taken into account when choosing between immediate and delayed reconstruction in breast cancer patients who will be receiving PMRT. Immediate reconstruction allows the preservation of the breast envelope and it is facilitated by SSM, since the goal is to replace the breast volume rather than to replace the missing skin. Conversely, in delayed breast reconstruction a substantial proportion of the skin below the mastectomy incision is often severely fibrotic after PMRT and needs to be replaced with healthy skin from a donor site to adequately reconstruct the breast contour and may therefore limit the amount of tissue available for reconstruction. These uncertainties emphasise the importance of a multidisciplinary approach to anticipating and planning for PMRT, particularly in women with clinical stage II breast cancer whose lymph node status (the main determinant for requiring PMRT) is either not known or has changed based on response to neoadjuvant chemotherapy.

Delayed–immediate reconstruction is an approach that involves placing tissue expanders at the time of mastectomy. After the need for PMRT is determined by the radiation oncologist, patients who will not receive PMRT will complete reconstruction with an implant or flap, whereas patients who will receive PMRT will typically undergo irradiation of the tissue expander followed by definitive reconstruction at a later time [42]. This option not only permits the opportunity to avoid RT to an autologous flap (in the event a flap reconstruction is planned), but also carries the benefits

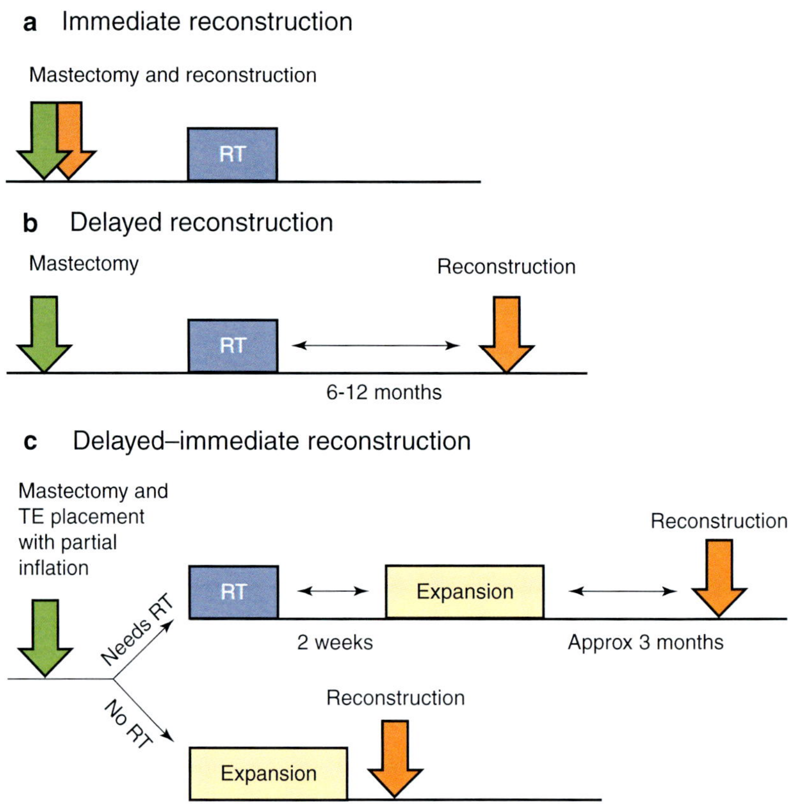

Fig. 34.3 Sequencing of breast reconstruction. *RT* radiotherapy, *TE* tissue expander. (**a**) Immediate reconstruction (**b**) Delayed reconstruction (**c**) Immediate - delayed

of providing an immediate breast mound for the patient after mastectomy.

34.8 Timing of PMRT in Two-Stage Expander/Implant Reconstruction

For patients who receive two-stage expander/implant reconstruction, the optimal timing of PMRT delivery (RT to the TE vs. RT to the PI; Figs. 34.3 and 34.4) continues to be a subject of considerable controversy, even following numerous large retrospective series and prospective trials specifically examining this question (Table 34.1 and Fig. 34.4).

The rate of reconstruction failures varies substantially from 0 to 40%, depending on whether PMRT was delivered to the tissue expander or to the permanent implant [43, 45–47]. While these retrospective studies provided some of the earliest evidence for increased rates of implant loss following radiation to the tissue expander (versus radiation to the permanent implant), we acknowledge that certain flaws limit interpretation of these findings. In the series by Nava and colleagues [44], 20 out of 50 patients (40%) had implant failures when RT was delivered to the tissue expander, compared with seven of 109 patients (6.4%) who were treated with RT to the permanent implant ($p < 0.0001$). Surgeons' assessment of the shape and symmetry of the reconstructed breast showed a higher incidence of good results in patients who received RT to the permanent implant than those who received RT to the tissue expander. The incidence of Baker grade IV capsular contracture was the highest in patients who received RT to the permanent implant, compared with those who received RT to the tissue expander (13.3% vs. 10.1% vs. 0% in the no RT group; $p = 0.0001$) [44]. A subsequent large Memorial Sloan-Kettering series corrobo-

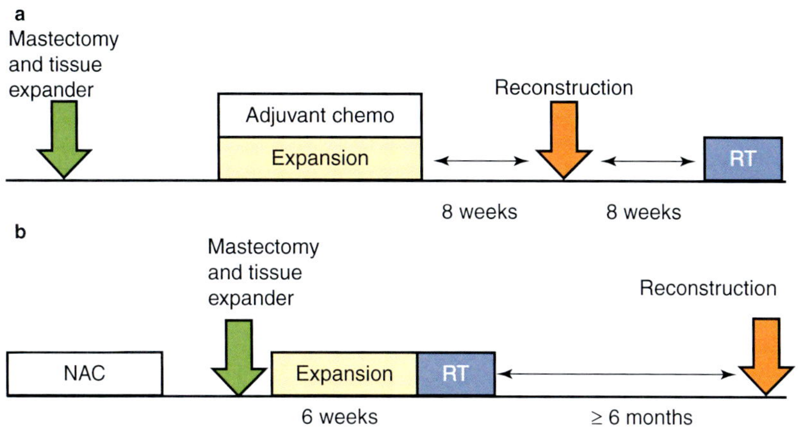

Fig. 34.4 Radiotherapy timing during two-stage tissue expander-permanent implant reconstruction. (**a**) Radiotherapy is delivered to the permanent implant. (**b**) Radiotherapy is delivered to the tissue expander, which is exchanged for a permanent implant more than 6 months after RT. *RT* radiotherapy, *chemo* chemotherapy, *NAC* neoadjuvant chemotherapy

Table 34.1 Reconstruction failure rates and the timing of radiotherapy treatment

	Total number of patients (*n*)	Median follow-up (months)	Failure rate
Anderson et al. [43]			
Permanent implant	12	48	0%
Tissue expander	62	48	4.8%
Nava et al. [44]			
Permanent implant	109	–[a]	6.4%
Tissue expander	50	–[a]	40.0%
Ho et al. [45]			
Permanent implant	151	86	13.3%
Hvilsom et al. [46]			
Permanent implant	49	–[a]	4.1%
Tissue expander	76	–[a]	13.2%
Baschnagel et al. [47]			
Permanent implant	4	24	18.0%[b]
Tissue expander	90	24	–[a]
Cordeiro et al. [48]			
Permanent implant	210	72	16.4%
Tissue expander	94	72	32.0%
Fowble et al. [49]			
Permanent implant	13	46	7.7%
Tissue expander	86	46	19.8%
Santosa et al. [50]			
Permanent implant	46	14	8.7%
Tissue expander	104	16	11.5%

[a]Not stated
[b]Of all patients

rated these findings, reporting a higher proportion of patients with reconstruction failure among patients receiving RT to the tissue expander compared with those patients receiving RT to the permanent implant, although this finding was not statistically significant (18·1% vs. 12·4%) [45]. An important finding was that the number of patients with moderate to severe capsular contracture was higher in patients who received radiation to the permanent implant, relative to those who received RT to the tissue expander, raising the issue of the "trade-off" of higher rates of capsular contracture, albeit reduced incidence of implant failures for those receiving RT to the permanent implant [45].

The "optimal" timing of PMRT in breast cancer patients receiving two-stage expander/implant reconstruction remains an elusive question even today, as the largest prospective study examining this very specific topic has reported no differences in the number of complications between the groups. A 2016 prospective study by the Mastectomy Reconstruction Outcomes (MROC) group showed no difference in outcomes between those patients who received RT delivered to the tissue expander and those who received RT to the permanent implant [50]. Endpoints included major complications, implant loss, and reconstruction failure, defined as removal of the tissue expander or permanent implant without subsequent replacement. All patients were followed for at least 2 years after reconstruction. The overall proportion of patients with reconstruction failure was 10.7%, with no significant difference between the two groups. Similarly, there was no difference in the proportion of patients who had major complications between the two groups, indicating that timing of RT was not a significant predictor of complications.

Although the incidence of capsular contracture varies substantially between studies [43, 45–47, 51], capsular contracture represents a significant long-term complication following radiation to an implant reconstruction and can lead to poor cosmesis, pain, and discomfort to the patient. In the absence of persuasive evidence to suggest that one timing of PMRT is superior to the other, choosing the option that minimises capsular contracture in weighing the risks and benefits of irradiating the expander or implant.

Clearly, high-quality evidence evaluating the type and timing of breast reconstruction in the setting of PMRT is still required [51]. Standardisation of outcome target delineation, standardisation of measures, more prospectively collected data on radiation technique-related risk factors (such as dosimetry, fractionation, and radiation modality), and the inclusion of patient-reported outcomes will accelerate progress in this important aspect of breast cancer therapy. For additional information, we recommend to read the Oncoplastic Breast Consortium (OPBC) recommendations for mastectomy and breast reconstruction in the setting of PMRT [52].

References

1. Eltahir Y, Werners LL, Dreise MM, et al. Quality-of-life outcomes between mastectomy alone and breast reconstruction: comparison of patient-reported BREAST-Q and other health-related quality-of-life measures. Plast Reconstr Surg. 2013;132:201e–9e.
2. Kaidar-Person O, Jones EL, Zagar TM. Team work: mastectomy, reconstruction, and radiation. Plast Reconstr Surg Glob Open. 2017;5:e1385.
3. Kaidar-Person O, Offersen BV, Hol S, et al. ESTRO ACROP consensus guideline for target volume delineation in the setting of postmastectomy radiation therapy after implant-based immediate reconstruction for early stage breast cancer. Radiother Oncol. 2019;137:159–66.
4. Kaidar-Person O, Boersma LJ, Poortmans P, et al. Residual glandular breast tissue after mastectomy: a systematic review. Ann Surg Oncol. 2020;27:2288–96.
5. Kaidar-Person O, Poortmans P, Offersen BV, et al. Spatial location of local recurrences after mastectomy: a systematic review. Breast Cancer Res Treat. 2020;183:263–73.
6. Kaidar-Person O, Hermann N, Poortmans P, et al. A multidisciplinary approach for autologous breast reconstruction: a narrative (re)view for better management. Radiother Oncol. 2021;157:263–71.
7. Kaidar-Person O, Offersen BV, Boersma LJ, et al. A multidisciplinary view of mastectomy and breast reconstruction: understanding the challenges. Breast. 2021;56:42–52.
8. Offersen BV, Boersma LJ, Kirkove C, et al. ESTRO consensus guideline on target volume delineation for elective radiation therapy of early stage breast cancer, version 1.1. Radiother Oncol. 2016;118:205–8.
9. Offersen BV, Boersma LJ, Kirkove C, et al. ESTRO consensus guideline on target volume delineation for elective radiation therapy of early stage breast cancer. Radiother Oncol. 2015;114:3–10.
10. Nielsen HM, Offersen BV. Regional recurrence after adjuvant breast cancer radiotherapy is not due to insufficient target coverage. Radiother Oncol. 2015;114:1–2.
11. Vargo JA, Beriwal S. RTOG chest wall contouring guidelines for post-mastectomy radiation therapy: is it evidence-based? Int J Radiat Oncol Biol Phys. 2015;93:266–7.
12. Vargo JA, Beriwal S. In reply to Chang et al.: Contouring guidelines for post-mastectomy radiotherapy a cry for international consensus. Radiother Oncol. 2017;123:483–4.
13. Noroozian M, Carlson LW, Savage JL, et al. Use of screening mammography to detect occult malignancy in autologous breast reconstructions: a 15-year experience. Radiology. 2018;289:39–48.
14. Slavin SA, Love SM, Goldwyn RM. Recurrent breast cancer following immediate reconstruction with myocutaneous flaps. Plast Reconstr Surg. 1994;93:1191–204; (discussion 1205–1197).
15. Gilliland MD, Barton RM, Copeland EM 3rd. The implications of local recurrence of breast cancer as the first site of therapeutic failure. Ann Surg. 1983;197:284–7.
16. Kaidar-Person O, Offersen BV, Poortmans P. Should risk-adapted delineation considered de-escalation of therapy? The ESTRO-ACROP radiation therapy guidelines after implant-based immediate reconstruction for early stage breast cancer. Radiother Oncol. 2019;141:327–8.
17. Komenaka IK, Bauer VP, Schnabel FR, et al. Interpectoral nodes as the initial site of recurrence in breast cancer. Arch Surg. 2004;139:175–8.

18. Tramm T, Zuckerman K, Tavassoli FA. Skip lesion of DIN (DCIS) in the nipple in a case of breast cancer. Int J Surg Pathol. 2011;19:817–21.
19. Eisenberg RE, Chan JS, Swistel AJ, Hoda SA. Pathological evaluation of nipple-sparing mastectomies with emphasis on occult nipple involvement: the Weill–Cornell experience with 325 cases. Breast J. 2014;20:15–21.
20. Caputo GG, Zingaretti N, Kiprianidis I, et al. Quality of life and early functional evaluation in direct-to-implant breast reconstruction after mastectomy: a comparative study between prepectoral versus dual-plane reconstruction. Clin Breast Cancer. 2020;21:344–51.
21. Sinnott CJ, Persing SM, Pronovost M, et al. Impact of postmastectomy radiation therapy in prepectoral versus subpectoral implant-based breast reconstruction. Ann Surg Oncol. 2018;25:2899–908.
22. Papassotiropoulos B, Guth U, Chiesa F, et al. Prospective evaluation of residual breast tissue after skin- or nipple-sparing mastectomy: results of the SKINI-trial. Ann Surg Oncol. 2019;26:1254–62.
23. Woitek R, Pfeiler G, Farr A, et al. MRI-based quantification of residual fibroglandular tissue of the breast after conservative mastectomies. Eur J Radiol. 2018;104:1–7.
24. Papassotiropoulos B, Guth U, Dubsky P, Tausch C. ASO author reflections: a call for surgeon experience and surgical radicality to prevent residual breast tissue after skin- and nipple-sparing mastectomy. Ann Surg Oncol. 2019;26:694–5.
25. Kaidar-Person O, Cardoso MJ. ASO author reflections: residual breast tissue after skin- and nipple-sparing mastectomies: a matter of concern or a point for improvement/action? Ann Surg Oncol. 2020;27:2297–8.
26. Kaidar-Person O, Kuhn T, Poortmans P. Should we worry about residual disease after mastectomy? Lancet Oncol. 2020;21:1011–3.
27. Chang JS, Byun HK, Kim JW, et al. Three-dimensional analysis of patterns of locoregional recurrence after treatment in breast cancer patients: validation of the ESTRO consensus guideline on target volume. Radiother Oncol. 2017;122:24–9.
28. Highton L, Johnson R, Kirwan C, Murphy J. Prepectoral implant-based breast reconstruction. Plast Reconstr Surg Glob Open. 2017;5:e1488.
29. Casella D, Di Taranto G, Marcasciano M, et al. Evaluation of prepectoral implant placement and complete coverage with TiLoop(R) bra mesh for breast reconstruction: a prospective study on long-term and patient reported BREAST-Q outcomes. Plast Reconstr Surg. 2018;143:1–9.
30. Kaidar-Person O, Nissen HD, Yates ES, et al. Postmastectomy radiation therapy planning after immediate implant-based reconstruction using the European Society for Radiotherapy and Oncology-Advisory Committee in radiation oncology practice consensus guidelines for target volume delineation. Clin Oncol. 2020;33:20–9.
31. Haviland JS, Owen JR, Dewar JA, et al. The UK standardisation of breast radiotherapy (START) trials of radiotherapy hypofractionation for treatment of early breast cancer: 10-year follow-up results of two randomised controlled trials. Lancet Oncol. 2013;14:1086–94.
32. Whelan T, MacKenzie R, Julian J, et al. Randomized trial of breast irradiation schedules after lumpectomy for women with lymph node-negative breast cancer. J Natl Cancer Inst. 2002;94:1143–50.
33. Burstein HJ, Curigliano G, Thürlimann B, Weber WP, Poortmans P, Regan MM, Senn HJ, Winer EP, Gnant M; Panelists of the St Gallen Consensus Conference. Customizing local and systemic therapies for women with early breast cancer: the St. Gallen International Consensus Guidelines for treatment of early breast cancer 2021. Ann Oncol. 2021;32(10):1216–35.
34. Meattini I, Becherini C, Boersma L, Kaidar-Person O, Marta GN, Montero A, Offersen BV, Aznar MC, Belka C, Brunt AM, Dicuonzo S, Franco P, Krause M, MacKenzie M, Marinko T, Marrazzo L, Ratosa I, Scholten A, Senkus E, Stobart H, Poortmans P, Coles CE. European Society for Radiotherapy and Oncology Advisory Committee in Radiation Oncology Practice consensus recommendations on patient selection and dose and fractionation for external beam radiotherapy in early breast cancer. Lancet Oncol. 2022 Jan;23(1):e21–e31.
35. Shiba S, Okamoto M, Kiyohara H, et al. Clinical advantage of chest-wall post-mastectomy radiation therapy without bolus. In Vivo. 2018;32:961–5.
36. Turner JY, Zeniou A, Williams A, Jyothirmayi R. Technique and outcome of post-mastectomy adjuvant chest wall radiotherapy—the role of tissue-equivalent bolus in reducing risk of local recurrence. Br J Radiol. 2016;89:20160060.
37. Yap ML, Tieu M, Sappiatzer J, et al. Outcomes in patients treated with post-mastectomy chest wall radiotherapy without the routine use of bolus. Clin Oncol (R Coll Radiol). 2018;30:427–32.
38. Nakamura N, Arahira S, Zenda S, et al. Post-mastectomy radiation therapy without usage of a bolus may be a reasonable option. J Radiat Res. 2017;58:66–70.
39. Aristei C, Kaidar-Person O, Tagliaferri L, et al. The Assisi think tank meeting and survey of post MAstectomy radiation therapy after breast reconstruction: the ATTM-SMART report. Eur J Surg Oncol. 2018;44:436–43.
40. Kaidar-Person O, Dahn HM, Nichol AM, Boersma LJ, de Ruysscher D, Meattini I, Pignol JP, Aristei C, Belkacemi Y, Benjamin D, Bese N, Coles CE, Franco P, Ho AY, Hol S, Jagsi R, Kirby AM, Marrazzo L, Marta GN, Moran MS, Nissen HD, Strnad V, Zissiadis Y, Poortmans PM, Offersen BV. A Delphi study and International Consensus Recommendations: The use

of bolus in the setting of postmastectomy radiation therapy for early breast cancer. Radiother Oncol. 2021;164:115–21.
41. Naoum GE, Salama L, Ho A, et al. The impact of chest wall boost on reconstruction complications and local control in patients treated for breast cancer. Int J Radiat Oncol Biol Phys. 2019;105:155–64.
42. Kronowitz SJ, Hunt KK, Kuerer HM, et al. Delayed-immediate breast reconstruction. Plast Reconstr Surg. 2004;113:1617–28.
43. Anderson PR, Freedman G, Nicolaou N, et al. Postmastectomy chest wall radiation to a temporary tissue expander or permanent breast implant—is there a difference in complication rates? Int J Radiat Oncol Biol Phys. 2009;74:81–5.
44. Nava MB, Pennati AE, Lozza L, et al. Outcome of different timings of radiotherapy in implant-based breast reconstructions. Plast Reconstr Surg. 2011;128:353–9.
45. Ho A, Cordeiro P, Disa J, et al. Long-term outcomes in breast cancer patients undergoing immediate 2-stage expander/implant reconstruction and postmastectomy radiation. Cancer. 2012;118:2552–9.
46. Hvilsom GB, Holmich LR, Steding-Jessen M, et al. Delayed breast implant reconstruction: is radiation therapy associated with capsular contracture or reoperations? Ann Plast Surg. 2012;68:246–52.
47. Baschnagel AM, Shah C, Wilkinson JB, et al. Failure rate and cosmesis of immediate tissue expander/implant breast reconstruction after postmastectomy irradiation. Clin Breast Cancer. 2012;12:428–32.
48. Cordeiro PG, Albornoz CR, McCormick B, et al. What is the optimum timing of postmastectomy radiotherapy in two-stage prosthetic reconstruction: radiation to the tissue expander or permanent implant? Plast Reconstr Surg. 2015;135:1509–17.
49. Fowble B, Park C, Wang F, et al. Rates of reconstruction failure in patients undergoing immediate reconstruction with tissue expanders and/or implants and postmastectomy radiation therapy. Int J Radiat Oncol Biol Phys. 2015;92:634–41.
50. Santosa KB, Chen X, Qi J, et al. Postmastectomy radiation therapy and two-stage implant-based breast reconstruction: is there a better time to irradiate? Plast Reconstr Surg. 2016;138:761–9.
51. Lee KT, Mun GH. Optimal sequencing of postmastectomy radiotherapy and two stages of prosthetic reconstruction: a meta-analysis. Ann Surg Oncol. 2017;24:1262–8.
52. Weber WP, Shaw J, Pusic A, et al. Oncoplastic breast consortium recommendations for mastectomy and whole breast reconstruction in the setting of post-mastectomy radiation therapy. Breast. 2022;63:123–39.

Oncoplastic Breast Conserving Surgery

35

Nicola Rocco, Naama Hermann, and Marco Bernini

35.1 Background

Oncoplastic breast conserving surgery (BCS) techniques for the treatment of breast cancer have been developed with the aim of providing better results in terms of cosmetic outcomes when compared with standard BCS, potentially improving postoperative quality of life (QoL), reducing positive margins and re-intervention rates [1]. This is especially useful in the case of a challenging position of the tumour within the breast (e.g. the upper-inner quadrant or at the lower pole) and in case of an unfavourable tumour/breast size ratio.

A consensus definition and classification system of oncoplastic BCS has been recently developed by the American Society of Breast Surgeons (ASBrS), deriving from a systematic review of the published literature [2]. The ASBrS defined oncoplastic BCS as "breast conservation surgery incorporating an oncologic partial mastectomy with ipsilateral defect repair using volume displacement or volume replacement techniques with contralateral surgery as appropriate" (Table 35.1).

35.1.1 Volume Displacement Techniques

Volume displacement is defined as closing the lumpectomy defect and redistributing the not-resected volume over the preserved breast. It is further divided into two levels according to the classification by Clough [3]: level I techniques consider the excision of less than 20% of breast volume without skin excision; level II techniques allow larger volume resections (20–50% of breast volume), encompassing more complex procedures deriving from breast reduction techniques, also called therapeutic mammoplasties, involving extensive skin excision and breast reshaping (Fig. 35.1).

Level I volume displacement techniques consist of glandular flap rearrangements around the defect caused by the lumpectomy without skin excision. These techniques are preferably used for premenopausal patients with a higher glandular component of the breast, therefore reducing the risks of fat necrosis postoperatively [4].

N. Rocco (✉)
G.Re.T.A. Group for Reconstructive and Therapeutic Advancements, Naples, Italy

Breast Surgery Unit, University of Naples "Federico II", Naples, Italy

N. Hermann
Department of Surgery B, Sheba Medical Center, Ramat Gan, Israel

Sackler Faculty of Medicine, Tel Aviv University, Tel Aviv, Israel
e-mail: Naama.Herman@sheba.health.gov.il

M. Bernini
Breast Surgery, Breast Unit, Oncology Department, Careggi University Hospital, Florence, Italy

© The Author(s), under exclusive license to Springer Nature Switzerland AG 2022

O. Kaidar-Person et al. (eds.), *Breast Cancer Radiation Therapy*,
https://doi.org/10.1007/978-3-030-91170-6_35

Table 35.1 Breast conserving oncoplastic surgery techniques

Oncoplastic technique	% Breast excised volume	Skin excision	Use of regional and distant flaps	Asymmetry to contralateral breast	Consider contralateral symmetrization surgery
Volume displacement					
Level I	<20	No	No	Slight	Rare
Level II	20–50	Yes	No	Noteable	Common
Volume replacement	20–50	Yes	Yes	Slight	Rare

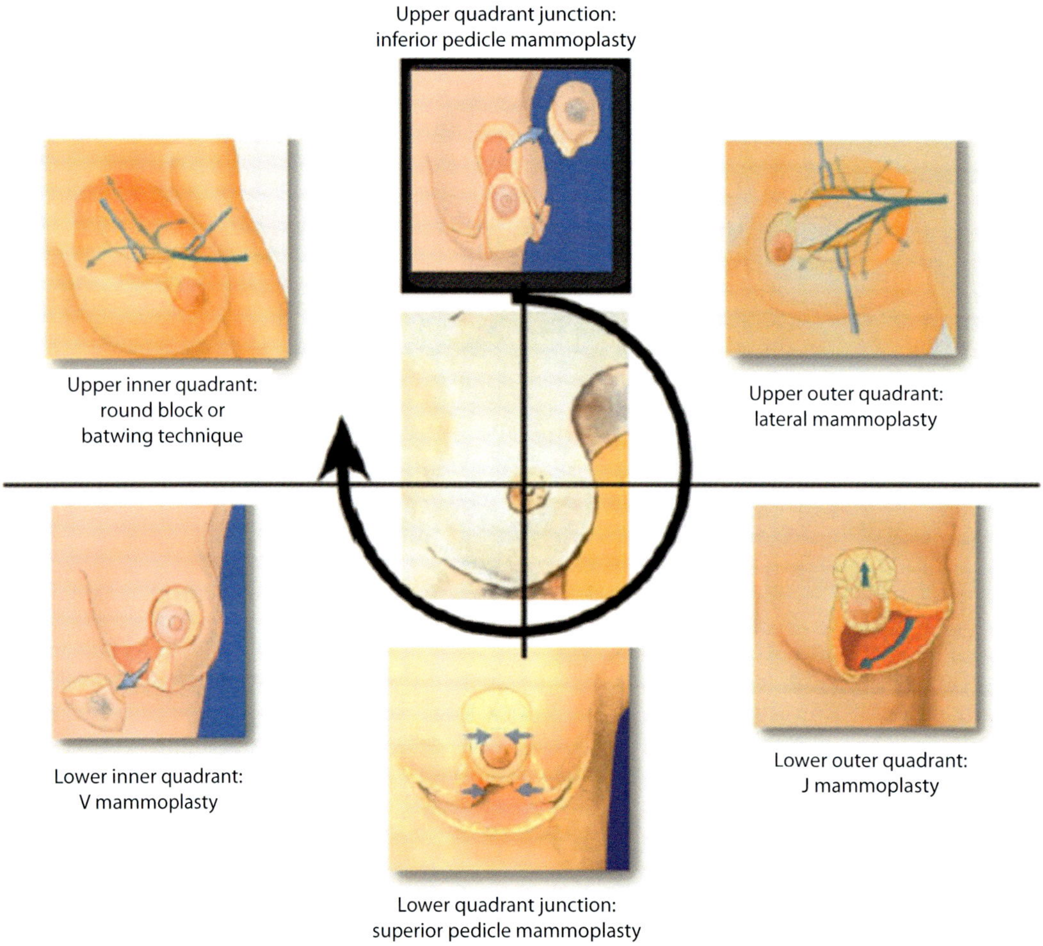

Fig. 35.1 Oncoplastic techniques for breast conservation (from Clough et al. [3])

Level II displacement techniques are mainly inspired by reduction mammoplasties techniques. In small or medium volume breasts with slight or medium ptosis, a complete peri-areolar approach could be considered according to the "round block" technique described by Benelli [5], with a major skin undermining, detaching the glandular tissue from the skin and chest wall. This technique could be used for tumours located in any quadrant of the breast.

In large volume breasts or medium volume breasts with severe ptosis, superior or inferior pedicle-based breast reduction techniques could be used for tumours located at the lower or upper quadrants, respectively. The techniques for treating tumours located at the lower quadrants are borrowed from aesthetic surgery [6, 7], with the use of superior vascular pedicles. The skin excess excision could follow a vertical or a Wise pattern [8] depending on the breast volume and ptosis, larger volumes, and higher degrees of ptosis requiring a Wise pattern rather than a vertical scar (Fig. 35.1).

The techniques for treating tumours located at the upper quadrants are based on inferior and posterior vascular pedicles as described by Ribeiro and Robbins [9, 10]. The choice of the skin excess excision pattern is made on the same considerations as for superior vascular pedicles techniques.

There are also other vascular pedicles that may be useful for treating tumours located in other quadrants, such as the medial [11, 12] and lateral pedicles [13, 14] and the vertical bi-pedicled flap (McKissock technique) [15].

Breast conserving oncoplastic techniques for tumours located in the central quadrant could be selected according to breast volume and ptosis. Centrally located tumours in medium/small breasts with slight/medium ptosis could be treated with the rotation of an infero-lateral dermo-glandular pedicle, preserving a skin island that replaces the NAC, a technique originally described by Grisotti [16]. Centrally located tumours in large volume breasts or medium volume with high degree of ptosis could be treated with breast reduction patterns as described above, preserving a skin pad for immediate NAC replacement.

35.1.2 Volume Replacement Techniques

Volume replacement techniques in oncoplastic BCS use local and regional flaps to correct the partial mastectomy defect. Defects in the lower quadrants of the breast can be addressed using local flaps such as abdominal adipo-fascial flaps or thoraco-epigastric perforator flaps. Defects in the lateral quadrants can be rebuilt with lateral chest wall perforator flaps including lateral intercostal artery perforator (LICAP) flap, lateral thoracic artery perforator (LTAP), and thoracodorsal artery perforator (TDAP) flap [17].

Distant flaps (latissimus dorsi miniflap, omental flap) used for partial volume replacement are most commonly pedicled and can be used to reconstruct infero-medial defects.

The use of free flap volume replacement techniques is also described after BCS [18]. They are adaptable to repair defects in any breast quadrant.

Some authors proposed algorithms and flow charts with the aim of helping breast surgeons in the choice of the best oncoplastic technique according to tumour location, breast volume, and ptosis [4, 19], some others developed and validated a decision support system also considering other decisional drivers as tumour stage, risk of positive margins, and patient wishes [20].

35.2 Oncoplastic Breast Conserving Surgery and Radiation Planning

When creating a radiation plan for patients who underwent oncoplastic surgery, teamwork and clear communication between the breast surgical oncologists and the radiation oncologists are of paramount importance.

Unlike after the so-called standard lumpectomies, when performing oncoplastic BCS the surgical incisions on the skin often do not directly overlay the tumour bed. In addition parenchymal flaps could be moved from other quadrants to fill the defect in the tumour bed or the tumour bed could be replaced with loco-regional or even distant flaps in cases of volume replacement techniques. Furthermore, the surgical cavity margins may be rotated and moved to other quadrants of the breast.

It is important for the radiation oncologists to understand the new arrangement of the breast tissue when evaluating margins and looking for the tumour cavity. Notably this is even more pronounced when a boost or partial breast irradiation (PBI) is considered, as in some cases the tumour bed may not be easy to identify, or simply no longer exists.

Cavity marking (thoroughly discussed in the next section) and detailed operation reporting might be of great help, but direct communication with the surgical oncologist who performed the surgery is probably the best way for the radiation oncologists to understand the breast tissue arrangement postoperatively.

35.3 Cavity Marking in Oncoplastic Breast Conserving Surgery

Breast radiation therapy (RT) is an essential companion of BCS [21, 22]. Randomised trials have demonstrated a significant reduction of local recurrence with an additional boost dose of 10–16 Gy or equivalent to the primary tumour bed [23, 24].

Therefore, in order to achieve an adequate tumour bed identification, placing surgical clips at the excision cavity has been recommended to improve the accuracy of boost field rather than clinical information only [25–27]. Despite the increasing trend for computed tomography (CT)-based target delineation, boost planning based on clips with conventional simulator still forms the base of most clinical practices [28].

There are many studies reporting that CT-based tumour bed definition, based on postoperative seroma and preoperative imaging, exceeds the clipped tumour (rather surgical) bed by a variable millimetre gap, outside the conventional boost field borders, which were simulated directly based on the clips [29–32]. Unfortunately, clips are not capable to demarcate very reliably the tumour bed but rather mark the surgical bed, not being the same as the tumour bed [33]. However, its role as an aid to assist in defining the excision cavity is widely recognised [34]. Nearly half of tumour beds on planning CT were unsatisfactorily visualised [29–32]. Under these circumstances, the routine use of clips and the way such clips are positioned by surgeons, in terms of number and sites, are definitely a topic to be considered in a teamwork between breast surgeons and their fellow radiation oncologists colleagues. Hence, a standardisation of clips placement should be regarded as an important part of surgical protocol [35].

More recently, the habit of "clipping" the surgical cavity should be regarded as essential due to the introduction of two independent revolutionary approaches in BCS, namely PBI and oncoplastic BCS. In External Beam Radiation Therapy (EBRT) PBI, the exact tumour bed definition is of utmost importance, considering that the RT will be aimed at the tissue surrounding the tumour area only and that there is not going to be a Whole Breast Irradiation (WBI). In the majority of trials, PBI was performed requiring clip positioning at the surgical site [35, 36]. For example, in the APBI (Accelerated Partial Breast Irradiation) - IMRT (Intensity Modulated Radiation Therapy) - Florence trial the positioning of at least 4 clips at tumour resection margins was required to draw the PBI-Clinical Target Volume (CTV) [36].

In the IMPORT trial's protocol the researchers suggested the routine use of paired 6 mm titanium clips around the tumour bed as follows [35]: 1—medial, lateral, superior and inferior: half-way between skin and fascia; 2—deep: mid-point, usually the pectoral fascia (posterior); 3—anterior: close to the suture line, avoiding skin dimpling.

Some studies, albeit few in literature, have found that clip placement is helpful in oncoplastic breast surgery and that 4 clips, on the glandular resection margins, are the minimum sufficient number effective for an adequate tumour bed identification in oncoplastic BCS [37–41]. For target volume definition and contouring of the tumour bed, please review the chapter entitled "Target volume definition and contouring-boost/SIB/PBI".

35.4 Oncoplastic Breast Conserving Surgery Versus Standard Breast Conserving Surgery: The Evidence

35.4.1 Patient-Reported Outcome Measures (PROMs)

The positive effects on PROMs are among the strongest supposed advantages of oncoplastic BCS compared to standard BCS. Currently this has not been thoroughly studied, and reports are mostly observational. Observational studies comparing QoL after oncoplastic or standard BCS did not show significant differences in terms of QoL (assessed with different tools) [42–44].

Observational studies comparing patients' satisfaction with aesthetic outcome after oncoplastic versus standard BCS show conflicting results [43–49].

Acosta-Marin [45], Di Micco [42], Lansu [50], Plasdottir [47], Rose [43], Santos [48], and Tenofsky et al. [49] did not report significantly different patient-reported cosmetic outcomes (assessed with different methods) between oncoplastic and standard BCS.

Schechter et al. [44] reported significantly better patient-reported cosmetic outcomes assessed with BREAST-Q [51] with oncoplastic BCS. Ojala et al. [46] reported significantly better patient-reported cosmetic outcomes assessed with BCTOS (Breast Cancer Treatment Outcome Scale) [52] with standard BCS.

Lansu et al. assessed the cosmetic outcome with a standardised objective tool (BCCT.core) showing better cosmetic results with standard BCS [50].

35.4.2 Surgical Outcomes

Oncoplastic BCS is not associated with significantly higher rates of surgical complications (infection, seroma, haematoma, bleeding, non-healing wound, wound dehiscence, skin necrosis, pain, abscess formation) compared to standard BCS, without any significant impact on timing to adjuvant treatments [44, 45, 47, 53–62].

Statistically significant lower rates of positive surgical margins are associated with oncoplastic BCS compared to standard BCS [42, 47, 54, 55, 58–60, 63–68], with significantly lower re-excision rates due to positive margins [42, 47, 49, 53, 58–61, 63, 67–69], despite the fact that patients treated by oncoplastic BCS had larger tumour size.

35.4.3 Oncological Outcomes

Loco-regional recurrences have been demonstrated to be not significantly reduced with oncoplastic BCS compared to standard BCS [53, 55, 58, 62], without any significant impact on disease-free and overall survival [54, 62, 64, 69–72].

35.5 Summary

Despite the low level of evidence supporting the use of oncoplastic BCS, these techniques are broadly accepted and used worldwide for the treatment of many breast cancer patients, extending the benefits of BCT for patients who might otherwise not be eligible for breast conservation. Oncoplastic BCS extends the role of BCS by enabling complete excision of a greater range of tumours, helping to achieve clear margins with acceptable cosmetic results without compromising oncological results. Conversely, oncoplastic BCS consumes more time and potentially more resources and today cost-effectiveness is a major concern. The application of oncoplastic BCS must be justified and this is why we need the production of more robust evidence, possibly in a randomised setting and using standardised tools for the assessment of outcomes.

Due to lack of evidence-based data, some unanswered questions remain about radiation planning after oncoplastic BCS. Not only is the tumour bed often quite more challenging to identify, but also it may no longer exist (neither as a potential space nor as a seroma field cavity), but rather be transferred to different quadrants of the breast as part of the volume displacement flaps. In that context, the use of radiation techniques that rely on identification of the tumour bed, such as PBI and tumour bed boost remains to be evaluated in this perspective. For both, intraoperative radiation therapy, delivered after tumourectomy and before oncoplastic tumour re-arrangement, seems an attractive approach to potentially overcome the challenges of identifying the tumour bed. However, this approach should be evaluated in a clinical study.

When planning RT after oncoplastic BCS, clear communication between the surgeon and the radiation oncologist is of paramount importance. While global standardisation is still lacking, understanding of the surgical procedure and identification of the tumour bed, when possible, should be part of the multidisciplinary care.

References

1. Clough KB, Kroll SS, Audretsch W. An approach to the repair of partial mastectomy defects. Plast Reconstr Surg. 1999;104(2):409–20.
2. Chatterjee A, Gass J, Patel K, Holmes D, Kopkash K, Peiris L, Peled A, Ryan J, El-Tamer M, Reiland J. A consensus definition and classification system of oncoplastic surgery developed by the American Society of Breast Surgeons. Ann Surg Oncol. 2019;26(11):3436–44.
3. Clough KB, Ihrai T, Oden S, Kaufman G, Massey E, Nos C. Oncoplastic surgery for breast cancer based on tumour location and a quadrant-per-quadrant atlas. Br J Surg. 2012;99(10):1389–95.
4. Urban C, Lima R, Schunemann E, Spautz C, Rabinovich I, Anselmi K. Oncoplastic principles in breast conserving surgery. Breast. 2011;20(Suppl 3):S92–5.
5. Benelli L. A new periareolar mammaplasty: the "round block" technique. Aesthetic Plast Surg. 1990;14(2):93–100.
6. Pitanguy I. Surgical treatment of breast hypertrophy. Br J Plast Surg. 1967;20(1):78–85.
7. Lejour M. Vertical mammaplasty: early complications after 250 personal consecutive cases. Plast Reconstr Surg. 1999;104(3):764–70.
8. Parsons RW, Burton FC, Shaw RC. The versatile mammaplasty pattern of wise. Plast Reconstr Surg. 1975;55(1):1–4.
9. Ribeiro L, Accorsi A Jr, Buss A, Marcal-Pessoa M. Creation and evolution of 30 years of the inferior pedicle in reduction mammaplasties. Plast Reconstr Surg. 2002;110(3):960–70.
10. Robbins TH. A reduction mammaplasty with the areola-nipple based on an inferior dermal pedicle. Plast Reconstr Surg. 1977;59(1):64–7.
11. Brown RH, Siy R, Khan K, Izaddoost S. The superomedial pedicle wise-pattern breast reduction: reproducible, reliable, and resilient. Semin Plast Surg. 2015;29(2):94–101.
12. Ron O, Inbal A, Arad E, Zaretski A, Leshem D, Yanko R, Gur E, Barnea Y. Superomedial pedicle vertical scar breast reduction: objective and subjective assessment of breast symmetry and aesthetics. Aesthetic Plast Surg. 2018;42(3):639–47.
13. Cárdenas-Camarena L, Vergara R. Reduction mammaplasty with superior-lateral dermoglandular pedicle: another alternative. Plast Reconstr Surg. 2001;107(3):693–9.
14. Blondeel PN, Hamdi M, Van de Sijpe KA, Van Landuyt KH, Thiessen FE, Monstrey SJ. The latero-central glandular pedicle technique for breast reduction. Br J Plast Surg. 2003;56(4):348–59.
15. McKissock PK. Reduction mammaplasty by the vertical bipedicle flap technique rationale and results. Clin Plast Surg. 1976;3(2):309–20.
16. Galimberti V, Zurrida S, Zanini V, Callegari M, Veronesi P, Catania S, Luini A, Greco M, Grisotti A. Central small size breast cancer: how to overcome the problem of nipple and areola involvement. Eur J Cancer. 1993;29A(8):1093–6.
17. Munhoz AM, Montag E, Arruda E, Brasil JA, Aldrighi JM, Gemperli R, Filassi JR, Ferreira MC. Immediate conservative breast surgery reconstruction with perforator flaps: new challenges in the era of partial mastectomy reconstruction? Breast. 2011;20(3):233–40.
18. McCulley SJ, Macmillan RD, Rasheed T. Transverse Upper Gracilis (TUG) flap for volume replacement in breast conserving surgery for medial breast tumours in small to medium sized breasts. J Plast Reconstr Aesthet Surg. 2011;64(8):1056–60.
19. Munhoz AM, Montag E, Arruda E, Pellarin L, Filassi JR, Piato JR, de Barros AC, Prado LC, Fonseca A, Baracat E, Ferreira MC. Assessment of immediate conservative breast surgery reconstruction: a classification system of defects revisited and an algorithm for selecting the appropriate technique. Plast Reconstr Surg. 2008;121(3):716–27.
20. Catanuto G, Pappalardo F, Rocco N, Leotta M, Ursino V, Chiodini P, Buggi F, Folli S, Catalano F, Nava MB. Formal analysis of the surgical pathway and development of a new software tool to assist surgeons in the decision making in primary breast surgery. Breast. 2016;29:74–81.
21. Fisher B, Anderson S, Bryant J, et al. Twenty-year follow-up of a randomized trial comparing total mastectomy, lumpectomy, and lumpectomy plus irradiation for the treatment of invasive breast cancer. N Engl J Med. 2002;347:1233–41.
22. Clarke M, Collins R, Darby S, et al. Effects of radiotherapy and of differences in the extent of surgery for early breast cancer on local recurrence and 15-year survival: an overview of the randomised trials. Lancet. 2005;366:2087–106.
23. Romestaing P, Lehingue Y, Carrie C, et al. Role of a 10-Gy boost in the conservative treatment of early breast cancer: results of a randomized clinical trial in Lyon, France. J Clin Oncol. 1997;15:963–8.
24. Bartelink H, Horiot JC, Poortmans PM, et al. Impact of a higher radiation dose on local control and survival in breast-conserving therapy of early breast can-

cer: 10-year results of the randomized boost versus no boost EORTC 22881–10882 trial. J Clin Oncol. 2007;25:3259–65.
25. Machtay M, Lanciano R, Hoffman J, et al. Inaccuracies in using the lumpectomy scar for planning electron boosts in primary breast carcinoma. Int J Radiat Oncol Biol Phys. 1994;30:43–8.
26. Harrington KJ, Harrison M, Bayle P, et al. Surgical clips in planning the electron boost in breast cancer: a qualitative and quantitative evaluation. Int J Radiat Oncol Biol Phys. 1996;34:579–84.
27. Ringash J, Whelan T, Elliott E, et al. Accuracy of ultrasound in localization of breast boost field. Radiother Oncol. 2004;72:61–6.
28. Wolmark N, Curran WJ. On behalf of NSABP and RTOG of the American College of Radiology (ACR). NSABP Protocol B-39. RTOG Protocol 0413. A randomized phase III study of conventional whole breast irradiation versus partial breast irradiation for women with stage 0, I, or II breast cancer. National surgical adjuvant breast and bowel project (NSABP). Trial protocol March 13; 2007. p. 1–132.
29. Yang Z, Chen J, Hu W, Pan Z, Cai G, Yu X, Mei X, Zhang Q, Liu T, Guo X. Planning the breast boost: how accurately do surgical clips represent the CT seroma? Radiother Oncol. 2010;97(3):530–4.
30. Goldberg H, Prosnitz RG, Olson JA, et al. Definition of post lumpectomy tumour bed for radiotherapy boost field planning: CT versus surgical clips. Int J Radiat Oncol Biol Phys. 2005;63:209–13.
31. van der Laan HP, Dolsma WV, Maduro JH, et al. Dosimetric consequences of the shift towards computed tomography guided target definition, planning for breast conserving radiotherapy. Radiat Oncol. 2008;3:6.
32. Harris EJ, Donovan EM, Yarnold JR, et al. Characterization of target volume changes during breast radiotherapy using implanted fiducial markers and portal imaging. Int J Radiat Oncol Biol Phys. 2009;73:958–66.
33. Bartelink H, Bourgier C, Elkhuizen P. Has partial breast irradiation by IORT or brachytherapy been prematurely introduced into the clinic? Radiother Oncol. 2012;104(2):139–42.
34. Aznar MC, Meattini I, Poortmans P, Steyerova P, Wyld L. To clip or not to clip. That is no question! Eur J Surg Oncol. 2017;43(7):1145–7.
35. Coles CE, Wilson CB, Cumming J, et al. Titanium clip placement to allow accurate tumour bed localisation following breast conserving surgery: audit on behalf of the IMPORT Trial Management Group. Eur J Surg Oncol. 2009;35:578–82.
36. Meattini I, Marrazzo L, Saieva C, Desideri I, Scotti V, Simontacchi G, Bonomo P, Greto D, Mangoni M, Scoccianti S, Lucidi S, Paoletti L, Fambrini M, Bernini M, Sanchez L, Orzalesi L, Nori J, Bianchi S, Pallotta S, Livi L. Accelerated partial-breast irradiation compared with whole-breast irradiation for early breast cancer: long-term results of the randomized phase III APBI-IMRT-Florence trial. J Clin Oncol. 2020;24:JCO2000650. https://doi.org/10.1200/JCO.20.00650.
37. Riina MD, Rashad R, Cohen S, Brownlee Z, Sioshansi S, Hepel J, Chatterjee A, Huber KE. The effectiveness of intraoperative clip placement in improving radiation therapy boost targeting after oncoplastic surgery. Pract Radiat Oncol. 2020;10(5):e348–56.
38. Pezner RD, Tan MC, Clancy SL, Chen YJ, Joseph T, Vora NL. Radiation therapy for breast cancer patients who undergo oncoplastic surgery: localization of the tumour bed for the local boost. Am J Clin Oncol. 2013;36(6):535–9.
39. Pezner RD. The oncoplastic breast surgery challenge to the local radiation boost. Int J Radiat Oncol Biol Phys. 2011;79(4):963–4.
40. Oden S, Thureau S, Baron M, Hanzen C. Conservative treatment for breast cancer: optimization of the tumour bed localization. Cancer Radiother. 2010;14(2):96–102.
41. Thomas K, Rahimi A, Spangler A, Anderson J, Garwood D. Radiation practice patterns among United States radiation oncologists for postmastectomy breast reconstruction and oncoplastic breast reduction. Pract Radiat Oncol. 2014;4(6):466–71.
42. Di Micco R, O'Connell RL, Barry PA, Roche N, MacNeill FA, Rusby JE. Standard wide local excision or bilateral reduction mammoplasty in large-breasted women with small tumours: surgical and patient-reported outcomes. Eur J Surg Oncol. 2017;43(4):636–41. https://doi.org/10.1016/j.ejso.2016.10.027.
43. Rose M, Svensson H, Handler J, Hoyer U, Ringberg A, Manjer J. Patient-reported outcome after oncoplastic breast surgery compared with conventional breast-conserving surgery in breast cancer. Breast Cancer Res Treat. 2020;180(1):247–56.
44. Shechter S, Friedman O, Inbal A, et al. Oncoplastic partial breast reconstruction improves patient satisfaction and aesthetic outcome for central breast tumours. ANZ J Surg. 2019;89(5):536–40. https://doi.org/10.1111/ans.15078.
45. Acosta-Marin V, Acosta-Freites V, Contreras A, et al. Oncoplastic breast surgery: initial experience at the Centro Clinico de Estereotaxia-CECLINES, Caracas, Venezuela. E Cancer Med Sci. 2014;8:470.
46. Ojala K, Meretoja TJ, Leidenius MH. Aesthetic and functional outcome after breast conserving surgery—comparison between conventional and oncoplastic resection. Eur J Surg Oncol. 2017;43(4):658–64.
47. Palsdottir EP, Lund SHL, Asgeirsson KSA. Oncoplastic breast-conserving surgery in Iceland: a population-based study. Scand J Surg. 2018;107(3):224–9.
48. Santos G, Urban C, Edelweiss MI, et al. Long-term comparison of aesthetical outcomes after oncoplastic

surgery and lumpectomy in breast cancer patients. Ann Surg Oncol. 2015;22(8):2500–8.

49. Tenofsky PL, Dowell P, Topalovski T, Helmer SD. Surgical, oncologic, and cosmetic differences between oncoplastic and nononcoplastic breast conserving surgery in breast cancer patients. Am J Surg. 2014;207(3):398–402.
50. Lansu JT, Essers M, Voogd AC, Luiten EJ, Buijs C, Groenendaal N, Poortmans PM. The influence of simultaneous integrated boost, hypofractionation and oncoplastic surgery on cosmetic outcome and PROMs after breast conserving therapy. Eur J Surg Oncol. 2015;41(10):1411–6.
51. Pusic AL, Klassen AF, Scott AM, Klok JA, Cordeiro PG, Cano SJ. Development of a new patient-reported outcome measure for breast surgery: the BREAST-Q. Plast Reconstr Surg. 2009;124(2):345–53.
52. Stanton AL, Krishnan L, Collins CA. Form or function? Part 1. Subjective cosmetic and functional correlates of quality of life in women treated with breast-conserving surgical procedures and radiotherapy. Cancer. 2001;91:2273–81.
53. Calì Cassi L, Vanni G, Petrella G, et al. Comparative study of oncoplastic versus non-oncoplastic breast conserving surgery in a group of 211 breast cancer patients. Eur Rev Med Pharmacol Sci. 2016;20(14):2950–4.
54. Carter SA, Lyons GR, Kuerer HM, et al. Operative and oncologic outcomes in 9861 patients with operable breast cancer: single-institution analysis of breast conservation with oncoplastic reconstruction. Ann Surg Oncol. 2016;23(10):3190–8.
55. Chauhan A, Sharma MM. Evaluation of surgical outcomes following oncoplastic breast surgery in early breast cancer and comparison with conventional breast conservation surgery. Med J Armed Forces India. 2016;72(1):12–8.
56. Cil TD, Cordeiro E. Complications of oncoplastic breast surgery involving soft tissue transfer versus breast-conserving surgery: an analysis of the NSQIP database. Ann Surg Oncol. 2016;23(10):3266–71.
57. Dolan R, Patel M, Weiler-Mithoff E, et al. Imaging results following oncoplastic and standard breast conserving surgery. Breast Care (Basel). 2015;10(5):325–9.
58. Down SK, Jha PK, Burger A, Hussien MI. Oncological advantages of oncoplastic breast-conserving surgery in treatment of early breast cancer. Breast J. 2013;19(1):56–63.
59. Giacalone PL, Roger P, Dubon O, et al. Comparative study of the accuracy of breast resection in oncoplastic surgery and quadrantectomy in breast cancer. Ann Surg Oncol. 2007;14(2):605–14.
60. Giacalone PL, Roger P, Dubon O, El Gareh N, Daurés JP, Laffargue F. Traitement conservateur des cancers du sein: zonectomie vs oncoplastie. Etude prospective à propos de 99 patientes [Lumpectomy vs oncoplastic surgery for breast-conserving therapy of cancer. A prospective study about 99 patients]. Ann Chir. 2006;131(4):256–61.
61. Jonczyk MM, Jean J, Graham R, Chatterjee A. Trending towards safer breast cancer surgeries? Examining acute complication rates from a 13-year NSQIP analysis. Cancers (Basel). 2019;11(2):253.
62. Kelemen P, Pukancsik D, Újhelyi M, et al. Comparison of clinicopathologic, cosmetic and quality of life outcomes in 700 oncoplastic and conventional breast-conserving surgery cases: a single-centre retrospective study. Eur J Surg Oncol. 2019;45(2):118–24.
63. Bali R, Kankam HKN, Borkar N, Provenzano E, Agrawal A. Wide local excision versus oncoplastic breast surgery: differences in surgical outcome for an assumed margin (0, 1, or 2 mm) distance. Clin Breast Cancer. 2018;18(5):e1053–7.
64. Gulcelik MA, Dogan L, Yuksel M, Camlibel M, Ozaslan C, Reis E. Comparison of outcomes of standard and oncoplastic breast-conserving surgery. J Breast Cancer. 2013;16(2):193–7.
65. Kaur N, Petit JY, Rietjens M, et al. Comparative study of surgical margins in oncoplastic surgery and quadrantectomy in breast cancer. Ann Surg Oncol. 2005;12(7):539–45.
66. Losken A, Pinell-White X, Hart AM, Freitas AM, Carlson GW, Styblo TM. The oncoplastic reduction approach to breast conservation therapy: benefits for margin control. Aesthet Surg J. 2014;34(8):1185–91.
67. Nisiri A, Pour RO, Zadeh HM, Ramim T. Comparison of surgical margin after breast cancer surgery between oncoplastic technique and conventional breast-conserving surgery. Int J Cancer Manag. 2018;11(4):e9696.
68. Wijgman DJ, Ten Wolde B, van Groesen NR, Keemers-Gels ME, van den Wildenberg FJ, Strobbe LJ. Short term safety of oncoplastic breast conserving surgery for larger tumours. Eur J Surg Oncol. 2017;43(4):665–71. https://doi.org/10.1016/j.ejso.2016.11.021.
69. Piper M, Peled AW, Sbitany H, Foster RD, Esserman LJ, Price ER. Comparison of mammographic findings following oncoplastic mammoplasty and lumpectomy without reconstruction. Ann Surg Oncol. 2016;23(1):65–71.
70. De Lorenzi F, Hubner G, Rotmensz N, et al. Oncological results of oncoplastic breast-conserving surgery: long term follow-up of a large series at a single institution: a matched-cohort analysis. Eur J Surg Oncol. 2016;42(1):71–7. https://doi.org/10.1016/j.ejso.2015.08.160.
71. Mansell J, Weiler-Mithoff E, Stallard S, Doughty JC, Mallon E, Romics L. Oncoplastic breast conservation surgery is oncologically safe when compared to wide local excision and mastectomy. Breast. 2017;32:179–85.
72. Rose M, Svensson H, Handler J, Hoyer U, Ringberg A, Manjer J. Oncoplastic breast surgery compared to conventional breast-conserving surgery with regard to oncologic outcome. Clin Breast Cancer. 2019;19(6):423–32.

36 Sequential Boost Versus SIB

Pierfrancesco Franco and Melanie Machiels

36.1 Background

Breast conserving therapy—consisting of BCS followed by whole breast irradiation (WBI)—has been well established by several randomised trials [1, 2]. An additional boost dose to the tumour bed has been shown to increase local relapse-free survival in selected patients [3].

With external beam RT, this extra dose to the tumour bed can be delivered either with a sequential boost approach or with a concomitant or simultaneous integrated boost (SIB). When delivering a sequential boost, treatment consists of two phases, the first being directed to the entire set of target volumes and the boost limited to the primary tumour bed with a margin, with a progressive shrinkage of target volumes.

In the context of breast cancer, a sequential boost is typically delivered in 4–8 extra fractions which prolong the overall treatment time by 1–2 weeks. Of note, the boost dose, together with other cofactors, negatively influences cosmetic outcomes, especially in case of large boost volumes [3–5].

P. Franco (✉)
Department of Translational Medicine, University of Eastern Piedmont, Novara, Italy

M. Machiels
Iridium Kankernetwerk/Universiteit Antwerpen, Wilrijk, Belgium
e-mail: Melanie.machiels@gza.be

Over the past few decades, there is a growing interest in the delivery of a concomitant or SIB for breast cancer. SIB is generally managed as a single treatment plan for the entire course of treatment with different radiation doses for the whole breast and tumour bed. The term 'simultaneous integrated boost' was introduced by Mohan et al. to describe the delivery of different doses per fraction to different target regions including an elective dose to the entire set of target volumes and a higher dose to the high risk volumes [6]. This allows to modulate dose levels depending on the specific risk of recurrence.

There are basically two different approaches to manage the delivery of a concomitant boost in this clinical setting.

1. The SIB employed as an additional dose given to a specific volume (the tumour bed in this case) on top of the dose received by the elective volumes (whole breast with/without lymph nodes). With this approach, the dose per fraction to the elective volumes can be given with conventional fractionation or hypofractionation, while the boost dose to the tumour bed is given as an extra dose in the same treatment fraction within the same treatment plan (SIB) or using a different set of calculations (concomitant boost). The overall treatment time is reduced compared to the delivery of a sequential boost (*model 2 in* Table 36.1).

© The Author(s), under exclusive license to Springer Nature Switzerland AG 2022
O. Kaidar-Person et al. (eds.), *Breast Cancer Radiation Therapy*,
https://doi.org/10.1007/978-3-030-91170-6_36

Table 36.1 Example for dose and fractionations of whole breast with/without simultaneous integrated boost

Type of SIB	Prescription	WBI Fraction size	Number of fractions	Total dose	Boost Fraction size	Number of fractions	Total dose	Total dose incl WBI
Model 1	No boost	2.67	15	40.05	0	0	0	40.05
	With boost	2.18	20	43.6	0.49	20	9.8	53.4
Model 2	No boost	2.67	15	40.05	0	0	0	40.05
	With boost	2.67	15	40.05	3.2	15	48	48

Fraction size (Gy), total dose (Gy)

2. The SIB combining a stable dose per fraction to the boost volume with a higher number of fractions, for which, at the same time, the dose to the elective volumes has to be decreased. The dose to the elective volumes can be delivered using conventional or hypofractionation (*model 1 in* Table 36.1).

Model 2 leads to a benefit in terms of patient's convenience and radiation oncology department throughput. For both, a significant dosimetric advantage is provided. This allows to be on the safer side with respect to the risk of increasing the rate of side effects (by decreased high-dose volume sizes while the maximal dose remains constant or lowered based on radiobiological calculations). In other settings, such as head and neck cancer, fractionations schemes usually employ lower dose per fraction (generally ≤1.8 Gy). This allows for a slight contraction in overall treatment time, to deliver the full dose to the high-dose volumes.

The use of SIB was significantly associated with improved patient compliance, health-related QoL, lowered patient-related costs, and increased utilisation of BCT [7, 8]. Tumour bed boost integration is also theorised to improve disease control due to the overall increased dose per fraction to the tumour bed in accelerated fractionation compared to sequential boost.

This chapter provides a critical appraisal of the available evidence of administration of a sequential boost as compared to a SIB in breast cancer patients who are planned for BCT.

36.2 Existing Literature

36.2.1 Dosimetry

Compared to the sequential delivery of a boost dose to the tumour bed, the use of SIB is based on the incorporation of the boost within the WBI and potentially provides a dosimetric advantage for both OARs and target volumes (Fig. 36.1). An example of a comparison between a sequential boost and SIB using a conventional 3DCRT technique is shown in Fig. 36.2. Several dosimetric comparison planning studies investigated the potential advantage of boost integration. Singla et al. compared SIB plans using IMRT versus a sequential boost using 3DCRT tangential fields to deliver a 16 Gy boost above 50.4 Gy of conventionally fractionated WBI. Albeit, 28 fractions to the whole breast plus 8 additional fractions to the tumour bed were given in the 3DCRT arm versus 28 fractions of 1.8 Gy were given to the whole breast and of 2.37 Gy to tumour bed in the IMRT SIB arm [9]. An improvement in target conformality (up to 67%) could be detected with IMRT SIB as a reduction in mean lung dose (MLD) and maximum heart dose. Hurkmans et al. performed a planning study of SIB using inverse optimisation vs a 3-field boost approach [10]. The comparison demonstrated a similar volume of whole breast and tumour bed receiving >95% of the prescribed dose and similar mean heart dose (MHD) and MLD. Interestingly, the SIB approach provided a reduction in the volume of whole breast (excluding the boost volume) receiving >95% of

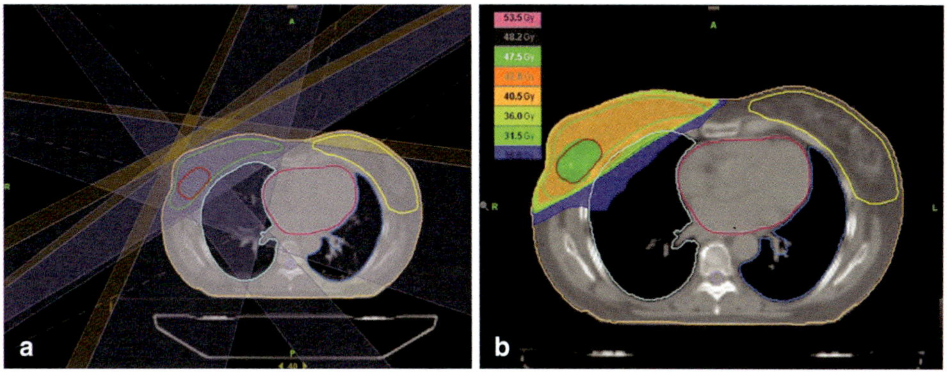

Fig. 36.1 Exemplary dose distribution of a SIB

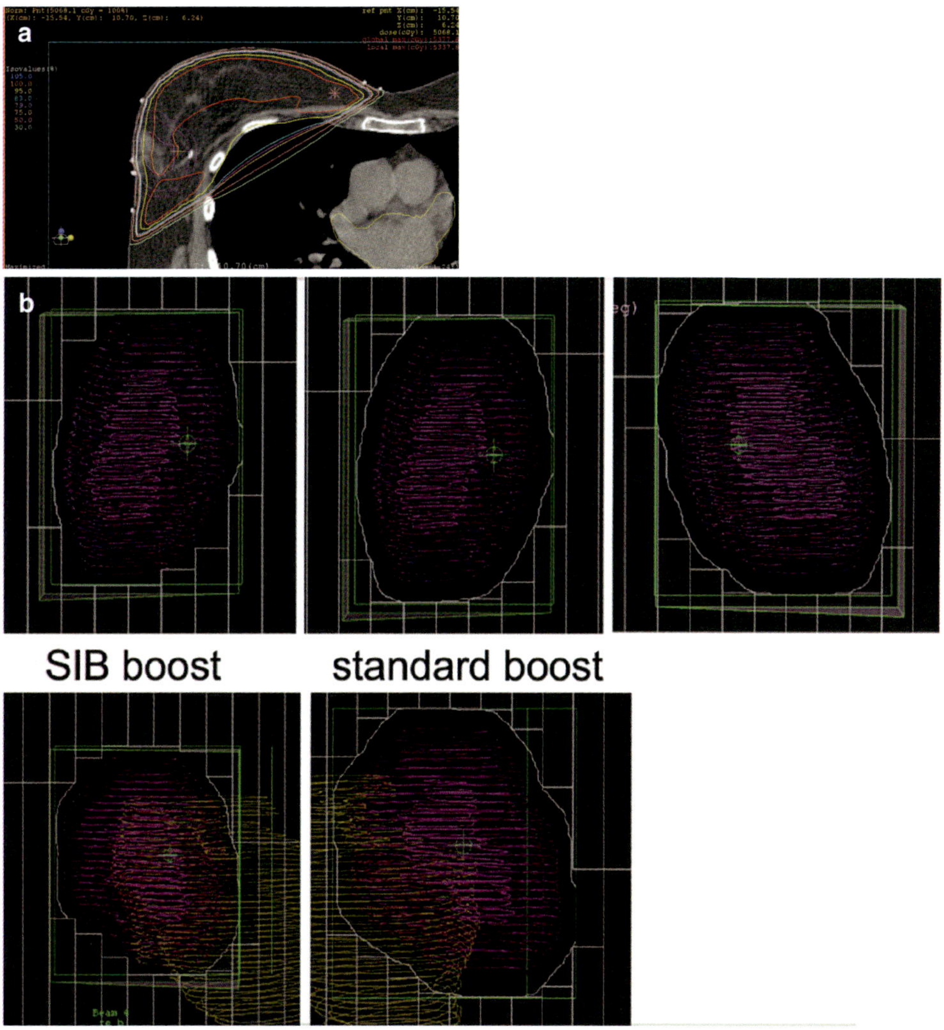

Fig. 36.2 Comparison between a sequential boost and SIB with a conventional 3D-CRT technique as used in 2012 (ESTRO course, courtesy S. Hol, Tilburg, NL). *Note: only the planning at the central axis through the PTV boost is shown. SIB = left; sequential = right.* (**a**) Breast treatment planning is identical for SIB compared to sequential. (**b**) For SIB the MLCs can be put at the PTV borders, while for sequential a 0.5–0.8 cm margin is required to obtain electronic equilibrium. (**c**) After summing both treatment plans further optimising can be done

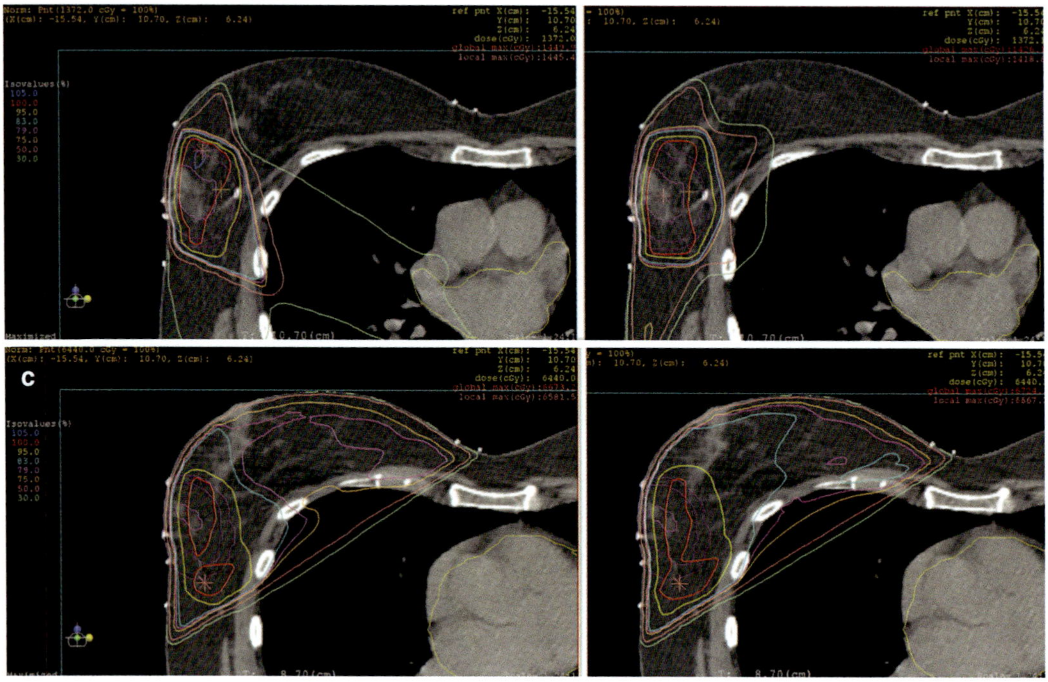

Fig. 36.2 (continued)

the prescribed dose, with hence a smaller volume receiving the high-boost dose and a better conformality [10]. This is in line with other findings. Van der Laan et al. reported on comparative planning study of SIB in 30 patients affected with left-sided breast cancer, comparing standard RT (50 Gy in 25 fractions +16 Gy in 8 fractions as a sequential boost versus a forward-planned 3DCRT WBI delivering 1.81 Gy × 28 fractions with a concomitant boost of another 0.49 Gy (2.3 Gy daily) [11]. With boost incorporation, the mean volume getting ≥107% of whole breast prescribed dose was reduced by 20%, the mean volume of breast tissue outside the tumour bed receiving ≥95% of the boost dose was reduced by 54% and MHD and MLD were reduced by 10%. More data about the use of this SIB technique with a slight reduction of the total number of fractions (28 vs. 33 and 31 vs. 38, respectively, for the standard and the high-boost dose with SIB vs. sequential boost) will become available soon after the analysis of the "Young Boost Trial" [12]. Consistently, in a comparison between 3DCRT and helical tomotherapy for WBI, Hijal et al. demonstrated that a tomotherapy-based SIB approach leads to the reduction in excess irradiation of the whole breast excluding the tumour bed. With 3DCRT, a large amount of breast tissue outside tumour bed was unnecessarily irradiated [13]. This issue has a clinical translation. It has been shown that, during the delivery of sequential boost, even if given with tomotherapy-based IMRT and steep dose gradients, the adjunctive dose received by the breast tissue outside the tumour bed may be correlated with acute skin toxicity [14]. On the same platform, but with the use of SIB, the authors were able to limit the unintended irradiation of breast tissue outside the tumour bed and to consequently reduce the acute skin profile toxicity as will be discussed hereafter [15]. However, when using VMAT/vIMRT techniques or any beam arrangement that is not aligned with the conventional tangential techniques for breast cancer, care must be given to identify RT doses to non-target tissue, e.g. contralateral breast, low doses to the lungs, liver, etc. The key of the dosimetry advantage of SIB compared to sequential boost is mainly due to smaller beam arrangement used in case of beam (see treatment planning section).

36.2.2 Toxicity

There are concerns that when using the SIB technique, a higher dose per fraction is administered to a part of the breast, which might increase the incidence of toxicity. However, better dose conformity can be reached if doses to the whole breast and to the boost volume are optimised simultaneously as demonstrated previously. Furthermore, when giving a sequential boost, hot spots of the WBI plan can coincide with hot spots in the boost plan, despite modern treatment planning systems allowing to take the dose delivered by the WBI plan into account when planning the boost, setup differences or anatomy changes are currently not considered.

Main toxicity data on the use of a SIB for BCT in early stage breast cancer consists of non-comparative series and has been thoroughly summarised in a systematic review published in 2016 [16]. In only ten studies grade 3 acute toxicities were observed and ranged from 1% to 7% [7, 15, 17]. It was noted that the incidence of acute radiation dermatitis across studies was reversible, with six studies (46%) reporting resolution of moderate to severe toxicities within 12 weeks of finishing RT. Considering late toxicity, largest experience comes from a large prospective cohort investigating 982 patients treated with normofractionated WBI with a SIB [18]. After 3 years, 8.5 and 3.7% of patients had grade ≥2 fibrosis in the boost area and grade ≥2 telangiectasia, respectively. In other smaller series, longest median follow-up reported was 5.1 years [19]. The incidence of moderate to severe late toxicities ranged from 1% to 9% and 0% to 9% for both breast fibrosis and telangiectasia, respectively [15, 19, 20].

More recently, Cante et al. published data from 178 patients treated with hypofractionated WBI (45 Gy total dose) and a concomitant boost to the tumour bed (50 Gy total dose) over 4 weeks [21]. With a median follow-up of 117 months (range 4–140), they reported grade 2 (fibrosis) and grade 3 (telangiectasia) skin toxicity in 7% and 5% of the patients, and good or excellent cosmesis in 87.8% of the patients. Lansu et al. retrospectively investigated and compared the cosmetic outcomes of a SIB versus a sequential boost, in the setting of hypofractionation in patients who underwent oncoplastic surgery [22]. The authors reported that the SIB and hypofractionation did not have an influence on cosmetic outcome but had a favourable influence on quality of life, while oncoplastic surgery negatively influenced cosmesis. Krug et al. demonstrated low acute toxicity (grade ≥2 skin toxicity of 14.7%) and high treatment adherence to hypofractionated WBI with SIB [23].

Comparative data are scarce, with only three randomised controlled trials found. A series of 400 patients treated to 40.05 Gy in 15 fractions to the breast in prone position and randomised between a daily SIB of 0.5 Gy (2.67 Gy + 0.5 Gy) or a weekly 2 Gy SIB demonstrated comparable acute grade 2 and long-term toxicity between both groups with a median follow-up of 45 months [24]. One randomised controlled trial in 69 patients showed less toxicity in the SIB arm after 1 year of follow-up, while heart and lung function were not impaired [25]. Results need to be interpreted with caution since in this trial other factors differed between the SIB and sequential boost arm. A more recent phase II randomised controlled trial evaluated whether the combination of a SIB with prone hypofractionated WBI would increase acute toxicity compared to the routinely used hypofractionation scheme of 40.05 Gy in15 fractions plus a sequential boost of 10 Gy in four fractions or 14.88 Gy in six fractions [26]. It was demonstrated that the rate of moist desquamation was not different between both treatment arms. In both arms, 7% of patients developed moist desquamation, nonetheless, the incidence of grade 2/3 dermatitis and pruritus was reduced by one-third in the SIB arm ($p = 0.037$ and $p = 0.015$, respectively).

An impact of used treatment planning technique also impacts toxicity as is demonstrated in Fig. 36.3. In the aforementioned systematic review, it was noted that only three of the five studies that employed IMRT (both forward-planned and inverse-planned-IMRT) or VMAT to deliver the boost dose concurrently reported incidences of grade 3 acute skin toxicity totalling three events representing 0.4% of the total cohort [16]. In contrast, concurrent boosts delivered

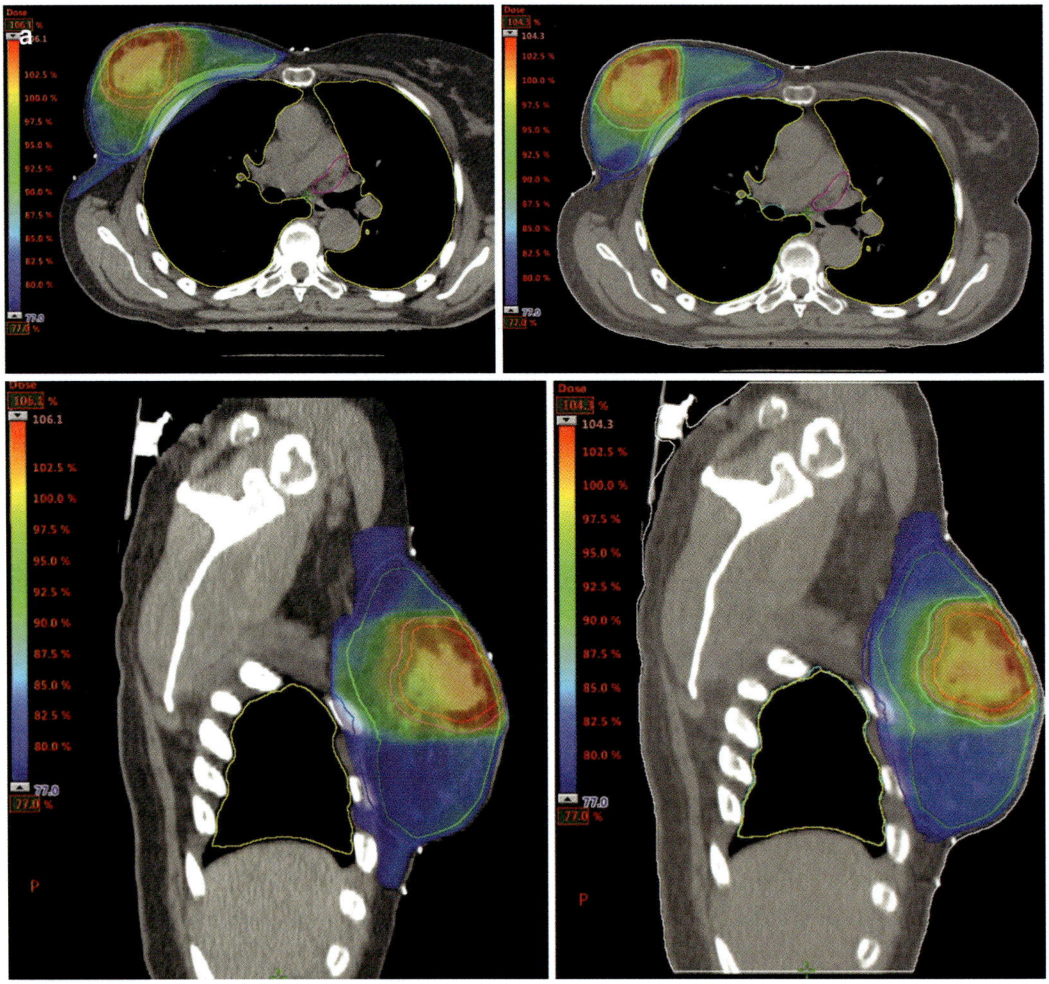

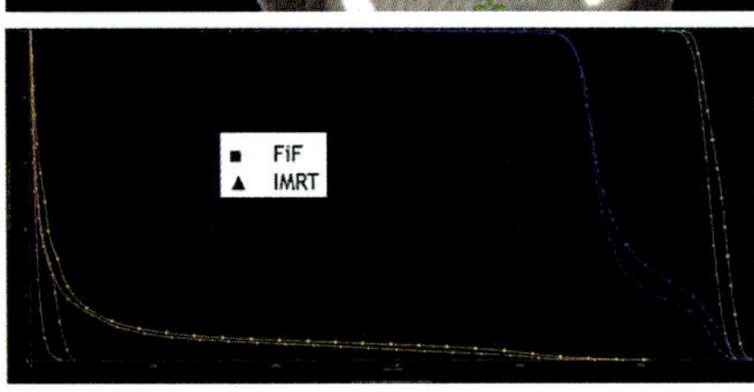

	Lungs		Heart			
	V20	MLD	V20	V10	V5	MHD
FiF	6,3	414	0	0	0	110
IMRT	5,3	331	0	0	0	53

Fig. 36.3 Comparisons between field-in-field and IMRT for SIB, as used in 2019 (ESTRO course, courtesy S. Hol, Tilburg, NL). *Note: only the planning at the central axis through the PTV boost is shown. FiF = left; IMRT = right. Dose prescription = 21*2.17 Gy on the whole breast and 21*2.66 Gy on boost.* (**a**) SIB right-sided breast cancer. (**b**) SIB left-sided breast cancer. Note: volumes dosimetry is expressed using percentage (%), mean heart and lung doses using cGy

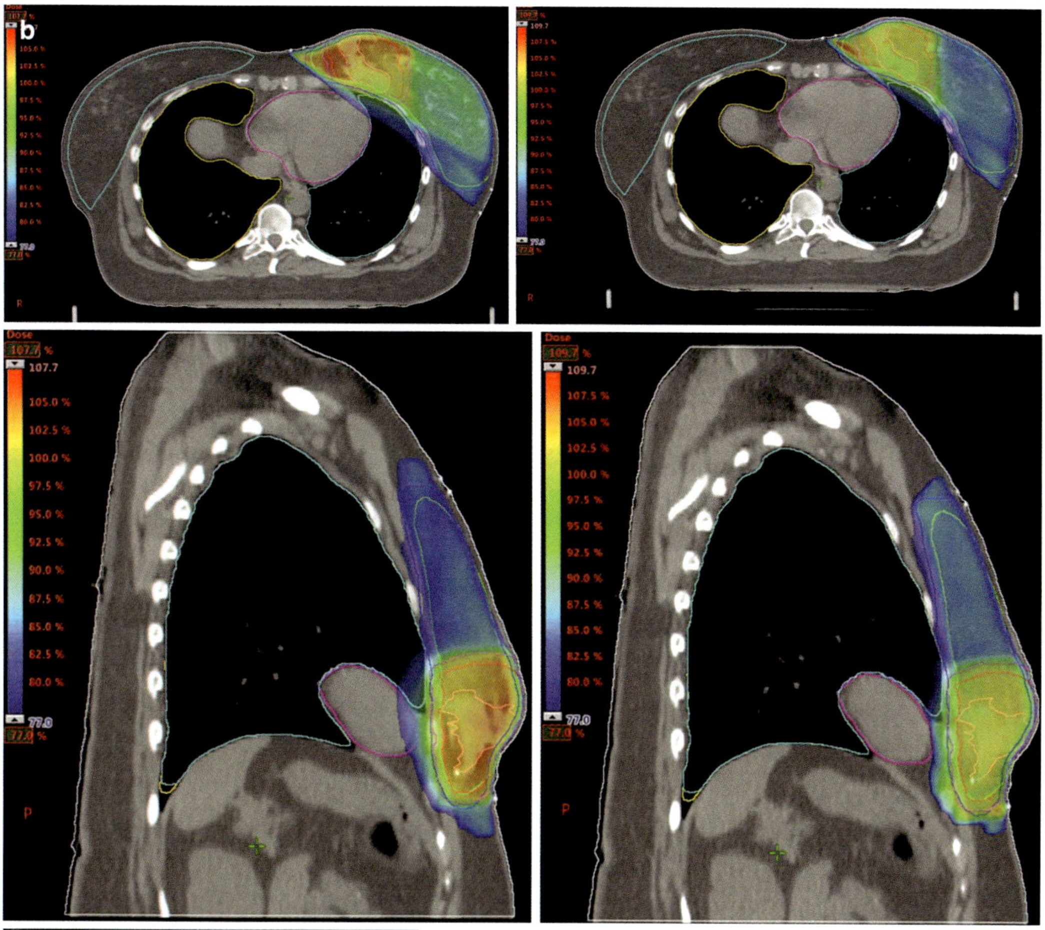

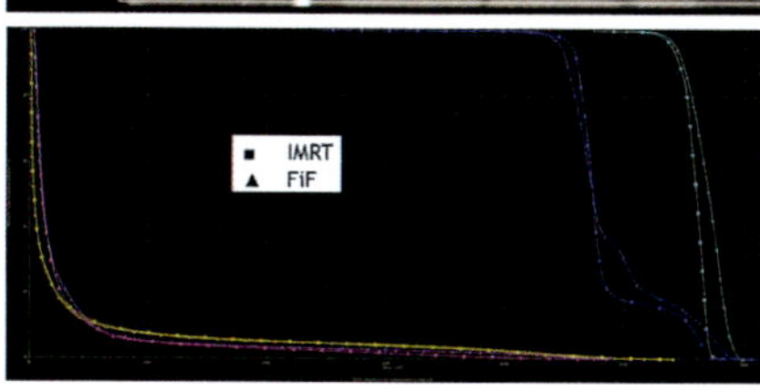

	Lungs		Heart			
	V20	MLD	V20	V10	V5	MHD
FiF	5,2	321	3,4	4,9	11,1	310
IMRT	5,2	321	2,9	4,9	10,3	278

Fig. 36.3 (continued)

using conventional 3DCRT techniques generally reported higher incidences of grade 3 toxicity. These results support previous studies proposing a correlation between IMRT and reduced incidence of acute radiation dermatitis [7, 27, 28].

In conclusion, randomised evidence on toxicity and cosmetic outcome is limited, but suggest that SIB gives at least comparable acute toxicity and, in some series, even less toxicity as compared to a sequential boost, independently of the WBI fractionation scheme. However, with current evolution towards ultra-hypofractionated WBI, these findings might need to be reassessed. Late toxicity profiles appear to be comparable to historical controls using a sequential boost.

36.3 Future Perspectives (and Unmet Needs)

Few prospective studies are currently investigating the role of boost integration during WBI employing hypofractionation and will help clarifying the clinical advantage of boost integration during WBI. The RTOG 1005 trial is a phase III prospective trial investigating accelerated WBI for early breast cancer, comparing standard RT (50 Gy/25 fractions) (with the hypofractionation option of 42.7 Gy in 16 fractions; 2.67 Gy daily) followed by a sequential boost of 12–14 Gy in 6–7 fractions vs a hypofractionated schedule of 40 Gy in 15 fractions (2.67 Gy daily) with a concomitant boost of 3.2 Gy to the tumour bed (up to 48 Gy in 15 fractions). This trial has been closed to accrual and results are eagerly awaited (RTOG 1005) [29]. The IMPORT High Trial testes dose escalated RT delivered with IMRT (both forward- and inverse-planned IMRT) in early breast cancer patients with higher than average risk of local recurrence, with the primary end-point of palpable induration inside boost volume of irradiated breast [30]. The standard arm comprises 40.5 Gy in 15 fractions and a sequential tumour bed boost of 16 Gy in 8 fractions for adjunctive 1.6 weeks (23 fractions for a total of 4.6 weeks). Two different experimental arms were chosen: in addition to 36 Gy in 15 fractions to the whole breast and 2.67 Gy × 15 fractions to the index quadrant, the first arm receives 3.2 Gy × 15 fractions (up to 48 Gy), while the second arm gets 3.53 Gy × 15 fractions (up to 53 Gy) to the tumour bed (Fig. 36.4). These schedules were calculated

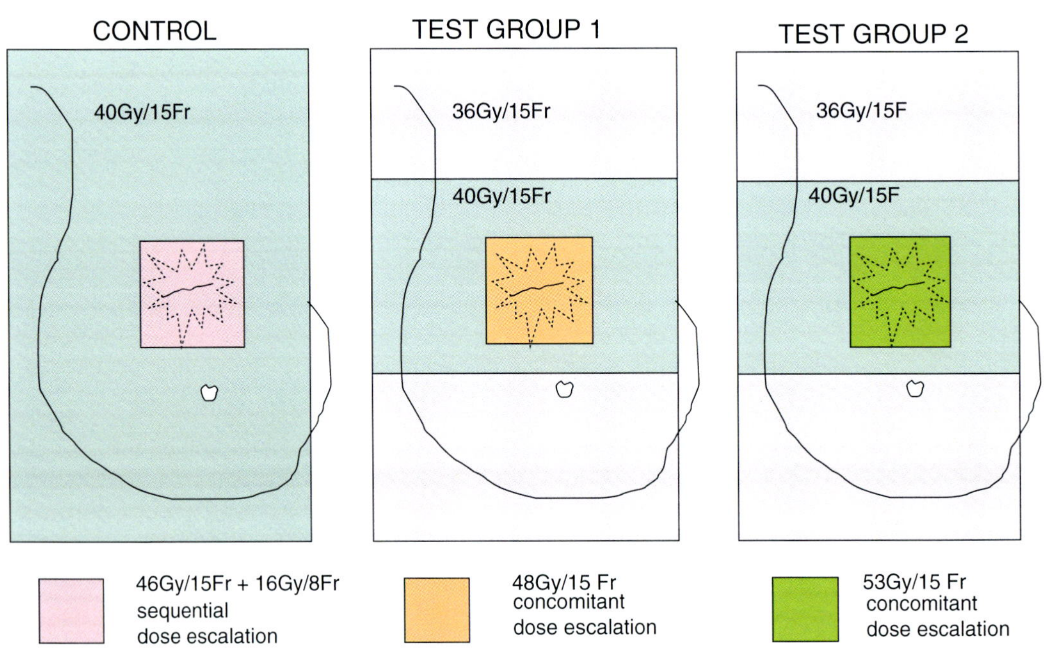

Fig. 36.4 Study design IMPORT HIGH trial (Full protocol available at https://www.isrctn.com/ISRCTN47437448; registered under NCT00818051)

(considering an α/β ratio = 3 Gy for tumour control) as isoeffective to 60 Gy and 69 Gy, respectively. The global sample size is 2568 patients.

Further, Skagen Trial 1 was initiated in 2015 to introduce hypofractionation and SIB as a Danish Breast Cancer Group standard for loco-regional treatment of early breast cancer. Eligible patients are women affected by pT1-3 pN0-N3 M0 breast cancer, treated with regional nodal RT after mastectomy or BCS. Patients are randomised to normofractionated (50 Gy/25 fractions) versus hypofractionated (40 Gy/15 fractions) RT on the whole breast/chest wall and regional nodes, and patients will receive SIB without any randomisation. The primary endpoint of the trial is the rate of lymph oedema on the treated side.

The aforementioned trials and others (Table 36.2) will provide evidence on boost integration during WBI after BCS for early breast cancer.

36.4 Summary

Tumour bed boost strategies in postoperative RT for breast cancer are considered an area of high investigational potential. A SIB approach provides a better conformality and a reduction in dose administered to the whole breast volume. Albeit evidence on toxicity and cosmetic outcome is limited, it suggests that SIB gives at least comparable acute toxicity and, in some series, even less toxicity as compared to a sequential boost. The success of SIB is however highly dependent on correct planning techniques and contoured target volumes, since no technique can correct for poor contouring. As there is currently no consensus on dose and fractionation, it is expected that results from ongoing randomised-controlled trials will further enhance the knowledge on this topic.

Table 36.2 Ongoing trials investigating the role of boost integration during WBI

				Dose and fractionation (experimental arm)		
Study	Country	Primary end-point	Target population (*n*)	*Whole breast*	*Index quadrant*	*Tumour bed*
RTOG 1005	USA	In-breast relapse	2300	40.05 Gy/15 fr (2.67 Gy daily)	/	48 Gy/15 fr (3.2 Gy daily)
IMPORT-HIGH	UK	Palpable induration	2568	36 Gy/15 fr (2.4 Gy daily)	40.05 Gy/15 fr (2.67 Gy daily)	I: 48 Gy/15 fr (3.2 Gy daily)
						II: 53 Gy/15 fr (3.53 Gy daily)
IMRT MC-2	Germany	Cosmesis	502	50.4 Gy/28 fr (1.8 Gy daily)	/	64.4 Gy/28 fr (2.3 Gy daily)
UZB trial	Belgium	Pulmonary-heart function	123	42 Gy/15 fr (2.8 Gy daily)	/	51/15 fr (3.4 Gy daily)
		Arm mobility and lymphoedema				
SKAGEN 1 trial	Denmark	Lymph oedema rate treated side	2000	40 Gy/15 fr (2.67 Gy daily)	/	I: 52.2 Gy/18 fr (2.9 Gy daily) II: 45.75 Gy/15 fr (3.05 Gy daily)

fr fractions

References

1. Fisher B, Anderson S, Bryant J, et al. Twenty-year follow-up of a randomized trial comparing total mastectomy, lumpectomy, and lumpectomy plus irradiation for the treatment of invasive breast cancer. N Engl J Med. 2002;347:1233–41.
2. Veronesi U, Cascinelli N, Mariani L, et al. Twenty-year follow-up of a randomized study comparing breast-conserving surgery with radical mastectomy for early breast cancer. N Engl J Med. 2002;347: 1227–32.
3. Bartelink H, Maingon P, Poortmans P, et al. Whole-breast irradiation with or without a boost for patients treated with breast-conserving surgery for early breast cancer: 20-year follow-up of a randomised phase 3 trial. Lancet Oncol. 2015;16:47–56.
4. Immink JM, Putter H, Bartelink H, et al. Long-term cosmetic changes after breast-conserving treatment of patients with stage I-II breast cancer and included in the EORTC "boost versus no boost" trial. Ann Oncol Off J Eur Soc Med Oncol. 2012;23:2591–8.
5. Borger JH, Kemperman H, Smitt HS, et al. Dose and volume effects on fibrosis after breast conservation therapy. Int J Radiat Oncol Biol Phys. 1994;30: 1073–81.
6. Mohan R, Wu Q, Manning M, Schmidt-Ullrich R. Radiobiological considerations in the design of fractionation strategies for intensity-modulated radiation therapy of head and neck cancers. Int J Radiat Oncol Biol Phys. 2000;46:619–30.
7. Teh AYM, Walsh L, Purdie TG, et al. Concomitant intensity modulated boost during whole breast hypofractionated radiotherapy--a feasibility and toxicity study. Radiother Oncol J Eur Soc Ther Radiol Oncol. 2012;102:89–95.
8. Osa E-OO, DeWyngaert K, Roses D, et al. Prone breast intensity modulated radiation therapy: 5-year results. Int J Radiat Oncol Biol Phys. 2014;89: 899–906.
9. Singla R, King S, Albuquerque K, Creech S, Dogan N. Simultaneous-integrated boost intensity-modulated radiation therapy (SIB-IMRT) in the treatment of early-stage left-sided breast carcinoma. Med Dosim Off J Am Assoc Med Dosim. 2006;31: 190–6.
10. Hurkmans CW, Meijer GJ, van Vliet-Vroegindeweij C, van der Sangen MJ, Cassee J. High-dose simultaneously integrated breast boost using intensity-modulated radiotherapy and inverse optimization. Int J Radiat Oncol Biol Phys. 2006;66:923–30.
11. van der Laan HP, Dolsma WV, Maduro JH, Korevaar EW, Hollander M, Langendijk JA. Three-dimensional conformal simultaneously integrated boost technique for breast-conserving radiotherapy. Int J Radiat Oncol Biol Phys. 2007;68:1018–23.
12. Brouwers PJAM, van Werkhoven E, Bartelink H, et al. Predictors for poor cosmetic outcome in patients with early stage breast cancer treated with breast conserving therapy: results of the young boost trial. Radiother Oncol J Eur Soc Ther Radiol Oncol. 2018;128: 434–41.
13. Hijal T, Fournier-Bidoz N, Castro-Pena P, et al. Simultaneous integrated boost in breast conserving treatment of breast cancer: a dosimetric comparison of helical tomotherapy and three-dimensional conformal radiotherapy. Radiother Oncol J Eur Soc Ther Radiol Oncol. 2010;94:300–6.
14. Franco P, Zeverino M, Migliaccio F, et al. Intensity-modulated adjuvant whole breast radiation delivered with static angle tomotherapy (TomoDirect): a prospective case series. J Cancer Res Clin Oncol. 2013;139:1927–36.
15. Franco P, Zeverino M, Migliaccio F, et al. Intensity-modulated and hypofractionated simultaneous integrated boost adjuvant breast radiation employing statics ports of tomotherapy (TomoDirect): a prospective phase II trial. J Cancer Res Clin Oncol. 2014;140:167–77.
16. Hamilton DG, Bale R, Jones C, et al. Impact of tumour bed boost integration on acute and late toxicity in patients with breast cancer: a systematic review. Breast. 2016;27:126–35.
17. Formenti SC, Gidea-Addeo D, Goldberg JD, et al. Phase I-II trial of prone accelerated intensity modulated radiation therapy to the breast to optimally spare normal tissue. J Clin Oncol Off J Am Soc Clin Oncol. 2007;25:2236–42.
18. Bantema-Joppe EJ, Schilstra C, De Bock GH, et al. Simultaneous integrated boost irradiation after breast-conserving surgery: physician-rated toxicity and cosmetic outcome at 30 months' follow-up. Int J Radiat Oncol Biol Phys. 2012;83:e471–7.
19. Raza S, Lymberis SC, Ciervide R, et al. Comparison of acute and late toxicity of two regimens of 3- and 5-week concomitant boost prone IMRT to standard 6-week breast radiotherapy. Front Oncol. 2012;2:44.
20. Alford SL, Prassas GN, Vogelesang CR, Leggett HJ, Hamilton CS. Adjuvant breast radiotherapy using a simultaneous integrated boost: clinical and dosimetric perspectives. J Med Imaging Radiat Oncol. 2013;57:222–9.
21. Cante D, Petrucci E, Sciacero P, et al. Ten-year results of accelerated hypofractionated adjuvant whole-breast radiation with concomitant boost to the lumpectomy cavity after conserving surgery for early breast cancer. Med Oncol. 2017;34:152.
22. Lansu JTP, Essers M, Voogd AC, et al. The influence of simultaneous integrated boost, hypofractionation and oncoplastic surgery on cosmetic outcome and PROMs after breast conserving therapy. Eur J Surg Oncol J Eur Soc Surg Oncol Br Assoc Surg Oncol. 2015;41:1411–6.
23. Krug D, Baumann R, Krockenberger K, et al. Adjuvant hypofractionated radiotherapy with simultaneous integrated boost after breast-conserving surgery: results of a prospective trial. Strahlenther Onkol. 2020;197:48–55.

24. Cooper BT, Formenti-Ujlaki GF, Li X, et al. Prospective randomized trial of prone accelerated intensity modulated breast radiation therapy with a daily versus weekly boost to the tumor bed. Int J Radiat Oncol Biol Phys. 2016;95:571–8.
25. Van Parijs H, Miedema G, Vinh-Hung V, et al. Short course radiotherapy with simultaneous integrated boost for stage I-II breast cancer, early toxicities of a randomized clinical trial. Radiat Oncol. 2012;7:80.
26. Paelinck L, Gulyban A, Lakosi F, et al. Does an integrated boost increase acute toxicity in prone hypofractionated breast irradiation? A randomized controlled trial. Radiother Oncol J Eur Soc Ther Radiol Oncol. 2017;122:30–6.
27. Pignol J-P, Olivotto I, Rakovitch E, et al. A multicenter randomized trial of breast intensity-modulated radiation therapy to reduce acute radiation dermatitis. J Clin Oncol Off J Am Soc Clin Oncol. 2008;26:v2085–92.
28. Freedman GM, Li T, Nicolaou N, Chen Y, Ma CC-M, Anderson PR. Breast intensity-modulated radiation therapy reduces time spent with acute dermatitis for women of all breast sizes during radiation. Int J Radiat Oncol Biol Phys. 2009;74:689–94.
29. RTOG 1005. A Phase III trial of accelerated whole breast irradiation with hypofractionation plus concurrent boost versus standard whole breast irradiation plus sequential boost for early-stage breast cancer.
30. Coles C, Yarnold J. The IMPORT trials are launched (September 2006). Clin Oncol (R Coll Radiol). 2006;18:587–90.

37 Partial Breast Irradiation

Indrani S. Bhattacharya and Charlotte E. Coles

37.1 Background

Data from >10,000 patients in randomised controlled trials (RCT) demonstrate whole-breast irradiation (WBI) following breast-conserving surgery (BCS) reduces local recurrence risk and breast cancer mortality [1]. However, radiation therapy (RT) is not without risk including normal tissue toxicities [2], cardiac effects, [3] and second cancers [4]. Improvements in breast cancer care have led to a substantial fall in local relapse rates over recent decades [5]. For example, in the UK, a breast radiotherapy trial conducted between 1986 and 1998 reported a 5-year local recurrence rate of 8.0% (95% CI 6.5–9.5%) [6]. In contrast, the START trials conducted between 1998 and 2002 had a 5-year local recurrence rate of 3.1% (95% CI 2.6–3.7%) [2]. Even lower levels of 5-year local recurrence have been reported in both the IMPORT LOW trial conducted between 2007 and 2010 [7] and FAST FORWARD trial conducted between 2011 and 2014 [8]. Although the relative benefit from breast RT remains the same, the absolute benefit is much smaller by virtue of the decreased local relapse rate. Furthermore, risks of RT remain the same regardless of the degree of benefit.

For some patients with a low-risk of local relapse, benefits of WBI may not outweigh the risks. Local relapse risk is highest in and around the tumour bed [9] meaning women with low-risk disease may not require WBI. In women with low-risk disease, the volume irradiated can be reduced to the area in and around the tumour bed, i.e. the partial breast, thereby reducing side-effects [10] and potentially treatment times [11].

However, partial breast irradiation (PBI) is not a new concept. PBI trials conducted in the 1980s showed local relapse rates in patients receiving PBI were significantly higher than those receiving WBI [12] which is likely related to older RT techniques as well as sub-optimal patient selection.

There has now been a resurgence in the interest in PBI with a range of trials being conducted internationally. Techniques employed to deliver PBI include intraoperative RT (IORT), brachytherapy, and external beam RT (EBRT). Accelerated PBI (APBI) is where the overall treatment time is shorter compared with 'standard' WBI. It should also be noted that 'standard' WBI was 5-weeks +/-boost for the vast majority of PBI trials. A major challenge in interpreting results of PBI studies is the vast heterogeneity between techniques in terms of the total dose, fractionation, overall treatment time, and

I. S. Bhattacharya (✉)
Addenbrooke's Hospital, Cambridge University Hospitals NHS Foundation Trust, Cambridge, UK
e-mail: indranisb@doctors.org.uk

C. E. Coles
Department of Oncology, University of Cambridge, Cambridge, UK
e-mail: colesc@doctors.org.uk

© The Author(s), under exclusive license to Springer Nature Switzerland AG 2022
O. Kaidar-Person et al. (eds.), *Breast Cancer Radiation Therapy*,
https://doi.org/10.1007/978-3-030-91170-6_37

irradiated volume. Furthermore, another challenge for PBI trials and trial design is the low event rate in early breast cancer.

Priorities include achieving at least as good and certainly no worse local control with reduced toxicity using an easily deliverable technique that is acceptable and convenient for patients.

37.2 Existing Literature

PBI may be delivered using a variety of techniques including IORT, brachytherapy, and EBRT. Technical details of IORT and brachytherapy are covered in detail elsewhere. In brief, IORT offers the potential for a rapid 'one-off' treatment without having to return for daily RT treatments, providing the histology is favourable. IORT has been delivered using electrons (IOeRT) and photons as per the ELIOT [13] and TARGIT [14, 15] trials, respectively. ELIOT randomised women to 50 Gy in 25 fractions over 5 weeks + boost versus IOeRT 21 Gy to tumour bed [13]. 5-year local relapse was 4.4% (95% CI 2.7–6.1) and 0.4% (95% CI 0.0–1.0) for the IOeRT and WBI groups, respectively [HR 9.3 (95% CI 3.3–26.3)] (Table 37.1). Although the local relapse rate in the IOeRT group was significantly greater than patients receiving WBI, the IOeRT local relapse was still within the pre-specified equivalence margin and there was no difference in overall survival. On review of the baseline characteristics, a considerable proportion had high-risk features (>25% were lymph node positive and 20% G3 tumours). This trial like many others began recruitment prior to the establishment of GEC-ESTRO/ASTRO guidelines [16, 17]. When the multivariable analysis was re-analysed according to GEC-ESTRO/ASTRO risk groups, local recurrence in the low-risk groups was similar highlighting the importance of patient selection. Although toxicity was not systematically recorded, a difference in skin toxicity favouring IOeRT was reported but IOeRT patients had increased fat necrosis [13].

TARGIT randomised women to IORT using 50 kV photons or WBI. The trial had two strata; pre-pathology given at time of BCS and post-pathology given after BCS where the wound was re-opened [14, 15] (Table 37.1). Local relapse rates in the control group were in fact much lower than originally anticipated at the time of trial development. Furthermore, 20% patients receiving IORT in the pre-pathology strata required additional WBI due to unfavourable histology results after definitive surgery [14]. There was also no systematic collection of toxicity data.

GEC-ESTRO randomly assigned women to APBI with interstitial brachytherapy; either high dose rate or pulsed dose rate versus WBI 50 Gy with a 10 Gy tumour bed boost [18]. At a median follow-up of 6.6 years, local recurrence was 1.44% (95% CI 0.51–2.38) with APBI and 0·92% (0.12–1.73) with WBI (difference 0.52%, 95% CI −0.72 to 1.75; $p = 0.42$). There was a comprehensive assessment of toxicity by patients and clinicians [19]. Overall toxicity was low in both groups but there was a statistically significant difference in favour of G2–3 skin toxicity for APBI at 5 years (10.7% [95% CI 8.0–13.4)] WBI vs 6.9% (4.8–9.0) APBI (difference -3.8%, 95% CI-7.2–0.4; $p = 0.020$) [20].

PBI trials delivered using EBRT include Florence [21], IMPORT LOW [7], RAPID, [22] and NSABP B-39/RTOG 0413 [23]. The smaller of these trials is Florence which randomised 520 women to APBI using IMRT 30 Gy in 5 fractions on alternate days versus conformal WBI 50 Gy in 25 fractions plus a boost [21]. At 10-years local recurrence rates were 3.7% and 2.5% [HR 1.56 (95% CI 0.55–4.37, $p = 0.40$)] in the APBI and WBI groups, respectively, with reduced toxicity in the APBI group. These results are reassuring in terms of safety of delivering PBI using EBRT although the small patient numbers should be interpreted with caution regarding efficacy of PBI.

IMPORT LOW randomised 2018 women to receive 40 Gy WBI (control), 36 Gy WBI, and 40 Gy to the partial breast (reduced-dose group), or 40 Gy to the partial breast only (partial breast group) in 15 daily treatment fractions using simple field in field (FiF) [7]. At a median follow-up of 72 months, local relapse rates were 1.1% (95% CI 0.5–2.3), 0.2% (0.02–1.2), and 0.5% (0.2–1.4) in the WBI, reduced-dose, and PBI groups,

Table 37.1 Summary of PBI trials

TRIAL	Patients recruited	Eligibility	Control group	Intervention group	Pre-specified margin	Local recurrence	Toxicity
ELIOT [13]	1305	48–75 years, ≤2.5 cm, G1–3 and N1–2	WBRT 50 Gy/25 F + boost	IORT 21 Gy to tumour bed-electrons	LRR of 7.5% for IORT (assumed LRR of 3% for WBRT)	5-years IORT 4.4%, WBRT 0.4% [HR 9.3 (3.3–26.3)]	Not systematically recorded. Statistically significant difference in skin toxicity favouring IORT but increase in fat necrosis in IORT
TARGIT [14, 15]	3451	≥45 years, IDC	WBRT 45-50 Gy/25 F +/ boost	18–20 Gy at applicator surface, attenuating to 5-7 cm at 1 cm	2.5% at 5 years	Pre-pathology strata 8.6 years IORT 167/1140 15% EBRT 147/1158 13% [HR 1.13 (0.91–1.41)] Post-pathology strata 9 years IORT 98/581,17% EBRT 72/572,13% [HR 0.75 (0.57–1.003)]	Not systematically recorded
FLORENCE [21]	520	>40 years, <25 mm, surgical margins ≥5 mm	WBRT 50 Gy/25 F + boost	IMRT 30 Gy in 5 F alternate days	2% non-inferiority margin assumed 3% LRR in control at 5 years, not to exceed 5% in APBI	10 years APBI 3.7%, WBRT 2.5% [1.56 (0.55–4.37)]	Systematic collection of toxicity data. Significantly less acute and late toxicity and improved cosmesis in APBI evaluated by clinicians and patients
IMPORT LOW [7]	2018	≥50 years, ≤3 cm, G1–3, pN0–1, surgical margins, ≥2 mm	WBRT 40.5 Gy/15 F	Reduced-dose group: IMRT 36 Gy to whole breast and 40.5 Gy to partial breast in 15 F, Partial breast group: IMRT 40.5 Gy/15 F to partial breast	2.5% at 5 years	5 years WBRT 1·1% (95% CI 0·5–2·3) Reduced-dose 0·2% (0·02–1·2) Partial breast 0·5% (0·2–1·4)	Systematic collection of toxicity data using patient-reported, clinician-reported outcomes and photographs. Reduced toxicity including less patient-reported breast firmness and appearance change in the reduced and partial-breast groups

(continued)

Table 37.1 (continued)

TRIAL	Patients recruited	Eligibility	Control group	Intervention group	Pre-specified margin	Local recurrence	Toxicity
RAPID [22]	2135	≥40 years, ≤3 cm, IDC/ DCIS, N0	WBRT 42.5 Gy/16 F or 50 Gy/25 F+/-boost	APBI 38.5 Gy/10 F twice daily-3DCRT/ IMRT	LRR of 2.75% for APBI (assumed LRR of 4% for WBRT at 5 years); adjusted sample on basis of expected 1.5% LRR at 5 years and 1.5% non-inferiority margin (HR < 2.02)	10 years APBI 3% WBRT 2.8% (1.27, 0.84–1.91)	Systematic collection of toxicity data using patient-reported, clinician-reported outcomes and photographs. Significantly worse toxicity and worse cosmetic outcome in ABPI
NSABP B-39/ RTOG 0413 [23]	4216	≥18 years, ≤3 cm, IDC/ DCIS, up to 3LN + ve	WBRT 50 Gy/25 F+/-boost	APBI 38.5/10 F twice daily-3DCRT/ IMRT APBI HDR brachytherapy: Multicatheter or single entry	50% increase of relative risk, HR < 1.5	10 years APBI 4.6% WBRT 3.9% (1.22, 0.94–1.58)	Similar between treatment groups but formal reports awaited
GEC-ESTRO [18]	1328	≥40 years, ≤3 cm, pN0, margins ≥2 mm, LVSI negative	WBRT 50 Gy/25 F+/-boost	APBI interstitial brachytherapy HDR: 8 × 4 Gy or 7 × 4.3 Gy PDR: 50 Gy	3% at 5 years	5 years 1.44% APBI 0.92% WBRT (0.52, (difference 0.52%, –0.72 to 1.75)	Systematic collection of toxicity data. Significantly less skin toxicity in APBI

respectively. IMPORT LOW provided a sole test of irradiated volume as the dose/fractionation in all groups was identical with regard to disease control and toxicity. Toxicity was significantly less in the reduced and PBI groups compared with the WBI group [7, 24] (Table 37.1).

Furthermore, it is now possible to deliver PBI in 1-week using the techniques in IMPORT LOW. The recently published FAST FORWARD [8] trial was designed in parallel with IMPORT LOW [7] with the same control group. FAST FORWARD (26 Gy in5 fractions) showed non-inferiority with 40 Gy in15 fractions for efficacy and similar toxicity, whilst IMPORT LOW showed non-inferiority with 40 Gy in15 fractions for efficacy and reduced toxicity. This has enabled the FAST FORWARD fractionation to be seamlessly adopted for PBI and has been approved by the UK community with >90% consensus [25]. It should be noted that an RCT of 1-week versus 3-weeks PBI would have required many thousands of patients given the very-low event rate with many years of follow-up. This would not be fundable or ethical hence both trials designed in parallel.

RAPID trial randomised women to WBI 42.5 Gy in 16 fractions or 50 Gy in25 fractions daily ±boost versus APBI 38.5 Gy in 10 fractions twice daily using 3DCRT/FIF [22]. At a median follow-up of 8·6 years, the cumulative incidence of local recurrence was 3.0% (95% CI 1.9–4.0) in the APBI group and 2.8% (1.8–3.9) in the WBI group (HR 1.27, 90% CI 0.84–1.91). This result was reported as meeting the pre-specified conditions of the trial for one-sided non-inferiority of the primary endpoint (to exclude HR >2.02 calculated from 5-year estimated recurrence rates).

In contrast, NSABP B-39/RTOG 0413 randomly assigned women to receive either APBI (via EBRT or brachytherapy) or WBI with an optional tumour bed boost [23]. APBI dosage regimens were 38.5 Gy with EBRT or 34 Gy for brachytherapy in 10 twice daily fractions over 1-week. At 10-years local recurrence was 4.6% (95% CI 3.7–5.7) for APBI and 3.9% (3.1–5.0) for whole-breast irradiation (HR 1.22, 90% CI 0.94–1.58), thus not meeting their pre-specified conditions for two-sided equivalence defined as a maximum 50% increase in relative risk (i.e. to exclude HR ≤0.677 or ≥1.50 irrespective of timepoint).

RAPID [22] and NSABP B-39/RTOG 0413 [23] raise an important point regarding non-inferiority and equivalence trials. Essentially non-inferiority trials aim to show that the intervention is no worse than standard treatment, whilst equivalence trials aim to show the intervention is no better and no worse than the standard treatment. Non-inferiority or equivalence boundaries must be specified beforehand. However, determining these boundaries is not always simple. The HRs reported show that both trials were similar in their estimates of relative effect of APBI compared with WBI. However, RAPID concluded that the non-inferiority conditions for local recurrence were met, whereas NSABP B-39/RTOG 0413 concludes that the equivalence conditions were not met. Clinically, the HRs and associated CI are similar between the two trials and any differences in interpretation are related to statistical design [26].

Regarding toxicity, NSABP B-39/RTOG 0413 reported similar toxicity between the treatment groups although detail was limited in the primary endpoint publication and a further toxicity publication is planned [23]. However, in RAPID cosmetic outcome was significantly worse in patients receiving ABPI [22]. This could be due to twice daily fractionation where the equivalent dose in 2 Gy per fraction (EQD2) is around 53 Gy; however, it may in fact be as high as 65 Gy if incomplete repair between fractions is considered [27]. Additional factors associated with adverse cosmesis in patients receiving APBI include tumour location, smoking, age, and seroma volume ($p < 0.05$) and smoking was associated with cosmetic deterioration ($p = 0.02$) [28]. We await further publications in order to understand the difference between these two trials.

From the studies described above, it is clear local relapse rates are low and PBI is suitable and safe for a subgroup of patients with low-risk breast cancer. Challenges regarding heterogeneity between techniques, total dose, fractionation, and irradiated volume still exist. More detail concerning how these individual techniques interact to cause normal tissue toxicities is required.

Regarding ongoing trials, The Danish Breast Cancer Group are conducting the Natural trial with low-risk patients being randomised to PBI (using EBRT 40 Gy/15 F) or no radiotherapy (including no endocrine treatment in some centres). Eligibility criteria include women with breast cancer ≥60 years having had breast-conserving surgery with pT1, pN0, ER ≥10%, HER2 neg, grade 1–2, non-lobular type, and margins ≥2 mm [29]. This is a non-inferiority trial recruiting 926 patients using a cut-off of an ipsilateral local recurrence rate of 4% in patients not having radiotherapy.

It should also be noted that as well as EBRT and other IORT techniques already described above, there are various other technologies available to deliver PBI, for example, the Mammosite Radiation Therapy System (RTS) [30] for which there are less data available but already in clinic use.

37.3 Patient Selection

Importance of patient selection for PBI is key as was highlighted in the ELIOT trial [13] where there was a significant increase in local relapse in high-risk patients. It is likely these patients were only included due to the lack of guidelines at the time of recruitment. PBI should be considered for those patients with low-risk disease especially outside the setting of a clinical trial. Overall the PBI guidelines are similar albeit with some differences [16, 17, 31–33] (Table 37.2). For example, in the ESTRO guidelines [16], eligible patients may have high grade or oestrogen receptor negative tumours in contrast to the UK guidelines [31, 32]. Furthermore, ESTRO guidance also has an intermediate-risk group who may receive PBI within a clinical study [16]. In contrast, the American Society for Radiation Oncology (ASTRO) defines three patient groups which include suitable, cautionary, and unsuitable [17]. Of note the ASTRO guidelines state that IORT using electrons should be restricted to patients in the 'suitable' category. In general, the guidelines described above reflect the majority of patients treated within the PBI trials but not necessarily meeting the criteria for the individual trials. The priority is to offer PBI to patients with low-risk disease. Patients with any high-risk features, e.g. Grade 3 tumours, triple negative subtype and those with a BRCA mutation should not be recommended PBI. The 2022 European Society for Radiotherapy and Oncology Advisory Committee in Radiation Oncology Practice (ESTRO-ACROP) consensus recommendations on patient selection and dose and fractionation for external beam radiotherapy in early breast cancer identified low risk-features suitable for PBI: luminal-like subtypes small tumour (≤3 cm), absence of lymph vascular space invasion, non-lobular invasive carcinoma, tumour grade 1–2, low-to-intermediate grade DCIS (sized ≤2.5 cm with clear surgical margins ≥3 mm), age at diagnosis 50 years or more, unicentric or unifocal lesion, clear surgical margins (>2 mm), node negative (including isolated tumour cells), and no use of primary systemic therapy and neoadjuvant chemotherapy [34].

It is likely these current guidelines will evolve further. Given the low local relapse rates there may be a group of patients where the risks of radiotherapy completely outweigh the benefits and RT can be safely avoided. The results of the omission of RT trials being conducted internationally are awaited [35–40].

37.4 Practical Suggestions When Implementing PBI Using EBRT

The following may be useful when considering PBI implementation *using EBRT*:

1. When selecting patients consider those with low-risk features including smaller, node-negative tumours with favourable histology and in older patients.

Table 37.2 Summary of PBI Guidelines

	ASTRO [17]	GEC-ESTRO [16]	NICE [31]	RCR consensus [32]	IOERT [33]
Age	≥50 years	>50 years	≥50 years	≥50 years	≥50 years
Tumour size	≤2 cm	≤3 cm	≤3 cm	≤3 cm	≤2 cm
Margins	≥2 mm	≥2 mm	Clear margins	≥1 mm	–
Grade	Any	Any	G1–2	G1–2	G1–2
LVSI	No	No	–	No	–
ER status	Positive	Any	Positive	Positive	Positive (luminal A)
Multifocality	Unifocal	Unifocal	–	–	Unifocal
Histology	IDC or other favourable sub-types	IDC, mucinous, tubular, medullary, and colloid	Invasive cancer, lobular excluded	Lobular excluded	Ductal and other favourable histologies
Pure DCIS	If screen detected, low-intermediate nuclear grade, ≤2.5 cm size, and resected with margins negative at ≥3 mm	Not allowed	Not allowed	Not allowed	–
N-stage	N0	N0	N0	N0	N0
Neo-adjuvant therapy	Not allowed	Not allowed	Not allowed	Not allowed	Not allowed

2. The technique used should be determined by local resource and expertise; for example, brachytherapy or IORT using electrons (for appropriate patients) may be preferable for some centres, whereas others will favour EBRT techniques.
3. When delivering EBRT, daily or alternate day treatments should be used as per the IMPORT LOW and FLORENCE trials, respectively, with 5 fractions being offered.
4. It is essential to minimise the heart dose in left-sided tumours; techniques such as deep inspiratory breath-hold (DIBH) can enable this, although may not be required if the tumour bed is in the upper half of the left breast.

37.5 Summary

RCT data demonstrates PBI using certain techniques can achieve at least as good and certainly no worse local recurrence rates as WBI with reduced toxicity and be delivered in shorter treatment times. Considerable heterogeneity exists between the techniques with a range of dose/fractionations being employed with differences in irradiated volume and treatment times. More detail regarding how these individual techniques interact to cause normal tissue toxicities is required. Selection of appropriate patients for PBI is key. Finally, patients must be fully informed regarding treatment options enabling them to actively participate in the shared decision-making process.

References

1. Darby S, McGale P, Correa C, et al. Effect of radiotherapy after breast-conserving surgery on 10-year recurrence and 15-year breast cancer death: meta-analysis of individual patient data for 10,801 women in 17 randomised trials. Lancet. 2011;378:1707–16.
2. Haviland JS, Owen JR, Dewar JA, et al. The UK Standardisation of Breast Radiotherapy (START) trials of radiotherapy hypofractionation for treatment of early breast cancer: 10-year follow-up results of two randomised controlled trials. Lancet Oncol. 2013;14:1086–94.
3. Darby SC, Ewertz M, McGale P, et al. Risk of ischemic heart disease in women after radiotherapy for breast cancer. N Engl J Med. 2013;368:987–98.
4. Grantzau T, Overgaard J. Risk of second non-breast cancer after radiotherapy for breast cancer: a system-

atic review and meta-analysis of 762,468 patients. Radiother Oncol. 2015;114:56–65.
5. Mannino M, Yarnold JR. Local relapse rates are falling after breast conserving surgery and systemic therapy for early breast cancer: can radiotherapy ever be safely withheld? Radiother Oncol. 2009;90:14–22.
6. Owen JR, Ashton A, Bliss JM, et al. Effect of radiotherapy fraction size on tumour control in patients with early-stage breast cancer after local tumour excision: long-term results of a randomised trial. Lancet Oncol. 2006;7:467–71.
7. Coles CE, Griffin CL, Kirby AM, et al. Partial-breast radiotherapy after breast conservation surgery for patients with early breast cancer (UK IMPORT LOW trial): 5-year results from a multicentre, randomised, controlled, phase 3, non-inferiority trial. Lancet. 2017;390:1048–60.
8. Murray Brunt A, Haviland JS, Wheatley DA, et al. Hypofractionated breast radiotherapy for 1 week versus 3 weeks (FAST-Forward): 5-year efficacy and late normal tissue effects results from a multicentre, non-inferiority, randomised, phase 3 trial. Lancet. 2020;395:1613–26.
9. Salvadori B, Marubini E, Miceli R, et al. Reoperation for locally recurrent breast cancer in patients previously treated with conservative surgery. BJS (Br J Surg). 1999;86:84–7.
10. Borger JH, Kemperman H, Smitt HS, et al. Dose and volume effects on fibrosis after breast conservation therapy. Int J Radiat Oncol Biol Phys. 1994;30:1073–81.
11. Rippy EE, Ainsworth R, Sathananthan D, et al. Influences on decision for mastectomy in patients eligible for breast conserving surgery. Breast. 2014;23:273–8.
12. Ribeiro GG, Magee B, Swindell R, et al. The Christie Hospital breast conservation trial: an update at 8 years from inception. Clin Oncol (R Coll Radiol). 1993;5:278–83.
13. Veronesi U, Orecchia R, Maisonneuve P, et al. Intraoperative radiotherapy versus external radiotherapy for early breast cancer (ELIOT): a randomised controlled equivalence trial. Lancet Oncol. 2013;14:1269–77.
14. Vaidya JS, Bulsara M, Baum M, et al. Long term survival and local control outcomes from single dose targeted intraoperative radiotherapy during lumpectomy (TARGIT-IORT) for early breast cancer: TARGIT-A randomised clinical trial. BMJ. 2020;370:m2836.
15. Vaidya JS, Bulsara M, Saunders C, et al. Effect of delayed targeted intraoperative radiotherapy vs whole-breast radiotherapy on local recurrence and survival: long-term results from the TARGIT-a randomized clinical trial in early breast cancer. JAMA Oncol. 2020;6:e200249.
16. Polgár C, Van Limbergen E, Pötter R, et al. Patient selection for accelerated partial-breast irradiation (APBI) after breast-conserving surgery: recommendations of the Groupe Européen de Curiethérapie-European Society for Therapeutic Radiology and Oncology (GEC-ESTRO) breast cancer working group based on clinical evidence (2009). Radiother Oncol. 2010;94:264–73.
17. Correa C, Harris EE, Leonardi MC, et al. Accelerated partial breast irradiation: executive summary for the update of an astro evidence-based consensus statement. Pract Radiat Oncol. 2017;7:73–9.
18. Strnad V, Ott OJ, Hildebrandt G, et al. 5-year results of accelerated partial breast irradiation using sole interstitial multicatheter brachytherapy versus whole-breast irradiation with boost after breast-conserving surgery for low-risk invasive and in-situ carcinoma of the female breast: a randomised, phase 3, non-inferiority trial. Lancet. 2016;387:229–38.
19. Schafer R, Strnad V, Polgar C, et al. Quality-of-life results for accelerated partial breast irradiation with interstitial brachytherapy versus whole-breast irradiation in early breast cancer after breast-conserving surgery (GEC-ESTRO): 5-year results of a randomised, phase 3 trial. Lancet Oncol. 2018;19(6):834–44.
20. Polgár C, Ott OJ, Hildebrandt G, et al. Groupe Européen de Curiethérapie of European Society for Radiotherapy and Oncology (GEC-ESTRO). Late side-effects and cosmetic results of accelerated partial breast irradiation with interstitial brachytherapy versus whole-breast irradiation after breast-conserving surgery for low-risk invasive and in-situ carcinoma of the female breast: 5-year results of a randomised, controlled, phase 3 trial. Lancet Oncol. 2017;18(2):259–68. https://doi.org/10.1016/S1470-2045173001l-6. Epub 2017 Jan 14. PMID: 28094198.
21. Meattini I, Marrazzo L, Saieva C, et al. Accelerated partial-breast irradiation compared with whole-breast irradiation for early breast cancer: long-term results of the randomized phase III APBI-IMRT-Florence trial. J Clin Oncol. 2020;38(35):4175–83.
22. Whelan TJ, Julian JA, Berrang TS, et al. External beam accelerated partial breast irradiation versus whole breast irradiation after breast conserving surgery in women with ductal carcinoma in situ and node-negative breast cancer (RAPID): a randomised controlled trial. Lancet. 2019;394:2165–72.
23. Vicini FA, Cecchini RS, White JR, et al. Long-term primary results of accelerated partial breast irradiation after breast-conserving surgery for early-stage breast cancer: a randomised, phase 3, equivalence trial. Lancet. 2019;394:2155–64.
24. Bhattacharya IS, Haviland JS, Kirby AM, et al. Patient-reported outcomes over 5 years after whole- or partial-breast radiotherapy: longitudinal analysis of the IMPORT LOW (CRUK/06/003) phase III randomized controlled trial. J Clin Oncol. 2018;37(4):305–17.
25. RCR https://www.rcr.ac.uk/publication/postoperative-radiotherapy-breast-cancer-hypofractionation-rcr-consensus-statements
26. Coles CE. Another piece in the jigsaw of accelerated partial breast irradiation. Lancet Oncol. 2017;18:168–9.
27. Yarnold J, Bentzen SM, Coles C, et al. Hypofractionated whole-breast radiotherapy for women with early breast cancer: myths and realities. Int J Radiat Oncol Biol Phys. 2011;79:1–9.

28. Peterson D, Truong PT, Parpia S, et al. Predictors of adverse cosmetic outcome in the RAPID trial: an exploratory analysis. Int J Radiat Oncol Biol Phys. 2015;91:968–76.
29. Natural Trial. https://clinicaltrials.gov/ct2/show/NCT03646955. Accessed 9 Mar 2021.
30. Zauls AJ, Watkins JM, Wahlquist AE, et al. Outcomes in women treated with MammoSite brachytherapy or whole breast irradiation stratified by ASTRO Accelerated Partial Breast Irradiation Consensus Statement Groups. Int J Radiat Oncol Biol Phys. 2012;82:21–9.
31. PBI. https://www.nice.org.uk/guidance/ng101/evidence/h-breast-radiotherapy-pdf-4904666613.
32. RCR. https://www.rcr.ac.uk/clinical-oncology/service-delivery/postoperative-radiotherapy-breast-cancer-uk-consensus-statements#Consensus%20statements.
33. Fastner G, Gaisberger C, Kaiser J, et al. ESTRO IORT Task Force/ACROP recommendations for intraoperative radiation therapy with electrons (IOERT) in breast cancer. Radiother Oncol. 2020;149:150–7.
34. Icro, Meattini Carlotta, Becherini Liesbeth, Boersma Orit, Kaidar-Person Gustavo Nader, Marta Angel, Montero Birgitte Vrou, Offersen Marianne C, Aznar Claus, Belka Adrian Murray, Brunt Samantha, Dicuonzo Pierfrancesco, Franco Mechthild, Krause Mairead, MacKenzie Tanja, Marinko Livia, Marrazzo Ivica, Ratosa Astrid, Scholten Elżbieta, Senkus Hilary, Stobart Philip, Poortmans Charlotte E, Coles. European Society for Radiotherapy and Oncology Advisory Committee in Radiation Oncology Practice consensus recommendations on patient selection and dose and fractionation for external beam radiotherapy in early breast cancer. The Lancet Oncology. 2022;23(1):e21–e31. https://doi.org/10.1016/S1470-2045(21)00539-8.
35. Meattini I, Poortmans PMP, Marrazzo L, Desideri I, Brain E, Hamaker M, et al. Exclusive endocrine therapy or partial breast irradiation for women aged ≥70 years with luminal A-like early stage breast cancer (NCT04134598 – EUROPA): Proof of concept of a randomized controlled trial comparing health related quality of life by patient reported outcome measures. J Geriatr Oncol. 2021;12(2):182–189. https://doi.org/10.1016/j.jgo.2020.07.013.
36. Kirwan CC, Coles CE, Bliss J. It's PRIMETIME. Postoperative avoidance of radiotherapy: biomarker selection of women at very low risk of local recurrence. Clin Oncol (R Coll Radiol). 2016;28:594–6.
37. LUMINA. https://clinicaltrials.gov/ct2/show/NCT01791829?term=LUMINA+breast+cancer&rank=1. Accessed 1 Aug 2018.
38. EXPERT. https://clinicaltrials.gov/ct2/show/NCT02889874?term=EXPERT+breast+cancer&rank=1. Accessed 6 Aug 2019.
39. IDEA. https://clinicaltrials.gov/ct2/show/NCT02400190?term=IDEA+breast+cancer&rank=1. Accessed 6 Aug 2019.
40. PRECISION. https://clinicaltrials.gov/ct2/show/NCT02653755?term=PRECISION+breast+cancer&rank=1. Accessed 1 Aug 2018.

Techniques to Reduce Dose to Organs at Risk

38

Marianne Camille Aznar and Livia Marrazzo

38.1 Introduction

As survival rates improve, increasing attention is paid to treatment toxicity, varying between potentially fatal side effects (e.g. second primary cancers, radiation-associated heart disease) and negative impacts on quality of life (e.g. pain, fatigue). Dose–effect relationships (DER) derived from large epidemiological studies have been established and suggest a linear relationship between dose and major coronary events [1] as well as second primary cancers [2]. However, it is unclear to which extent DERs established for average dose to a whole organ and 3DCRT tangential treatments can help us optimise dose deposition in modern, often inverse-modulated treatments. Though this is an active ongoing field of research, the evidence available to date suggests that reducing the dose to OARs should have a clinically relevant impact on toxicity reduction.

Efforts have predominantly focussed on the dose to the heart and lungs [3, 4]. In a systematic review of the literature published between 2003 and 2013, Taylor et al. [3] report that an MHD of around 4 Gy for left-sided breast/chest wall irradiation, is increasing to 8 Gy when the IMNs are included. Doses to the ipsilateral lung published between 2010 and 2015 suggest an MLD ranging from 8 Gy for the breast/chest wall alone, to 14 Gy when nodal regions where included in the target volume [4]. However, it should be noted that both systematic reviews report large variations between studies, and that other large studies suggest lower doses may be delivered in clinical practice [5] or in recent years [6] thanks to the increased awareness and improved tools to lower doses to OARs.

In this section, we review some of the approaches developed to decrease the dose delivered to OARs in breast cancer irradiation. Some of these techniques are widely implemented, others have been only investigated in selected centres or in academic settings, and their large-scale implementation remains to be investigated.

38.2 Improved Delineation

Target volume delineation is a crucial step in radiation treatment planning and is widely recognised to be particularly sensitive to uncertainties [7]. Consensus guidelines are available to reduce this uncertainty [8, 9], but still require a certain degree of experience and interpretation. Feng et al. [10] produced an atlas for contouring the heart and coronary arteries, and Duane et al. [11]

M. C. Aznar (✉)
Manchester Cancer Research Center, University of Manchester, Manchester, UK
e-mail: marianne.aznar@manchester.ac.uk

L. Marrazzo (✉)
Medical Physics Unit, Careggi University Hospital, Florence, Italy
e-mail: livia.marrazzo@unifi.it

© The Author(s), under exclusive license to Springer Nature Switzerland AG 2022
O. Kaidar-Person et al. (eds.), *Breast Cancer Radiation Therapy*,
https://doi.org/10.1007/978-3-030-91170-6_38

have suggested an atlas of cardiac segments for use in retrospective studies of radiation-associated cardiac toxicity. However, in clinical practice, such extensive contouring is too time-consuming, and hinders a full optimisation of treatment delivery taking into account the dose to cardiac substructures.

Automatic contouring has been suggested as a solution not only to save time and improve the clinical workflow but also as a tool to increase consistency, and thereby possibly reduce delineation uncertainties. Several commercial solutions are available, often based on either a) "template" patients followed by deformable image registration and contour propagation or b) artificial intelligent approaches, such as deep learning (DL). There is a clear trend of improvement (i.e. automatic solutions becoming closer and closer to the quality of manual contouring) in the published literature [12]. Though small structures in low-contrast regions (e.g. coronary arteries) are still challenging for both algorithms [13] and human observers [14] alike, this is an area of continuous development. For example, Morris et al. [15] have suggested that training a neural network on both CT and MRI significantly improved performance for the segmentation of coronary arteries.

As algorithms improve, the potential of dose reduction to cardiac substructures could be considerable. In Hodgkin lymphoma patients, Levis et al. [16] have shown that the dose to coronary arteries and the left ventricle can be reduced considerably by including constraints in the optimisation, without a significant increase in dose to other OARs.

However, without the knowledge and experience of the treating team (RTT, radiation oncologist, etc.) of proper delineation, one cannot reliably supervise and correct the automatic delineation. Therefore, it is recommended that teams will have proper teaching for target volume and OARs delineation, which can be done in various settings including by national and international courses (such as ASTRO and ESTRO courses) and ESTRO's FALCON online fellowship.

38.3 Breathing Adaptation

The use of moderate DIBH is arguably the most common approach to reduce the dose to the heart in breast cancer but is also used in other patient groups (e.g. Hodgkin lymphoma, lung cancer). The recent survey on "Patterns Of Practice in Adaptive and Real-Time Radiotherapy" ("POP-ART RT") [17] revealed that out of 200 responding centres, over 50% offered some form of breathing adaptation (breath-hold or gating in deep inspiration) to their breast cancer patients. However, the percentage of breast cancer benefitting from this approach varied widely between institutions.

By inflating the lungs and increasing the distance between the heart and the chest wall, deep inspiration offers a more favourable irradiation geometry (see Fig. 38.1).

Compliance is generally very high (>90%) and the dosimetric impact can be considerable, especially for patients where the IMNs are irradiated [3]. However, breathing adaptation often requires an investment in time (to coach patients prior to treatment simulation) and training (communication between the patient and the treatment personnel is crucial to ensure a good compliance and reproducibility) (see Chap. 18). Following the popularity of DIBH, many reports are available reviewing the dosimetric benefits [18, 19] and the comparative advantages of different technical approaches (see Figs. 38.2 and 38.3) [20, 21].

It is worth highlighting that DIBH does not necessarily require a technical investment, and that equipment-free solutions have been proposed [22]. Though this approach is breast-specific and does not have the advantage of translation to other patient groups (as commercial solutions do), it offers to possibility to rapidly "scale up" and offer DIBH to a large number of patients [23].

There has been a recent interest in techniques which could assist patients in achieving a deep inspiration or holding it for longer. For example, CPAP, often used in individuals suffering from sleep apnoea, has been successfully used in

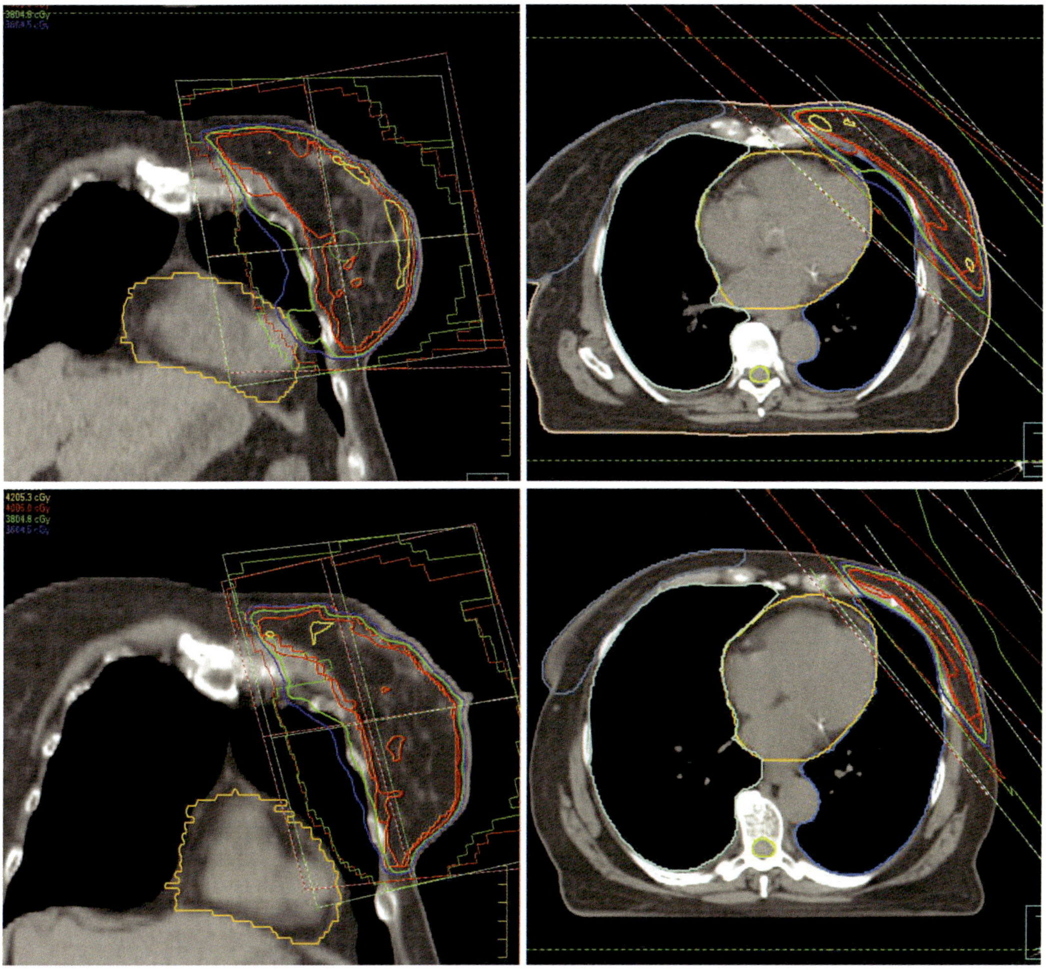

Fig. 38.1 Anatomical changes and heart sparing in Deep Inspiration Breath Hold (DIBH).Top row: free breathing scan in coronal (left) and transaxial (right) views. A portion of the heart (outlined orange) is included in the tangential fields (red and green beam lines). Bottom row: DIBH and the inflation of the lungs push the heart in the inferior, medial and posterior direction (clearly visible in the coronal view- left). The distance from the chest wall is increased (right: transaxial view at the same heart level as in the top row)

breast cancer RT (see Fig. 38.4) [24]. More technologically intensive approaches such as mechanical ventilation, with or without oxygen, have led to long breath holds of up to >5 min in healthy volunteers [25]. Though more research is needed regarding the potential clinical benefit of prolonged breath hold, and its safety in cancer patients, it could potentially be beneficial in longer treatments, such as proton beam radiation therapy.

38.4 Planning Considerations

As mentioned in Chap. 26, different treatment planning techniques will be appropriate for different target volumes. Before considering the technical approaches used to reduce the dose to the heart and lungs, it is worth noting that two non-technical factors will arguably have the largest influence. The first one is the extent and thereby size and geometry of target volumes:

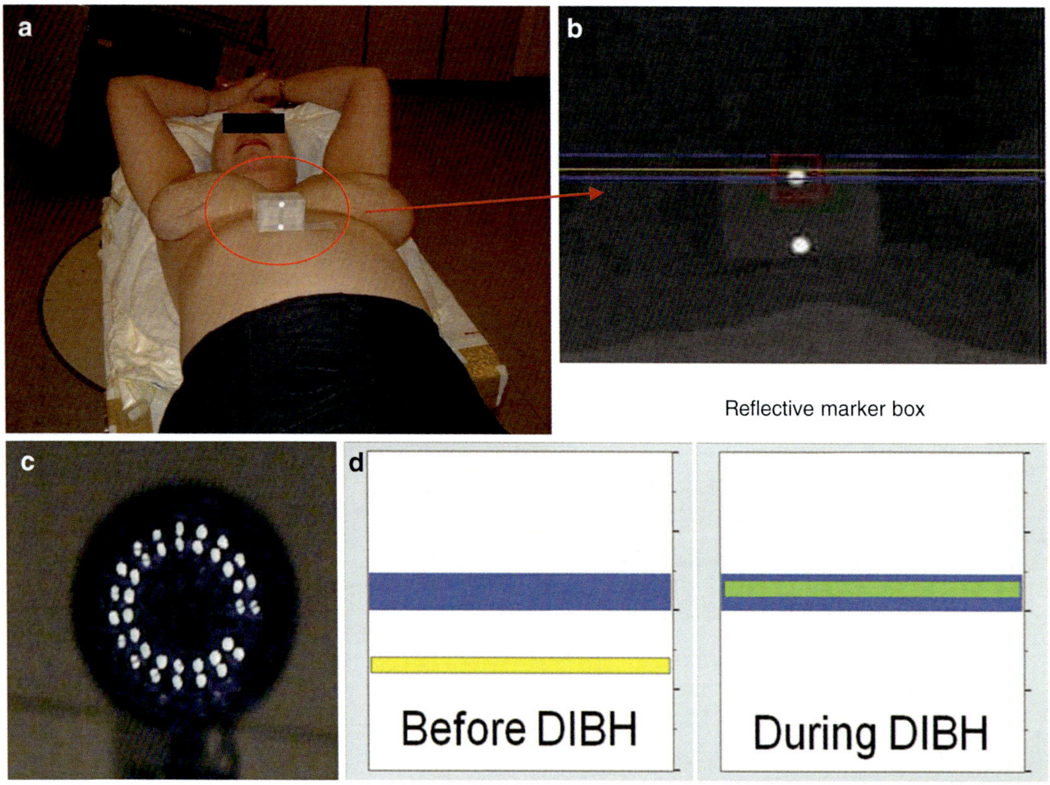

Fig. 38.2 Example of DIBH guidance equipment: here, the RPM ™ from Varian Medical Systems (Palo Alto, USA). With the patient in treatment position (**a**), a small marker box is placed on the sternum or the abdomen. The reflective markers on box (**b**) are tracked by an infrared camera (**d**). In (**d**) the visual guidance given to the patient is shown

breast alone vs nodal region, whole breast vs partial breast. The second one is the prescription dose: the shift from 50 Gy in 25 fractions to mild hypofractionation regimens (e.g. 40 Gy in 15 fractions) probably explains the trend in decreased physical dose to the heart in recent years [3, 6]. This trend will be even more pronounced with the adoption of the FAST FORWARD regimen [26]. However, it is important to note that, though the physical dose is reduced, the relative biological effect of those newer regimens on the heart remain unknown. While the transition from 50 Gy in 25 fractions to 40 Gy in 15 fractions is likely to even reduce the radiobiological equivalent dose to the heart and lungs [27], the same needs to be confirmed for the 26 Gy in 5 fractions schedule.

In the systematic reviews cited previously [3, 4], several technical factors systematically reduced the dose to the heart and lungs: irradiation with protons, use of DIBH, prone or lateral positioning (see Fig. 38.5). Proton therapy is discussed in a dedicated section within this book, but its limited availability, complexity and price means it will be necessary to collect strong evidence about its clinical benefits in breast cancer patients. Prone positioning is used in few institutions and requires dedicated equipment to keep the patient in a stable position (see Chap. 17). Though it can be combined with regional node irradiation [28], the data is relatively sparse. Lateral positioning faces the same issues and is used even more rarely [29]. The data on the positive impact of DIBH is particularly clear, as highlighted by the breast cancer expert panel of the DEGRO [30]. However, the role of VMAT/IMRT was less clear [31]. Though studies diverge, there seems to be a consensus that IMRT/VMAT can

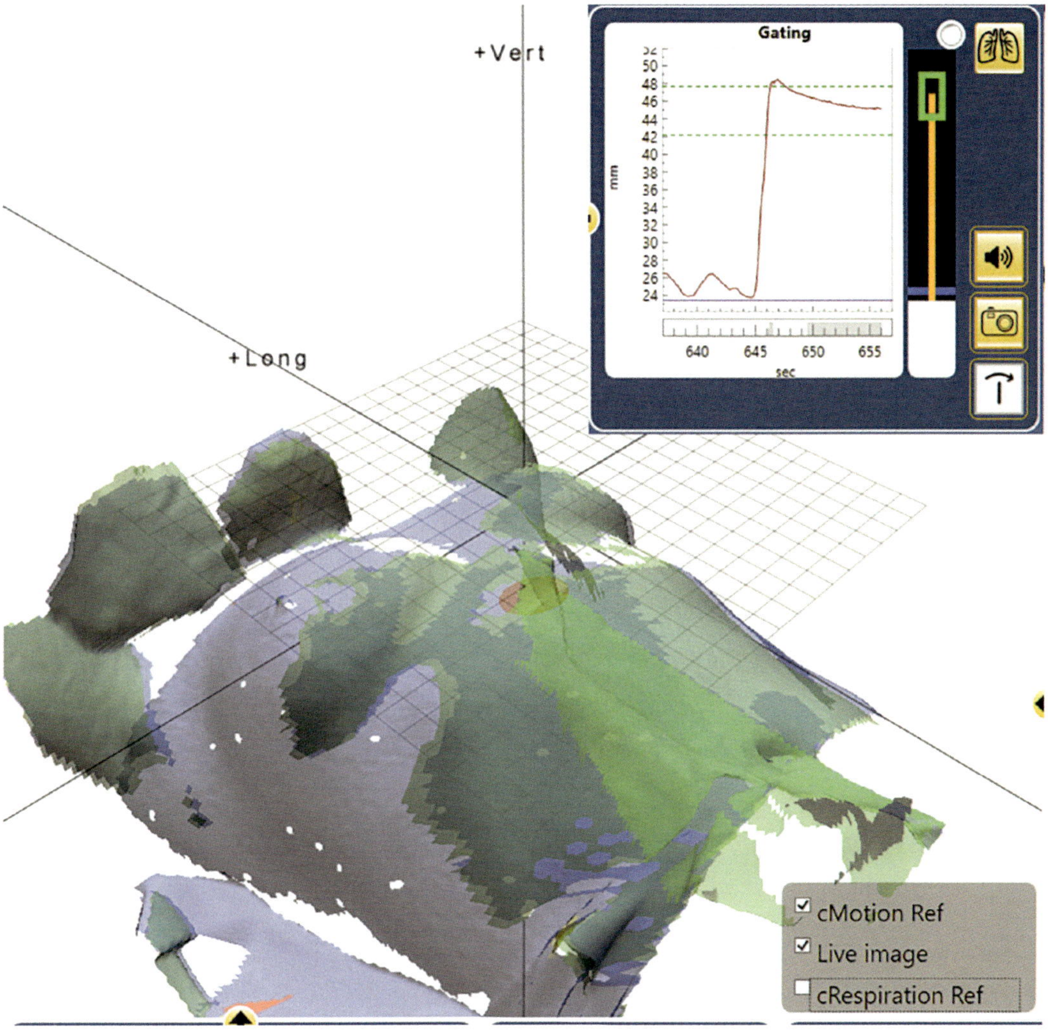

Fig. 38.3 Example of DIBH guidance equipment: here, the Catalyst system (C-RAD, Uppsala, Sweden). The surface of the patient is tracked and followed by the radiation therapist (RTT) on a monitoring screen. The respiratory signal is measured as the motion of a "primary point" (in red in the image). The beam is automatically switched on when the patient is in the correct "gating window" (see insert top right)

further reduce high OAR dose (e.g. in case of MHD >3 Gy) but will have no effect or even increase moderate to low OAR doses [32]. Though synchronous bilateral breast cancer is rare, many studies have reported the advantages of IMRT/VMAT in this challenging situation, both in terms of target volume coverage and homogeneity as well as OAR dose [33–35].

At the opposite end of the spectrum, VMAT could also have a role in case of smaller target volumes, where conformality is especially important, for example, APBI [36]. Hybrid techniques, that is, the combination of open tangential fields with modulated fields, are also increasingly used: their advantage is to enhance the robustness of VMAT/IMRT, while still providing some modulation and targeted avoidance of OARs.

As a general role in RT planning, the OARs that need to be delineated are the ones that are in the range/path of the radiation beams. With the use of VMAT these may need to be adapted compared to tangential beam arrangements as this

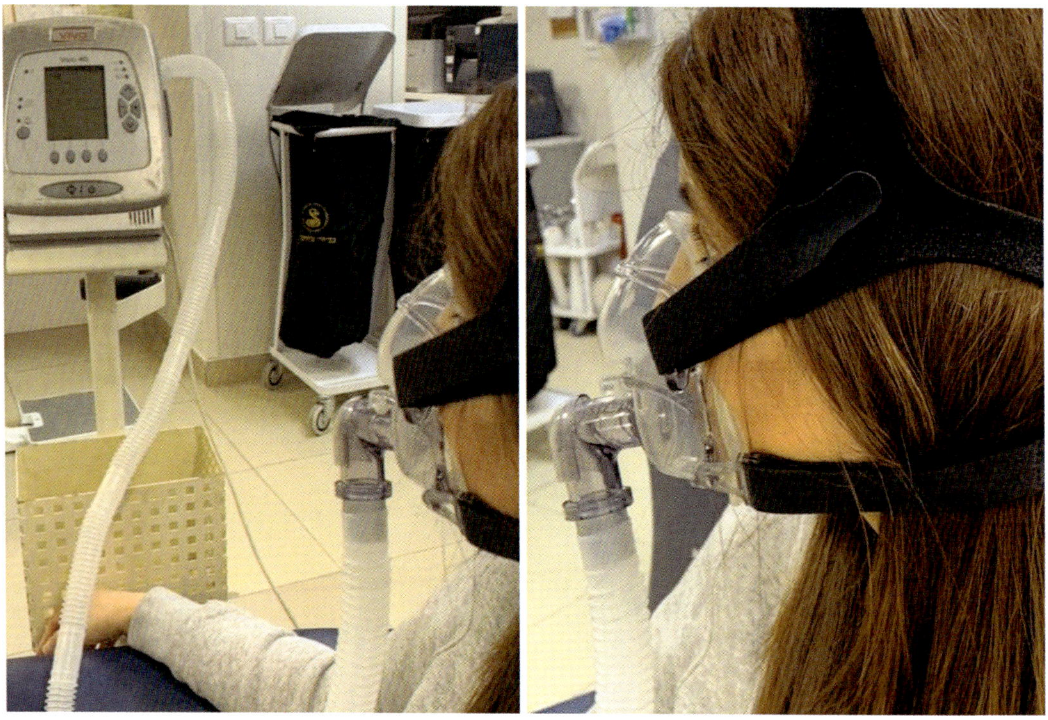

Fig. 38.4 Example of DIBH guidance equipment: here, the Continous Positive Airway Pressure (C-PAP) equipment used at the Sheba Medical centre. C-PAP machines (left) are widely used to treat sleep apnea, and are available from many manufacturers. The patient is fitted with a mask (right) and air pressure encourages the inflation of the lungs during treatment

can result in different dose distribution to OARs (e.g. dose to contralateral breast, low doses to the liver).

38.5 Alternative Delivery Systems

As mentioned in Chap. 26, changes in the shape or volume of the target volume may require adaptive re-planning. MR-guided RT delivery systems (i.e. "MR-linacs" or MR-Cobalt systems, see Fig. 38.6) have been designed to facilitate frequent online re-planning (while the patient lies on the treatment couch), and some versions allow gating (e.g. in deep inspiration). In addition, the superior soft tissue of MR imaging may enable better visualisation of some structures (e.g. breast glandular tissue; lumpectomy cavity) [37] inter- and intra-fractions. Those monitoring abilities might even enable the delivery of one-fraction treatments, for example, for APBI [38]. In theory, the possibility of daily adaptation could enable the use of tighter CTV-PTV margins [37] and thereby reduce the dose to OARs.

38.6 Gaps in Knowledge, Future Research

Though reports of dose reduction have generally concentrated on the heart and lungs, other OARs such as the oesophagus, thyroid or liver may be increasingly relevant when large volumes are irradiated with inverse-modulated approaches. Retrospective evaluations of volumetric IMRT for breast cancer patients suggest an larger low dose bath and an increased risk of nausea [39] or dysphagia [40]. Though retrospective toxicity studies are notoriously difficult to interpret, often are based on erroneous (excessively large) target

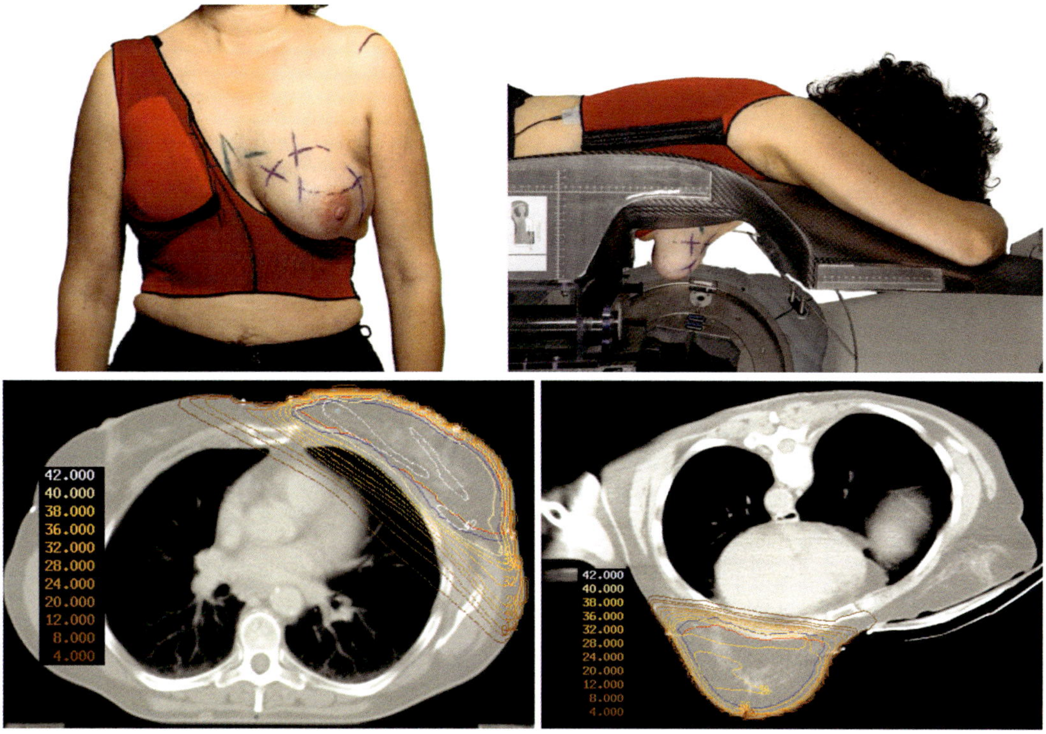

Fig. 38.5 Prone treatment using the "crawl position" at Ghent University Hospital. Top row: patient set up. Bottom row: isodose for left-breast irradiation in supine (left) and prone position (right). Images courtesy of Vincent Vakaet and Bruno Speleers, Ghent University, Dept. of Human Structure and Repair, Ghent, Belgium

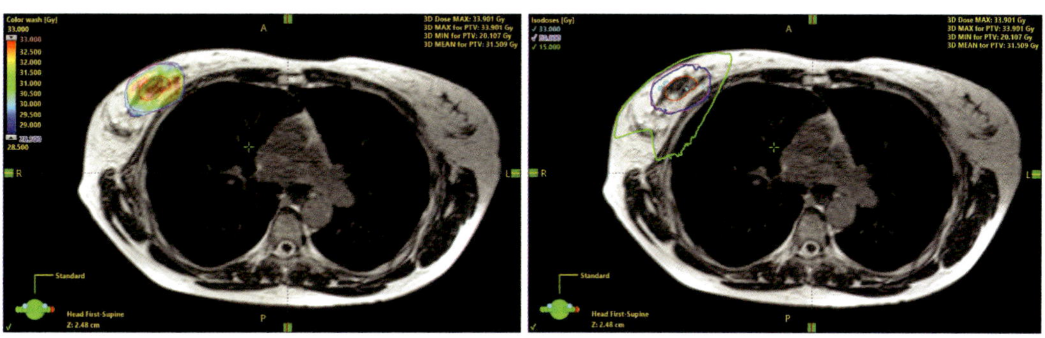

Fig. 38.6 Partial Breast Irradiation on the ViewRay Mridian™. Images courtesy of Dr. Jennifer Dolan, Henry Ford Health Systems (Michigan, USA)

volumes, especially for the chest wall, and some sub-optimal results might result from a "learning curve" in the sue of newer technologies, these concerns should not be dismissed. It is well acknowledged that "moderate" toxicities are under-reported, though they could have at least a temporary significant effect on the quality of life of patients.

38.7 Summary

As we move towards more individualised treatments, and the possibility of irradiating larger volumes in some patients, it becomes increasingly important to develop dose response relationship figures related to the dose to OARs beside heart and lungs, such as the thyroid, the oesophagus, or even the liver when necessary. While we await these data, awareness of the dose deposition outside of commonly delineated OARs is warranted.

References

1. Darby S, Blom-goldman U, Brønnum D, Correa C, Cutter D, Gagliardi G, et al. Risk of is che mic heart disease in women after radiotherapy for breast cancer. New. 2013;368:987–98. https://doi.org/10.1056/NEJMoa1209825.
2. Morton LM, Gilbert ES, Hall P, Andersson M, Joensuu H, Vaalavirta L, et al. Risk of treatment-related esophageal cancer among breast cancer survivors. Ann Oncol. 2012;23:3081–91. https://doi.org/10.1093/annonc/mds144.
3. Taylor CW, Zhe W, Macaulay E, Jagsi R, Duane F, Darby SC. Exposure of the heart in breast cancer radiation therapy: a systematic review of heart doses published during 2003 to 2013. Int J Radiat Oncol Biol Phys. 2015;93:845–53. https://doi.org/10.1016/j.ijrobp.2015.07.2292.
4. Aznar MC, Duane FK, Darby SC, Wang Z, Taylor CW. Exposure of the lungs in breast cancer radiotherapy: a systematic review of lung doses published 2010-2015. Radiother Oncol. 2017;126(1):148–54. https://doi.org/10.1016/j.radonc.2017.11.022.
5. Pierce LJ, Feng M, Griffith KA, Jagsi R, Boike T, Dryden D, et al. Recent time trends and predictors of heart dose from breast radiation therapy in a large quality consortium of radiation oncology practices. Int J Radiat Oncol Biol Phys. 2017;99:1154–61. https://doi.org/10.1016/j.ijrobp.2017.07.022.
6. Drost L, Yee C, Lam H, Zhang L, Wronski M, Mccann C, et al. Review a systematic review of heart dose in breast radiotherapy. Clin Breast Cancer. 2018;18:e819–24. https://doi.org/10.1016/j.clbc.2018.05.010.
7. Vinod SK, Jameson MG, Min M, Holloway LC. Uncertainties in volume delineation in radiation oncology: a systematic review and recommendations for future studies. Radiother Oncol. 2016;121:169–79. https://doi.org/10.1016/j.radonc.2016.09.009.
8. Offersen BV, Boersma LJ, Kirkove C, Hol S, Aznar MC, Biete Sola A, et al. ESTRO consensus guideline on target volume delineation for elective radiation therapy of early stage breast cancer. Radiother Oncol. 2015;114:3–10. https://doi.org/10.1016/j.radonc.2014.11.030.
9. Offersen BV, Boersma LJ, Kirkove C, Hol S, Aznar MC, Sola AB, et al. ESTRO consensus guideline on target volume delineation for elective radiation therapy of early stage breast cancer, version 1.1 Radiother Oncol. 2016;118. https://doi.org/10.1016/j.radonc.2015.12.027.
10. Feng M, Moran J, Koelling T, Chughtai A, Chan J, Reedman LAF, et al. Development and validation of a heart atlas to study cardiac exposure to radiation following treatment for breast cancer. Cardiac Atlas. 2011;79:10–8. https://doi.org/10.1016/j.ijrobp.2009.10.058.
11. Duane F, Aznar MC, Bartlett F, Cutter DJ, Darby SC, Jagsi R, et al. A cardiac contouring atlas for radiotherapy. Radiother Oncol. 2017;122:416–22. https://doi.org/10.1016/j.radonc.2017.01.008.
12. Poortmans PMP, Takanen S, Nader G, Meattini I. Winter is over: the use of artificial intelligence to individualise radiation therapy for breast cancer. Breast. 2020;49:194–200. https://doi.org/10.1016/j.breast.2019.11.011.
13. Loap P, Tkatchenko N, Kirova Y. Evaluation of a delineation software for cardiac atlas-based autosegmentation: an example of the use of artificial intelligence in modern radiotherapy. Cancer Radiother. 2020;24(8):826–33.
14. Lorenzen EL, Taylor CW, Maraldo M, Nielsen MH, Offersen BV, Andersen MR, et al. Inter-observer variation in delineation of the heart and left anterior descending coronary artery in radiotherapy for breast cancer: a multi-centre study from Denmark and the UK. Radiother Oncol. 2013;108:254–8. https://doi.org/10.1016/j.radonc.2013.06.025.
15. Morris ED, Ghanem AI, Pantelic MV, Walker EM. Cardiac substructure segmentation with deep learning for improved cardiac sparing. Med Phys. 2020;47(2):576–86. https://doi.org/10.1002/mp.13940.
16. Levis M, Riccardo A, Fiandra C, De Luca V, Bartoncini S, Vella D, et al. Inclusion of heart substructures in the optimization process of volumetric modulated arc therapy techniques may reduce the risk of heart disease in Hodgkin ' s lymphoma patients. Radiother Oncol. 2019;138:52–8. https://doi.org/10.1016/j.radonc.2019.05.009.
17. Anastasi G, Bertholet J, Poulsen P, Roggen T, Garibaldi C, Tilly N, et al. Patterns of practice for adaptive and real-time radiation therapy (POP-ART RT) part I: intra-fraction breathing motion management. Radiother Oncol. 2020;153:79–87.
18. Smyth LM, Rt M, Knight KA, Rt M, Rt B, Aarons YK, et al. The cardiac dose-sparing benefits of deep inspiration breath-hold in left breast irradiation: a systematic review. J Med Radiat Sci. 2015;62(1):66–73. https://doi.org/10.1002/jmrs.89.
19. Bergom C, Currey A, Desai N, Tai A, Strauss JB, Bergom C. Deep inspiration breath hold: techniques and advantages for cardiac sparing during breast cancer irradiation. Front Oncol. 2018;8:1–10. https://doi.org/10.3389/fonc.2018.00087.
20. Boda-Heggemann J, Walter C, Mai S, Dobler B, Dinter D, Wenz F, et al. Frameless stereotactic radiosurgery of a solitary liver metastasis using active breathing control and stereotactic ultrasound. Strahlenther Onkol. 2006;182:216–37. https://doi.org/10.1007/s00066-006-1453-8.

21. Latty D, Stuart KE, Wang W, Ahern V. Review of deep inspiration breath-hold techniques for the treatment of breast cancer. J Med Radiat Sci. 2015;62:74–81. https://doi.org/10.1002/jmrs.96.
22. Bartlett FR, Colgan RM, Donovan EM, Carr K, Landeg S, Clements N, et al. Voluntary breath-hold technique for reducing heart dose in left breast radiotherapy. J Vis Exp. 2014;(89):51578. https://doi.org/10.3791/51578.
23. Estoesta RP, Attwood L, Naehrig D, Claridge-mackonis E, Odgers D, Martin D, et al. Assessment of voluntary deep inspiration breath-hold with CINE imaging for breast radiotherapy. J Med Imaging Radiat Oncol. 2017;61:689–94. https://doi.org/10.1111/1754-9485.12616.
24. Allen AM, Ceder YK, Shochat T, Fenig E, Popovtzer A, Bragilofsky D, et al. CPAP (Continuous Positive Airway Pressure) is an effective and stable solution for heart sparing radiotherapy of left sided breast cancer. Radiat Oncol. 2020;15:59.
25. Parkes M, Green S, Kilby W, Cashmore J, Ghafoor Q, Clutton-brock TH. The feasibility, safety and optimization of multiple prolonged breath-holds for radiotherapy. Radiother Oncol. 2019;141:296–303. https://doi.org/10.1016/j.radonc.2019.06.014.
26. Brunt AM, Haviland JS, Wheatley DA, Sydenham MA, Alhasso A, Bloomfield DJ, et al. Articles Hypofractionated breast radiotherapy for 1 week versus 3 weeks (FAST-Forward): 5-year efficacy and late normal tissue effects results from a multicentre, non-inferiority, randomised, phase 3 trial. Lancet. 2020;395:1613–26. https://doi.org/10.1016/S0140-6736(20)30932-6.
27. Yarnold J, Bentzen SM, Coles C, Haviland JS. Hypofractionated whole-breast radiotherapy for women with early breast cancer: myths and realities. Int J Radiat Oncol Biol Phys. 2011;79:1–9. https://doi.org/10.1016/j.ijrobp.2010.08.035.
28. Deseyne P, Speleers B, De Neve W, Boute B, Paelinck L, Van Hoof T, et al. Whole breast and regional nodal irradiation in prone versus supine position in left sided breast cancer. Radiat Oncol. 2017;12(1):89. https://doi.org/10.1186/s13014-017-0828-6.
29. Aznar MC, Duane FK, Darby SC, Wang Z, Taylor CW. Exposure of the lungs in breast cancer radiotherapy: a systematic review of lung doses published 2010–2015. Radiother Oncol. 2018;126:148–54.
30. Duma M, Wilfried B, Jürgen B, Petra D, Rainer F, Haase W, et al. Heart-sparing radiotherapy techniques in breast cancer patients: a recommendation of the breast cancer expert panel of the German society of radiation oncology (DEGRO). Strahlenther Onkol. 2019;195:861–71. https://doi.org/10.1007/s00066-019-01495-w.
31. Ashby O, Bridge P. Radiography late effects arising from volumetric modulated arc therapy to the breast: a systematic review. Radiography. 2020;27(2):650–3. https://doi.org/10.1016/j.radi.2020.08.003.
32. Osman SOS, Hol S, Poortmans PM, Essers M. Volumetric modulated arc therapy and breath-hold in image-guided locoregional left-sided breast irradiation. Radiother Oncol. 2014;112:17–22. https://doi.org/10.1016/j.radonc.2014.04.004.
33. Alongi F, Fogliata A, Clerici E, Navarria P, Tozzi A, Comito T, et al. Volumetric modulated arc therapy with flattening filter free beams for isolated abdominal/pelvic lymph nodes: report of dosimetric and early clinical results in oligometastatic patients. Radiat Oncol. 2012;7:204. https://doi.org/10.1186/1748-717X-7-204.
34. Cho Y, Cho YJ, Chang WS, Kim JW, Choi WH, Lee IJ. Evaluation of optimal treatment planning for radiotherapy of synchronous bilateral breast cancer including regional lymph node irradiation. Radiat Oncol. 2019;14:56.
35. Sun T, Lin X, Tong Y, Liu X, Pan L, Tao C, et al. Heart and cardiac substructure dose sparing in synchronous bilateral breast radiotherapy: a dosimetric study of proton and photon radiation. Therapy. 2020;9:1–11. https://doi.org/10.3389/fonc.2019.01456.
36. Essers M, Osman SOS, Hol S, Donkers T, Philip M. Accelerated partial breast irradiation (APBI): are breath-hold and volumetric radiation therapy techniques useful? Acta Oncolog (Stockholm, Sweden). 2014; 53(6). https://doi.org/10.3109/0284186X.2014.887226.
37. Koerkamp MLG, Vasmel JE, Russell NS, Shaitelman SF, Anandadas CN, Currey A, et al. Optimizing MR-guided radiotherapy for breast cancer patients. Front Oncol. 2020;10:1107. https://doi.org/10.3389/fonc.2020.01107.
38. Kennedy WR, Thomas MA, Stanley JA, Luo J, Ochoa LL, Clifton KK, et al. Single-institution phase 1/2 prospective clinical trial of single-fraction, high-gradient adjuvant partial-breast irradiation for hormone sensitive stage 0-I breast cancer. Radiat Oncol Biol. 2020;107:344–52. https://doi.org/10.1016/j.ijrobp.2020.02.021.
39. Lazzari G, Terlizzi A, Leo MG, Silvano G. VMAT radiation-induced nausea and vomiting in adjuvant breast cancer radiotherapy: the incidental effect of low-dose bath exposure. Clin Transl Radiat Oncol. 2017;7:43–8. https://doi.org/10.1016/j.ctro.2017.09.009.
40. Kaidar-Person O, Meattini I, Aznar MC, Poortmans P. Breast cancer outcomes and toxicity reduction with SGRT. In: Surface guided radiation therapy, vol. 227; 2020.

39 Particle Therapy

Anna M. Kirby and Liesbeth J. Boersma

39.1 Background

39.1.1 Rationale for Particle Therapy in Breast Cancer

Particle therapy is a form of radiation therapy in which high energy ionised particles, most commonly protons or neutrons, are aimed at the target tissue. In the context of breast cancer treatment, proton beam therapy (PBT) is the most commonly used particle therapy and is therefore the focus of this section. In contrast to standard external beam radiation therapy delivery using photons and/or electrons in which the highest dose is deposited within centimetres of the entry point of the beam into the body, PBT delivers most of the dose over a narrow-defined depth (known as a Bragg peak) within the tissue. By changing the energy of the delivered protons, radiation dose can be distributed within the patient such that there is a much sharper fall off in dose between especially the dorsal edge of the target volume and the adjacent non-target tissues than there would be with standard photon therapy. In certain clinical situations, this might facilitate the delivery of radiation to target tissues whilst delivering lower doses to neighbouring tissues such as heart and lung. Since the costs of PBT are, however, much higher than of photon therapy, proper selection of those patients that are expected to derive a clinically relevant benefit is crucial. Here, we discuss the clinical scenarios that might benefit most from the use of PBT, the clinical and technical literature around the use of PBT in breast cancer and currently recruiting PBT trials.

39.1.2 Potential Applications of PBT in Breast Cancer

The two main areas of interest in applying PBT to breast cancer have been partial breast irradiation and locoregional irradiation. For partial breast irradiation, in the light of a non-randomised comparative study showing higher skin toxicity in PBT patients than in those treated with photons [1], and given more recent data showing the efficacy and relatively low toxicity of other partial breast irradiation techniques [2, 3], it seems unlikely that PBT will prove advantageous enough over current evidence-based partial breast irradiation techniques to become a cost-effective standard of care.

A. M. Kirby
Royal Marsden NHS Foundation Trust and Institute of Cancer Research, Sutton, UK
e-mail: anna.kirby@rmh.nhs.uk

L. J. Boersma (✉)
Department of Radiation Oncology (Maastro), GROW School for Oncology and Reproduction, Maastricht University Medical Center, Maastricht, The Netherlands
e-mail: liesbeth.boersma@maastro.nl

© The Author(s), under exclusive license to Springer Nature Switzerland AG 2022
O. Kaidar-Person et al. (eds.), *Breast Cancer Radiation Therapy*,
https://doi.org/10.1007/978-3-030-91170-6_39

In the context of locoregional irradiation for breast cancer, however, there may be more to be gained. The organs that are expected to benefit most from PBT are heart, lungs and contralateral breast, with most studies focussing on prevention of cardiac injury [4]. Several recent trials have shown disease-free and overall survival benefits from inclusion of the internal mammary nodes chain (IMN) in the radiation therapy target volume [5–8]. However, given the proximity of the IMN to the heart, and given that irradiation of the IMN can therefore increase the radiation dose to the heart, there are concerns over increased risks of late cardiac toxicity [9] which may be greater in younger women and persist for decades after treatment [10]. Whilst the benefits of IMN-RT will significantly outweigh the risks for many patients, there is likely to be a relatively small subgroup of women in whom, due to chest wall shape and/or cardiovascular risk factors, even the most advanced photon technique of volumetric modulated arc therapy (VMAT) in combination with deep-inspiration breath-hold (DIBH) would struggle to cover the target volume, especially the IMN, without unacceptably increasing the risk of late cardiac effects [11]. In this group of women, PBT could be advantageous by more precisely targeting the target tissues with a steep fall off in dose between the target volume and heart such that both target and normal tissue constraints are met with consequent lower long-term risk of cardiac damage. The steep fall off in dose also reduces dose to lung and contralateral breast tissues with consequent lower risks of second primary cancers in either of these organ systems [12–15].

39.1.3 Dosimetric, Clinical and Technical Literature

At present there are no data from randomised clinical trials to support the use of PBT outside a clinical trial. There is, however, a growing literature on dosimetric gains of PBT, early clinical outcomes and technical aspects.

Dosimetry studies in the locoregional breast radiation therapy setting show reductions in dose to normal tissues for PBT. One study of 14 patients scanned in free-breathing and breath-hold and planned for radiation therapy to the breast/chest wall and locoregional lymph nodes including the IMC, demonstrated that PBT achieved lower doses than the best-performing photon technique of VMAT in DIBH to heart (median mean heart dose 0.5–1.0 Gy for PBT in DIBH and free-breathing versus 2.6 Gy for VMAT-DIBH), ipsilateral lung (ipsi lung V17 Gy 16–19% versus 28%) and contralateral breast (mean dose 0.2 Gy versus 1.5 Gy) [16]. A similar dosimetry study in 20 breast/chest wall patients planned for VMAT in DIBH versus intensity-modulated PBT also reported lower doses for PBT versus VMAT in heart (3.9 Gy PBT versus 0.4 Gy VMAT), ipsilateral lung (ipsi lung V_{20Gy} 18% versus 12%) and contralateral breast (mean dose 3.1 Gy versus 0.3 Gy) [12]. The latter paper suggests that such dose reductions could translate to an order of magnitude lower risk of second malignancies in contralateral breast and lung. Other groups suggested that the use of PBT in young women (instead of VMAT and DIBH) would reduce the risk of a radiation-induced contralateral breast cancer by sixfold [14] and for lung cancer two-fold [17].

Whilst dosimetry studies show lower physical doses from PBT on paper, it should be borne in mind that the biological effects of PBT are less well understood than the biological effects of standard photon radiation therapy. Current PBT planning systems assume the biological effect of PBT to be around 10% higher than that of photons (expressed as a relative biological effectiveness (RBE) of 1.1). In reality, RBE depends on a number of factors including the dose per fraction, the responsiveness of the tissue to radiation (expressed as alpha–beta ratio) and the linear energy transfer (LET) which increases along the path of the PBT beam peaking just beyond the Bragg peak. A number of models (known as variable RBE models) have been developed to take account of these factors albeit that clinical validation of the models is difficult outside the context of a randomised controlled trial. Variations in patient position on a day-to-day (interfraction) and intrafraction basis could also affect the delivered dose with particular concern over where the higher dose at the end of the Bragg peak is deposited. Consequences of inaccuracies in either the estimation of biological effect and/or the consistency of patient position and shape could include significant increases in delivered PBT dose to critical structures distal to the beam edge (including the ribs and/or the left anterior descending coronary artery). To counteract these uncertainties, PBT planning techniques [12, 18], algorithms for calculating biological dose [19], and methods for set-up verification [20] are continually being optimised. Nevertheless, caution is therefore advised in applying the results of dosimetric studies outside the context of a clinical trial.

Whilst efforts to better predict the biological consequences of PBT are ongoing, data from more recent clinical studies using the most modern PBT techniques in breast patients are relatively reassuring. Jimenez and colleagues at Massachusetts General reported outcomes in 69 breast cancer patients requiring radiation therapy to breast/chest wall and locoregional lymph nodes treated with PBT between 2011 and 2016 [21]. Patients early in the trial were treated with 3D-passively scattered proton therapy and later on with pencil beam scanning (PBS). Patients were prescribed 45 to 50.4 Gy (RBE) in 1.8 to 2.0 Gy per fraction. Maximum toxicities were grade 3 skin dermatitis in 3 (2%) patients, and grade 2 radiation pneumonitis in one (1%) patient. Grade 1 telangiectasia were reported in 16 patients (11%) but all were in the earlier 3D-passively scattered PBT group with no cases in the PBS group. Seven patients (5%) experienced grade 1 rib fractures, slightly higher than reported in the photon literature [22]. In view of this, ongoing PBT studies referred to below include rib toxicity as endpoints. Smith and colleagues at the Mayo Clinic reported outcomes in 51 patients who received intensity-modulated PBT to the chest wall and implant-based reconstructions between 2015 and 2017 [23]. A total of 37 patients were treated to 50 Gy in 25 fractions and 14 patients to 40 Gy in 15 fractions. Maximal acute dermatitis was grade 1 in 63% patients, grade 2 in 33% and grade 3 in 4% patients. In 8 out of 51 irradiated reconstructed breasts, the reconstruction failed (comparing favourably with the 20–30% implant failure rates reported in the photon literature [24–26]). Five out of 14 patients treated with 40 Gy in 15 fractions experienced reconstruction failure compared with three out of 37 patients treated with 50 Gy in 25 fractions. Although this was statistically significant, the authors acknowledge that the numbers are small. Indeed it would be expected that 40 Gy in 15 fractions should be gentler on late-reacting tissues than 50 Gy in 25 fractions. Going forward, prospective (including (randomised) controlled) trials will be invaluable to furthering our understanding of all oncological and normal tissue outcomes following PBT.

Parallel to the development of randomised clinical trials (RCTs) of PBT, the technical literature around PBT planning and delivery in breast cancer patients is increasing. PBT techniques have advanced considerably over the last 10–20 years with more modern intensity-modulated proton therapy (IMPT) delivered using PBS techniques allowing for modification of the skin dose to meet pre-specified constraints reflected in lower skin toxicity rates using IMPT as compared to older PBT techniques. Optimisation of planning approaches using multiple beams will reduce the likelihood of depositing higher doses beyond the edge of the Bragg peak at the same spots in crucial organs such as the ribs and LAD. Meanwhile, approaches to deal with the effects of set-up errors and changes in patient shape on PBT delivery are also being standardised through methods such as uncertainty analysis [27]. These entail evaluating the PBT plan under different uncertainty scenarios to check that the PBT plan would meet target and normal tissue constraints under a range of conditions [12, 18, 27]. Such approaches also require evaluation in the clinic, ideally in the context of RCTs or controlled prospective cohort studies.

39.1.4 Current Clinical Trials in PBT

As mentioned above, level one clinical evidence for the benefit of proton therapy over photon therapy in breast cancer patients is still lacking. Two large randomised clinical trials are currently recruiting patients aiming to fill this knowledge gap: the RADCOMP trial (NCT02603341) and the DBCG trial (NCT04291378). The RADCOMP trial aims to randomise 1278 patients, between PBT (either PBS or passively scattered PBT) and photon therapy to at least the internal mammary chain, with conventional fractionation schemes (1.8–2.0 Gy per fraction). The trial is powered to detect a reduction in major cardiac events at 10 years after radiation therapy from 6.3% to 3.5% with a power of 80% and a one-sided alpha of 0.05 [28]. The other endpoints include oncological control, other normal tissue toxicities and quality of life. The trial aims to complete accrual between 2016 and 2020; by 2019, 700 patients had been accrued.

The DBCG trial has a similar primary endpoint, that is, radiation associated ischaemic and valvular heart disease 10 years after RT. This trial aims to randomise 1502 patients with a photon-based mean heart dose ≥4 Gy or $V_{17/20Gy}$ to the ipsilateral lung ≥37%, between photon therapy and PBT, using 50 Gy in 25 fractions with or without a boost. Assuming that the mean heart dose will be reduced from 4 Gy with photons to 0.5 Gy with PBT, and assuming an excess relative risk of 20% per Gy MHD [29], the trial is powered to detect a reduction from 10.2% risk of cardiac events 10 years after photon therapy to 6.3% after PBT. The trial aims to complete recruitment by 2027.

Although RCTs are still considered the most valuable evidence by most medical doctors, it has also been argued that RCTs evaluating technological improvements are not always required, or even suitable [30]. The pitfall of the above-mentioned trials is that the results may be affected by the learning curve inherent in a trial of new technology [31]. In addition, patient selection may be too broad, for example, all patients undergoing IMN treatment, or all patients with a MHD ≥4 Gy from their photon plan. Whilst PBT is likely to deliver lower MHDs in the majority of patients, in only a subgroup will the MHD reduction be large enough (depending on other cardiac risk factors) to deliver a clinically meaningful reduction in risk of late cardiac effects. Furthermore, PBT is only expected to be cost-effective if patients are selected on the basis of expected better outcome [32]. It has been argued that if the dosimetric advantages are expected to translate into a clinical benefit, it may not be ethical anymore to randomise patients. Therefore, in the Netherlands, PBT for breast cancer patients is reimbursed if the predicted reduction in the lifetime risk of acute coronary events (ACE) is larger than 2%, provided that prospective data-registration is ensured with the aim of validating the applied predictive model [33]. This approved predictive model to estimate the lifetime risk of ACE is based on the model of Darby et al. [9]. Darby et al. found a relative increase in ACE of 7% per Gy MHD (in contrast to the 20% increase in ACE per Gy MHD in the DBCG data [29]). The absolute incidence of ACE is estimated by applying the relative risk of ACE of Darby to the absolute incidence of ACE in the Dutch population, for male and female patients, for all ages between 40 and 70 years of age, and for patients with and without cardiovascular risk factors. From January 2019 until October 2020 more than 200 breast cancer patients have been treated with PBT, in the Netherlands, based on this selection procedure, using a moderate hypofractionation scheme (15–22 fractions of 2.67 Gy [34]).

Finally, the Mayo Clinic randomised 15 vs 25 fractions PBT after mastectomy recruiting 109 patients during 2016–2020, with a primary endpoint of grade 3 late effects (NCT 02783690). A follow-on study in which patients are randomised between 15 fractions photon therapy vs. 5 fractions PBT is now recruiting aiming to recruit 98 patients between June 2020 and June 2022, with the primary endpoint being ≥ Grade 3 complication rate at 2 years (NCT04443413).

39.2 Summary

PBT is currently a rapid evolving technique, with assumed clinical benefits in a small subset of patients, which should be carefully selected. Sound clinical data of large RCTs and cohorts of patients, treated with contemporary proton therapy techniques are therefore eagerly awaited.

References

1. Galland-Girodet S, Pashtan I, MacDonald SM, Ancukiewicz M, Hirsch AE, Kachnic LA, Specht M, Gadd M, Smith BL, Powell SN, Recht A, Taghian AG. Long-term cosmetic outcomes and toxicities of proton beam therapy compared with photon-based 3-dimensional conformal accelerated partial-breast irradiation: a phase 1 trial. Int J Radiat Oncol Biol Phys. 2014;90(3):493–500. https://doi.org/10.1016/j.ijrobp.2014.04.008.
2. Coles CE, Griffin CL, Kirby AM, Titley J, Agrawal RK, Alhasso A, Bhattacharya IS, Brunt AM, Ciurlionis L, Chan C, Donovan EM, Emson MA, Harnett AN, Haviland JS, Hopwood P, Jefford ML, Kaggwa R, Sawyer EJ, Syndikus I, Tsang YM, Wheatley DA, Wilcox M, Yarnold JR, Bliss JM, IMPORT Trialists. Partial-breast radiotherapy after breast conservation surgery for patients with early breast cancer (UK IMPORT LOW trial): 5-year results from a multicentre, randomised, controlled, phase 3, non-inferiority trial. Lancet. 2017;390(10099):1048–60. https://doi.org/10.1016/S0140-6736(17)31145-5.
3. Strnad V, Ott OJ, Hildebrandt G, Kauer-Dorner D, Knauerhase H, Major T, et al. Groupe Européen de Curiethérapie of European Society for Radiotherapy and Oncology (GEC-ESTRO). 5-year results of accelerated partial breast irradiation using sole interstitial multicatheter brachytherapy versus whole-breast irradiation with boost after breast-conserving surgery for low-risk invasive and in-situ carcinoma of the female breast: a randomised, phase 3, non-inferiority trial. Lancet. 2016;387(10015):229–38. https://doi.org/10.1016/S0140-6736(15)00471-7.
4. Braunstein LZ, Cahlon O. Potential morbidity reduction with proton radiation therapy for breast cancer. Semin Radiat Oncol. 2018;28(2):138–49. https://doi.org/10.1016/j.semradonc.2017.11.009.
5. Whelan TJ, Olivotto IA, Parulekar WR, Ackerman I, Chua BH, Nabid A, et al. Regional nodal irradiation in early-stage breast cancer. NEJM. 2015;373:307–16.
6. Poortmans PM, Collette S, Kirkove C, Van Limbergen E, Budach V, Struikmans H, et al. Internal mammary and medial supraclavicular irradiation in breast cancer. NEJM. 2015;373:317–27.
7. Poortmans PM, Weltens C, Fortpied C, Kirkove C, Peignaux-Casasnovas K, Budach V, et al. Internal mammary and medial supraclavicular lymph node chain irradiation in stage I-III breast cancer (EORTC 22922/10925): 15-year results of a randomised, phase 3 trial. Lancet Oncol. 2020;21(12):1602–10.
8. Thorsen LB, Offersen BV, Dano H, Berg M, Jensen I, Pedersen AN, et al. DBCG-IMN: a population-based cohort study on the effect of internal mammary node irradiation in early node-positive breast cancer. JCO. 2016;34:314–20.
9. Darby SC, Ewertz M, McGale P, Bennet AM, Blom-Goladman U, Bronnum D, et al. Risk of ischaemic heart disease in women after radiotherapy for breast cancer. NEJM. 2013;368:987–98.
10. Henson KE, McGale P, Darby SC, Parkin M, Wang Y, Taylor CW. Cardiac mortality after radiotherapy, chemotherapy and endocrine therapy for breast cancer: cohort study of 2 million women from 57 cancer registries in 22 countries. Int J Cancer. 2020;147(5):1437–49.
11. Stick L, Lorenzen EB, Yates ES, Anandadas C, Andersen K, et al. Selection criteria for early breast cancer patients in the DBCG proton trial – the randomised phase III strategy. Clin Transl Radiat Oncol. 2021;27:126–31.
12. De Rose F, Cozzi L, Meattini I, Fogliata A, Franceschini D, Franzese C, et al. The potential role of intensity-modulated proton therapy in the regional nodal irradiation of breast cancer: a treatment planning study. Clin Oncol (R Coll Radiol). 2020;32:26–34.
13. Stovall M, Smith SA, Langholz BM, Boice JD Jr, Shore RE, Andersson M, et al. Dose to the contralateral breast from radiotherapy and risk of second primary breast cancer in the WECARE study. Int J Radiat Oncol Biol Phys. 2008;72:1021–30.
14. Settatree S, Brand D, Ranger A, Dunlop A, Harris E, Gulliford S, Kirby A. Estimating contralateral breast cancer risk from photons versus protons in patients undergoing internal mammary nodal breast cancer radiotherapy. Clin Onc (R Coll Radiol). 2019;32:342–5.
15. Paganetti H, DePauw N, Johnson A, Forman RB, Lau J, Jimenez R. The risk for developing a secondary cancer after breast radiation therapy: comparison of photon and proton techniques. Radiother Oncol. 2020;149:212–8.
16. Ranger A, Dunlop A, Hutchinson K, Convery H, Maclennan MK, Chantler H, et al. A dosimetric comparison of breast radiotherapy techniques to treat locoregional lymph nodes including the internal mammary chain. Clin Oncol (RCR). 2018;30(6):346–53.
17. Cartechini G, Fracchiolla F, Menegotti L, Scifoni E, La Tessa C, Schwarz M, et al. Proton pencil beam scanning reduces secondary cancer risk in breast cancer patients with internal mammary chain involvement compared to photon radiotherapy. Radiat Oncol. 2020;15:228.
18. Korevaar EW, Habraken SJM, Scandurra D, Kierkels RGJ, Unipan M, Eenink MGC, Steenbakkers RJHM. Practical robustness evaluation in radiotherapy- a photon and proton-proof alternative

to PTV-based plan evaluation. Radiother Oncol. 2019;141:267–74.
19. Wang CC, McNamara AL, Shin J, Schuemann J, Grassberger C, Taghian AG, et al. End-of-range radiobiological effect on rib fractures in patients receiving proton therapy for breast cancer. Int J Radiat Oncol Biol Phys. 2020;107(3):449–54.
20. Liang X, Vega RBM, Li Z, Zeng D, Mendenhall N, Bradley JA. Dosimetric consequences of image guidance techniques on robust optimized intensity-modulated proton therapy for treatment of breast cancer. Radiat Oncol. 2020;15(1):47.
21. Jimenez RB, Hickey S, DePauw N, Yeap BY, Batin E, Gadd MA, et al. Phase II study of proton beam radiation therapy for patients with breast cancer requiring regional nodal irradiation. J Clin Oncol. 2019;37(30):2778–85.
22. Smith GL, Xu Y, Buchholz TA, et al. Association between treatment with brachytherapy vs whole-breast irradiation and subsequent mastectomy, complications, and survival among older women with invasive breast cancer. JAMA. 2012;307:1827–37.
23. Smith NL, Jethwa KR, Viehman JK, Harmsen WS, Gonuguntla K, Elswick SM, et al. Post-mastectomy intensity modulated proton therapy after immediate breast reconstruction: initial report of reconstruction outcomes and predictors of complications. Radiother Oncol. 2019;140:76–83.
24. Khan AJ, Poppe MM, Goyal S, et al. Hypofractionated postmastectomy radiation therapy is safe and effective: first results from a prospective phase II trial. J Clin Oncol. 2017;35:2037–43.
25. Whitfield GA, Horan G, Irwin MS, Malata CM, Wishart GC, Wilson CB. Incidence of severe capsular contracture following implant-based immediate breast reconstruction with or without postoperative chest wall radiotherapy using 40 gray in 15 fractions. Radiother Oncol. 2009;90(1):141–7.
26. Momoh AO, Ahmed R, Kelley BP, Aliu O, Kidwell KM, Kozlow JH, Chung KC. A systematic review of complications of implant-based reconstruction with prereconstruction and postreconstruction radiotherapy. Ann Surg Oncol. 2014;21:118–24.
27. Lowe M, Gosling A, Nichols O, Underwood T, Miles E, Chang YC, et al. Comparing proton to photon radiotherapy plans: UK consensus guidance for reporting under uncertainty for clinical trials. Clin Oncol (R Coll Radiol). 2020;32(7):459–66. https://doi.org/10.1016/j.clon.2020.03.014.
28. Bekelman JE, Lu H, Pugh S, Baker K, Berg CD, Berrington de Gonzalez A, Braunstein LZ, Bosch W, Chauhan C, Ellenberg S, Fang LC, Freedman GM, Hahn EA, Haffty BG, Khan AJ, Jimenez RB, Kesslering C, Ky B, Lee C, Lu H-M, Mishra MV, Mullins CD, Mutter RW, Nagda S, Pankuch M, Powell SN, Prior FW, Schupak K, Taghian AG, Wilkinson JB, MacDonald SM, Cahlon O, RadComp (Radiotherapy Comparative Effectiveness Consortium). Pragmatic randomised clinical trial of proton versus photon therapy for patients with non-metastatic breast cancer: the Radiotherapy Comparative Effectiveness (RadComp) Consortium trial protocol. BMJ Open. 2019;9(10):e025556. https://doi.org/10.1136/bmjopen-2018-025556.
29. Lorenzen EL, Rehammar JC, Jensen M-B, Ewertz M, Brink C. Radiation-induced risk of ischemic heart disease following breast cancer radiotherapy in Denmark, 1977–2005. Radiother Oncol. 2020;152:103–10. https://doi.org/10.1016/j.radonc.2020.08.007.
30. Goitein M, Cox JD. Should randomized clinical trials be required for proton radiotherapy? J Clin Oncol. 2008;26(2):175–6.
31. Liao Z, Lee J, Komaki R, Gomez DR, O'Reilly MS, Fossella FV, Blumenschein GR, Heymach JV, Vaporciyan AA, Swisher SG, Allen PK, Choi NC, DeLaney TF, Hahn SM, Cox JD, Lu CS, Mohan R. Bayesian adaptive randomization trial of passive scattering proton therapy and intensity-modulated photon radiotherapy for locally advanced non–small-cell lung cancer. J Clin Oncol. 2018;36(18):1813–22.
32. Ramaekers BLT, Grutters JPC, Pijls-Johannesma M, Lambin P, Joore MA, Langendijk JA. Protons in head-and-neck cancer: bridging the gap of evidence. Int J Radiat Oncol Biol Phys. 2013;85(5):1282–8.
33. Langendijk JA, Boersma LJ, Rasch CRN, van Vulpen M, Reitsma JB, van der Schaaf A, Schuit E. Clinical trial strategies to compare protons with photons. Semin Radiat Oncol. 2018;28(2):79–87.
34. Haviland JS, Owen JR, Dewar JA, Agrawal RK, Barrett J, Barrett-Lee PJ, Dobbs HJ, Hopwood P, Lawton PA, Magee BJ, Mills J, Simmons S, Sydenham MA, Venables K, Bliss JM, Yarnold JR, START Trialists' Group. The UK Standardisation of Breast Radiotherapy (START) trials of radiotherapy hypofractionation for treatment of early breast cancer: 10-year follow-up results of two randomised controlled trials. Lancet Oncol. 2013;14(11):1086–94.

40 Preoperative Radiation

Sara Lightowlers and Yazid Belkacemi

40.1 Background

40.1.1 Rationale and Objectives

40.1.1.1 Downstaging Tumours to Facilitate Breast-Conserving Surgery

After Whole Breast Irradiation

For women with breast tumours too large for BCS, it is possible to downstage the tumour using PST [1]. However, low-grade ER-positive cancers frequently poorly respond to chemotherapy [2] and are less likely to be amenable to conservative surgery [2]. In certain cases primary endocrine therapy may be used; however, this is often reserved for elderly or frail patients [3]. Experience from other tumour sites suggests that RT could potentially be used to downstage a locally advanced cancer prior to surgery [4]. There is some limited evidence from historical series to support this approach in breast cancer.

S. Lightowlers (✉)
Department of Oncology, University of Cambridge, Cambridge, UK
e-mail: Sara.lightowlers@cruk.cam.ac.uk

Y. Belkacemi
Department of Radiation Oncology and Henri Mondor Breast Center, INSERM Unit 955, Team 21, IMRB, University of Paris-Est (UPEC), Creteil, France
e-mail: Yazid.belkacemi@aphp.fr

Calitchi et al. [5] reported a series of 75 women with T2/T3 N0–2 tumours diagnosed between 1977 and 1992, initially unsuitable for conservative surgery due to breast–tumour volume ratio. Receptor status was not reported, but the majority of patients (61%) had well-moderately differentiated infiltrating ductal carcinoma. Following treatment with preoperative RT to a dose of 45 Gy over 5 weeks, BCS (lumpectomy or reduction mammaplasty) was successfully performed in all patients; 55% had good or excellent cosmetic results. In another series [6] of 41 women with ER-positive breast tumours treated with primary RT and endocrine therapy, 45% underwent BCS, having previously been judged ineligible for surgery.

After Partial Breast Irradiation

PBI is currently an accepted treatment option for selected patients in the postoperative setting and is recommended in multiple national and international guidelines for tumours [7–9]. PBI may be indicated for comparable tumours in the preoperative setting and delivering this treatment prior to surgery also has potential advantages. The postoperative primary tumour bed may be difficult to define (see Chap. 20); reports have found high interobserver variability amongst oncologists delineating the clinical target volume in this setting [10]. Modern oncoplastic techniques further complicate this; oncologists' defined tumour bed volumes have been reported to be significantly

© The Author(s), under exclusive license to Springer Nature Switzerland AG 2022
O. Kaidar-Person et al. (eds.), *Breast Cancer Radiation Therapy*,
https://doi.org/10.1007/978-3-030-91170-6_40

different from those defined by surgeons [11] (see Chap. 35). Irradiating the tumour prior to surgery likely reduces the risk of geographic miss of the target. It may also reduce the irradiated volume, as it avoids the need to irradiate the complex and large tumour bed following oncoplastic surgery including possible postoperative seroma or haematoma. The tissue irradiated to a high dose is then removed surgically, limiting the risk of fibrosis and poor cosmesis. The PAPBI I trial of preoperative PBI, in which 100% of patients had a good or excellent cosmetic outcome at 3 years, supporting the concept requiring further study [12] (Table 40.1).

Improving Survival Outcomes

The overall survival benefit of systemic treatment is established in adjuvant and preoperative settings [13]. An advantage of the preoperative approach lies in risk stratification, with the aim of further improving outcomes. For example, the pathologic response to PST in HER2 positive and triple-negative subtypes provides predictive and prognostic information that can be used to direct the subsequent treatment strategy; non-responders may benefit from T-DM1 [14] and capecitabine [15] respectively. In addition, pCR in triple-negative and HER2-positive subtypes is reported as a surrogate marker for better survival [16]. Thus, increasing local response rates is an attractive target for further research for all breast cancer subtypes.

A large number of phase 1–2 studies are currently exploring combinations with targeted drugs or immunotherapy to look for increased response signals. The idea of enhancing the immune effect of radiation to the primary tumour in situ is of particular interest; the pre-clinical and clinical rationale for combining immunotherapy and RT in breast cancer is thoroughly reviewed by Formenti and Ye [17]. This increasing understanding of the breast cancer biological response to radiation could be used to direct precision medicine approaches for RT and drug–irradiation combinations.

40.2 Existing Literature

40.2.1 Whole Breast Radiation Therapy Alone

Early data on preoperative WBI comes from retrospective and single arm studies from the 1970s, 80s and 90s, in a variety of patient populations [5, 18–20]. Those reporting on locoregional control found rates between 76% and 91% at 10–15 years. pCR rates were likewise inconsistently recorded, but were found to be between 8% and 19% in those studies that did so. Retrospective pathological review in the study by Riet et al. [20] allowed analysis of response to preoperative radiation by breast cancer subtype. This series of 187 patients treated between 1970 and 1984 with 45Gy to whole breast and regional nodes reported an overall pCR rate of 10% in the whole population and 26% in triple-negative tumours. After a median follow-up of 32 years, locoregional control rates were 89% at 20 and 30 years, with DFS rates of 35% and 27% at 20 and 30 years.

The only randomised trial of preoperative RT reported in the historical literature is the Swedish breast cancer trial [21]. The 960 patients with early breast cancer diagnosed between 1977 and 1992 were treated with either mastectomy alone or mastectomy with postoperative or preoperative RT. At 16-year median follow-up, no difference in overall survival was observed between patients irradiated pre- or postoperatively.

40.2.2 Partial Breast Irradiation Alone

The first trials of PBI in the preoperative setting are now reported. The Dutch PAPBI study [12, 22] is a phase 2 trial of accelerated PBI (either 4Gy in 10 fractions over 2 weeks or 6 Gy in 5 fractions over 1 week), in low-risk node-negative breast cancers (<3 cm on MRI and pathologically node negative on pre-treatment SLNB). The trial reported four local recurrences in the 70 patients

Table 40.1 Early phase trials involving preoperative breast radiotherapy, currently in set up or recruiting patients

Trial name	Planned enrolment	Trial design	Patient population	RT target volume	RT schedule Total dose/# fx	PST
PRADA (NCT02771938)	60	Non-randomised interventional trial	Breast cancer requiring mastectomy	Whole breast	42.72 Gy/16 OR 40 Gy/15 over 3 weeks	Sequential chemotherapy
NeoRT (NCT03818100)	43	Phase I non-randomised feasibility trial	ER+ HER2− with tumour >2cm	Whole breast ± boost	40 Gy/15 ± SIB to 48 Gy OR sequential boost over 3 weeks OR 26 Gy/5 ± sequential boost over 1 week	Sequential endocrine therapy
Feasibility Study of Accelerated Preoperative Radiotherapy for Early Breast Cancer (NCT02858934)	24	Non-randomised interventional trial	Unifocal cT1-2N0 ER+	Whole breast + boost	25 Gy/5 + SIB to 30 Gy over 1 week	None
MRI Based Preoperative Accelerated Partial Breast Irradiation (NCT02728076)[a]	40	Phase II non-randomised trial	Unifocal ER+ with tumour <3 cm	Partial breast	Not specified	None
Néo-APBI-01 (NCT02806258)	362	Phase I and Phase II randomised trial	Intermediate and high-risk luminal B-like and TNBC	Partial breast	25 Gy/10 over 1 week	Sequential anthracycline and/or taxane based chemotherapy
PRECISE (NCT03359954)	25	Phase II non-randomised trial	ER+/HER2−	Tumour	Not specified	None
CBCV (NCT03804944)	100	Phase II randomised trial	Clinical stage II-III,ER+HER2−	Tumour	24 Gy/3 over 1 week	None/pembrolizumab/Flt-3 ligand/ pembrolizumab + Flt-3 ligand (concurrent)

(continued)

Table 40.1 (continued)

Trial name	Planned enrolment	Trial design	Patient population	RT target volume	RT schedule Total dose/# fx	PST
NeoCheckRay (NCT03875573)	147	Phase II randomised trial	ER+ HER2− with high-risk MammaPrint genomic score	Tumour	24 Gy/3 over 3 days	Taxane and anthracycline chemotherapy/ chemotherapy + durvalumab/ chemotherapy + durvalumab plus oleclumab (anti-CD73)
PANDoRA (NCT03872505)	140	Phase II randomised trial	Clinical stage II-III TNBC	Tumour	24 Gy/3 over 1 week	Carboplatin, paclitaxel and durvalumab
ROCK (NCT03520894)	25	Non-randomised interventional trial	T1 ER+HER2-	Tumour[b]	21 Gy single fraction	None

PST primary systemic therapy
[a]MRI planning
[b]Target not clearly defined

treated, three of which were thought to be related to the biopsy track. As stated above, cosmetic outcome was good or excellent in 89% at 1-year, and 100% at 3-year. In contrast, the United States APBI feasibility study of 27 patients reported by Nichols et al. [23], in which patients received 3.85Gy in 10 fractions (two fractions a day) over 1 week, reported no local recurrences but a lower rate of good/ex cellent cosmetic outcome: 79% at 1-year. Rates of pCR were 10% and 15% respectively; the United States trial also reported a drop in Ki67%, taken as a surrogate of radiation response, in an additional 19 patients. The hypofractionation of preoperative PBI is taken further by Horton et al. [24], who report preoperative delivery of single fraction SBRT up to 21 Gy to 32 patients with low-risk breast cancers less than 2 cm in size, without dose limiting toxicity.

40.2.3 Whole Breast Radiation Therapy with Systemic Therapy

The historical literature also includes several series of preoperative RT delivered concurrently with chemotherapy [18, 25–33]. The acute toxicity described in these reports is consistent with the increase in toxicity found with concurrent chemoradiation in the postoperative setting [34]. In some cases, this resulted in delays to surgery and in problems with wound healing. Oncologic outcomes, again, were inconsistently reported, but rates of pCR up to 45% have been observed [30]. More recently, in the phase 2, S14 study [35, 36], 60 patients ineligible for breast-conserving surgery were treated with 4 cycles of 5-FU and vinorelbine and concurrent radiation (50 Gy to whole breast and 46 Gy to regional nodes, over 5 weeks). Following this preoperative treatment, 69% went on to have conservative surgery, with 27% having had a pCR. However, 36% of patients experienced G3–4 toxicity. Five-year overall survival, and distant-disease free survival were 88% and 83%, respectively.

40.2.4 Partial Breast Radiation Therapy with Systemic Therapy

Bondiau et al. [37] combined SBRT with systemic treatments in a phase 1 study dose escalation study: 25 breast tumours were treated with 3 fractions of preoperative SBRT delivered alongside docetaxel chemotherapy. Nine patients (36%) achieved a pCR, and 23 (92%) underwent breast-conserving surgery despite having initially been thought to require mastectomy. Grade 3 skin toxicity was experienced by one patient who received 28.5 Gy in 3 fractions, but no other dose limiting toxicities were observed. The authors conclude safety of SBRT up to a dose of 31.5 Gy, but recommend, based on efficacy-toxicity tradeoff, that the schedule of 25.5 Gy in 3 fractions be taken forward to phase 2. The preoperative radiation is considered as a boost dose; all subjects in the trial also received 50 Gy in 25 fractions postoperative RT to the whole breast and regional lymph nodes following surgery. No update has been published to date.

40.3 Ongoing Trials

40.3.1 Open Phase 3 Trials

The follow on to the PAPBI study, PAPBI-II (NCT02913729) [38], is a phase 3 trial recruiting since 2016. Low-risk patients (grade 1 or 2 tumours that are ER-positive and HER2-negative, with size <3 cm) are randomised between pre- and postoperative PBI (28.5 Gy in 5 fractions). The primary endpoint in this trial is cosmetic outcome, secondary endpoints include tumour response and postoperative complications. The German phase 3 trial NEORAD (NCT04261244) [39] opened in July 2020, aiming to recruit 1826 patients. A higher risk patient population with indications for preoperative chemotherapy will be enrolled in this trial and randomised to either WBI (40.5 Gy in 15 fractions) given preoperatively following systemic treatment, or postoperatively. The primary outcome measure will be DFS.

40.3.2 Ongoing Early Phase Trials

Phase 1–2 trials of preoperative breast radiation therapy are in progress in a diversity of settings. Those delivering WBRT include the UK PRADA trial (NCT02771938) [40] in patients requiring mastectomy following preoperative systemic therapy and wishing to have immediate breast reconstruction. The UK feasibility study Neo-RT (NCT03818100) [41] is recruiting patients with low-grade ER-positive and HER2-negative tumours greater than 2 cm in size, for whom RT may facilitate breast-conserving surgery. Following WBI (40 Gy in 15 fractions or 26.5 Gy in 5 fractions with or without SIB) patients receive 20 weeks endocrine therapy, allowing time for tumour regression in response to treatment.

The Belgian trial Feasibility Study of Accelerated Preoperative Radiotherapy for Early Breast Cancer (NCT02858934) [42] is another single-arm trial, of accelerated whole breast preoperative radiation (25 Gy in 5 fractions, plus SIB to the tumour) in patients with low-grade ER-positive and HER2-negative tumours. Preoperative accelerated PBI also continues to be investigated in the United States study MRI-Based Preoperative Accelerated Partial Breast Irradiation (NCT02728076) [43], recruiting patients with clinical stage I–II ER-positive breast cancers, in which MRI imaging is used in the planning procedure. Postoperative complications is the primary outcome measure, and secondary outcome measures include feasibility of MRI-based treatment planning.

Early phase trials of preoperative breast irradiation with sequential systemic therapy include the French study Néo-APBI-01 (NCT02806258) [44], a phase 1/2 trial randomising between the control arm 6–8 cycles of primary systemic therapy, and primary systemic therapy with the addition of accelerated PBI planned between cycles. The patients recruited are those with higher risk luminal B-like and triple-negative cancers, for whom chemotherapy prior to breast surgery is indicated; the primary outcome is pCR rate. The Phase I trial fixed the tumour dose to 25 Gy in 10 twice daily fractions Translational research on predictive parameters of pCR is planned.

Building on the data from Horton et al. [24] and Bondiau et al. [37], a number of early phase trials investigating the use of preoperative RT to a boost tumour volume only, with or without systemic therapy, are also in progress. The PRECISE trial (NCT03359954) [45] is a single arm trial of preoperative boost alone in ER-positive and HER2-negative breast cancer, with the primary objective of evaluating the change in tumour-infiltrating lymphocytes before and after the boost. In ER-positive HER2-negative cancers, the CBCV trial (NCT03804944) [46] is randomising patients receiving preoperative letrozole between boost radiation alone (24 Gy in 3 alternate day fractions), in combination with pembrolizumab, recombinant FLT-3 ligand, or both. The European trial NeoCheckRay (NCT03875573) [47] delivers preoperative boost SBRT (24 Gy in 3 daily fractions) in combination with paclitaxel, with or without the addition of the anti-PDL1 durvalumab and the anti-CD73 antibody oleclumab. In triple-negative breast cancer, the PANDoRA trial (NCT03872505)l [48] will randomise 140 patients between preoperative systemic therapy (carboplatin, paclitaxel and durvalumab) alone, or with the addition of boost SBRT (24 Gy in 3 alternate day fractions). All of these trials for which radiation dose is available deliver a moderately hypofractionated preoperative radiotherapy schedule similar to that recommended by Formenti [17] and by Bondiau [37], and patients in these trials also go on to receive standard of care postoperative radiation therapy at the discretion of the treating clinician. In contrast, the Italian single arm ROCK trial (NCT03520894) [49] is aiming to treat 25 patients with low-grade, ER-positive and HER2-negative breast cancer with a single preoperative 21 Gy fraction to a partial breast volume.

40.4 Summary

A significant number of ongoing studies investigating preoperative RT approaches in breast cancer as well as recently completed trials is available, with modern RT techniques including PBI and SBRT being included in preoperative research. Moreover, dedicated studies according to breast cancer subtype are set up. Preliminary results indicate that these concepts are both feasible and safe. The introduction of preoperative irradiation directed to the primary tumour could offer a number of opportunities to increase our knowledge of tumour biology, including immunology, response to RT in breast cancer, and improve not only quality of life for patients, but also potentially survival outcomes.

References

1. Fisher B, et al. Effect of preoperative chemotherapy on local-regional disease in women with operable breast cancer: findings from National Surgical Adjuvant Breast and Bowel Project B-18. J Clin Oncol. 1997;15:2483–93.
2. Loibl S, et al. Response and prognosis after neoadjuvant chemotherapy in 1,051 patients with infiltrating lobular breast carcinoma. Breast Cancer Res Treat. 2014;144:153–62.
3. Morgan J, Wyld L, Collins KA, Reed MW. Surgery versus primary endocrine therapy for operable primary breast cancer in elderly women (70 years plus). Cochrane Database Syst Rev. 2014;(1):CD004272.
4. Renehan AG, et al. Watch-and-wait approach versus surgical resection after chemoradiotherapy for patients with rectal cancer (the OnCoRe project): a propensity-score matched cohort analysis. Lancet Oncol. 2016;17:174–83.
5. Calitchi E, et al. Long-term results of neoadjuvant radiation therapy for breast cancer. Int J Cancer. 2001;259:253–9.
6. Bollet MA, et al. Responses to concurrent radiotherapy and hormone-therapy and outcome for large breast cancers in post-menopausal women. Radiother Oncol. 2007;85(3):336–45. https://doi.org/10.1016/j.radonc.2007.10.003.
7. Postoperative radiotherapy for breast cancer: UK consensus statements. 2016. www.rcr.ac.uk.
8. Strnad V, et al. DEGRO practical guideline for partial-breast irradiation. Strahlenther Onkol. 2020;196:749–63.
9. Correa C, et al. Accelerated partial breast irradiation: executive summary for the update of an ASTRO evidence-based consensus statement. Pract Radiat Oncol. 2017;7:73–9.
10. Yang TJ, et al. Tumor bed delineation for external beam accelerated partial breast irradiation: a systematic review. Radiother Oncol. 2013;108:181–9.
11. Garreffa E, Hughes-Davies L, Russell S, Lightowlers S, Agrawal A. Definition of tumor bed boost in oncoplastic breast surgery: an understanding and approach. Clin Breast Cancer. 2020;20:e510–5.
12. Van Der Leij F, et al. First results of the preoperative accelerated partial breast irradiation (PAPBI) trial. Radiother Oncol. 2015;114:322–7.
13. Asselain B, et al. Long-term outcomes for neoadjuvant versus adjuvant chemotherapy in early breast cancer: meta-analysis of individual patient data from ten randomised trials. Lancet Oncol. 2018;19:27–39.
14. von Minckwitz G, et al. Trastuzumab emtansine for residual invasive HER2-positive breast cancer. N Engl J Med. 2019;380:617–28.
15. Masuda N, et al. Adjuvant capecitabine for breast cancer after preoperative chemotherapy. N Engl J Med. 2017;376:2147–59.
16. Spring LM, et al. Pathologic complete response after neoadjuvant chemotherapy and impact on breast cancer recurrence and survival: a comprehensive meta-analysis. Clin Cancer Res. 2020;26:2838–48.
17. Ye JC, Formenti SC. Integration of radiation and immunotherapy in breast cancer - treatment implications. Breast. 2018;38:66–74.
18. Semiglazov VF, et al. Primary (neoadjuvant) chemotherapy and radiotherapy compared with primary radiotherapy alone in stage IIb-IIIa breast cancer. Ann Oncol Off J Eur Soc Med Oncol. 1994;5:591–5.
19. Touboul E, et al. Possibility of conservative local treatment after combined chemotherapy and preoperative irradiation for locally advanced noninflammatory breast cancer. Int J Radiat Oncol Biol Phys. 1996;34:1019–28.
20. Riet FG, et al. Preoperative radiotherapy in breast cancer patients: 32 years of follow-up ScienceDirect. Eur J Cancer. 2017;76:S62–9.
21. Rutqvist LE, Pettersson D, Johansson H. Adjuvant radiation therapy versus surgery alone in operable breast cancer: long-term follow-up of a randomized clinical trial. Radiother Oncol. 1993;26:104–10.
22. Bosma SCJ, et al. Five-year results of the preoperative accelerated partial breast irradiation (PAPBI) trial. Int J Radiat Oncol Biol Phys. 2020;106:958–67.
23. Nichols E, et al. Preoperative accelerated partial breast irradiation for early-stage breast cancer: preliminary results of a prospective, phase 2 trial. Int J Radiat Oncol Biol Phys. 2017;97:747–53.
24. Horton JK, et al. Preoperative single-fraction partial breast radiation therapy: a novel phase 1, dose-escalation protocol with radiation response

biomarkers. Int J Radiat Oncol Biol Phys. 2015;92:846–55.
25. Skinner KA, et al. Pre-operative 5-fluorouracil and radiation therapy for locally advanced breast cancer. Am J Surg. 1997;174:705–8.
26. Skinner KA, et al. Preoperative paclitaxel and radiotherapy for locally advanced breast cancer: surgical aspects. Ann Surg Oncol. 2000;7:145–9.
27. Formenti SC, et al. Concurrent paclitaxel and radiation therapy for breast cancer. Semin Radiat Oncol. 1999;9:34–42.
28. Lerouge D, et al. Combined chemotherapy and preoperative irradiation for locally advanced noninflammatory breast cancer: updated results in a series of 120 patients. Int J Radiat Oncol. 2004;59:1062–73.
29. Chakravarthy AB, et al. Neoadjuvant concurrent paclitaxel and radiation in stage II/III breast cancer. Clin Cancer Res. 2006;12:1570–6.
30. Shanta V, Swaminathan R, Rama R, Radhika R. Retrospective analysis of locally advanced noninflammatory breast cancer from Chennai, South India, 1990-1999. Int J Radiat Oncol Biol Phys. 2008;70:51–8.
31. Alvarado-Miranda A, et al. Concurrent chemoradiotherapy following neoadjuvant chemotherapy in locally advanced breast cancer. Radiat Oncol. 2009;4:24.
32. Adams S, et al. Preoperative concurrent paclitaxel-radiation in locally advanced breast cancer: pathologic response correlates with five-year overall survival. Breast Cancer Res Treat. 2010;124:723–32.
33. Matuschek C, et al. Long-term outcome after neoadjuvant radiochemotherapy in locally advanced noninflammatory breast cancer and predictive factors for a pathologic complete remission. Strahlenther Onkol. 2012;188:777–81.
34. Fernando IN, et al. Synchronous versus sequential chemo-radiotherapy in patients with early stage breast cancer (SECRAB): a randomised, phase III, trial. Radiother Oncol. 2020;142:52–61.
35. Bollet MA, et al. Pathological response to preoperative concurrent chemo-radiotherapy for breast cancer: results of a phase II study. Eur J Cancer. 2006;42:2286–95.
36. Bollet MA, et al. Preoperative radio-chemotherapy in early breast cancer patients: long-term results of a phase II trial. Radiother Oncol. 2012;102:82–8.
37. Bondiau PY, et al. Phase 1 clinical trial of stereotactic body radiation therapy concomitant with neoadjuvant chemotherapy for breast cancer. Int J Radiat Oncol Biol Phys. 2013;85:1193–9.
38. Pre- versus postoperative accelerated partial breast irradiation. Full text view.ClinicalTrials.gov. https://clinicaltrials.gov/ct2/show/NCT02913729.
39. No title. https://clinicaltrials.gov/ct2/show/NCT04261244.
40. No title. https://clinicaltrials.gov/ct2/show/NCT02771938.
41. https://clinicaltrials.gov/ct2/show/NCT03818100.
42. No title. https://clinicaltrials.gov/ct2/show/NCT02858934.
43. No title. https://clinicaltrials.gov/ct2/show/NCT02728076.
44. Comparing sequential neoadjuvant treatment including chemotherapy and accelerated radiation focused to the tumor bed vs neoadjuvant chemotherapy alone. Full text view. ClinicalTrials.gov. https://clinicaltrials.gov/ct2/show/NCT02806258.
45. No title. https://clinicaltrials.gov/ct2/show/NCT03359954.
46. No title. https://clinicaltrials.gov/ct2/show/NCT03804944.
47. No title. https://clinicaltrials.gov/ct2/show/NCT03875573.
48. No title. https://clinicaltrials.gov/ct2/show/NCT03872505.
49. No title. https://clinicaltrials.gov/ct2/show/study/NCT03520894.

41 Brachytherapy

Vratislav Strnad

41.1 Background

Brachytherapy as a minimal invasive technique of RT that allows for delivering a high-RT dose in a precise, small in-breast target volume avoiding to the greatest extent the exposure of adjacent OARs and thereby radiation side effects. It results in excellent local control with low rates of side effects. Thus, brachytherapy is commonly used in the treatment of patients with low-risk breast cancer as APBI—or by patients with defined risk factors as a RT boost in addition to WBI [1–10]. As logical consequence, brachytherapy represents one of the most reported irradiation techniques for APBI or for salvage APBI after in case of recurrence after BCT [1, 11, 12]. Importantly and as general rule applies that PBI trials using multicatheter brachytherapy demonstrated identical long-term results as the PBI trials using EBRT [1, 13–18]. In contrast to it, the published data about brachytherapy as a boost are limited and not distinct from results using different EBRT techniques [19–22]. Until now, no significant differences have been reported in terms of local control, late side effects and cosmesis between brachytherapy and other boost techniques. However, prospective head-to-head comparison is missing. Due to the fact that as well different boost techniques as different APBI techniques result in similar excellent oncological outcomes, the current challenge is to define factors that could guide treatment decisions.

The point is that interstitial brachytherapy as boost or APBI is a technique with high precision, which make possible to easily shape the reference isodose respecting as well individual anatomy of tumour and breast, as the individual different resection margins in different directions. Moreover, brachytherapy as APBI in comparison to all other available techniques of EBRT including CyberKnife® based techniques, reduces significantly radiation dose in the majority of clinical scenarios to all surrounding tissues and organs, especially to the lung [2, 23, 24]. In this context, the recently published detailed dosimetric analysis by Hoekstra et al. plays a role of some nontrivial consequence [24]. First not surprisingly, this dosimetric analysis demonstrates impressively that in general PBI using multicatheter brachytherapy reduces significantly dose to all surroundings OARs compared not only to WBI but also to all other techniques of PBI. Beyond that, what is remarkably and clinically important, are the results regarding secondary cancer. It is know that PBI may have a favourable impact on risk of second cancer in the contra-lateral breast and lung for older patients at low risk of recurrence [25] and simultaneously that lung cancer accounted for 75–97% of secondary malignancies by breast cancer patients

V. Strnad (✉)
Department of Radiation Oncology, University Hospital Erlangen, Erlangen, Germany
e-mail: vratislav.strnad@uk-erlangen.de

© The Author(s), under exclusive license to Springer Nature Switzerland AG 2022
O. Kaidar-Person et al. (eds.), *Breast Cancer Radiation Therapy*,
https://doi.org/10.1007/978-3-030-91170-6_41

[24]. Calculating "Secondary cancers Lifetime Attributable Risks" with modified BEIR-VII formalism for the specific survival of breast cancer patients for a typical early stage patient irradiated at 50 year old, the excess risks of secondary lung cancer were 1.1% for multicatheter HDR-brachytherapy, between 2.2% and 2.5% for 3DCRT or CyberKnife®, 3.5% for VMAT for APBI, and 3.8% for WBI [24]. Similar differences have been observed also for other age groups. Finally, based on this analysis, it seems evident that APBI using multicatheter brachytherapy among others has the potential to reduce risk of secondary cancer of the lung twofold to fourfold compared to WBI and onefold to threefold compared to other APBI techniques. With other words, multicatheter brachytherapy reflects very well the ALARA ("as low as reasonably achievable") principle of radiation protection of surrounding structures. As a consequence, we as breast experts have to consider this advantage of brachytherapy as well by indication of boost techniques as by indication of APBI technique by patients with breast cancer.

41.2 Key Information for Clinical Practice

Numerous brachytherapy techniques are available to deliver APBI or a boost. Interstitial multicatheter brachytherapy represents the most investigated brachytherapy technique to deliver both APBI and tumour bed boost [1, 5, 6, 10, 11, 20, 26]. However, to make brachytherapy for APBI easier, in North America single-entry devices were developed as an alternative, with the first being the single-lumen MammoSite® applicator [27, 28], followed by multi-lumen and strut applicators [29–31]. The MammoSite device consists of inflatable balloon catheter that is placed after open cavity surgery in the tumourectomy cavity. Typically, the MamoSite® fills the tumourectomy cavity, giving a spherical or ellipsoid dose distribution. The main limitation of MammoSite® device is the extraordinary restricted possibility to vary the shape and size of reference isodose and as a consequence lack of possibility to adapt the shape and size of reference isodose respecting most usual resection margins in different directions. Simultaneously the possibility to avoid OAR as skin is very limited. To overcome these problems encountered with MammoSite® were developed other single-entry devices as Contura®, ClearPath®, SAVI® and the electronic brachytherapy [29, 31, 32]. The Contura® is very similar to the MammoSite® device with additional catheters inside of balloon to be able to steer radiation dose on the surface of inflatable balloon. The other devices—ClearPath® and SAVI®—use instead inflatable balloon dispersed source catheter with different architectures. Finally, electronic brachytherapy device such as the Axxent® system have been proposed—a miniature X-ray tube that steps through a catheter similar as an Ir-source. This X-ray tube operates with 50 kV and the dose distribution is similar that of J-125. Importantly all these single-entry devices request as obligate precondition that BCS be performed as open cavity surgery and this fact poses an important limitation for using single-entry devices. Finally, no randomised trials are available evaluating specific single-entry applicator-based brachytherapy alone for PBI. Both these facts limit substantial possible use and as consequence, the clinical use of single-entry devices for PBI is limited to North America. Additionally, for single-entry devices no international guideline is currently available. Hence, in following we describe the clinical practice merely for multicatheter brachytherapy.

Worthy of mention is also the fact that as well multicatheter brachytherapy as the single-entry devices can be used in the time of breast-conserving surgery or in a separate procedure later. While stressing that we strictly recommend and prefer to perform PBI procedure as separate procedure after BCS (typically after 8–10 weeks) for the simple reason that only in such time schedule it is possible to respect all key requested information as tumour size, resection margins, and related prognostic factors needed for medical indication for PBI [12].

41.3 Treatment Planning and Catheter Insertion

In order to plan treatment, the radiation oncologist needs for appropriate treatment planning to have a detailed surgical and pathological report including size of resection margins in six directions, knowledge about number and position of surgical clips, images of preoperative mammography, ultrasound and, where necessary and available, magnetic resonance imaging (MRI). The standard procedure for catheter insertion for multicatheter brachytherapy (Figs. 41.1 and 41.2) is to insert appropriate number of catheters trans-

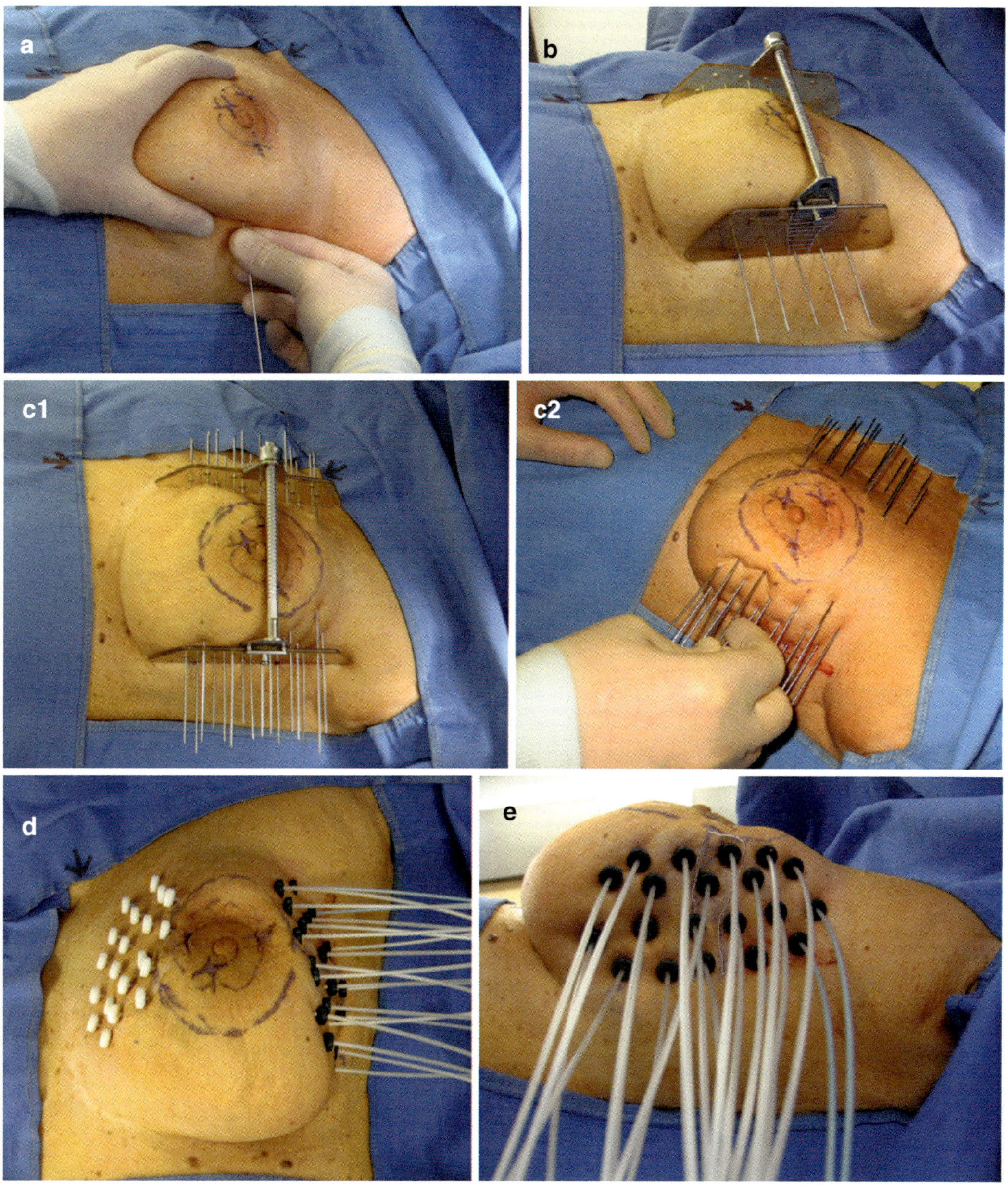

Fig. 41.1 Typical sequence of insertion of single-leader catheters for APBI using multicatheter brachytherapy: (**a**) Insertion of guide needle, (**b**) Projection of in-breast scare on template with inserted guide needle and needles of lower row, (**c**) Final arrangement of needles with and without template, (**d**) Final arrangement of catheters, (**e**) Final arrangement of catheters with visualisation of in-breast scar on skin surface

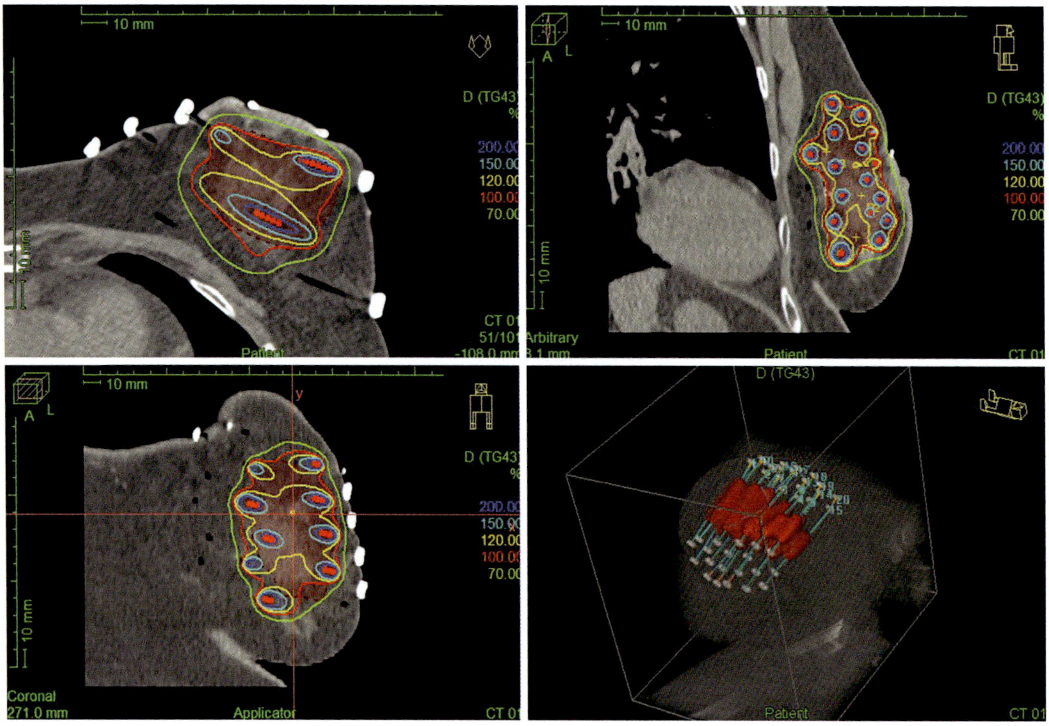

Fig. 41.2 An example of typical dose distribution of APBI with multicatheter brachytherapy

cutaneous and image-guided—with the help of computed tomography, ultrasound or X-ray monitoring and preferably using template guidance. A square or triangular arrangement of all catheters is reasonable [12, 33]. When open cavity surgical technique has been used, it is mostly very easy to identify the seroma cavity and to decide suitable arrangement of needles. After closed cavity surgery or oncoplastic surgery, the marks on the skin scar and surgical clips in tumour bed region are important prerequisite for adequate identification of tumour bed location. Notably, in any case the radiation oncologist has to visualise the estimated localisation and size of CTV before insertion of the first guide needle and has to check continuously the position of all catheters during insertion to guarantee accuracy, appropriate size and shape of implant volume. For CT-based pre-implant treatment planning and consecutive insertion of catheters after open or closed cavity surgery various policies exist, but in general the catheter positions are at first determined using the 3D rendering of the target volume, patient anatomy and virtual simulation of optimal catheter positions during pre-implant CT-imaging. Catheter insertion follows later, using predefined skin marks and identical template parameters. Ultrasound based pre-implant treatment planning and catheter insertion is particularly suitable for patients with seroma after open cavity surgery. X-ray based pre-implant treatment planning and catheter insertion after closed or open cavity surgery can be performed in a similar manner as the CT-based procedure, but an important precondition is that the resection margins of the surgical bed inside the breast must be marked with appropriate number of surgical marker clips (at least 4, ideally 6 clips). For more details, please see corresponding guideline [12]. Furthermore, we strictly recommend defining the target in accordance with current published guidelines [34, 35]—for more details see Chapter Target volume definition and contouring-boost/SIB/PBI.

41.4 Treatment Schedules

First, we recommend that the selected fractionation for PBI correspond to a biologically equivalent total dose EQD2 ($\alpha/\beta = 4$–5 Gy) in the range of 42–45 Gy. As consequence the most common prescription utilised for PBI with HDR-brachytherapy and validated in prospective trials are 32 Gy in 8 fractions, 30.1 Gy in 7 fractions, 34.2 Gy in 9 fractions or v 34 Gy in 10 fractions. The HDR-brachytherapy for APBI is typically scheduled twice a day, with an interval between fractions of at least 6 h, and with a total treatment time of 4–5 days. For PBI with PDR-brachytherapy pulsed-dose 0.5–0.8 Gy/pulse, and a total dose 50 Gy, scheduled every hour, 24 h per day with total treatment time 4–5 days is a typical regime.

The current recommended schedules for boost with HDR-Brachytherapy is 8 to 12 Gy in 2 fractions, or 9 to 15 Gy in 3 fractions, scheduled twice a day, with an interval between fractions of at least 6 hours, and a total treatment time of 1–2 days, or a single fraction of 7–10 Gy, depending on the preferred total EQD2 [12, 26]. The recommended total dose for boost with PDR-Brachytherapy is 10–20 Gy arranged identical as for APBI.

41.5 Dose–Volume Parameters and Dose Constraints

For an appropriate objective assessment of any treatment plan of breast brachytherapy, quantitative parameters have to be analysed, considered and documented. Based on the ESTRO-ACROP guideline [12] and NSABP Protocol B-39/RTOG 0413 [36], we recommend the following dose–volume limits.

1. Coverage index (CI): V100 ≥90–95% (i.e. at least 90% of the CTV/PTV had to receive the prescription dose)
2. V_{150} <65 cm^3
3. V_{200} <15 cm^3
4. Absolute volume irradiated by prescription dose ≤300 cm^3
5. Dose non-uniformity ratio (DNR) ≤35
6. Conformal index (COIN) ≥65

Table 41.1 Recommended dose–volume limits for organ at risk (modified according to [12, 24])

Organ	Constraints
Ipsilateral non-target breast	V_{90} <10% V_{50} <40–50%
Skin	D_{1cm3} <90% $D_{0.2cm3}$ <100%
Rib	$D_{0,1cm3}$ <90% D_{1cm3} <80%
Heart	MHD <2.5 Gy
Lung	Stochastic effects: MLD <1–1,5 Gy Deterministic effects: MLD <3–4 Gy

MHD mean heart dose, *MLD* mean lung dose

The current recommended dose–volume limits for OARs [12, 24, 36], according the published data and guidelines, which should be in each PBI-patient documented and respected, are summarised in Table 41.1.

41.6 Summary

Breast brachytherapy is an interventional technique of RT requiring local or general anaesthesia, which make possible to deliver very precisely the prescribed dose in strictly limited in-breast target volume and simultaneously to avoid of the utmost significance the radiation exposure of lung, hearth and skin. Nevertheless, the related recent standards and guidelines must be respected to assure optimal results.

References

1. Strnad V, Ott OJ, Hildebrandt G, et al. 5-year results of accelerated partial breast irradiation using sole interstitial multicatheter brachytherapy versus whole-breast irradiation with boost after breast-conserving surgery for low-risk invasive and in-situ carcinoma

of the female breast: a randomised, phase 3, non-inferiority trial. Lancet. 2016;387(10015):229–38.
2. Lettmaier S, Kreppner S, Lotter M, et al. Radiation exposure of the heart, lung and skin by radiation therapy for breast cancer: a dosimetric comparison between partial breast irradiation using multicatheter brachytherapy and whole breast teletherapy. Radiother Oncol. 2011;100(2):189–94.
3. Major T, Gutierrez C, Guix B, et al. Interobserver variations of target volume delineation in multicatheter partial breast brachytherapy after open cavity surgery. Brachytherapy. 2015;14(6):925–32.
4. Ott OJ, Schulz-Wendtland R, Uter W, et al. Fat necrosis after conserving surgery and interstitial brachytherapy and/or external-beam irradiation in women with breast cancer. Strahlenther Onkol. 2005;181(10):638–44.
5. Strnad V, Hildebrandt G, Potter R, et al. Accelerated partial breast irradiation: 5-year results of the German-Austrian multicenter phase II trial using interstitial multicatheter brachytherapy alone after breast-conserving surgery. Int J Radiat Oncol Biol Phys. 2011;80(1):17–24.
6. Polgar C, Major T, Fodor J, et al. Accelerated partial-breast irradiation using high-dose-rate interstitial brachytherapy: 12-year update of a prospective clinical study. Radiother Oncol. 2010;94(3):274–9.
7. Polgar C, Fodor J, Major T, Sulyok Z, Kasler M. Breast-conserving therapy with partial or whole breast irradiation: ten-year results of the Budapest randomized trial. Radiother Oncol. 2013;108(2):197–202.
8. Rabinovitch R, Winter K, Kuske R, et al. RTOG 95-17, a Phase II trial to evaluate brachytherapy as the sole method of radiation therapy for Stage I and II breast carcinoma--year-5 toxicity and cosmesis. Brachytherapy. 2014;13(1):17–22.
9. Khan AJ, Arthur D, Vicini F, et al. Six-year analysis of treatment-related toxicities in patients treated with accelerated partial breast irradiation on the American Society of Breast Surgeons MammoSite Breast Brachytherapy registry trial. Ann Surg Oncol. 2012;19(5):1477–83.
10. Hepel JT, Arthur D, Shaitelman S, et al. American Brachytherapy Society consensus report for accelerated partial breast irradiation using interstitial multicatheter brachytherapy. Brachytherapy. 2017;16(5):919–28.
11. Hannoun-Levi JM, Resch A, Gal J, et al. Accelerated partial breast irradiation with interstitial brachytherapy as second conservative treatment for ipsilateral breast tumour recurrence: multicentric study of the GEC-ESTRO Breast Cancer Working Group. Radiother Oncol. 2013;108(2):226–31.
12. Strnad V, Major T, Polgar C, et al. ESTRO-ACROP guideline: interstitial multi-catheter breast brachytherapy as Accelerated Partial Breast Irradiation alone or as boost - GEC-ESTRO Breast Cancer Working Group practical recommendations. Radiother Oncol. 2018;128(3):411–20.
13. Coles CE, Griffin CL, Kirby AM, et al. Partial-breast radiotherapy after breast conservation surgery for patients with early breast cancer (UK IMPORT LOW trial): 5-year results from a multicentre, randomised, controlled, phase 3, non-inferiority trial. Lancet. 2017;390(10099):1048–60.
14. Livi L, Meattini I, Marrazzo L, et al. Accelerated partial breast irradiation using intensity-modulated radiotherapy versus whole breast irradiation: 5-year survival analysis of a phase 3 randomised controlled trial. Eur J Cancer. 2015;51(4):451–63.
15. Vicini FA, Cecchini RS, White JR, et al. Long-term primary results of accelerated partial breast irradiation after breast-conserving surgery for early-stage breast cancer: a randomised, phase 3, equivalence trial. Lancet. 2019;394(10215):2155–64.
16. Bhattacharya IS, Haviland JS, Kirby AM, et al. Patient-reported outcomes over 5 years after whole- or partial-breast radiotherapy: longitudinal analysis of the IMPORT LOW (CRUK/06/003) phase III randomized controlled trial. J Clin Oncol. 2019;37(4):305–17.
17. Polgar C, Ott OJ, Hildebrandt G, et al. Late side-effects and cosmetic results of accelerated partial breast irradiation with interstitial brachytherapy versus whole-breast irradiation after breast-conserving surgery for low-risk invasive and in-situ carcinoma of the female breast: 5-year results of a randomised, controlled, phase 3 trial. Lancet Oncol. 2017;18(2):259–68.
18. Schafer R, Strnad V, Polgar C, et al. Quality-of-life results for accelerated partial breast irradiation with interstitial brachytherapy versus whole-breast irradiation in early breast cancer after breast-conserving surgery (GEC-ESTRO): 5-year results of a randomised, phase 3 trial. Lancet Oncol. 2018;19(6):834–44.
19. Poortmans P, Bartelink H, Horiot JC, et al. The influence of the boost technique on local control in breast conserving treatment in the EORTC 'boost versus no boost' randomised trial. Radiother Oncol. 2004;72(1):25–33.
20. Kindts I, Laenen A, Christiaens M, Janssen H, Van Limbergen E, Weltens C. Comparison of brachytherapy and external beam radiotherapy boost in breast-conserving therapy: patient-reported outcome measures and aesthetic outcome. Strahlenther Onkol. 2019;195(1):21–31.
21. Polgar C, Major T, Fodor J, et al. High-dose-rate brachytherapy alone versus whole breast radiotherapy with or without tumor bed boost after breast-conserving surgery: seven-year results of a comparative study. Int J Radiat Oncol Biol Phys. 2004;60(4):1173–81.
22. Guinot JL, Baixauli-Perez C, Soler P, et al. High-dose-rate brachytherapy boost effect on local tumor control in young women with breast cancer. Int J Radiat Oncol Biol Phys. 2015;91(1):165–71.
23. Major T, Frohlich G, Lovey K, Fodor J, Polgar C. Dosimetric experience with accelerated partial breast irradiation using image-guided interstitial brachytherapy. Radiother Oncol. 2009;90(1):48–55.

24. Hoekstra N, Fleury E, Merino Lara TR, et al. Long-term risks of secondary cancer for various whole and partial breast irradiation techniques. Radiother Oncol. 2018;128(3):428–33.
25. Donovan EM, James H, Bonora M, Yarnold JR, Evans PM. Second cancer incidence risk estimates using BEIR VII models for standard and complex external beam radiotherapy for early breast cancer. Med Phys. 2012;39(10):5814–24.
26. Polo A, Polgar C, Hannoun-Levi JM, et al. Risk factors and state-of-the-art indications for boost irradiation in invasive breast carcinoma. Brachytherapy. 2017;16(3):552–64.
27. Benitez PR, Keisch ME, Vicini F, et al. Five-year results: the initial clinical trial of MammoSite balloon brachytherapy for partial breast irradiation in early-stage breast cancer. Am J Surg. 2007;194(4):456–62.
28. Shah C, Badiyan S, Ben Wilkinson J, et al. Treatment efficacy with accelerated partial breast irradiation (APBI): final analysis of the American Society of Breast Surgeons MammoSite((R)) breast brachytherapy registry trial. Ann Surg Oncol. 2013;20(10):3279–85.
29. Arthur DW, Vicini FA, Todor DA, Julian TB, Cuttino LW, Mukhopadhyay ND. Contura Multi-Lumen Balloon breast brachytherapy catheter: comparative dosimetric findings of a phase 4 trial. Int J Radiat Oncol Biol Phys. 2013;86(2):264–9.
30. Yashar C, Attai D, Butler E, et al. Strut-based accelerated partial breast irradiation: report of treatment results for 250 consecutive patients at 5 years from a multicenter retrospective study. Brachytherapy. 2016;15(6):780–7.
31. Cuttino LW, Arthur DW, Vicini F, Todor D, Julian T, Mukhopadhyay N. Long-term results from the Contura multilumen balloon breast brachytherapy catheter phase 4 registry trial. Int J Radiat Oncol Biol Phys. 2014;90(5):1025–9.
32. Yashar CM, Scanderbeg D, Kuske R, et al. Initial clinical experience with the Strut-Adjusted Volume implant (SAVI) breast brachytherapy device for accelerated partial-breast irradiation (APBI): first 100 patients with more than 1 year of follow-up. Int J Radiat Oncol Biol Phys. 2011;80(3):765–70.
33. Pierquin B, Wilson JF, Chassagne D. The Paris system. In: Modern brachytherapy. Masson Publishing; 1987.
34. Major T, Gutierrez C, Guix B, et al. Recommendations from GEC ESTRO Breast Cancer Working Group (II): target definition and target delineation for accelerated or boost partial breast irradiation using multicatheter interstitial brachytherapy after breast conserving open cavity surgery. Radiother Oncol. 2016;118(1):199–204.
35. Strnad V, Hannoun-Levi JM, Guinot JL, et al. Recommendations from GEC ESTRO Breast Cancer Working Group (I): target definition and target delineation for accelerated or boost Partial Breast Irradiation using multicatheter interstitial brachytherapy after breast conserving closed cavity surgery. Radiother Oncol. 2015;115(3):342–8.
36. RTOG. NSABP PROTOCOL B-39/RTOG PROTOCOL 0413: a randomized phase III study of conventional whole breast irradiation (WBI) versus partial breast irradiation (PBI) for women with stage 0, I, or II breast cancer. 2007. https://www.atc-wustledu/protocols/nsabp/b-39/0413.pdf. Accessed 31 Jan 2018.

42 Intraoperative Radiation Therapy

Gerd Fastner, Douglas Zippel, and Vered Noy

42.1 Background

In the case of breast conserving therapy, RT delivered as WBI has been shown to be an indispensable therapeutical component following BCS, in order to significantly reduce the local recurrence risk by two-thirds as well as for an appreciable benefit in long-term survival [1]. An additional dose escalation to the tumour bed as a boost (10–16 Gy), has contributed a further increase in local breast control (LC), with the absolute highest benefit demonstrated for younger patients [2]. For such a dose augmentation, different techniques such as brachytherapy and IORT were suggested for tumour bed boost (see Chap. 41) [3] with favourable LC rates in numerous oncological risk constellations.

Supplementary Information The online version contains supplementary material available at [https://doi.org/10.1007/978-3-030-91170-6_42].

G. Fastner
Department of Radiotherapy and Radio-Oncology, Paracelsus Medical University Hospital Salzburg, Salzburg, Austria
e-mail: g.fastner@salk.at

D. Zippel (✉) · V. Noy
Meirav Breast Health Center and the Department of Surgery C, Chaim Sheba Medical Center, Tel Hashomer, Israel
e-mail: Dov.Zippel@sheba.health.gov.il; vered.noy@sheba.health.gov.il

In addition, in selected subgroups with a low local recurrence risk, PBI to the affected index breast quadrant after BCS, has been confirmed to be a feasible treatment option either by external photons [4], brachytherapy [5] or IORT [6]. APBI is defined as accelerated PBI in which the overall treatment duration is shortened significantly (as opposed to PBI protocol used in the IMPROT LOW trial [4]. All methods for APBI have the aim of decreasing the treatment burden for appropriate patients by reducing both treated volumes and duration. IORT can be done by low energy photon IORT device (50 kV X-ray device) [7] or electrons (IOeRT) [8].

Mobile IORT technology led to increased use of IORT-PBI, mostly 50 kV low-energy X-rays [9] and IOeRT [8] However, these techniques are not identical, with large differences concerning surgical techniques, dose distributions, dose homogeneity and skin doses [10]. The 50 kV spherical applicator is relatively easy to use. It is positioned within the lumpectomy cavity without special preparations other than haemostasis. The applicator provides the therapeutic dose around at the applicator surface (the size of the applicator can be adjusted to the surgical cavity), with a steep dose gradient and leading to only 25% of the prescribed dose at 1 cm distance from the applicator (Supplement Fig. 1 [7]). Complete haemostasis is needed as bleeding in the lumpectomy cavity during the procedure will reduce the RT dose to the cavity. The applicator should be

© The Author(s), under exclusive license to Springer Nature Switzerland AG 2022
O. Kaidar-Person et al. (eds.), *Breast Cancer Radiation Therapy*, https://doi.org/10.1007/978-3-030-91170-6_42

applied in an adequate distance from the skin, as a distance of less than 1 cm can lead to significant skin doses and complications [11]. The 50 kV low-energy X-rays IORT results for APBI were reported in a large randomised clinical trial; however, it failed to demonstrate non-inferiority to WBI. Therefore, per guidelines it is not approved for clinical use outside a clinical trial or prospective registries [12].

This chapter highlights IOeRT, given as a boost and as APBI. On the basis of recently published recommendations of the ESTRO Task Force group for IORT [8] a detailed overview will be given on the available literature, patient selection criteria, surgical, technical and physical aspects of IOeRT, in order to enable an implementation of this technique in daily clinical practice.

42.2 Rationale and Clinical Results

42.2.1 IOeRT as a Boost

In regard to treatment accuracy as well as to minimise the risk for a higher grade of late normal tissue effects, IOeRT provided as a circumscribed Boost of 10–11 Gy (D_{max}) to the tumour bed has reported to offer some advantages during clinical practice: avoidance of geographic as well as temporal misses of the verified target tissue, complete skin protection and tight treatment volumes [3, 13]. From a biological point of view, IOeRT might increase anti-tumour effects by blocking a potential stimulation of cell proliferation by the wound exudate, which was reported after application of higher singles doses several times [14–21]. In retrospective unselected large cohort analyses, boost-IOeRT has demonstrated a high LC, with actuarial 6- and 10-year LR rates of 0.8% and 2.7%, respectively [13, 22]. Also, in subgroup analyses of patients at "higher risk" for in-breast LR, such as after preoperative chemo−/immunotherapy of locally advanced breast cancer or triple-negative subtypes, IOeRT has shown favourable results at least comparable to conventional boost methods [23, 24]. Additionally, the combination of boost-IOeRT with moderate hypofractionated WBI, seems to be feasible in terms of acute/subacute toxicity as well as breast cosmesis outcome [25].

42.2.2 IOeRT as APBI

For APBI, IOeRT was investigated in the randomised prospective ELIOT trial with a single-dose of 21 Gy. After a mid-term follow-up period, patients treated with IOeRT demonstrated higher LR rates compared to those after WBI (4.4% vs. 0.4%, $p < 0.0001$) but with no significant differences in survival [6]. Importantly, for the 69.5% of the patients in the experimental arm that were classified as low-risk (i.e. none of the following risk factors: ≥4 positive lymph nodes, grade 3 tumours, tumour size >2 cm and triple-negative subtype), an LR-rate of only 1.5% was observed, which is in line with the 5-year data for "suitable" APBI-patients according to current ASTRO guidelines [26, 27]. A classification by GEC-ESRTO [28] was performed for 1822 patients, who were treated with full dose IOeRT outside the ELIOT trial [29]., Accordingly, 32% ($n = 573$) of these patients could be classified as "good candidates" for an APBI approach with a 5-year LR rate of 1.9% [30]. Moreover, a similar exercise for the same cohort revealed in 16% ($n = 294$) patients rated as "suitable" according to ASTRO-criteria with a 5-year LR of 1.5%, respectively [26]. Furthermore, the guideline classification for APBI-patients by ASTRO [26] and ESTRO [30] recommendations was supported by several other published clinical data sets [31, 32].

42.3 Toxicity and Cosmetic Outcome (Boost and APBI)

42.3.1 Acute Toxicity and Late Normal Tissue Effects

Wound complications (infection, haematoma, delayed wound healing and seroma) were reported for boost-IOeRT between 3% and 4.9% and after APBI between 1% and 16% [13, 25, 29, 31, 33–41]. Grade 3 fibrosis as a subacute/late reaction following APBI was observed in the range of 2–6% and as grade 2 fibrosis in up to 30% of cases [33, 39, 40, 42]. After IOeRT as a boost, grade 3 fibrosis occurred in less than 2% and grades 1–2 in between 10% and 25% of cases, respectively [25, 43–45]. These data on acute and late toxicity after IOeRT, do not seem to be inferior from those by means of standard WBI. In the ELIOT-trial acute skin reactions were rarely observed and turned out to be superior compared to those verified after WBI, but with no differences in terms of for late reactions (fibrosis, retraction, pain or burning sensation) [6]. However, fat necrosis were detected significantly more frequently after IOeRT than with WBI ($p = 0.04$) [6]. Furthermore, IORT as APBI with 50-kv X-rays, investigated within the TARGIT-trail, has not demonstrated to initiate a higher rate of wound complications compared to standard EBRT [46], Some single institutional experiences, which performed IORT either as Boost or as APBI, reported rates for seroma, haematoma and perioperative infections in the range of 11–15.8%, 5.8% and 2–3%, respectively [47–49]. Ebner F et al. observed no differences in terms of postoperative seroma compared to a control group without IORT [50]. Additional reports after IORT along the "TARGIT-concept" about late toxicity was published by then Mannheim-group in 2012 [11]. Accordingly, IORT as APBI or applicated as a Boost followed by WBI was not observed to initiate a higher rate of radiotherapy-related late side effects (i.e. pain, fibrosis, breast oedema ulceration, retraction hyperpigmentation and lymphoedema) compared to conventional WBI alone, which was accompanied with significant more telangiectasia ($p = 0.049$). Of note, within a treatment related subanalysis, a higher grade (2/3) of fibrosis occurred more frequently after IORT as a boost plus WBI (37.5%) compared to WBI (18.4%) or IORT (5.9%) alone, respectively [11].

42.3.2 Breast Cosmesis

First experiences for objective breast cosmesis after boost IOeRT reported excellent/good results in 86% of cases [51] or as clinical overall impression after long term observation [45]. After median follow-up periods of 45 and 56 months, including 261–583 analysed patients, excellent/good results rated by doctors and patients were reported in 64–75% and in 86–91%, respectively [13, 25]. Objective scorings done by doctors were performed on the basis of photographs in predefined positions. Breast cosmesis was evaluated using an international scoring-system [52] and did not demonstrate a remarkable difference between baseline and annual evaluations thereafter [25]. Cosmesis after APBI was also assessed by doctors and patients and were implemented using different scoring systems with excellent/good ratings in more than 90% for both groups [36, 37, 53–55]. However, there was some differences in cosmesis assessment between patient and doctors in some analyses [36, 37]. The current literature on clinical outcome data of IOeRT adopted as boost or APBI is summarised in Table 42.1 [13, 22–25, 43–45, 51, 54, 56] and Table 42.2 [6, 26, 29–38, 40–42, 57–60].

42.4 Patient Selection (Boost and APBI)

Patient eligibility for primarily boost or PBI and subsequently for performing this with an IOeRT technique, is determined within a multidisciplinary tumour board according to international guidelines and recommendations [8, 12]. If IOeRT will be performed as APBI, as definitive pathology is missing at the time of treatment, additional breast MRI has turned out to be advantageous in order to get some more clinical information about obvious contraindications [e.g. multifocality or suspicious lymph nodes) rendering such patients as ineligible in up 12.5% of cases [61, 62] especially with risk factors such as tumour sizes larger than T2, invasive lobular histology or premenopausal status [62]. For APBI, the following criteria for patient selection are listed [27, 28, 63]: age 50 years or older, unicentric tumours 2 cm or smaller, hormone positive and HER2-negative receptor status, tumour grade 1–2 with ductal or other favourable histological types and a negative nodal status (pN0 (i−/i+)). Please refer for additional reading in the PBI and omission of radiation sections.

Table 42.1 Evidence on IOeRT-Boost (reused with the agreement of Elsevier on 22nd of September 2020, G et al., Radiother Oncol 2020; 249:150–157, page 153)

Author	FUP	Patients	Patient selection	Technology	IORT dose (range)	EBRT	LC	OS/DFS
Merrick et al. [44]	[a]71 mo (up to 144)	21	Stage I–II	IOERT	D_{max}: 10–15 Gy	45–50 Gy Fx: 1.7-2 Gy	Crude 100%	OS: Crude 90.5%
Dubois et al. [54]	Min. 24mo	101 51/50	Stage I–II (III)	IOERT/no	D90%: 10 Gy	45 Gy Fx:2 Gy	Crude 100% vs nc	nc
Lemanski et al. [45]	[a]109 mo (60–180)	50	Stage I–II	IOERT	D90%: 9–20 Gy	50 Gy Fx:2 Gy	Crude 96%	nc
Ciabattoni et al. [51]	nc	234 (122/112)	Stage I–II	IOERT/ ext. e	D_{max}: 10 Gy	50 Gy Fx: nc	Crude 100% vs 98.2% (nc)	nc
Reitsamer et al. [56]	[a]51/81 mo	378 (190/188)	Stage I–II	IOERT/ ext. e	D_{max}: 10 Gy	51–56 Gy Fx: 1.7 Gy	[b]100% vs 95.7% (ss)	nc
Ivaldi GB et al. [43]	[a]8.9 mo (0.8–32.4)	204	Stage (0) I–III	IOERT	D_{max}: 13.3 Gy	37.05 Gy Fx: 2.85	[c]100%	nc
Fastner et al. [22]	[a]72.4 mo (0.8–239)	1109	Stage I–III	IOERT	D_{max}: 6–15 Gy	50–54 Gy Fx: 1.7–2 Gy	[d]99.2%	OS: [d]91.4%
Fastner et al. [23]	[a]59/67.5 mo (3–120)	107 (81/26)	Stage II–III	IOERT/ ext. e	D_{max}: 10 Gy	51–57 Gy Fx: 1.7–1.8 Gy	[d]98.5% vs 88.1% (ns)	OS: [d]86.4% vs 92% (ns)
Fastner et al. [24]	[a]97 mo (20–170)	71	Stage I–II	IOERT	D_{max}: 7–12 Gy	[a]54 Gy Fx:1.6–1.85 Gy	[e]89%	OS: [e]69%
Kaiser et al. [13]	[a]121 mo (4–200)	770	Stage I–III	IOERT	D_{max}: 5–12 Gy	[a]54 Gy Fx:1.6–2 Gy	[f]97.2%	OS: [f]85.7%
Fastner et al. [25]	[a]45 mo (0–74)	583	Stage I–II	IOERT	D_{max}: 11 Gy	40.5 Gy Fx: 2.7 Gy	Crude 100%	DFS: [g]97.8%

mo months, *LC* local control, *OS* overall survival, *nc* no comments, *ss* statistically significant, *ns* not significant, *D90%* 90%-reference-isodose, *Fx* dose per fraction, *OS* overall survival, *LC* local control, *FUP* follow-up
[a]Median
[b]Actuarial 5-year rate
[c]Actuarial 9-months rate
[d]Actuarial 6-year rate
[e]Actuarial 8-year rate
[f]Actuarial 10-year rate
[g]Actuarial 3-year rate ext

For both IOeRT treatment options, as a boost and APBI, invasive breast cancer has to be confirmed by a biopsy before BCS. However, IOeRT applied as a boost should be especially considered after histopathological proof of malignancies with a high potential to locally recur as well as for patients with one or more of several risk factors according to national and international guidelines like: younger age (at least <50 years), tumour grading 3, the absence of positive hormonal receptors, confirmed triple negative, positivity for Her2, lymphovascular invasion (LVI), no clear resection margins, extensive intraductal component (EIC) and tumour sizes >2 cm, respectively [64–67].

Table 42.2 Evidence on full-dose IOeRT (reused with the agreement of Elsevier on 22nd of September 2020, Fastner G et al., Radiother Oncol 2020; 249:150–157, page 153, page 152)

Author	Study period	Follow-up (months)	Patients	Patient selection	WBI	Local recurrences (%)	DFS (%)	Overall Survival (%)	Comments
Mussari et al. [33]	10/2000–11/2002	Median 48	47	>45 years, size≤2 cm, N0, G1-G2, positive oestrogen receptors, no EIC on biopsy,	No	0%	–	100%	Phase I-II trial, lobular histology included (13%)
VanderWalde et al. [57], Ollilla et al. [34], Kimple et al. [37]	3/2003–7/2007	Median 69	71	>48 years, IDC, size ≤3 cm, cN0	11 (46 Gy/2 Gy/fx)	15% (5 true, 3 elsewhere)	–	94.4%	Phase II study of pre-excision IOERT
Lemanski et al. [35, 36]	11/2004–11/2007	Median 72	42	≥65 years, IDC, size≤2 cm, N0, free margin>2 mm, positive oestrogen receptors. No LVI or EIC in the primary biopsy	No	9.5% (3 true, 1 elsewhere)	92.7%	100%	Phase II trial
Veronesi et al. [29], Leonardi et al. [26, 30]	1/2000–12/2008	Median 36.1	1822	Median age 58 years, median size 1.3 cm, 71.4% cN0	No	3.3% (2.3% true, 1% elsewhere); according to ASTRO-GEC-ESTRO subgroups: 1.5% (low risk)–8.8% (high risk)	–	94.4%; According to ASTRO-GEC-ESTRO subgroups: 98.6% (low risk)–94.4% (high risk)	Out-trial patients 22 pts included in the dose escalation studies. The same population was categorised according to ASTRO and GEC-ESTRO guidelines
Maluta et al. [31, 38]	6/2006–12/2009	Median 62	226	≥50 years, IDC, size ≤3 cm, no EIC,	No	1.8%	–	100%	–
Osti et al. [40]	6/2007–10/2011	Median 27 months	110	>48 years, size <2.5 cm, cN0, no EIC	No	2.7% (2 true, 1 elsewhere)	92.9%	97.3	–
Veronesi et al. [6]	11/2000–12/2007	Median 69.6	1305 (654 WBI and 651 IOERT)	>48–75 years, ≤2.5 cm, cN0	WBI in the control arm (50 Gy/2 Gy/fx)	4.4% vs. 0.4% in the WBI arm, ($p < 0.0001$)	.	96.8%	Randomised controlled equivalence trial

(continued)

Table 42.2 (continued)

Author	Study period	Follow-up (months)	Patients	Patient selection	WBI	Local recurrences (%)	DFS (%)	Overall Survival (%)	Comments
Hanna et al. [58], Barros et al. [59]	5/2004–7/2012	Median 50.7	187	>40 years (modified ≥50), IDC, size <3 cm (modified ≤2 cm), cN0	No	3.7% (4 true and 1 elsewhere)	92.5%	97.8%	Preoperative MRI; intraoperative IORT feasibility: 81.2%; Portal film to check collimator-shield alignment; eligibility modified after ASTRO/GEC-ESTRO guidelines
Cedolini et al. [60]	1/2005–12/2009	Mean 69.46	77	≥48 years, IDC, size <3 cm, N0, N1mi, free margin>5 mm	4 pts. < 48 years	2% (0% in IOERT +EBRT group)	–	98.7%	Intraoperative IORT feasibility was 95.1%; 5 pts. re-excised for positive margins
Philippson et al. [42]	2/2010–2/2012	Median 23.3	200	≥40 years, IDC and other favourable, size ≤2 cm, pN0 (SN), free margin≥1 mm, no EIC	No	0.5%	97.6%	98.9%	Risk adapted treatment volume: Field diameter at least 40 mm larger than the tumour size
Kawamura et al. [41]	12/2007–3/2010	Median 72	38	>50 years, size <2.5 cm, negative margins, cN0 since 2/2009	No	0%	100%	100% (BCSS)	Phase I/II dose escalation study Intraoperative IORT feasibility: 84,2%
Takanen et al. [32]	2/2006–1/2016	Median 62.4	758	Median age 64; T1-T2, any N, any grade, any margin status, any histology, uni- and multi-focal tumours	No	1.2% (low risk)–13.5% (high risk)	–	99% (low risk)–90.8% (high risk)	Patients' categorisation according to ASTRO and GEC-ESTRO guidelines

LR local recurrence, *BCSS* breast cancer specific survival, *OS* overall survival, *LRFS* local recurrence free survival, *DFS* disease free survival, *ASTRO* American Society for Radiation Oncology, *GEC-ESTRO* The Groupe Européen de Curiethérapie and the European Society for Radiotherapy and Oncology, *MRI* Magnetic Resonance, *WBI* whole-breast irradiation, *IOERT* intraoperative radiotherapy with electrons, *EIC* extensive intraductal component, *LVI* lymphovascular invasion; IDC: invasive ductal carcinoma

42.5 IOeRT Surgical and Technical Procedures (Boost and APBI)

IOeRT can be delivered using mobile or standard linear accelerators (Fig. 42.1) within a dedicated operating theatre. The tumour should be preoperatively localised if not clearly palpable, and the sentinel lymph node, if SLNB performed, is labelled with isotope mapping. The operating room is set up to facilitate easy access of the accelerator to the patient lying prone with the affected side's arm extended at 90°. In addition, the bed must be positioned to allow a radiation beam absorber to be inserted below the surgical table, to prevent dissemination of any radiation beyond the floor of the operating room. Surgery commences with an axillary sentinel lymph node biopsy which will be sent for frozen section pathology analysis prior to RT in order to confirm a nodal negative status. This allows for time to proceed with the surgical procedure as well as for docking the accelerator to the applicator tube. The lumpectomy is performed in a standard manner with emphasis on achieving clean resection margins and removing the breast mass down to the fascia of the pectoral muscle. Site and length of the incision, are selected in accordance to the affected breast quadrant and tumour size, respectively. Notably, in situations where the tumour is detected in a very peripheral or inferior breast site, the ability to mobilise sufficient tissue for sub dermal flaps may be compromised, and therefore may be less suitable for IOeRT. The incision should be wide enough, in order to insert tube applicators and/or shielding discs with a minimum diameter of at least 3–4 cm. After surgical tumour removal, subdermal flaps are mobilised in all directions and fixed with temporary sutures to create a tumour bed as target volume for irradiation. Considering that 90% of subclinical tumour cells are scattered within a circumferential distance of 4 cm from the macroscopic index tumour [68], the following margin-distance—for an appropriate CTV-definition could be recommended: By taking into account the amount of tumour free resections margins provided by the surgeon a CTV of least 2 cm calculated from the macroscopic tumour edge has to be considered in all directions and encompassed by the 90% isodose (boost and APBI) To achieve this from a technical standpoint, appropriate sizes of electron tubes (diameters of 3–12 cm with bevel angles of 0°, 15°, 30° and 45°) and energies (4 and 12 MeV) are essential. From a practical point of view, for APBI, a tube diameter of 4 cm larger than the macroscopic tumour diameter was reported [42]. Furthermore, the thickness of the defined tumour bed can be evaluated either by ultrasound measurement or by inserting a needle probe until it touches the protective disc at four points (12, 3, 6 and 9 o'clock) (Supplement Figs. 2, 3, and 4 [8]) and then measuring the distance with a sterile ruler.

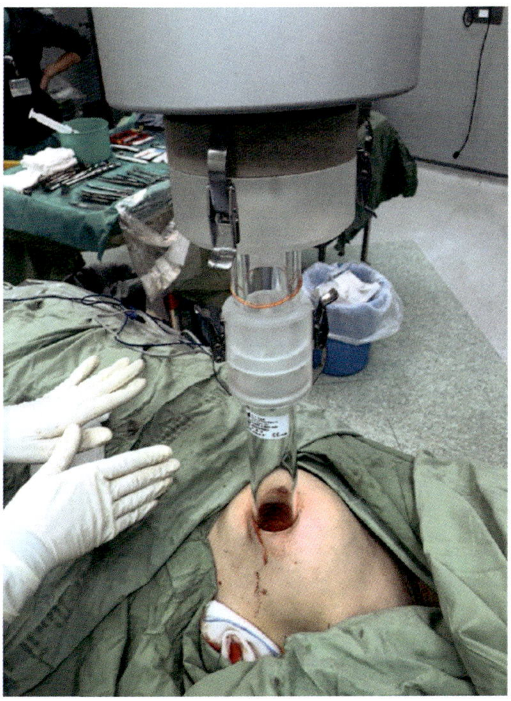

Fig. 42.1 IOeRT as "hard-docking" technique uisng LIAC HWL® accelerator, Sordina Technologies, Vicenza, Italy (as an alternative "soft-docking" technique provided by Mobetron-system®,IntraOp Medical,Sunnyvale, United States, is available)

At this point the accelerator can be moved towards the patient. If the "hard-docking" system is used, the upper part of the applicator is coupled directly to the head of the accelerator, and this connection is accomplished with three metallic clasps. Please note that the accelerator head can be rotated to allow straight docking between the upper connector and the lower applicator tube. In addition, the surgical table can also be tilted to achieve better alignment for docking. The lower tube is inserted into the wound cavity, such that it fits snugly within the incision confines, anterior to the sutured flaps. A second technical option to provide a correct positioning between the electron-tube and the accelerator's head but without a direct rigid fixation is feasible by a "soft-docking" system on the basis of laser-light alignment (Fig. 42.1) A bevelled applicator end may be selected if the curvature of the chest wall does not allow for direct coverage of the flaps. When the upper connector and the lower tube have docked, this is reinforced with another set of metallic clips and the patient is ready for treatment. The position of the beam absorber underneath the table is verified by a shield positioning device to ensure that it effectively blocks the path of radiation towards the operating room floor. At the time of RT, all operating room personnel are to leave to a safely shielded location within or outside the operating room. Delivery of radiation takes typically about 1–2 min. When the treatment is concluded, the accelerator is undocked from the applicator. The applicator tube is removed from the surgical wound, the subdermal flaps are opened, and the protective disc is also removed, which is followed by closing the incision in the usual manner [6].

To assure the safety of the procedure and staff, we recommend that prior to starting this technique, the teams need to have training and a written protocol for the preparations needed prior to each case. Each case should be documented including the depth, dose, bevel, angle, energy, and other relevant treatment features. Moreover, the operating theatre should be arranged that all of the applicators and instruments are easily available.

42.6 Physical Aspects and Dose Recommendations

In general, for boost IOeRT proceeding WBI a dose range of 9–10 Gy as 90% isodose (D90) can be recommended for all clinical risk constellations [13] with a defined dose limitation of 5 (7) Gy (D45) at bony structures, (Supplement Fig. 2). For this dose prescription, the application of a prepectoral shielding disc is not mandatory.

If IOeRT is indicated as APBI, usually single doses of 21 Gy (D90) are applied as "full-dose" RT. In this case, the rib surface is usually protected by a lead shielding (Fig. 42.1), which is temporarily fixed to the chest wall, with the plastic side up—to absorb scattered dose—and the metallic side down to the chest wall. The diameter of such a shielding disc should be selected as 1–2 cm larger than the appropriate tube sizes, in order to avoid any mismatch during the irradiation procedure.

42.7 Whole-Breast Irradiation After Definitive IORT

A particular case is when IORT was given for PBI (21 Gy), like with IOeRT, and the final pathology reports showed unexpected adverse factors, requiring re-excision or further RT, like WBI (e.g. lymph node tumour involvement)). In the latter, WBI with relative sparing of the already irradiated tissue (like an "inverse SIB") could be administered using volumetric IMRT, delivering full-dose RT to the breast while limiting the dose to the irradiated tissue (in the case of IOeRT often around 100 cc) to 70–80% of the prescribed dose.

42.8 Summary

In summary, there are different APBI methods. IOeRT is one of the techniques, when available and well-prepared, that provides sufficient covering of the target volume while sparing OARs.

Also, according to the ESTRO Task Force group for IORT [8], IOeRT as a boost enables excellent LC in several high-risk groups. IOeRT as APBI is now recommended as an alternative to WBI for highly selected low-risk breast cancer patients [8], estimated to being at least about 15–25% of all BCT cases [69].

References

1. Correa C, McGale P, Taylor C, Wang Y, Clarke M, Davies C, et al. Overview of the randomized trials of radiotherapy in ductal carcinoma in situ of the breast. J Natl Cancer Inst Monogr. 2010;2010:162–77.
2. Bartelink H, Maingon P, Poortmans P, Weltens C, Fourquet A, Jager J, et al. Whole-breast irradiation with or without a boost for patients treated with breast-conserving surgery for early breast cancer: 20-year follow-up of a randomised phase 3 trial. Lancet Oncol. 2015;16:47–56.
3. Kaiser J, Reitsamer R, Kopp P, Gaisberger C, Kopp M, Fischer T, et al. Intraoperative electron radiotherapy (IOERT) in the treatment of primary breast cancer. Breast Care (Basel, Switzerland). 2018;13:162–7.
4. Coles CE, Griffin CL, Kirby AM, Titley J, Agrawal RK, Alhasso A, et al. Partial-breast radiotherapy after breast conservation surgery for patients with early breast cancer (UK IMPORT LOW trial): 5-year results from a multicentre, randomised, controlled, phase 3, non-inferiority trial. Lancet. 2017;390:1048–60.
5. Strnad V, Ott OJ, Hildebrandt G, Kauer-Dorner D, Knauerhase H, Major T, et al. 5-year results of accelerated partial breast irradiation using sole interstitial multicatheter brachytherapy versus whole-breast irradiation with boost after breast-conserving surgery for low-risk invasive and in-situ carcinoma of the female breast: a randomised, phase 3, non-inferiority trial. Lancet. 2016;387:229–38.
6. Veronesi U, Orecchia R, Maisonneuve P, Viale G, Rotmensz N, Sangalli C, et al. Intraoperative radiotherapy versus external radiotherapy for early breast cancer (ELIOT): a randomised controlled equivalence trial. Lancet Oncol. 2013;14:1269–77.
7. Vaidya JS, Tobias JS, Baum M, Keshtgar M, Joseph D, Wenz F, et al. Intraoperative radiotherapy for breast cancer. Lancet Oncol. 2004;5:165–73.
8. Fastner G, Gaisberger C, Kaiser J, Scherer P, Ciabattoni A, Petoukhova A, et al. ESTRO IORT Task Force/ACROP recommendations for intraoperative radiation therapy with electrons (IOERT) in breast cancer. Radiother Oncol. 2020;149:150–7.
9. Vaidya JS, Bulsara M, Baum M, Wenz F, Massarut S, Pigorsch S, et al. Long term survival and local control outcomes from single dose targeted intraoperative radiotherapy during lumpectomy (TARGIT-IORT) for early breast cancer: TARGIT-A randomised clinical trial. BMJ. 2020;370:m2836.
10. Kaidar-Person O, Meattini I, Zippel D, Poortmans P. Apples and oranges: comparing partial breast irradiation techniques. Rep Pract Oncol Radiother. 2020;25:780–2.
11. Sperk E, Welzel G, Keller A, Kraus-Tiefenbacher U, Gerhardt A, Sütterlin M, et al. Late radiation toxicity after intraoperative radiotherapy (IORT) for breast cancer: results from the randomized phase III trial TARGIT a. Breast Cancer Res Treat. 2012;135:253–60.
12. Strnad V, Krug D, Sedlmayer F, Piroth MD, Budach W, Baumann R, et al. DEGRO practical guideline for partial-breast irradiation. Strahlenther Onkol. 2020;196:749–63.
13. Kaiser J, Kronberger C, Moder A, Kopp P, Wallner M, Reitsamer R, et al. Intraoperative tumor bed boost with electrons in breast cancer of clinical stages I through III: updated 10-year results. Int J Radiat Oncol Biol Phys. 2018;102:92–101.
14. Belletti B, Vaidya JS, D'Andrea S, Entschladen F, Roncadin M, Lovat F, et al. Targeted intraoperative radiotherapy impairs the stimulation of breast cancer cell proliferation and invasion caused by surgical wounding. Clin Cancer Res. 2008;14:1325–32.
15. Veldwijk MR, Neumaier C, Gerhardt A, Giordano FA, Sütterlin M, Herskind C, et al. Comparison of the proliferative and clonogenic growth capacity of wound fluid from breast cancer patients treated with and without intraoperative radiotherapy. Transl Cancer Res. 2015;4:173–7.
16. Kulcenty K, Piotrowski I, Rucinski M, Wroblewska JP, Jopek K, Murawa D, et al. Surgical wound fluids from patients with breast cancer reveal similarities in the biological response induced by intraoperative radiation therapy and the radiation-induced bystander effect-transcriptomic approach. Int J Mol Sci. 2020;21(3):1159.
17. Kulcenty K, Piotrowski I, Wróblewska JP, Wasiewicz J, Suchorska AWM. The composition of surgical wound fluids from breast cancer patients is affected by intraoperative radiotherapy treatment and depends on the molecular subtype of breast cancer. Cancers. 2019;12:11.
18. Kulcenty K, Piotrowski I, Zaleska K, Wichtowski M, Wróblewska J, Murawa D, et al. Wound fluids collected postoperatively from patients with breast cancer induce epithelial to mesenchymal transition but intraoperative radiotherapy impairs this effect by activating the radiation-induced bystander effect. Sci Rep. 2019;9:7891.
19. Kulcenty KI, Piotrowski I, Zaleska K, Murawa D, Suchorska WM. Wound fluids collected from patients after IORT treatment activates extrinsic apoptotic pathway in MCF7 breast cancer cell line. Ginekol Pol. 2018;89:175–82.
20. Piotrowski I, Kulcenty K, Murawa D, Suchorska W. Surgical wound fluids from patients treated with

intraoperative radiotherapy induce radiobiological response in breast cancer cells. Medical Oncol (Northwood, London, England). 2018;36:14.
21. Zaleska K, Przybyła A, Kulcenty K, Wichtowski M, Mackiewicz A, Suchorska W, et al. Wound fluids affect miR-21, miR-155 and miR-221 expression in breast cancer cell lines, and this effect is partially abrogated by intraoperative radiation therapy treatment. Oncol Lett. 2017;14:4029–36.
22. Fastner G, Sedlmayer F, Merz F, Deutschmann H, Reitsamer R, Menzel C, et al. IORT with electrons as boost strategy during breast conserving therapy in limited stage breast cancer: long term results of an ISIORT pooled analysis. Radiother Oncol. 2013;108:279–86.
23. Fastner G, Reitsamer R, Ziegler I, Zehentmayr F, Fussl C, Kopp P, et al. IOERT as anticipated tumor bed boost during breast-conserving surgery after neoadjuvant chemotherapy in locally advanced breast cancer--results of a case series after 5-year follow-up. Int J Cancer. 2015;136:1193–201.
24. Fastner G, Hauser-Kronberger C, Moder A, Reitsamer R, Zehentmayr F, Kopp P, et al. Survival and local control rates of triple-negative breast cancer patients treated with boost-IOERT during breast-conserving surgery. Strahlenther Onkol. 2016;192:1–7.
25. Fastner G, Reitsamer R, Urbański B, Kopp P, Murawa D, Adamczyk B, et al. Toxicity and cosmetic outcome after hypofractionated whole breast irradiation and boost-IOERT in early stage breast cancer (HIOB): first results of a prospective multicenter trial (NCT01343459). Radiother Oncol. 2020;146:136–42.
26. Leonardi MC, Maisonneuve P, Mastropasqua MG, Morra A, Lazzari R, Rotmensz N, et al. How do the ASTRO consensus statement guidelines for the application of accelerated partial breast irradiation fit intraoperative radiotherapy? A retrospective analysis of patients treated at the European Institute of Oncology. Int J Radiat Oncol Biol Phys. 2012;83:806–13.
27. Correa C, Harris EE, Leonardi MC, Smith BD, Taghian AG, Thompson AM, et al. Accelerated partial breast irradiation: executive summary for the update of an ASTRO evidence-based consensus statement. Pract Radiat Oncol. 2017;7:73–9.
28. Polgár C, Van Limbergen E, Pötter R, Kovács G, Polo A, Lyczek J, et al. Patient selection for accelerated partial-breast irradiation (APBI) after breast-conserving surgery: recommendations of the Groupe Européen de Curiethérapie-European Society for Therapeutic Radiology and Oncology (GEC-ESTRO) breast cancer working group based on clinical evidence (2009). Radiother Oncol. 2010;94:264–73.
29. Veronesi U, Orecchia R, Luini A, Galimberti V, Zurrida S, Intra M, et al. Intraoperative radiotherapy during breast conserving surgery: a study on 1,822 cases treated with electrons. Breast Cancer Res Treat. 2010;124:141–51.
30. Leonardi MC, Maisonneuve P, Mastropasqua MG, Morra A, Lazzari R, Dell'Acqua V, et al. Accelerated partial breast irradiation with intraoperative electrons: using GEC-ESTRO recommendations as guidance for patient selection. Radiother Oncol. 2013;106:21–7.
31. Maluta S, Dall'Oglio S, Marciai N, Gabbani M, Franchini Z, Pietrarota P, et al. Accelerated partial breast irradiation using only intraoperative electron radiation therapy in early stage breast cancer. Int J Radiat Oncol Biol Phys. 2012;84:e145–52.
32. Takanen S, Gambirasio A, Gritti G, Kalli M, Andreoli S, Fortunato M, et al. Breast cancer electron intraoperative radiotherapy: assessment of preoperative selection factors from a retrospective analysis of 758 patients and review of literature. Breast Cancer Res Treat. 2017;165:261–71.
33. Mussari S, Sabino Della Sala W, Busana L, Vanoni V, Eccher C, Zani B, et al. Full-dose intraoperative radiotherapy with electrons in breast cancer. First report on late toxicity and cosmetic results from a single-institution experience. Strahlenther Onkol. 2006;182:589–95.
34. Ollila DW, Klauber-DeMore N, Tesche LJ, Kuzmiak CM, Pavic D, Goyal LK, et al. Feasibility of breast preserving therapy with single fraction in situ radiotherapy delivered intraoperatively. Ann Surg Oncol. 2007;14:660–9.
35. Lemanski C, Azria D, Gourgon-Bourgade S, Gutowski M, Rouanet P, Saint-Aubert B, et al. Intraoperative radiotherapy in early-stage breast cancer: results of the Montpellier phase II trial. Int J Radiat Oncol Biol Phys. 2010;76:698–703.
36. Lemanski C, Azria D, Gourgou-Bourgade S, Ailleres N, Pastant A, Rouanet P, et al. Electrons for intraoperative radiotherapy in selected breast-cancer patients: late results of the Montpellier phase II trial. Radiat Oncol. 2013;8:191.
37. Kimple RJ, Klauber-DeMore N, Kuzmiak CM, Pavic D, Lian J, Livasy CA, et al. Cosmetic outcomes for accelerated partial breast irradiation before surgical excision of early-stage breast cancer using single-dose intraoperative radiotherapy. Int J Radiat Oncol Biol Phys. 2011;79:400–7.
38. Maluta S, Dall'Oglio S, Goer DA, Marciai N. Intraoperative electron radiotherapy (IOERT) as an alternative to standard whole breast irradiation: only for low-risk subgroups? Breast Care (Basel, Switzerland). 2014;9:102–6.
39. Leonardi MC, Ivaldi GB, Santoro L, Lazzari R, Ferrari A, Morra A, et al. Long-term side effects and cosmetic outcome in a pool of breast cancer patients treated with intraoperative radiotherapy with electrons as sole treatment. Tumori. 2012;98:324–30.
40. Osti MF, Carnevale A, Bracci S, Amanti C, Lombardi A, Maggi S, et al. Exclusive electron intraoperative radiotherapy in early-stage breast cancer: a monoinstitutional experience. Anticancer Res. 2013;33:1229–35.
41. Kawamura M, Itoh Y, Sawaki M, Kikumori T, Tsunoda N, Kamomae T, et al. A phase I/II trial of intraoperative breast radiotherapy in an Asian population: 5-year results of local control and cosmetic outcome. Radiat Oncol. 2015;10:150.

42. Philippson C, Simon S, Vandekerkhove C, Hertens D, Veys I, Noterman D, et al. Early invasive cancer and partial intraoperative electron radiation therapy of the breast: experience of the jules bordet institute. Int J Breast Cancer. 2014;2014:627352.
43. Ivaldi GB, Leonardi MC, Orecchia R, Zerini D, Morra A, Galimberti V, et al. Preliminary results of electron intraoperative therapy boost and hypofractionated external beam radiotherapy after breast-conserving surgery in premenopausal women. Int J Radiat Oncol Biol Phys. 2008;72:485–93.
44. Merrick HW 3rd, Battle JA, Padgett BJ, Dobelbower RR Jr. IORT for early breast cancer: a report on long-term results. Front Radiat Ther Oncol. 1997;31:126–30.
45. Lemanski C, Azria D, Thezenas S, Gutowski M, Saint-Aubert B, Rouanet P, et al. Intraoperative radiotherapy given as a boost for early breast cancer: long-term clinical and cosmetic results. Int J Radiat Oncol Biol Phys. 2006;64:1410–5.
46. Vaidya JS, Wenz F, Bulsara M, Tobias JS, Joseph DJ, Keshtgar M, et al. Risk-adapted targeted intraoperative radiotherapy versus whole-breast radiotherapy for breast cancer: 5-year results for local control and overall survival from the TARGIT-A randomised trial. Lancet. 2014;383:603–13.
47. Falco M, Masojć B, Rolla M, Czekała A, Pietruszewska J, Rubik-Leszczyńska A, et al. Risk factors for seroma evacuation in breast cancer patients treated with intraoperative radiotherapy. Rep Pract Oncol Radiother. 2016;21:225–31.
48. Ahn SG, Bae SJ, Lee HW, Yoon CI, Kim JW, Lee IJ, et al. A phase II study investigating the acute toxicity of targeted intraoperative radiotherapy as tumor-bed boost plus whole breast irradiation after breast-conserving surgery in Korean patients. Breast Cancer Res Treat. 2019;174:157–63.
49. Tejera Hernández AA, Vega Benítez VM, Rocca Cardenas JC, Ortega Pérez N, Rodriguez Ibarria N, Díaz Chico JC, et al. Complications and local relapse after intraoperative low-voltage X-ray radiotherapy in breast cancer. Ann Surg Treat Res. 2020;98:299–306.
50. Ebner F, Schramm A, Bottke D, Friedl TW, Wiegel T, Fink V, et al. Comparison of seroma production in breast conserving surgery with or without intraoperative radiotherapy as tumour bed boost. Arch Gynecol Obstet. 2016;294:861–6.
51. Ciabattoni A, Fortuna G, Ciccone V, Drago S, Grassi G, Consorti R, et al. IORT in breast cancer as boost: preliminary results of a pilot randomized study on use of IORT for stage I and II breast cancer. Radiother Oncol. 2004;73:35–6.
52. Van Limbergen E, van der Schueren E, Van Tongelen K. Cosmetic evaluation of breast conserving treatment for mammary cancer. 1. Proposal of a quantitative scoring system. Radiother Oncol. 1989;16:159–67.
53. Beal K, McCormick B, Zelefsky MJ, Borgen P, Fey J, Goldberg J, et al. Single-fraction intraoperative radiotherapy for breast cancer: early cosmetic results. Int J Radiat Oncol Biol Phys. 2007;69:19–24.
54. Dubois JB, Hay M, Gely S, Saint-Aubert B, Rouanet P, Pujol H. IORT in breast carcinomas. Front Radiat Ther Oncol. 1997;31:131–7.
55. Wazer DE, DiPetrillo T, Schmidt-Ullrich R, Weld L, Smith TJ, Marchant DJ, et al. Factors influencing cosmetic outcome and complication risk after conservative surgery and radiotherapy for early-stage breast carcinoma. J Clin Oncol. 1992;10:356–63.
56. Reitsamer R, Sedlmayer F, Kopp M, Kametriser G, Menzel C, Deutschmann H, et al. The Salzburg concept of intraoperative radiotherapy for breast cancer: results and considerations. Int J Cancer. 2006;118:2882–7.
57. Vanderwalde NA, Jones EL, Kimple RJ, Moore DT, Klauber-Demore N, Sartor CI, et al. Phase 2 study of pre-excision single-dose intraoperative radiation therapy for early-stage breast cancers: six-year update with application of the ASTRO accelerated partial breast irradiation consensus statement criteria. Cancer. 2013;119:1736–43.
58. Hanna SA, de Barros AC, de Andrade FE, Bevilacqua JL, Piato JR, Pelosi EL, et al. Intraoperative radiation therapy in early breast cancer using a linear accelerator outside of the operative suite: an "image-guided" approach. Int J Radiat Oncol Biol Phys. 2014;89:1015–23.
59. Barros AC, Hanna SA, Carvalho HA, Martella E, Andrade FE, Piato JR, et al. Intraoperative full-dose of partial breast irradiation with electrons delivered by standard linear accelerators for early breast cancer. Int J Breast Cancer. 2014;2014:568136.
60. Cedolini C, Bertozzi S, Seriau L, Londero AP, Concina S, Moretti E, et al. Feasibility of concervative breast surgery and intraoperative radiation therapy for early breast cancer: a single-center, open, non-randomized, prospective pilot study. Oncol Rep. 2014;31:1539–46.
61. Paudel N, Bethke KP, Wang LC, Strauss JB, Hayes JP, Donnelly ED. Impact of breast MRI in women eligible for breast conservation surgery and intra-operative radiation therapy. Surg Oncol. 2018;27:95–9.
62. Di Leo G, Trimboli RM, Benedek A, Jereczek-Fossa BA, Fossati P, Leonardi MC, et al. MR imaging for selection of patients for partial breast irradiation: a systematic review and meta-analysis. Radiology. 2015;277:716–26.
63. Smith BD, Arthur DW, Buchholz TA, Haffty BG, Hahn CA, Hardenbergh PH, et al. Accelerated partial breast irradiation consensus statement from the American Society for Radiation Oncology (ASTRO). Int J Radiat Oncol Biol Phys. 2009;74:987–1001.
64. Wöckel A, Festl J, Stüber T, Brust K, Krockenberger M, Heuschmann PU, et al. Interdisciplinary screening, diagnosis, therapy and follow-up of breast cancer. Guideline of the DGGG and the DKG (S3-Level, AWMF Registry number 032/045OL, December 2017) - Part 2 with recommendations for the therapy of primary, recurrent and advanced breast cancer. Geburtshilfe Frauenheilkd. 2018;78:1056–88.
65. Smith BD, Bellon JR, Blitzblau R, Freedman G, Haffty B, Hahn C, et al. Radiation therapy for the

whole breast: executive summary of an American Society for Radiation Oncology (ASTRO) evidence-based guideline. Pract Radiat Oncol. 2018;8:145–52.
66. Burstein HJ, Curigliano G, Loibl S, Dubsky P, Gnant M, Poortmans P, et al. Estimating the benefits of therapy for early-stage breast cancer: the St. Gallen International Consensus Guidelines for the primary therapy of early breast cancer 2019. Ann Oncol. 2019;30:1541–57.
67. Cardoso F, Kyriakides S, Ohno S, Penault-Llorca F, Poortmans P, Rubio IT, et al. Early breast cancer: ESMO Clinical Practice Guidelines for diagnosis, treatment and follow-up†. Ann Oncol. 2019;30:1194–220.
68. Holland R, Veling SH, Mravunac M, Hendriks JH. Histologic multifocality of Tis, T1-2 breast carcinomas. Implications for clinical trials of breast-conserving surgery. Cancer. 1985;56:979–90.
69. Wenz F, Sedlmayer F, Herskind C, Welzel G, Sperk E, Neumaier C, et al. Accelerated partial breast irradiation in clinical practice. Breast Care (Basel, Switzerland). 2015;10:247–52.

Part IX

Specific Disease Topics

43 Defining the Target Volumes and Radiation Doses after Primary Systemic Therapy

Shira L. Galper, Galia Jacobson, and Angel Montero

43.1 Radiation Therapy after Primary Systemic Treatment

Breast cancer is treated with a multimodal approach including the combination of systemic treatment, surgery and RT. In recent years, it has become increasingly common to administer primary systemic treatment (PST) prior to surgery and RT. An analysis based on 5,500 women included in different randomised studies comparing primary versus adjuvant systemic treatment showed equivalent results in terms of survival. However, PST could prevent mastectomy in 25% of patients unsuitable for conservative surgery upfront, while <5% of patients initially eligible for conservative surgery required a mastectomy due to disease progression under PST [1].

Currently, PST is progressively being used for patients affected by breast tumours with unfavourable prognostic factors. A pCR has been recognised as a predictive prognostic factor for survival, especially in HER2-positive (HER2+)/hormone receptor–negative and triple-negative (TNBC) breast cancer patients [2, 3].

S. L. Galper (✉) · G. Jacobson
Department of Radiation Oncology, Sheba Medical Center, Ramat Gan, Israel
e-mail: Shira.galper@sheba.health.gov.il; Galia.jacobson@sheba.health.gov.il

A. Montero
Department of Radiation Oncology, HM Hospitales, Madrid, Spain

After PST, consensus exists in favour of postoperative WBI after BCS, regardless of the pathological response. In contrast, the role of RT after PST and mastectomy requires further investigations due to the absence of high-level evidence. Since data from randomised trials answering this question is lacking, guidelines are based on available evidence coming from retrospective studies, several using data from prospective studies addressing systemic therapy questions, characterised by heterogeneity in the sample sizes, stages at diagnosis, older chemotherapy schedules and non-uniform criteria for PMRT administration. Table 43.1 summarises clinical and pathologic risk factors for LRF in various studies of PST followed by mastectomy with or without PMRT [4–27]. Identifying a subgroup of breast cancer patients with LRF risk after PST and mastectomy being low enough to avoid PMRT remains a challenge [28] (please refer to the section about omission of radiation therapy, Chap. 45).

43.2 Tumour Bed Boost after PST

After BCS, postoperative RT to the whole breast is standard treatment for most patients irrespective of PST. Tumour bed boost has been shown to be beneficial in all patients undergoing breast conserving treatment, with a similar proportional effect independent of the absolute recurrence risk. Therefore, the largest absolute benefit is

© The Author(s), under exclusive license to Springer Nature Switzerland AG 2022
O. Kaidar-Person et al. (eds.), *Breast Cancer Radiation Therapy*,
https://doi.org/10.1007/978-3-030-91170-6_43

Table 43.1 Impact of different clinical and pathological risk factors in locoregional risk relapse after primary systemic treatment and mastectomy

Author	Type of study	Objective	*N*	MFU (months)	PMRT	Factors associated with increased risk of locoregional failure
Stage IIB (cT3N0)						
Garg 2004 [4]	Retrospective	Clinical and pathologic predictors of LRF in early breast cancer after PST and mastectomy w/o PMRT	132	46	0	cT3 ($p = 0.0057$)
Huang 2004 [5]	Retrospective	Role of PMRT after PST	676	69	80%	cT3 ($p = 0.002$)
Nagar 2011 [6]	Retrospective	Role of PMRT after PST in cT3N0	162	75	73.45%	cT3 ($p < 0.001$)
Meattini 2014 [7]	Retrospective	Role of PMRT after PST	170	92.4	57.6%	cT3 ($p = 0.015$)
ypN0						
Le Scodan 2012 [9]	Retrospective	Role of PMRT in stage II-III breast cancer patients ypN0 after PST	134	91.4	58.2%	No increased LRF risk when PMRT was omitted in ypN0 ($p = 0.18$)
Shim 2014 [10]	Retrospective	Role of PMRT after PST and ypN0	151	59	69.5%	No increased LRF risk when PMRT was omitted in ypN0 ($p = 0.148$)
Rong 2017 [13]	Retrospective	Role of PMRT after PST and ypN0	185	70	48%	No increased LRF risk when PMRT was omitted in ypN0 ($p = 0.071$)
Cao 2018 [14]	Retrospective	Role of PMRT in clinical T1-2N1 after PST	88	67	85.2%	PMRT decreases LRF risk in ypN0 (94.7% vs. 72.9%, p = NR)
Krug 2019 [15]	Retrospective	Role of PMRT after PST	817	51.5	82.7%	No increased LRF risk when PMRT was omitted in ypN0 ($p = 0.06$)
Miyashita 2019 [25]	Retrospective	Role of PMRT after PST	3226	>60	30.7%	No increased LRF risk when PMRT was omitted in ypN0 ($p = 0.81$)
Zhang 2020 [16]	Retrospective	Which patients benefit from PMRT after PST	4236	NR	69%	PMRT decreased LRF risk in ypN0 ($p = 0.0003$)
Wang 2020 [18]	Retrospective	Role of PMRT h T1-2N1M0 achieving ypN0 after PST	142	72	77.5	PMRT decreased LRF risk in ypN0 ($p = 0.006$)
Molecular subtypes						
Wright 2013 [19]	Retrospective	Identify predictors of LRF after PST and PMRT	464	50.5	100%	TNBC ($p < 0.0001$)

(continued)

Table 43.1 (continued)

Author	Type of study	Objective	*N*	MFU (months)	PMRT	Factors associated with increased risk of locoregional failure
Yang (2015) [20]	Retrospective	Contribution of biologic subtype to LRF after PST, mastectomy and PMRT	233	62	100%	TNBC ($p = 0.003$)
Arsenault 2015 [21]	Retrospective	Prognostic factors for LRF in HER2+ treated with PST	157 (142 mastectomy)	43	79.6%	ER negative ($p = 0.006$)
Cho 2019 [24]	Retrospective	Role of PMRT after ypN0 following PST according to molecular subtype	189	78	58.7%	No significance of molecular subtype in LRF ($p = 0.708$)
Age						
Garg 2004 [4]	Retrospective	Clinical and pathologic predictors of LRF in early breast cancer after PST and mastectomy w/o PMRT	132	46	0	Age < 40 (p = 0.0001)
Garg 2007 [26]	Retrospective	Role of PMRT in patients <35 years old after PST	107	72	75%	PMRT decreased LRF risk in age < 35 (p = 0.001)

PMRT post-mastectomy radiation therapy, *PST* primary systemic treatment, *MFU* median follow-up, *LRF* locoregional failure, *pCR* pathologic complete response, *ER* oestrogen receptor, *PR* progesterone receptor, *TNBC* triple-negative breast cancer, *NR* not reported

reported in young women or tumours with grade 3 disease, large tumour size, presence of LVI, or TNBC breast cancer [29–31].

Data regarding the benefits of a tumour bed boost largely comes from studies where chemotherapy was offered in the adjuvant setting. There is limited data regarding the benefit or omission of a tumour bed boost in patients who have undergone PST. Cho et al. reported on boost outcomes in patients who had a pCR on the KROG12–05 and 16–16 trials [24]. 180 patients had pCR, 12.2% of whom who did not receive a primary tumour bed boost. Despite having more aggressive disease with more N2–3 disease and more patients receiving RNI, the patients who had breast boost omitted faired equally as well regarding LRC, DFS, and OS at 5 years. This study has its limitations given its unplanned analysis nature and the limited number of patients who had boost omitted preventing its generalizability. In a study including 1082 patients with HER2+ breast cancer who participated in the HERA trial and received trastuzumab, local control at 11 years was not improved with delivery of a boost (93% vs. 91%, $p = 0.33$), suggesting a lack of benefit for a tumour bed boost in this subgroup of patients [32]. At present, one should consider omitting the boost to the primary tumour bed for those who did achieve a pCR and offer a boost for those not in pCR in patients for whom one would offer a postoperative boost including young age, grade 3 disease, and large tumour size, and/or TNBC breast cancer [33–35]. (Please refer to the section about target volume definition and contouring-boost/SIB).

43.3 Regional Nodal Irradiation after PST

Lymphatic drainage of the breast includes the axillary levels 1–4 and the IMN. In the case of pre-PST cN+ disease, SLNB alone with dual tracer and harvesting >2 LN, combined or not with a targeted LN dissection of the clipped node, can be performed after a complete response on imaging with an acceptably low false negative rate of less than <10% [33, 34]. If a pre-PST cN+ patient is found to be ypN0 in this setting, no further surgery is required and RNI nodal volumes should include all axillary levels and, especially in case of centrally or medially located primary tumours, the IMN. The NSABP 51 trial investigates the omission of RNI is this clinical situation for stage IB-II breast cancer patients (https://clinicaltrials.gov/ct2/show/NCT01872975).

ALND is typically performed for anyone with positive nodes by clinical examination or imaging tests after PST. The omission of ALND with residual nodal disease only on pathological examination of the SLNB after PST is controversial and currently under investigation. The ALLIANCE A011202 trial is comparing results of ALND versus axillary RT when a positive SLNB is found after PST with a nodal cCR (https://clinicaltrials.gov/ct2/show/NCT01901094).

In the setting of ALND and ypN+, RT treatment volumes should include the breast/CW and all axillary levels including, especially in case of centrally or medially located primary tumours, the IMN. The dissected axilla, typically levels 1 and part of 2, should not be included in the treatment field, except in case of incomplete dissection, to decrease the risk of lymphoedema [35–37].

43.3.1 Boost to Positive Non-resected LN

Advances in imaging techniques, with the increasing use of PET-CT and MRI, make it possible to identify the existence of metastatic involvement in the axillary or IMN nodes. Often, these lymph node regions are not suitable for surgical resection, in which cases one can consider regional nodal irradiation with a boost to the affected nodes [38, 39].

IMN involvement is a known as a poor prognostic factor for survival in patients with breast cancer [40]. Recent studies in which contemporary imaging modalities such as CT, MRI or PET-CT were performed, showed incidences of imaging-based IMN involvement ranging between 11 and 16% in breast cancer patients with advanced nodal disease (cN2-N3) [41, 42]. In the past, radical mastectomy and IMN dissection were performed for patients with IMN involvement, with surgical IMN treatment being abandoned because of high morbidity without survival benefit [43]. In recent years, multimodal treatments including breast surgery without IMN dissection, systemic therapy, and RT have been administered for patients with IMN positive breast cancer. Data on the long-term treatment outcomes of clinically IMN-positive patients who receive RT to the involved area without surgical dissection are scarce. Moreover, whether boost irradiation is beneficial and what dose should be administered remains unknown. Few studies have assessed the clinical outcomes of IMN boost irradiation and the optimal radiation dose to radiologically apparent IMN at diagnosis in breast cancer patients (Table 43.2) [41, 44–49].

As seen on Table 43.2, with multimodal treatment, the IMN control rates are excellent, with an IMN recurrence rate of 0–11%. In these studies, boosts with 6–16 Gy have been administered to the IMN region. See Fig. 43.1 illustrating an electron-based IMN boost.

Several retrospective studies showed PST followed by surgery and postoperative RT achieving acceptable in-field regional control rates in patients with extensive nodal involvement. A higher RT boost dose was associated with worse DFS in these patients [45, 50, 51], a fact that could be explained in part because patients with a higher tumour burden in the lymph nodes are more likely to receive higher doses of RT. However, the major patterns of failure were distant metastases, suggesting that the burden of residual disease after preoperative chemotherapy is a prognostic factor for LRC, as well as for DFS [50]. While controversial, some recommend boosting the involved nodes because of the difficulty of treating persistent LN disease. In those cases, it is important to contour the OAR such as the brachial plexus and remain below tolerance levels.

Table 43.2 Summary of studies in which multimodal treatment was performed without dissection of the internal mammary lymph node for patients with breast cancer and internal mammary lymph node metastases [48]. Table adopted from open-access publication: K. Yang, H. Kim, D.H. Choi, W. Park, J.M. Noh, W.K. Cho, Optimal radiotherapy for patients with internal mammary lymph node metastasis from breast cancer, Radiation Oncology 15(1) (2020) 1–12

Authors	No. of patients	Median FU (months)	Pathologic confirmation of IMN+	Chemotherapy regimen	Median IMN RT dose (range)	IMN recurrence	5-year survival rates
Zhang et al. [16]	96	41	9%	AT-based (100%)	60.0 Gy (50.0–72.0 Gy)	11%	DFS 56%, OS 76%
Joo et al. [44]	70	51	57%	T-based (94%)	60.0 Gy (56.0–66.0 Gy)	2.9%	DFS 72%, OS 77%
Park et al. [45]	15	38	0%	T-based (73%), A based (20%)	50.4 Gy (50.4–55.8 Gy)	6.7%	DFS 67%, OS 79%
Noh et al. [46]	45	57	40%	AT (54.5%), AC (29.1%)	50.0–50.4 Gy +/− boost	0%	DFS 66%, OS 76%
Sachdev et al. [47]	25	38	Not reported	Not reported	50.4 Gy (45.0–64.4 Gy)	0%	Not reported
Yang et al. [48]	84	58	48%	T-based (100%)	62.5 Gy (50.0–66.5 Gy)	2.4%	DFS 72%, OS 81%
Kim et al. [49]	95	43	2%	Not reported	50.0 Gy +/− boost	3.2%	DFS 70%, OS 84%

FU Follow-up, *IMN+* Metastasis to the internal mammary lymph nodes, *IMN* Internal mammary node, *RT* Radiation therapy, *A* Adriamycin, *T* Taxane, *DFS* Disease-free survival, *OS* Overall survival

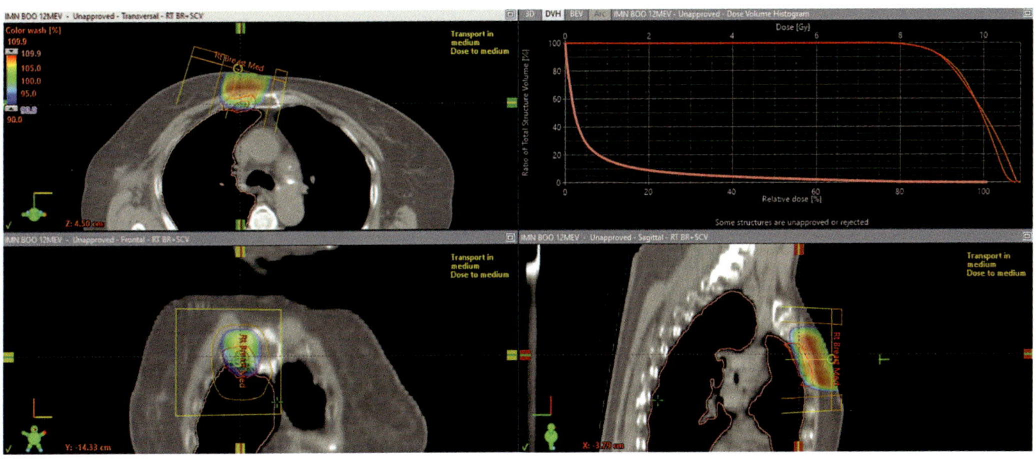

Fig. 43.1 IMN Boost following chest wall irradiation to an IMN node that was PET positive prior to PST and had a complete response on PET following PST. Treatment with a direct 12 MeV field with 10 Gy in 5 fractions

43.4 Doses

Recommended doses to the breast/CW should have an EDQ2 of 44–50 Gy. This corresponds to historical conventional fractionation doses of 45–50 Gy in 25–28 fractions (protracted regimen) and hypofractionation doses of 40–42.56 Gy in 15–16 fractions. RT to the regional nodes with protracted fractionation should be 45–50 Gy in 25–28 fractions and with hypofractionation

37.5–42.56 Gy in 15–16 fractions [52]. General recommendations regarding the tumour bed boost dose are 10–16 Gy for those receiving protracted fractionation. For those using hypofractionation, boosts of 10–12.5 Gy in 4–5 fractions have been used as well as simultaneous integrated boosts with doses up to 3–3.4 Gy per fraction [48].

A reasonable treatment approach for determining the indication and RT dose for a nodal boost would be to reimage patients after PST with PET-CT. If the originally positive unresectable node lost FDG avidity, one can consider an EDQ2 dose of 10 Gy boost. If the involved node is still FDG avid, one can consider an EQD2 dose of at least 16 Gy boost to the involved node.

43.5 Summary

Systemic therapy, once administered solely in the adjuvant setting, is progressively being offered in the preoperative setting. While postoperative RT to the breast after PST and BCS is always recommended, prospective studies are evaluating the value for RNI after PST. In this section, we presented the evidence for potential omission of PMRT in certain subsets of patients deriving from the existing literature. We also presented recommendations for target coverage after PST including when and what type of RNI should be offered.

References

1. van der Hage JH, van de Velde CC, Mieog SJ. Preoperative chemotherapy for women with operable breast cancer. Cochrane Database Syst Rev. 2007;2:CD005002.
2. Broglio KR, Quintana M, Foster M, Olinger M, McGlothlin A, Berry SM, Boileau J-F, Brezden-Masley C, Chia S, Dent S. Association of pathologic complete response to neoadjuvant therapy in HER2-positive breast cancer with long-term outcomes: a meta-analysis. JAMA Oncol. 2016;2(6):751–60.
3. Li J, Chen S, Chen C, Di G, Liu G, Wu J, Shao Z. Pathological complete response as a surrogate for relapse-free survival in patients with triple negative breast cancer after neoadjuvant chemotherapy. Oncotarget. 2017;8(11):18399.
4. Garg AK, Strom EA, McNeese MD, Buzdar AU, Hortobagyi GN, Kuerer HM, Perkins GH, Singletary SE, Hunt KK, Sahin A. T3 disease at presentation or pathologic involvement of four or more lymph nodes predict for locoregional recurrence in stage II breast cancer treated with neoadjuvant chemotherapy and mastectomy without radiotherapy. Int J Radiat Oncol Biol Phys. 2004;59(1):138–45.
5. Huang EH, Tucker SL, Strom EA, McNeese MD, Kuerer HM, Buzdar AU, Valero V, Perkins GH, Schechter NR, Hunt KK. Postmastectomy radiation improves local-regional control and survival for selected patients with locally advanced breast cancer treated with neoadjuvant chemotherapy and mastectomy. J Clin Oncol. 2004;22(23):4691–9.
6. Nagar H, Mittendorf EA, Strom EA, Perkins GH, Oh JL, Tereffe W, Woodward WA, Gonzalez-Angulo AM, Hunt KK, Buchholz TA. Local-regional recurrence with and without radiation therapy after neoadjuvant chemotherapy and mastectomy for clinically staged T3N0 breast cancer. Int J Radiat Oncol Biol Phys. 2011;81(3):782–7.
7. Meattini I, Cecchini S, Di Cataldo V, Saieva C, Francolini G, Scotti V, Bonomo P, Mangoni M, Greto D, Nori J. Postmastectomy radiotherapy for locally advanced breast cancer receiving neoadjuvant chemotherapy. Biomed Res Int. 2014;2014:719175.
8. Liu J, Mao K, Jiang S, Jiang W, Chen K, Kim BY, Liu Q, Jacobs LK. The role of postmastectomy radiotherapy in clinically node-positive, stage II-III breast cancer patients with pathological negative nodes after neoadjuvant chemotherapy: an analysis from the NCDB. Oncotarget. 2016;7(17):24848.
9. Le Scodan R, Selz J, Stevens D, Bollet MA, de la Lande B, Daveau C, Lerebours F, Labib A, Bruant S. Radiotherapy for stage II and stage III breast cancer patients with negative lymph nodes after preoperative chemotherapy and mastectomy. Int J Radiat Oncol Biol Phys. 2012;82(1):e1–7.
10. Shim SJ, Park W, Huh SJ, Choi DH, Shin KH, Lee NK, Suh C-O, Keum KC, Kim YB, Do Ahn S. The role of postmastectomy radiation therapy after neoadjuvant chemotherapy in clinical stage II-III breast cancer patients with pN0: a multicenter, retrospective study (KROG 12-05). Int J Radiat Oncol Biol Phys. 2014;88(1):65–72.
11. Rusthoven C, Rabinovitch R, Jones B, Koshy M, Amini A, Yeh N, Jackson M, Fisher C. The impact of postmastectomy and regional nodal radiation after neoadjuvant chemotherapy for clinically lymph node-positive breast cancer: a National Cancer Database (NCDB) analysis. Ann Oncol. 2016;27(5):818–27.
12. Kantor O, Pesce C, Singh P, Miller M, Tseng J, Wang CH, Winchester DJ, Yao K. Post-mastectomy radiation therapy and overall survival after neoadjuvant chemotherapy. J Surg Oncol. 2017;115(6):668–76.
13. Rong Q, Wang S, Tang Y, Jin J, Song Y, Wang W, Liu Y, Fang H, Ren H, Liu X. The role of postmastectomy radiotherapy in clinical T1-3N1M0 breast cancer patients with pathological negative lymph nodes

after neoadjuvant chemotherapy and mastectomy. Zhonghua Zhong liu za zhi [Chinese Journal of Oncology]. 2017;39(6):445–52.
14. Cao L, Ou D, Shen K-W, Cai G, Cai R, Xu F, Zhao S-G, Xu C, Adedjouma NG, Kirova Y. Outcome of postmastectomy radiotherapy after primary systemic treatment in patients with clinical T1-2N1 breast cancer. Cancer/Radiothérapie. 2018;22(1):38–44.
15. Krug D, Lederer B, Seither F, Nekljudova V, Ataseven B, Blohmer J-U, Costa SD, Denkert C, Ditsch N, Gerber B. Post-mastectomy radiotherapy after neoadjuvant chemotherapy in breast cancer: a pooled retrospective analysis of three prospective randomized trials. Ann Surg Oncol. 2019;26(12):3892–901.
16. Zhang J, Lu C-Y, Chen C-H, Chen H-M, Wu S-Y. Effect of pathologic stages on postmastectomy radiation therapy in breast cancer receiving neoadjuvant chemotherapy and total mastectomy: a cancer database analysis. Breast. 2020;54:70–8.
17. Shah R, Hunter-Smith AE, Botes A, Rayter Z. Does post mastectomy radiotherapy reduce loco-regional recurrence rates in all clinical stages of breast cancer following a complete pathological response to neoadjuvant chemotherapy? A systematic review and meta-analysis of the literature. Breast Cancer Manag. 2020;9:2.
18. Wang Q, Zhao J, Han X, Er P, Meng X, Shi J, Sun H, Zhu J, Zhu L, Wu S. Is there a role for postmastectomy radiotherapy for T1-2N1 breast cancers with node-positive pathology after patients become node-negative pathology following neoadjuvant chemotherapy? Front Oncol. 2020;10:892.
19. Wright JL, Takita C, Reis IM, Zhao W, Saigal K, Wolfson A, Markoe A, Moller M, Hurley J. Predictors of locoregional outcome in patients receiving neoadjuvant therapy and postmastectomy radiation. Cancer. 2013;119(1):16–25.
20. Yang TJ, Morrow M, Modi S, Zhang Z, Krause K, Siu C, McCormick B, Powell SN, Ho AY. The effect of molecular subtype and residual disease on locoregional recurrence in breast cancer patients treated with neoadjuvant chemotherapy and postmastectomy radiation. Ann Surg Oncol. 2015;22(3):495–501.
21. Arsenault D, Hurley J, Takita C, Reis IM, Zhao W, Rodgers S, Wright JL. Predictors of locoregional outcome in HER2-overexpressing breast cancer treated with neoadjuvant chemotherapy. Am J Clin Oncol. 2015;38(4):348–52.
22. Chen X, Xia F, Luo J, Ma J, Yang Z, Zhang L, Feng Y, Shao Z, Yu X, Guo X. Postmastectomy radiotherapy reduces locoregional and disease recurrence in patients with stage ii–iii triple-negative breast cancer treated with neoadjuvant chemotherapy and mastectomy. Onco Targets Ther. 2018;11:1973.
23. Fowble B, Jairam AK, Wang F, Peled A, Alvarado M, Ewing C, Esserman L, Park C, Lazar A. Indications for postmastectomy radiation after neoadjuvant chemotherapy in ypN0 and ypN1-3 axillary node-positive women. Clin Breast Cancer. 2018;18(1):e107–13.
24. Cho WK, Park W, Choi DH, Kim YB, Kim JH, Kim SS, Kim K, Kim JH, Ahn S-J, Lee SY. The benefit of post-mastectomy radiotherapy in ypN0 patients after neoadjuvant chemotherapy according to molecular subtypes. J Breast Cancer. 2019;22(2):285–96.
25. Miyashita M, Niikura N, Kumamaru H, Miyata H, Iwamoto T, Kawai M, Anan K, Hayashi N, Aogi K, Ishida T. Role of postmastectomy radiotherapy after neoadjuvant chemotherapy in breast cancer patients: A study from the Japanese breast cancer registry. Ann Surg Oncol. 2019;26(8):2475–85.
26. Garg AK, Oh JL, Oswald MJ, Huang E, Strom EA, Perkins GH, Woodward WA, Yu TK, Tereffe W, Meric-Bernstam F. Effect of postmastectomy radiotherapy in patients< 35 years old with stage II-III breast cancer treated with doxorubicin-based neoadjuvant chemotherapy and mastectomy. Int J Radiat Oncol Biol Phys. 2007;69(5):1478–83.
27. Fowble BL, Einck JP, Kim DN, McCloskey S, Mayadev J, Yashar C, Chen SL, Hwang ES, A.B.H. Network, role of postmastectomy radiation after neoadjuvant chemotherapy in stage II-III breast cancer. Int J Radiat Oncol Biol Phys. 2012;83(2):494–503.
28. Montero Á, Ciérvide R, Poortmans P. When can we avoid postmastectomy radiation following primary systemic therapy? Curr Oncol Rep. 2019;21(11):1–10.
29. Romestaing P, Lehingue Y, Carrie C, Coquard R, Montbarbon X, Ardiet J-M, Mamelle N, Gerard J-P. Role of a 10-Gy boost in the conservative treatment of early breast cancer: results of a randomized clinical trial in Lyon, France. J Clin Oncol. 1997;15(3):963–8.
30. Bartelink H, Horiot J-C, Poortmans P, Struikmans H, Van den Bogaert W, Barillot I, Fourquet A, Borger J, Jager J, Hoogenraad W. Recurrence rates after treatment of breast cancer with standard radiotherapy with or without additional radiation. N Engl J Med. 2001;345(19):1378–87.
31. Jones HA, Antonini N, Hart A, Peterse JL, Horiot J-C, Collin F, Poortmans PM, Oei SB, Collette L, Struikmans H. Impact of pathological characteristics on local relapse after breast-conserving therapy: a subgroup analysis of the EORTC boost versus no boost trial. J Clin Oncol. 2009;27(30):4939–47.
32. Abi Jaoude J, Kayali M, de Azambuja E, Makki M, Tamim H, Tfayli A, El Saghir N, Geara F, Piccart M, Poortmans P. De-intensifying radiation therapy in HER-2 positive breast cancer: to boost or not to boost? Int J Radiat Oncolgy Biol Phys. 2020;108(4):1040–6.
33. Kuehn T, Bauerfeind I, Fehm T, Fleige B, Hausschild M, Helms G, Lebeau A, Liedtke C, von Minckwitz G, Nekljudova V. Sentinel-lymph-node biopsy in patients with breast cancer before and after neoadjuvant chemotherapy (SENTINA): a prospective, multicentre cohort study. Lancet Oncol. 2013;14(7):609–18.
34. Caudle AS, Yang WT, Krishnamurthy S, Mittendorf EA, Black DM, Gilcrease MZ, Bedrosian I, Hobbs BP, DeSnyder SM, Hwang RF. Improved axillary evaluation following neoadjuvant therapy for patients with node-positive breast cancer using selective eval-

uation of clipped nodes: implementation of targeted axillary dissection. J Clin Oncol. 2016;34(10):1072.
35. Boughey JC, Suman VJ, Mittendorf EA, Ahrendt GM, Wilke LG, Taback B, Leitch AM, Kuerer HM, Bowling M, Flippo-Morton TS. Sentinel lymph node surgery after neoadjuvant chemotherapy in patients with node-positive breast cancer: the ACOSOG Z1071 (Alliance) clinical trial. JAMA. 2013;310(14):1455–61.
36. Ling DC, Iarrobino NA, Champ CE, Soran A, Beriwal S. Regional recurrence rates with or without complete axillary dissection for breast cancer patients with node-positive disease on sentinel lymph node biopsy after neoadjuvant chemotherapy. Adv Radiat Oncol. 2020;5(2):163–70.
37. Riogi B, Sripadam R, Barker D, Harris O, Innes H, Chagla L. Management of the axilla following neoadjuvant chemotherapy for breast cancer-A change in practice. Surgeon. 2020;19:1–7.
38. Davidson T, Ben-David M, Galper S, Haskin T, Howes M, Scaife R, Kanana N, Amit U, Weizman N, Chikman B. Use of 18F-FDG PET-CT imaging to determine internal mammary lymph node location for radiation therapy treatment planning in breast cancer patients. Pract Radiat Oncol. 2017;7(6):373–81.
39. Wu S-G, Sun J-Y, Zhou J, Li F-Y, Lin Q, Lin H-X, He Z-Y. The value of radiotherapy in breast cancer patients with isolated ipsilateral supraclavicular lymph node metastasis without distant metastases at diagnosis: a retrospective analysis of Chinese patients. Onco Targets Ther. 2014;7:281.
40. Sugg SL, Ferguson DJ, Posner MC, Heimann R. Should internal mammary nodes be sampled in the sentinel lymph node era? Ann Surg Oncol. 2000;7(3):188–92.
41. Zhang Y-J, Oh JL, Whitman GJ, Iyengar P, Yu T-K, Tereffe W, Woodward WA, Perkins G, Buchholz TA, Strom EA. Clinically apparent internal mammary nodal metastasis in patients with advanced breast cancer: incidence and local control. Int J Radiat Oncol Biol Phys. 2010;77(4):1113–9.
42. Jochelson MS, Lebron L, Jacobs SS, Zheng J, Moskowitz CS, Powell SN, Sacchini V, Ulaner GA, Morris EA, Dershaw DD. Detection of internal mammary adenopathy in patients with breast cancer by PET/CT and MRI. Am J Roentgenol. 2015;205(4):899–904.
43. Lacour J, Le M, Caceres E, Koszarowski T, Veronesi U, Hill C. Radical mastectomy versus radical mastectomy plus internal mammary dissection. Ten year results of an international cooperative trial in breast cancer. Cancer. 1983;51(10):1941–3.
44. Joo JH, Kim SS, Ahn S-D, Choi EK, Jung JH, Jeong Y, Ahn SH, Son BH, Lee JW, Kim HJ. Impact of pathologic diagnosis of internal mammary lymph node metastasis in clinical N2b and N3b breast cancer patients. Breast Cancer Res Treat. 2017;166(2):511–8.
45. Park HJ, Shin KH, Cho KH, Park IH, Lee KS, Ro J, Jung S-Y, Lee S, Kim SW, Kang H-S. Outcomes of positron emission tomography–staged clinical N3 breast cancer treated with neoadjuvant chemotherapy, surgery, and radiotherapy. Int J Radiat Oncol Biol Phys. 2011;81(5):e689–95.
46. Noh JM, Kim KH, Park W, Suh CO, Huh SJ, Choi DH, Keum KC, Kim YB. Prognostic significance of nodal involvement region in clinical stage IIIc breast cancer patients who received primary systemic treatment, surgery, and radiotherapy. Breast. 2015;24(5):637–41.
47. Sachdev S, Goodman CR, Neuschler E, Kalakota K, Cutright D, Donnelly ED, Hayes JP, Prescott AE, Mirabelli G, Strauss JB. Radiotherapy of MRI-detected involved internal mammary lymph nodes in breast cancer. Radiat Oncol. 2017;12(1):1–7.
48. Yang K, Kim H, Choi DH, Park W, Noh JM, Cho WK. Optimal radiotherapy for patients with internal mammary lymph node metastasis from breast cancer. Radiat Oncol. 2020;15(1):1–12.
49. Kim J, Chang JS, Choi SH, Kim YB, Keum KC, Suh C-O, Yang G, Cho Y, Kim JW, Lee IJ. Radiotherapy for initial clinically positive internal mammary nodes in breast cancer. Radiat Oncol J. 2019;37(2):91.
50. Huang EH, Strom EA, Valero V, Fornage B, Perkins GH, Oh JL, Yu T-K, Tereffe W, Woodward WA, Hunt KK. Locoregional treatment outcomes for breast cancer patients with ipsilateral supraclavicular metastases at diagnosis. Int J Radiat Oncol Biol Phys. 2007;67(2):490–6.
51. Kim K, Jeong Y, Shin KH, Kim JH, Do Ahn S, Kim SS, Suh C-O, Kim YB, Choi DH, Park W. Impact of regional nodal irradiation for breast cancer patients with supraclavicular and/or internal mammary lymph node involvement: a multicenter, retrospective study (KROG 16-14). Cancer Res Treat. 2019;51(4):1500.
52. Koulis TA, Phan T, Olivotto IA. Hypofractionated whole breast radiotherapy: current perspectives. Breast Cancer: Targets and Therapy. 2015;7:363.

Lymph Nodes Volumes

44

Giulio Francolini, Sileida Oliveros, and David Dodwell

44.1 Background

In 2005, data from 8,500 patients treated with mastectomy plus axillary lymph node dissection (ALND) for node positive (LN+) early breast cancer were included in an EBCTCG meta-analysis of post-mastectomy irradiation (PMRT) to the chest wall and regional lymph nodes vs no PMRT. Absolute reductions of 17%, 5.4%, and 4.4% in locoregional recurrence, 15-year breast cancer mortality, and overall mortality respectively were reported [1]. However, the effects of PMRT in patients with 1–3 positive lymph nodes after ALND were not separately reported. A further EBCTCG meta-analysis involving 8,135 women, of which 3,786 women had a mastectomy with at least ALND up to level 2 with zero (N0), 1–3, or ≥4 positive nodes, was performed. Patients were enrolled in trials assessing locoregional RT, including the chest wall and the axillary and internal mammary nodes (IMNs). Improvements in locoregional recurrence and breast cancer mortality were identified for women with positive nodes. These effects were independent of the number of involved nodes and of the use of adjuvant chemotherapy [2].

G. Francolini
Radiation Oncology Unit, Oncology Department, Azienda Ospedaliero-Universitaria Careggi, Florence, Italy

S. Oliveros
Oxford University Hospitals, Oxford, UK
e-mail: Sileida.Oliveros@ouh.nhs.uk

D. Dodwell (✉)
Nuffield Department of Population Health, University of Oxford, Oxford, UK
e-mail: david.dodwell@ndph.ox.ac.uk

44.2 Evidence Base for Regional Nodal Irradiation (RNI)

Prior to the publication of the four key studies described below, evidence for RNI was derived from the EBCTCG meta-analysis and a large number of retrospective studies. However, due to fear for late morbidity and lacking evidence of the contribution of the individual lymph node areas, clinical practice varied broadly.

The EORTC 22922 trial enrolled 4,004 patients with stage I-III early breast cancer, either centrally/medially located (irrespective of axillary involvement) or externally located with axillary involvement. After BCS or mastectomy, patients were randomised to receive whole-breast or chest wall irradiation with or without RNI. A modest but statistically significant improvement in breast cancer mortality and any breast cancer recurrence but not in overall survival after RNI was seen [3].

The MA.20 trial enrolled 1,832 patients with node-positive or high-risk node negative early breast cancer treated with BCS and adjuvant systemic therapy. Patients were randomised to undergo whole breast irradiation with or without

© The Author(s), under exclusive license to Springer Nature Switzerland AG 2022
O. Kaidar-Person et al. (eds.), *Breast Cancer Radiation Therapy*,
https://doi.org/10.1007/978-3-030-91170-6_44

RNI. After 10 years of follow-up, RNI was reported to improve DFS, but there was no significant impact on overall survival (OS) [4].

In a randomised controlled trial of IMN-RT, Hennequin and colleagues did not demonstrate an OS benefit for IMN-RT in trial of 1,334 patients. This study was not powered to exclude a modest benefit of IMN-RT and breast cancer mortality and recurrence outcomes were not available [5].

A prospective population-based cohort study was conducted in Denmark between 2003 and 2007. Patients with node-positive early breast cancer received IMN-RT if they had right-sided breast cancer but not if they had left sided breast cancer. After a median follow-up of 9 years OS was significantly better in patients with right-sided cancer who received IMN-RT (HR 0.82; $p = 0.005$) [6].

44.3 Target Volume Selection in RNI

In 2013/14 the EORTC carried out the NORA survey, to explore patterns of practice among affiliated centres.

- After BCS and ALND in patients with macrometastatic nodal involvement, 13%, 65%, and 2% of centres recommended target coverage of IMN, infra/supraclavicular (axilla levels 3–4), and axillary (level 1–2) nodes, respectively, while this was 15%, 65%, and 57%, respectively, after SLNB without ALND.
- After mastectomy and ALND, axillary levels 3–4 nodes in pN0 (i+), pN (mi), and LN+ were treated in 6%, 63%, and 61% of centres, respectively, and extracapsular extension was considered the most important factor to recommend axillary nodal RT. Moreover, axillary nodes were treated in 40% of centres in patients with ≥3 positive nodes, regardless of the number of examined nodes [7].

As evidence for RNI derives mostly from RCTs involving the irradiation of both the IMN and axillary nodes it is reasonable to state that RNI should in most circumstances include all nodal volumes, only excluding the part removed by ALND [8] (Table 44.1).

44.4 Level 1–2 of the Axilla

Close liaison between radiology, surgery and oncology services is needed to manage the lower part of the axilla, with the aim of obtaining prognostic information while minimising the risk of recurrence and treatment-related morbidity. The use of SLNB for the clinically and radiologically node negative axilla is now the key to modern axillary management.

If the SLNB is pathologically negative, positive with isolated tumour cells (ITCs) or with micrometastatic disease (<2 mms) only, no further axillary treatment is required.

After an SLNB for a macrometastasis in 1–2 nodes, then there are a number of reasonable options including observation, ALND or axillary irradiation. RCTs including the AMAROS and OTOASAR studies and the older Edinburgh trials have confirmed that in the clinically node negative (cN0) axilla with a positive SLNB or axillary node sample, axillary irradiation is as effective in preventing recurrence as ALND and has a significantly lower risk of lymphoedema [13–16]. As a consequence, axillary RT in these circumstances is increasingly preferred.

If ≥3 nodes are involved with macrometastatic disease, then ALND is often still recommended. Following ALND the operated axilla should not be irradiated routinely but this could be considered if there is macroscopic residual disease as defined by the surgeon, the pathologist or on the basis of imaging.

44.5 Patient Selection and Guidelines

Currently patient selection for RNI is dominated by traditional prognostic factors (stage and grade) and site of tumour within the breast as central/medial tumours are more likely to be associated with involved IMNs. An interim analysis of the

Table 44.1 Patient selection for RNI in available international guidelines

International Consensus Guideline	4 or more positive axillary nodes (usually after ALND)	1–3 positive axillary nodes (after ALND or SLNB)	N0—central or medially located tumours or other high risk factors
ESMO [9][a]	Comprehensive nodal RT L1–4, IMN	Comprehensive nodal RT L1–4, IMN	Not routinely recommended
Royal College of Radiologists (UK) [10]	Should be considered, particularly N2-N3 (>3 + LNs) disease	Should be considered, particularly central/medial tumours	Considered for T4N0 Not routinely recommended
NCCN [11]	Recommended RNI including SCF, infraclavicular (IFC), IMN and any part of the axillary bed at risk	Strongly considered RNI including SCF, infraclavicular (IFC), IMN and any part of the axillary bed at risk	After mastectomy - Tumours >5 cm or margin positive: Consider RT to CW +/– RNI. Tumour ≤5 cm and negative margins but <1 mm: Consider RT to CW +/– RNI in high risk features Tumour ≤5 cm and negative margins >1 mm - RT not recommended After BCS - high risk features
ASCO 2016 [12][b]	Recommended RNI (SCF, IFC, axillary apical node and IMN	Recommended RNI (SCF, IFC, axillary apical node and IMN, even in T1-T2 disease	Not routinely recommended

In node positive axillary disease after ALND, RNI is indicated but excluding the resected part of the axilla which should not be irradiated as risk of lymphoedema after ANC and axillary RT increases up to 40%

SCF supraclavicular region (axilla level 4), *IFC* intraclavicular region (axilla level 3), *IMN* internal mammary node chain

PMRT reduces the risks of LRF, any recurrence, and breast cancer mortality for patients with T1–2 breast cancer with one to three positive axillary nodes after ALND

[a]ESMO guidelines [9]: After SLNB without subsequent ALND, comprehensive RNI is recommended for patients with involved lymph nodes and it is difficult to discriminate which component of the RNI is more important to irradiate. After ALND, routine axillary irradiation should not be given to the operated part of the axilla

[b]ASCO guidelines: the prognostic and therapeutic impacts of a particular number of positive nodes may be different in patients who undergo SLNB without ALND than in those who undergo ALND, because the total number of positive nodes may only be inferred if only SLNB is performed

EBCTCG meta-analysis of RNI demonstrated a greater absolute benefit of RNI according to the burden of pathological axillary nodal involvement although the proportional effects of RNI were not significantly different between groups defined by the degree of nodal involvement (pN0, pN1-3, and pN4+) or site of tumour within the breast [17].

Table 44.1 summarises RNI recommendations from different international guidelines. See also the sections about breast and lymph node anatomy and target volume delineation (Chaps. 11 and 19).

An approach of recommending RNI based on number of involved lymph nodes cannot be applied to patients in whom ALND has not been performed and it is an increasingly common practice to advise axillary RT or no further axillary treatment after a SLNB has identified macrometastatic (≥2 mms) pN-positive disease [13, 18]. The use of nomograms and predictive tools to predict the risk of further nodal involvement could inform decision-making concerning RNI if ALND is not performed [19].

Tailored approaches based on molecular characterisation in this population are currently the object of ongoing trials and are not ready to be incorporated in current practice [20].

44.6 Dose Fractionation

Moderate hypofractionation schedules (15–16 fractions of 2.6–2.7 Gy/fraction) are recommended for routine postoperative RT of most if not all breast cancer patients. The very recent adoption of a daily, 5-fraction schedule of 26 Gy for whole breast and chest wall irradiation [21]

has led to consideration of this schedule in RNI and the result of the FAST Forward nodal subgroup study results are awaited.

44.7 RNI after Primary Systemic Therapy (PST)

There is no robust prospective evidence to inform decisions about RNI after PST. Many guidelines urge caution when making decisions about RT tailored by response to PST and decisions based on clinical and radiological staging and histological confirmation of axillary nodal status prior to systemic therapy are commonly used. Trials of postoperative locoregional radiation therapy after PST are a priority (see section on RT after PST, Chap. 43).

44.8 Clinical Target Volume (CTV) Delineation

Historically, anatomic boundaries have been used to define two-dimensional fields aimed to cover regional nodal volumes. Up to date delineation of target volumes is a critical part of contemporary RT planning workflow. For this reason, ESTRO and RTOG [22, 23] developed contouring guidelines aimed to define nodal CTVs for modern 3D volume-based conformal radiation therapy. An overview of suggested anatomical descriptions/boundaries for nodal CTV definition in the ESTRO and RTOG atlases is discussed in section on delineation (Chap. 19).

44.9 RNI Related Toxicity

The EBCTCG reported non-breast cancer mortality risks from 28 trials of PMRT. The odds ratio for non-breast cancer death was 1.54 in trials including IMN irradiation vs 1.22 in trials without [24]. This finding, although not a direct finding from randomised evidence naturally heightened concerns about cardiac toxicity. Direct randomised evidence is however preferable to quantify toxicity. In the EORTC 22922/10925 trial, there was a significant increase in pulmonary fibrosis (4.4% vs 1.7%), but no increase in cardiac events. With current RT, allowing to adapt the lung constraints based on correct delineation of lymph nodes CTV and chest wall/breast CTV, these rates are expected to be lower. The MA.20 trial reported an increase in acute radiation dermatitis (49.5% vs 40.1%), pneumonitis (1.2% vs 0.2%), lymphoedema (6.9% vs 4.5%), telangiectasia (8.4% vs 4.5%), and subcutaneous fibrosis (4.1% vs 2%) with RNI. Risks of brachial neuropathy and cardiac disease were equivalent [4]. Of note, no increased rates of lymphoedema were seen in the EORTC trial, likely because irradiation of the axillary part removed by ALND was explicitly not allowed. The AMAROS trial of ALND vs. axillary radiation therapy incorporated an estimation of lymphoedema and shoulder mobility. At 5 years the risk of lymphoedema was significantly lower in patients treated by axillary radiation therapy. Shoulder mobility was not significantly different between treatment groups but within the quality-of-life assessment shoulder abduction was more difficult in patients who had axillary radiation therapy. This was of borderline significance. The ESTRO guidelines advise shielding of the humeral head and this may further reduce the risk of impaired shoulder movements.

44.10 Summary

Further follow-up of the trials of RNI and patient-level meta-analysis will elaborate on the therapeutic index of RNI. Modern RT techniques including Volumetric Modulated Arc Therapy-VMAT and breath hold techniques, can significantly reduce irradiation of organs at risk and have the potential to reduce the risk of toxicity from modern RNI providing target volume irradiation is not compromised [25, 26]. Given all these factors it is likely that modern RNI carries a very low risk of serious toxicity. Recent trials confirm an acceptable toxicity profile for RNI compared to the benefits that this treatment provides.

References

1. Clarke M, Collins R, Darby S, Davies C, Elphinstone P, Evans V, Godwin J, Gray R, Hicks C, James S, MacKinnon E, McGale P, McHugh T, Peto R, Taylor C, Wang Y, Early Breast Cancer Trialists' Collaborative Group (EBCTCG). Effects of radiotherapy and of differences in the extent of surgery for early breast cancer on local recurrence and 15-year survival: an overview of the randomised trials. Lancet. 2005;366(9503):2087–106.
2. EBCTCG (Early Breast Cancer Trialists' Collaborative Group), McGale P, Taylor C, Correa C, Cutter D, Duane F, Ewertz M, Gray R, Mannu G, Peto R, Whelan T, Wang Y, Wang Z, Darby S. Effect of radiotherapy after mastectomy and axillary surgery on 10-year recurrence and 20-year breast cancer mortality: meta-analysis of individual patient data for 8135 women in 22 randomised trials. Lancet. 2014;383(9935):2127–35.
3. Poortmans PM, Weltens C, Fortpied C, Kirkove C, Peignaux-Casasnovas K, Budach V, van der Leij F, Vonk E, Weidner N, Rivera S, van Tienhoven G, Fourquet A, Noel G, Valli M, Guckenberger M, Koiter E, Racadot S, Abdah-Bortnyak R, Van Limbergen EF, Engelen A, De Brouwer P, Struikmans H, Bartelink H, European Organisation for Research and Treatment of Cancer Radiation Oncology and Breast Cancer Groups. Internal mammary and medial supraclavicular lymph node chain irradiation in stage I-III breast cancer (EORTC 22922/10925): 15-year results of a randomised, phase 3 trial. Lancet Oncol. 2020;21(12):1602–10.
4. Whelan TJ, Olivotto IA, Parulekar WR, Ackerman I, Chua BH, Nabid A, Vallis KA, White JR, Rousseau P, Fortin A, Pierce LJ, Manchul L, Chafe S, Nolan MC, Craighead P, Bowen J, McCready DR, Pritchard KI, Gelmon K, Murray Y, Chapman JA, Chen BE. Levine MN; MA.20 study investigators. Regional nodal irradiation in early-stage breast cancer. N Engl J Med. 2015;373(4):307–16.
5. Hennequin C, Bossard N, Servagi-Vernat S, Maingon P, Dubois JB, Datchary J, Carrie C, Roullet B, Suchaud JP, Teissier E, Lucardi A. Ten-year survival results of a randomized trial of irradiation of internal mammary nodes after mastectomy. Int J Radiat Oncol Biol Phys. 2013;86(5):860–6.
6. Thorsen LB, Offersen BV, DanøH BM, Jensen I, Pedersen AN, Zimmermann SJ, Brodersen HJ, Overgaard M, Overgaard J. DBCG-IMN: a population-based cohort study on the effect of internal mammary node irradiation in early node-positive breast cancer. J Clin Oncol. 2016;34(4):314–20.
7. Belkacemi Y, Kaidar-Person O, Poortmans P, Ozsahin M, Valli MC, Russell N, Kunkler I, Hermans J, Kuten A, van Tienhoven G, Westenberg H, Breast Working Party of the EORTC Radiation Oncology Group (ROG). Patterns of practice of regional nodal irradiation in breast cancer: results of the European Organization for Research and Treatment of cancer (EORTC) NOdal radiotherapy (NORA) survey. Ann Oncol. 2015;26(3):529–35.
8. Haussmann J, Budach W, Tamaskovics B, Bölke E, Corradini S, Djiepmo-Njanang FJ, Kammers K, Matuschek C. Which target volume should be considered when irradiating the regional nodes in breast cancer? Results of a network-meta-analysis. Radiat Oncol. 2019;14(1):102.
9. Cardoso F, Kyriakides S, Ohno S, Penault-Llorca F, Poortmans P, Rubio IT, Zackrisson S, Senkus E, ESMO Guidelines Committee. Early breast cancer: ESMO clinical practice guidelines for diagnosis, treatment and follow-up. Ann Oncol. 2019;30(10):1674.
10. Royal College of Radiologists (UK) (n.d.). https://www.rcr.ac.uk/clinical-oncology/service-delivery/postoperative-radiotherapy-breast-cancer-uk-consensus-statements.
11. NCCN (2022). https://www.nccn.org/professionals/physician_gls/pdf/breast.pdf.
12. Recht A, Comen EA, Fine RE, Fleming GF, Hardenbergh PH, Ho AY, Hudis CA, Hwang ES, Kirshner JJ, Morrow M, Salerno KE. Postmastectomy radiotherapy: an american society of clinical oncology, american society for radiation oncology, and society of surgical oncology focused guideline update. Pract Radiat Oncol. 2016;6(6):e219–34.
13. Donker M, van Tienhoven G, Straver ME, Meijnen P, van de Velde CJ, Mansel RE, Cataliotti L, Westenberg AH, Klinkenbijl JH, Orzalesi L, Bouma WH. Radiotherapy or surgery of the axilla after a positive sentinel node in breast cancer (EORTC 10981-22023 AMAROS): a randomised, multicentre, open-label, phase 3 non-inferiority trial. Lancet Oncol. 2014;15(12):1303–10.
14. Sávolt Á, Péley G, Polgár C, Udvarhelyi N, Rubovszky G, Kovacs E, Győrffy B, Kasler M, Matrai Z. Eight-year follow up result of the OTOASOR trial: the optimal treatment of the axilla–surgery or radiotherapy after positive sentinel lymph node biopsy in early-stage breast cancer: a randomized, single centre, phase III, non-inferiority trial. Eur J Surg Oncol. 2017;43(4):672–9.
15. Forrest AP, Everington D, McDonald CC, Steele RJ, Chetty U, Stewart HJ. The Edinburgh randomized trial of axillary sampling or clearance after mastectomy. Br J Surg. 1995;82(11):1504–8.
16. Chetty U, Jack W, Prescott RJ, Tyler C, Rodger A. Management of the axilla in operable breast cancer treated by breast conservation: a randomized clinical trial. Br J Surg. 2000;87(2):163–9.
17. Early Breast Cancer Trialists' Collaborative Group; Dodwell D, Taylor CW, McGale P, Kühn T, Poortmans PM, Whelan T, et al. Regional lymph node irradiation in early stage breast cancer: an EBCTCG meta-analysis of 13,000 women in 14 trials. San Antonio Breast Cancer Symp; 2018 Dec 4–8; San Antonio, USA.
18. Giuliano AE, Ballman KV, McCall L, Beitsch PD, Brennan MB, Kelemen PR, Ollila DW, Hansen

NM, Whitworth PW, Blumencranz PW, Leitch AM, Saha S, Hunt KK, Morrow M. Effect of axillary dissection vs no axillary dissection on 10-year overall survival among women with invasive breast cancer and sentinel node metastasis: the ACOSOG Z0011 (Alliance) Randomized Clinical Trial. JAMA. 2017;318(10):918–26.
19. Dingemans SA, de Rooij PD, van der Vuurst de Vries RM, Budel LM, Contant CM, van der Pool AE. Validation of six nomograms for predicting non-sentinel lymph node metastases in a Dutch breast cancer population. Ann Surg Oncol. 2016;23(2):477–81.
20. Algara López M, Rodríguez García E, Beato Tortajada I, Martínez Arcelus FJ, Salinas Ramos J, Rodríguez Garrido JR, Sanz Latiesas X, Soler Rodríguez A, Juan Rijo G, Flaquer García A. OPTimizing irradiation through molecular assessment of lymph node (OPTIMAL): a randomized open label trial. Radiat Oncol. 2020;15(1):229.
21. Brunt AM, Haviland JS, Wheatley DA, Sydenham MA, Alhasso A, Bloomfield DJ, Chan C, Churn M, Cleator S, Coles CE, Goodman A. Hypofractionated breast radiotherapy for 1 week versus 3 weeks (FAST-forward): 5-year efficacy and late normal tissue effects results from a multicentre, non-inferiority, randomised, phase 3 trial. Lancet. 2020;395:1613.
22. Offersen BV, Boersma LJ, Kirkove C, et al. ESTRO consensus guideline on target volume delineation for elective radiation therapy of early stage breast cancer. Radiother Oncol. 2015;114:3–10.
23. White et al. https://www.nrgoncology.org/Portals/0/Scientific%20Program/CIRO/Atlases/BreastCancerAtlas_corr.pdf?ver=2018-04-18-144201-270. Accessed 1.11.2020 2018.
24. Early Breast Cancer Trialists' Collaborative Group. Effects of radiotherapy and surgery in early breast cancer. N Engl J Med. 1995;333:1444–55.
25. Duma MN. An update on regional nodal irradiation: indication, target volume delineation, and radiotherapy techniques. Breast Care (Basel). 2020;15(2):128–35.
26. Osman SO, Hol S, Poortmans PM, Essers M. Volumetric modulated arc therapy and breath-hold in image-guided locoregional left-sided breast irradiation. Radiother Oncol. 2014;112(1):17–22.

45 Omission of Radiation

Elisabetta Bonzano and Icro Meattini

45.1 Background

45.1.1 Radiation Therapy Omission after BCS in Low-Risk Breast Cancer

Whole breast irradiation (WBI) represents the standard of care for most of postoperative patients receiving a BCS, significantly reducing both the rate of ipsilateral breast tumour recurrence and breast cancer death [1].

The first generation of prospective randomised phase III clinical trials, conducted in the 1980s–1990s to identify a low-risk group of patients in whom WBI might be safely omitted after BCS, used very broad inclusion criteria and obtained a consequent vague profile of patients at low risk of recurrence [2].

E. Bonzano
PhD School in Experimental Medicine, University of Pavia, Pavia, Italy

Department of Radiation Oncology, IRCCS San Matteo Polyclinic Foundation, Pavia, Italy

I. Meattini (✉)
Department of Experimental and Clinical Biomedical Sciences "M. Serio", University of Florence, Florence, Italy

Radiation Oncology Unit, Oncology Department, Azienda Ospedaliero-Universitaria Careggi, Florence, Italy
e-mail: icro.meattini@unifi.it

The Ontario Clinical Oncology Group (OCOG) trial (1984–1989) randomised 837 node-negative (up to 4 cm) breast cancer patients to receive WBI (416 patients) or no RT (421 patients). A dose of 42.5 Gy in 16 fractions over 3 weeks was given for WBI, followed by a 12.5 Gy boost dose to the tumour bed in 5 fractions. No endocrine therapy was used. After a median follow-up of 43 months, LR rate was 5.5% with WBI and 25.7% without. After a median follow-up of 91 months, LR rate was 11% with WBI and 35% without, while no difference in OS was observed. Young age (<50 years), tumour size (>2 cm) and higher tumour grade were found to be predictors of LR [3].

The Milan III trial (1987–1989) enrolled a total of 567 patients (aged <71 years; tumour size <25 mm), to receive WBI (294 patients) or no RT (273 patients). RT consisted of 50 Gy in 25 fractions WBI followed by a boost up to 10 Gy in 5 fractions. Node-positive patients received adjuvant chemotherapy in case of ER-negative tumours (17%) or endocrine therapy if ER-positive (12%). Long-term results showed a 10-year LR incidence of 23.5% with WBI as compared to 5.8% without. No 10-year OS difference was observed, while age was found to be a significant factor affecting LR rate [4–5].

A relevant study accounting for tumour size is the NSABP B-21 trial (1989–1998), which enrolled 1009 patients with invasive node-negative breast tumours sized equal or less than

© The Author(s), under exclusive license to Springer Nature Switzerland AG 2022
O. Kaidar-Person et al. (eds.), *Breast Cancer Radiation Therapy*,
https://doi.org/10.1007/978-3-030-91170-6_45

1 cm. Patients were randomised to receive adjuvant endocrine therapy only (336 patients), WBI (50 Gy in 25 fractions with or without a boost) and placebo (336 patients), or WBI plus endocrine therapy (337 patients). The cumulative 8-year IBTR rate was 16.5% for tamoxifen only, 9.3% for WBI only, and 2.8% for WBI plus tamoxifen arm. WBI benefit in LR occurrence was observed independently of ER status, while no difference in OS rate was shown [6].

The SweBCG 91 RT trial (1991–1997) randomised 1187 T1-2N0 patients to receive (593 patients) or not (594 patients) WBI (48–54 Gy in 24–27 fractions). Adjuvant endocrine therapy or chemotherapy were prescribed in stage II patients. The 5-year LR was 14% for no-RT patients and 4% for those receiving RT, while at a median follow-up of 15.6 years the LR rate was 23.9% and 11.5%, respectively. OS did not significantly differ between arms [7, 8].

Patient enrolment was heterogeneous, mainly based on the tumour size, negative axillary nodes, free-resection margins after BCS, and age criteria were often quite broad, resulting in the inability to clearly identify a subset of patients at very low-risk of recurrence eligible for a de-escalation of postoperative treatments [9–12]. Although clinical features of breast cancer at diagnosis still represent major prognostic factors for early breast cancer, it is clear nowadays that they could not represent anymore the only assessed factors to correctly stratify patients for the risk of relapse and allocate them to the optimal postoperative treatment approach.

Trials of second generation tried to create a more reliable profile of low-risk patients, with a systematic use of age thresholds, hormonal receptor status, and tumour biology factors for precise allocation. Strict selection criteria allow to better target the patient population in order to perform reliable subset analyses.

The Toronto and British Columbia trial (1992–2000), randomised 769 T1-2 patients aged more than 50 years to receive adjuvant endocrine therapy alone (386 patients) or endocrine therapy plus WBI (383 patients) [13].

WBI consisted of a moderate hypofractionated schedule of 40 Gy in 16 fractions, followed by a boost of 12.5 Gy in 5 fractions. Five-year LR rate was 7.7% in the exclusive endocrine therapy arm and 0.6% in WBI plus endocrine therapy arm. At 8-year, LR rates increased to 17.6% and 3.5%, respectively. Five-year DFS was in favour of combined treatments arm (91% vs 84%), while OS did not significantly differ.

According to an increased percentage of hormone receptor-positive tumours in the elderly, the biology of breast cancer in this population setting may be less aggressive. Based on data from Early Breast Cancer Trialists' Collaborative Group (EBCTCG) meta-analysis, where patients aged ≥70, with small and ER-positive tumours receiving tamoxifen, showed relatively less benefit from RT in terms of OS, several studies have been conducted to establish if RT omission was possible for a very low-risk group of patients [1, 13–16]. According to health conditions, comorbidities, and poor compliance, the balance between receive or not RT in older adults with early breast cancer is still a matter of constant debate and ongoing investigations. Therefore, minimising treatment in older adult patients to warrant a good profile of health-related QoL without compromising survival represents a key-point [17].

Two randomised clinical trials investigated RT omission in elder women at low LR risk after BCS followed by endocrine therapy: PRIME II [18] and CALGB 9343 [19] studies.

The PRIME II trial, enrolling ER-positive women, aged >65 years, with a low risk of local recurrence (cT1-T2N0 tumour sized ≤3 cm, with clear resection margins and hormonal receptor positive status). RT was given to the whole breast up to 40–50 Gy in 15–25 fractions over 3–5 weeks. A boost to the tumour bed was allowed up to 10–15 Gy. The study showed a 5-year LR rate of 3.3% in the RT omission group versus 1.2% in the RT group, a rate low enough to consider the omission of postoperative RT in a well-selected group of patients [18]. No risk factors predictive for LR were found except for the omission of WBI (HR: 4.87). At the recent 10-year follow-up update [20]. LR rate was further reduced by RT, with a significant difference found in regional recurrence (9.8% vs 0.9% rate in favour of RT arm; $P = 0.00008$); in the subgroup of patients omitting RT with low ER status, the 10-year LR rate was 18.8% ($P = 0.007$). As regard the secondary endpoints of distant metastases, contralateral breast cancer or OS, no differences were found.

In the CALGB 9343 trial a total of 636 clinical ER-positive stage I patients aged more than 70 were randomised after BCS and axillary sampling or dissection to receive adjuvant tamoxifen alone (319 patients) or with WBI (317 patients) [19]. WBI was delivered up to 45 Gy in 25 fractions over 5 weeks, including level I-II axillary nodes. A sequential electron boost of 14 Gy in 7 fractions was given. Tamoxifen was administered for 5 years. The 5-year IBTR rate was 1% in the WBI and tamoxifen arm and 4% in the tamoxifen alone arm [21], while at a median follow-up of 12.6 years it was 2% and 9%, respectively [19]. No significant difference in terms of OS, time to distant metastasis, or ultimate breast preservation was observed between arms [19].

It should be note that these were both negative trials for their primary endpoints (LR rate) and they were under powered for secondary survival outcomes. Moreover, CALBG 9343 did not report histologic tumour grade and in PRIME II study only 3% of patients had a grade 3 tumour. Also, information on comorbidity in both trials was not reported. Depending on the value placed on the LR event occurrence, omission of RT could be considered only in selected patients and after a careful multifactorial and multidisciplinary evaluation.

The British Association of Surgical Oncology (BASO) II study was a randomised clinical trial with a 2x2 factorial design evaluating the effect of the addition of WBI or endocrine therapy or both in early breast cancer after BCS. Eligibility criteria included patients <70 years of age with node negative invasive breast cancer sized <20 mm, with histological grade 1 or specific good prognosis histology, and no evidence of lymph vascular invasion [14]. The four treatment arms included BCS only, BCS plus WBI, BCS plus endocrine therapy or BCS plus WBI plus endocrine therapy. At a median follow-up time of 10 years, the cumulative incidence of LR was 10.2% for patients not receiving RT (both BCS only and BCS plus endocrine therapy groups), 3.9% for those receiving RT (BCS plus WBI and BCS plus WBI plus endocrine therapy groups), 11.7% for those not receiving endocrine therapy (BCS and BCS plus WBI groups) and 4.2% for patients receiving tamoxifen (BCS plus endocrine therapy and BCS plus WBI plus endocrine therapy groups). The annual rate of LR was 0.4% in patients receiving WBI or endocrine therapy, 1.2% and 1.3% in those having WBI or tamoxifen omitted, respectively. The risk of LR was reduced by both WBI or endocrine therapy, with a non-significant improvement in terms of OS.

Main studies investigating the omission of RT in selected patients affected by early breast cancer are reported in Table 45.1.

Patients selection is therefore of utmost importance. There is a growing burden of knowledge concerning the impact of tumour's biology on disease outcome. Biology signature might not be able to overcome the impact on prognosis of clinical features but should be strongly integrated in the decision-making process, in order to avoid over- or under-treatment and to implement personalised RT approaches. In order to help physicians and patients to make treatment decisions, also nomograms based on prognostic factors are becoming widely applied to quantify the likelihood of the specific events of interest. At the MD Anderson Cancer Center, a specific nomogram was developed to assess the benefit of RT for older patients with breast cancer treated with BCS. It is based on age (range from 66 to 79 year), ethnicity, tumour size, ER and nodal status [24].

A nomogram was also developed and validated to assess the benefit of RT after BCS in older adult patients who do not meet the CALGB 9343 criteria. ER, PR, grade, ethnicity, T-stage, and N-stage were included as predictors [25].

45.1.2 Interaction between Postoperative RT and Adjuvant Endocrine Therapy

Frailty represents a risk factor for mortality and the knowledge of pre-existing frailty is a crucial factor in the treatment decision of older adults. For patients older than 70 years affected by low-risk, hormone-positive breast cancer, the chance to de-escalate systemic therapy is currently investigated.

Table 45.1 Main studies investigating the omission of radiation therapy in selected patients affected by early breast cancer. Failure rates referred to median follow-up when not otherwise specified

Study	Years	Patients	Age, year	Stage	HR status	Size (mm)	Margins	Study design	LR	OS	DSS	Median FU (year)
Fisher et al. [6]	1989–1994 1996–1998	673	Any	T1N0	Any	<10	Negative	ET vs ET + RT vs RT + placebo	16.5% vs 9.3% vs 2.8	93% vs 94% vs 93%	NR	8
Fyles et al. Toronto-BC [13, 22]	1992–2000	769	>50 (mean 68)	T1–2N0	NR	<50	Negative	ET + RT vs ET	5.1% vs 13.7%	84%	NR	10
Potter et al. ABCSG 8A [16, 23]	1996–2004	869	Postmenopausal (mean 66)	T1–2N0	ER+/PR+ or both+	<31	Negative	ET + RT vs ET	2.2% vs 7.2%	87.6% vs 86.6%	94.5% vs 88.4	9.9
Blamey et al. BASO II [14]	1992–2000	1135	<70 (mean 57)	T1N0	ER/PR+	<20	Negative	BCS only vs BCS + ET vs BCS + RT vs BCS + ET + RT	2.2%/year (BCS) 0.8%/year (RT or ET) 0.2%/year (ET + RT)	96%	NR	10
Hughes et al. CALGB 9343 [19]	1994–1999	636	≥70	T1N0	Er+	<20	Negative	ET + RT vs ET	2% vs 9%[a]	67% vs 66%[a]	97% vs 98%[a]	12.6
Kunkler et al. PRIME II [20]	2003–2009	1326	≥65	T1N0	ER/PR+ or both+	<30	>0.9 mm	ET + RT vs ET	1.3% vs 4.1% 0.9% vs 9.8%[a, b]	93.9% vs 93.9%	97.6% vs 94.5%	5[b]

HR hormonal receptors, *LR* local relapse, *OS* overall survival, *DSS* disease-specific survival, *FU* follow-up, *BCS* breast-conserving surgery, *ER* oestrogen receptor, *PR* progesterone receptor, *NR* not reported, *ET* endocrine therapy, *RT* radiation therapy

[a]At 10-year

[b]10-year results presented at virtual San Antonio Breast Cancer Symposium 2020

Ferreira and colleagues [26], reported how endocrine therapy might have a major detrimental impact on health-related QoL scores, especially in postmenopausal women. Estimation models predicted how for healthy older women with biologically favourable disease, postoperative RT or endocrine therapy was related with not different 5-year survival rates [27]. Therefore, to capture the side-effect profile of RT alone or when combined with other therapies represents an important issue for older adults' patients. Furthermore, due to the wide spectrum of potential adverse events of endocrine therapy (i.e. bone fragility, thromboembolic events, sexual and cognitive dysfunctional, arthralgia/myalgia) in elder patients the adherence rate to therapy declines over time [28].

The adherence to adjuvant endocrine therapy is of utmost importance. It should be considered that poor compliance with endocrine therapy in elderly women is common, and long treatment gaps may be frequent [29]. The BIG 1–98 prospective trial (a four-arm, phase III, double-blind, RCT, comparing adjuvant letrozole versus tamoxifen) showed that the proportions of treatment discontinuation were 38.4% in patients aged over 75 years [30]. Advances in RT techniques, which allow even shorter treatment schedule with both moderate and ultra-hypofractionation, and the reduction of target volumes using partial breast irradiation, make adjuvant breast RT well tolerated by most of the patients [31–32]. Moreover, duration of endocrine therapy is increasing, so QoL should be considered when weighing this against the omission of RT [33]. Information about the pros and cons of all options and the balance risk of local recurrence against the burden of different treatments should be provided to patients to make themselves take an informed decision.

45.1.3 Radiation Therapy Omission after Primary Systemic Therapy (PST) in High-Risk Breast Cancer

PST is a standard of care in selected breast cancer treatment, historically aimed to achieve resectability converting inoperable tumours to operable, downstaging the primary tumour and providing prognostic information based on pathological response. However, currently an increased number of patients are candidate to receive a PST even when not locally advances, due to the predictive value of response to PST in specific tumours profiles. As a result, an increased number of relatively high-risk but early breast cancer patients will be treated with a preoperative systemic treatment. Nevertheless, the indication of adjuvant RT after PST represents an area of constant debate [34, 35]. The crucial point is to establish whether the extent and the intensity of RT should be based on clinical tumour stage, as historically recommended, or on the tumour extent after PST or both [34, 36].

Indeed, there may be a subgroup of high-risk women affected by breast cancer for whom the benefit of RT is small and for whom the omission of RT does not affect survival outcomes [37]. Several research aiming to establish the effect of RT in women with a pathologic complete response (pCR) to PST after BCS are still ongoing [34, 35]. Clinical tumour stage and tumour biology are the most important predictors of pCR in breast cancer patients receiving PST: lower clinical T-stages correlated with a higher pCR rates [38], and a pCR seems to be also a strong prognostic factor, especially in triple-negative or human epidermal growth factor receptor 2 (HER2)-overexpressing breast tumours [36].

Concerning de-escalation of RT treatment, a consistent burden of data derived from MD Anderson studies. Huang et al. in 2004 reported data on 676 patients, stage I-IV, who underwent mastectomy after PST with or without PMRT. As regard patients initially staged with clinical stage I-IIB, who had a pCR, and patients who had stage II disease with ypN1a (1–3 involved lymph nodes) found out there was no significant difference in 10-year LRR rates [39]. In 2007, McGuire et al. confirm these data, analysing 106 pts. stage I-III, one-third were clinical stage I or II who developed pCR after PST, none of 32 patients who had clinical stage I or II diseases at presentation had an LRR, the 10-year LRR rates were 0% regardless of whether PMRT was delivered [40]. Both mention that a benefit in terms of LRR with

PMRT was seen with clinical stage III, or greater, breast cancer presentations only.

However, it should be taken into account that the vast majority of patients included in the above-mentioned studies was treated at same institution, with overlapping observation time periods. Hence, there is a concrete risk of patients' cohorts overlap and selection biases due to the retrospective nature of these analysis.

In 2012, Mamounas and colleagues, combining data from the NSABP B-18 and from NSABP B-27, corroborated results from the MD Anderson studies, demonstrating that stage II disease patients that achieved a pCR following PST had an overall low risk of LRR [35]. Overall, these data suggest that the initial pre-chemotherapy burden of disease is crucial when making decisions regarding the benefit of postoperative RT [36] (Table 45.2).

Furthermore, Krug el al. conducted a retrospective explorative analysis of three large prospective randomised phase III trials (GeparTrio, GeparQuattro, and GeparQuinto) to analyse the impact of postoperative PMRT on LRR and survival [46]. In 3481 patients with a median follow-up of 55.9 months, RT use as compared with no RT, showed to improve 5-year LRR-free survival, without an improvement in DFS. It has to be considered that 61.3% of patients had clinically positive lymph nodes and 45.6% had clinical T3–4 tumours. Both subgroups had a significantly lower risk of LRR when treated with RT in the absence of a DFS benefit, while patients with cN0 had no benefit from RT and showed a worse DFS [46].

45.1.4 Ongoing Trials and Future Prospects

Several trials are currently investigating optimising de-escalation approaches according to the strategy of precision medicine for low-risk patients (i.e. EUROPA NCT04134598, EXPERT NCT02889874, NATURAL NCT03646955, PRECISION NCT02653755, PRIMETIME ISRCTN41579286, IDEA NCT02400190, LUMINA NCT01791829) (Table 45.3).

Notably, all published studies investigating on this subset of patients were designed and performed in order to evaluate RT omission, regardless of utilisation of and compliance to ET. The only exception is represented by the ongoing EUROPA trial, focussing on older adults (≥70 years) affected by good prognosis primary BC, evaluating if postoperative RT-alone is able to avoid the long-term toxicity of endocrine therapy and favourably impact on health-related QoL in this potentially frail population [47].

The IDEA (Individualized Decisions for Endocrine Therapy) trial (NCT02400190) is a multicentric prospective single-arm observational study (University of Michigan Cancer Center) assessing loco-regional relapse rate after BCS in post-menopausal women (aged 50–69), planned to undergo postoperative endocrine therapy. Inclusion criteria include unifocal T1N0 hormonal receptor-positive HER2-mbatgive patients stratified by a gene expression signature based on the 21-gene recurrence score assay OncotypeDX (Genomic Health Inc., Redwood City, CA), able to estimate the risk of LR [52].

The PRECISION (Profiling Early Breast Cancer for Radiotherapy Omission) trial is a non-randomised phase II trial (Dana Farber Cancer Institute-NCT02653755), evaluating the omission of WBI after BCS in patients aged 50–75 at low-risk receiving adjuvant endocrine therapy. Patients over 75 are excluded due to potential competing causes of death. The trial relies on Prosigna Breast Cancer Assay (NanoString Technologies Inc., Seattle, WA) for gene expression profiling using PAM50 gene signature. This test measures the transcriptional profile of 50 classifier genes to generate a clinically validated score for the 10-year risk of distant recurrence [50].

The EXPERT (Examining PErsonalised Radiation Therapy for Low-risk Early Breast Cancer) phase 3 trial, run by the Breast Cancer Trial Group in Australia and New Zealand, with inclusion criteria similar to the PRECISION trial, will employ Prosigna in order to identify low-risk breast cancer patients (aged more than 50 years, Stage I, ER positive, HER2 negative) [48].

Table 45.2 Main studies investigating radiation therapy after PST

Study	Years	Patients	CT-based regimen	Stage	pCR (%)	PMRT (%)	Study design	LRR with PMRT (pCR)	LRR without PMRT (pCR)	Median FU (year)
Huang et al. (2004) [39]	1974–2000	744	Anthra 100% Tax 15%	Stage I 0.15% Stage IIA 4.3% Stage IIB 18.9% Stage IIIA 28.5% Stage IIIB 39.2% Stage IV 8.8%	86	74	Retrospective, single centre	3% (stage III/IV)	33% (stage III/IV)	5.75
McGuire et al. (2007) [40]	1982–2002	106	Anthra 92% Tax 38%	Stage I 2% Stage II 31% Stage IIIA 30% Stage IIIB 25% Stage IIIC 11%	106	68	Retrospective, single centre	0% (stage I/II) 7.3% (stage III)	0% (stage I/II) 17.7% (stage III)	5.2
Le Scodan et al. (2011) [41]	1990–2004	134	Anthra 100% Tax 9.7%	Stage I 0.74% Stage II 61.9% Stage III 37.3%	24	58	Retrospective, single centre	NR	NR	7.6
Mamounas et al. (2012) [35]	1988–1993	1122	Anthra+tax	Stage IIA 36.4% Stage IIB 41.8% Stage IIIA 18.9%	94	NR	Pooled analysis of NSABP B18 and B27 trials	NR	6.5% (stage IIA) 8.1% (stage IIB)	11.7
Shim et al. (2014) [42]	1998–2009	151	Anthra 38.4% Tax 6% Anthra+tax 55.6%	Stage IIA 4.6% Stage IIB 55.6% Stage IIIA 31.1% Stage IIIB 8.6%	36	70	Retrospective, multicentre	0%	0%	4.8
Meattini et al. (2014) [43]	1997–2011	170	Anthra 40% Anthra+tax 54%	Stage IIA 10% Stage IIB 30% Stage IIIA 21% Stage IIIB 37% Stage IIIC 2%	NR	58	Retrospective, single centre	16.7% (stage III)	38.7% (stage III)	7.7
Nagar et al. (2015) [44]	2003–2010	161	Anthra 93% Tax 80%	Stage I 8.4% Stage II 44.8% Stage III 28.6%	33	73	Retrospective, single centre	0%	2.3%	4
Fowble et al. (2017) [45]	2004–2013	81	Anthra+tax	Stage I 7.4% Stage IIA 49.3% Stage IIB 28.9% Stage IIIA 14.8%	35	0	Retrospective, single centre	NR	3%	4.9

CT chemotherapy, *pCR* pathological complete response, *PMRT* postmastectomy radiation therapy, *LRR* locoregional relapse, *FU* follow-up, *antra* anthracycline-based, *tax* taxane-based, *anthra + tax* anthracycline and taxane-based, *NR* not reported

Table 45.3 Ongoing studies on optimisation of treatments for very low-risk breast cancer population

Name	EUROPA [47]	EXPERT [48]	NATURAL [49]	PRECISION [50]	PRIMETIME [51]	IDEA [52]	LUMINA [53]
Trial number	NCT04134598	NCT02889874	NCT03646955	NCT02653755	ISRCTN: 41579286	NCT02400190	NCT01791829
Study type	Randomised	Randomised	Randomised	Single arm	Single arm	Single arm	Single arm
Age (years)	≥70	≥50	≥60	≥50 and ≤ 75	≥60	≥50 and ≤ 69 (postmenopausal)	≥55
Stage	pT1 N0	pT1 N0	pT1 N0	pT1 N0	pT1 N0	pT1 N0	pT1 N0
Grade and histology	Any grade (pT ≤10 mm) Grade 1–2 (pT = 11–19 mm)	Grade 1–2 Non multifocal or multicentric invasive	Grade 1–2 Non-lobular unifocal unilateral histology	Grade 1–2 Non multicentric Invasive	Grade 1–2	Any grade Non multicentric and multifocal	Grade 1–2 Non-lobular multiple foci multicentric No EIC
Subtype	Luminal A	Luminal A	Luminal A	Luminal A	Very low risk patients (based on IHC4 + C)	Recurrence score ≤ 18	Luminal A
Assessment method	IHC FISH for HER2 Score 2+	PAM 50 FISH for HER2 2+	IHC FISH for HER2 2+	PAM 50 FISH for HER2 2+	IHC4 + C FISH for HER2 2+	Oncotype-DX FISH for HER2 2+	IHC FISH for HER2 2+
Biology	ER ≥10%; PR ≥10%; HER2 negative; Ki67 ≤20%	ER/PR ≥10%; HER2 negative; ROR score ≤ 60	ER ≥10%; HER2 negative	ER/PR ≥10%; HER2 negative	ER/PR positive; HER2 negative	ER/PR positive; HER2 negative	ER ≥1%; PR >20%; HER2 negative
Surgical margins	Negative	Negative	≥2 mm	Negative	≥1 mm	≥2 mm	≥1 mm
Interventions	ET vs RT (exp)	ET + RT vs ET (exp)	ET + APBI vs ET (exp)	ET only	ET only	ET only	ET only
Primary endpoint(s)	LR (equivalence) HRQoL (superiority)	LR (equivalence)	LR (equivalence)	LRR (equivalence)	LR	LRR	LR
Number of patients	926	1167	926	690	2400	202	500

LR local recurrence, *LRR* locoregional recurrence, *ET* endocrine therapy, *IHC* immunohistochemistry, *FISH* fluorescence in situ hybridization, *HRQoL* health-related quality of life, *APBI* accelerated partial breast irradiation, *EIC* extensive intraductal component, *IHC4 + C* immunohistochemistry biomarkers plus clinical information, *ER* oestrogen receptor, *PR* progesterone receptor, *ROR score* risk of recurrence score, *exp* experimental arm

The LUMINA study is a multicentric single-arm prospective cohort trial (Ontario Clinical Oncology Group-OCOG), investigating the hypothesis that Immunohistochemical 4 (IHC4) positive clinical factors may be able to identify low-risk patients. The trial evaluates the risk of IBTR after BCS and in patients aged more than 55 years receiving adjuvant endocrine therapy. The low-risk population is characterised by negative axilla, Luminal A-like subtype, size less than 2 cm, free margins, and no Grade 3 nor lymph vascular invasion or extensive intraductal component tumours. IHC4 score is an inexpensive tool predicting risk of distant recurrence in women with early breast cancer based on ER, PR, HER2, and Ki67 index [53].

In the UK, the PRIMETIME trial is a prospective biomarker-directed case-cohort study that plans to enrol 2400 women aged more than 60 affected by T1N0 tumours, having positive hormonal receptors, negative HER2, and Grade 1–2. Patients are planned to be scored according to IHC4 + clinical factors with a dedicated calculation algorithm. Those stratified in the "very low risk" category, will be spared WBI [51]. In Denmark, based on results from the UK IMPORT LOW and the DBCG RT PBI trials, 40 Gy/15 fr EBRT-PBI is standard since April 2016 for selected low risk breast cancer patients. Currently, a prospective randomised trials tests whether PBI can be safely omitted in selected low risk breast cancer patients without causing unacceptable high risk of local failure. The trial started on 5 September 2018, aims to accrue 926 participants, and should be completed by 2035 (NCT03646955) [49].

The future of precision medicine will be based on the integration of clinical features (patient- and disease-related) with biomarkers and gene-signatures. Another interesting example is the genomic-adjusted RT dose (GARD) score, which employs the gene expression–based radiosensitivity index and the linear quadratic model to determine the therapeutic effect of RT. This score showed also to be an independent predictor of RT-specific outcomes and to be able to estimate the probability for both relapse- and distant metastasis-free survival [54]. However, the cost-effectiveness and the reliability of this multimodal assessment has to be carefully evaluated within clinical trials.

Concerning high-risk patients, the NSABP B51/RTOG 1304 phase 3 trial should clarify the optimal locoregional strategy after PST. The primary aim is to evaluate whether the addition of regional nodal RT will improve invasive DFS rates in clinical node-positive patients who convert to ypN0 disease. Patients with clinical T1-3 N1 breast cancer receiving PST, with pathological negative lymph nodes (either by SLNB or ALND) are randomly assigned for WBI with or without RNI, including the IMN. Mastectomy patients will be randomised to PMRT, including RNI or no RT. The primary endpoint is 5-year invasive breast cancer recurrence-free interval with a superiority margin of 4.6% and a planned sample size of 1636 patients. The first results will be expected in July 2023. The results of the NSABP-B51 trial will provide prospective randomised data to delineate future PMRT recommendations in the setting of a pCR or ypN0 status after PST [55].

45.2 Summary

We should definitely favour to adopt the term of optimisation of the extent of, rather than merely searching for de-escalation of treatments, since the latter is a term easily misunderstood and comparable to the concept of over- and under-treatment. Strong evidence is needed to identify an optimised, cost-effective, and personalised treatment for patients affected by breast cancer. However, we undoubtedly support the worthwhile value of personalising RT for each unique breast cancer patient.

References

1. Early Breast Cancer Trialists' Collaborative Group (EBCTCG), Darby S, Mc Gale P, Correa C, et al. Effects of radiotherapy after breast-conserving surgery on 10-year recurrence and 15-year breast cancer death: meta-analysis of individual patient data for 10,801 women in 17 randomised trials. Lancet. 2011;378:1707–16.

2. Clark RM, McCulloch PB, Levine MN, et al. Randomized clinical trial to assess the effectiveness of breast irradiation following lumpectomy and axillary dissection for node-negative breast cancer. J Natl Cancer Inst. 1992;84:683–9.
3. Clark RM, Whelan T, Levine M, et al. Randomized clinical trial of breast irradiation following lumpectomy and axillary dissection for node-negative breast cancer: an update. J Natl Cancer Inst. 1996;88:1659–64.
4. Veronesi U, Luini A, Del Vecchio M, et al. Radiotherapy after breast-preserving surgery in women with localized cancer of the breast. N Engl J Med. 1993;328:1587–91.
5. Veronesi U, Marubini E, Mariani L, et al. Radiotherapy after breast-conserving surgery in small breast carcinoma: long-term results of a randomized trial. Ann Oncol. 2001;12:997–1003.
6. Fisher B, Bryant J, Dignam JJ, et al. Tamoxifen, radiation therapy, or both for prevention of ipsilateral breast tumor recurrence after lumpectomy in women with invasive breast cancers of one centimeter or less. J Clin Oncol. 2002;20:4141–9.
7. Malmstrom P, Holmberg L, Anderson H, et al. Breast conserving surgery, with and without radiotherapy, in women with lymph node-negative breast cancer: a randomised clinical trial in a population with access to public mammography screening. Eur J Cancer. 2003;39:1690–7.
8. Killander F, Karlsson P, Anderson H, et al. No breast cancer subgroup can be spared postoperative radiotherapy after breast-conserving surgery. Fifteen year results from the Swedish Breast Cancer Group randomised trial, SweBCG 91 RT. Eur J Cancer. 2016;67:57–65.
9. Uppsala-Orebro Breast Cancer Study Group. Sector resection with or without postoperative radiotherapy for stage I breast cancer: a randomized trial. J Natl Cancer Inst. 1990;82:277–82.
10. Liljegren G, Holmberg L, Adami HO, et al. Sector resection with or without postoperative radiotherapy for stage I breast cancer: five-year results of a randomized trial. J Natl Cancer Inst. 1994;86:717–22.
11. Liljegren G, Holmberg L, Bergh J, et al. Ten-year results after sector resection with or without postoperative radiotherapy for stage I breast cancer: a randomized trial. J Clin Oncol. 1999;17:2326–33.
12. Liljegren G, Lindgren A, Bergh J, et al. Risk factors for local recurrence after conservative treatment in stage I breast cancer. Definition of a subgroup not requiring radiotherapy. Ann Oncol. 1997;8:235–41.
13. Fyles AW, McCready DR, Manchul LA, et al. Tamoxifen with or without breast irradiation in women 50 years or older with early breast cancer. N Engl J Med. 2004;351:963–70.
14. Blamey RW, Bates T, Chetty U, et al. Radiotherapy or tamoxifen after conserving surgery for breast cancer of excellent prognosis: British Association of Surgical Oncology (BASO) II trial. Eur J Cancer. 2013;49:2294–302.
15. Chesney TR, Yin JX, Rajaee N, Tricco AC, Fyles AW, Acuna SA, Scheer AS. Tamoxifen with radiotherapy compared with tamoxifen alone in elderly women with early-stage breast cancer treated with breast conserving surgery: a systematic review and meta-analysis. Radiother Oncol. 2017;123(1):1–9. https://doi.org/10.1016/j.radonc.2017.02.019.
16. Potter R, Gnant M, Kwasny W, et al. Lumpectomy plus tamoxifen with or without whole breast irradiation in women with favourable breast cancer. Int J Radiat Oncol Biol Phys. 2007;68:334–40.
17. Poortmans PMP, Arenas M, Livi L. Over-irradiation. Breast. 2017;31:295–302. https://doi.org/10.1016/j.breast.2016.07.022. Epub 2016 Aug 10
18. Kunkler IH, Williams LJ, Jack WJL et al. Breast-conserving surgery with or without irradiation in women aged 65 years or older with early breast cancer (PRIME II): a randomised controlled trial. https://doi.org/10.1016/S1470-2045(14)71221-5.
19. Hughes KS, Schnaper LA, Bellon JR, et al. Lumpectomy plus tamoxifen with or without irradiation in women age 70 years or older with early breast cancer: long-term follow-up of CALGB 9343. doi: https://doi.org/10.1200/JCO.2012.45.2615.
20. Kunkler IH, Williams LJ, Jack WJL, et al; PRIME 2 Trial Investigators. PRIME 2 randomized trial (Postoperative Radiotherapy in Minimum-Risk Elderly): wide local excision and adjuvant hormonal therapy +/− whole breast irradiation in women ≥65 years with early invasive breast cancer: 10 year results. Presented at: 2020 San Antonio Breast Cancer Symposium; December 8–12, 2020; Virtual. Abstract GS2–03.
21. Hughes KS, Schnaper LA, Berry D, et al. Lumpectomy plus tamoxifen with or without irradiation in women 70 years of age or older with early breast cancer. N Engl J Med. 2004;351(10):971–7.
22. Liu FF, Shi W, Done SJ, Miller N, et al. Identification of a low-risk luminal a breast cancer cohort that may not benefit from breast radiotherapy. J Clin Oncol. 2015;33(18):2035–40. https://doi.org/10.1200/JCO.2014.57.7999. Epub 2015 May 11
23. Fastner G, Sedlmayer F, Widder J et al. Endocrine therapy with or without whole breast irradiation in low-risk breast cancer patients after breast-conserving surgery: 10-year results of the Austrian Breast and Colorectal Cancer Study Group 8A trial. https://doi.org/10.1016/j.ejca.2019.11.024.
24. Albert JM, Liu DD, Shen Y, Pan IW, Shih YC, Hoffman KE, Buchholz TA, Giordano SH, Smith BD. Nomogram to predict the benefit of radiation for older patients with breast cancer treated with conservative surgery. J Clin Oncol. 2012;30(23):2837–43.
25. Chen K, Su F, Jacobs LK. A nomogram to predict the benefit of radiation therapy after breast-conserving surgery in elderly patients with stage I & ER-negative, or stage II/III disease. Ann Surg Oncol. 2015;22:3497–503. https://doi.org/10.1245/s10434-015-4393-7.
26. Ferreira AR, Di Meglio A, Pistilli B, Gbenou AS, El-Mouhebb M, Dauchy S, et al. Differential impact of endocrine therapy and chemotherapy on qual-

ity of life of breast cancer survivors: a prospective patient-reported outcomes analysis. Ann Oncol. 2019;30:1784–95.
27. Ward MC, Vicini F, Chadha M, Pierce L, Recht A, Hayman J, et al. Radiation therapy without hormone therapy for women age 70 or above with low-risk early breast cancer: a microsimulation. Int J Radiat Oncol Biol Phys. 2019;105:296–306.
28. Brett J, Fenlon D, Boulton M, Hulbert-Williams NJ, Walter FM, Donnelly P, et al. Factors associated with intentional and unintentional non-adherence to adjuvant endocrine therapy following breast cancer. Eur J Cancer Care (Engl). 2018;27:1.
29. Nekhlyudov L, Li L, Ross-Degnan D, Wagner AK. Five-year patterns of adjuvant hormonal therapy use, persistence, and adherence among insured women with early-stage breast cancer. Breast Cancer Res Treat. 2011;130(2):681–9. https://doi.org/10.1007/s10549-011-1703-z. Epub 2011 Aug 13
30. Crivellari D, Sun Z, Coates AS, Price KN, Thürlimann B, Mouridsen H, Mauriac L, Forbes JF, Paridaens RJ, Castiglione-Gertsch M, Gelber RD, Colleoni M, Láng I, Del Mastro L, Gladieff L, Rabaglio M, Smith IE, Chirgwin JH, Goldhirsch A. Letrozole compared with tamoxifen for elderly patients with endocrine-responsive early breast cancer: the BIG 1-98 trial. J Clin Oncol. 2008;26(12):1972–9. https://doi.org/10.1200/JCO.2007.14.0459. Epub 2008 Mar 10
31. Escott CE, Zaenger D, Switchencko JM, Lin JY, Abugideiri M, Arciero CA, Pfister NT, Xu KM, Meisel JL, Subhedar P, Torres M, Curran WJ, Patel PR. The influence of histologic grade on outcomes of elderly women with early stage breast cancer treated with breast conserving surgery with or without radiotherapy. Clin Breast Cancer. 2020;20(6):e701–10. https://doi.org/10.1016/j.clbc.2020.05.007. Epub 2020 May 13
32. Franco P, Iorio GC, Bartoncini S, et al. De-escalation of breast radiotherapy after conserving surgery in low-risk early breast cancer patients. Med Oncol. 2018;35:62. https://doi.org/10.1007/s12032-018-1121-8.
33. Davies C, Pan H, Godwin J, et al. Long-term effects of continuing adjuvant tamoxifen to 10 years versus stopping at 5 years after diagnosis of oestrogen receptor-positive breast cancer: ATLAS, a randomised trial. Lancet. 2013;381:805–16.
34. Mandish SF, Gaskins JT, Yusuf MB, Amer YM, Eldredge-Hindy H. The effect of omission of adjuvant radiotherapy after neoadjuvant chemotherapy and breast conserving surgery with a pathologic complete response. Acta Oncol. 2020;59(10):1210–7. https://doi.org/10.1080/0284186X.2020.1797161. Epub 2020 Jul 27
35. Mamounas EP, Anderson SJ, Dignam JJ, et al. Predictors of locoregional recurrence after neoadjuvant chemotherapy: results from combined analysis of National Surgical Adjuvant Breast and bowel project B-18 and B-27. J Clin Oncol. 2012;30(32):3960–6.
36. Morrow M, Khan AJ. Locoregional management after neoadjuvant chemotherapy. J Clin Oncol. 2020;38(20):2281–9.
37. Esposito AC, Crawford J, Sigurdson ER, et al. Omission of radiotherapy after breast conservation surgery in the postneoadjuvant setting. J Surg Res. 2018;221:49–57. https://doi.org/10.1016/j.jss.2017.08.008.
38. Goorts B, van Nijnatten TJ, de Munck L, Moossdorff M, Heuts EM, de Boer M, Lobbes MB, Smidt ML. Clinical tumor stage is the most important predictor of pathological complete response rate after neoadjuvant chemotherapy in breast cancer patients. Breast Cancer Res Treat. 2017;163(1):83–91. https://doi.org/10.1007/s10549-017-4155-2. Epub 2017 Feb 15. PMID: 28205044; PMCID: PMC5387027
39. Huang EH, Tucker SL, Strom EA, McNeese MD, Kuerer HM, Buzdar AU, Valero V, Perkins GH, Schechter NR, Hunt KK, Sahin AA, Hortobagyi GN, Buchholz TA. Postmastectomy radiation improves local-regional control and survival for selected patients with locally advanced breast cancer treated with neoadjuvant chemotherapy and mastectomy. J Clin Oncol. 2004;22(23):4691–9. https://doi.org/10.1200/JCO.2004.11.129. Erratum in: J Clin Oncol 2005 Jan 1;23(1):248
40. McGuire SE, Gonzalez-Angulo AM, Huang EH, et al. Postmastectomy radiation improves the outcome of patients with locally advanced breast cancer who achieve a pathologic complete response to neoadjuvant chemotherapy. Int J Radiat Oncol Biol Phys. 2007;68(4):1004–9. https://doi.org/10.1016/j.ijrobp.2007.01.023.
41. Le Scodan R, Bruant S, Selz J, et al. Rôle de l'irradiation locorégionale adjuvante en l'absence d'envahissement ganglionnaire après chimiothérapie néoadjuvante, mastectomie totale et lymphadénectomie axillaire pour un cancer du sein. Expérience de l'hôpital René-Huguenin-institut Curie [Role of locoregional radiation therapy in breast cancer patients with negative lymph nodes after preoperative chemotherapy and mastectomy. The Institut Curie-Hôpital René-Huguenin experience]. Cancer Radiother. 2011;15(8):675–82. https://doi.org/10.1016/j.canrad.2011.04.004. French. Epub 2011 Aug 9
42. Shim SJ, Park W, Huh SJ, et al. The role of postmastectomy radiation therapy after neoadjuvant chemotherapy in clinical stage II-III breast cancer patients with pN0: a multicenter, retrospective study (KROG 12-05). Int J Radiat Oncol Biol Phys. 2014;88(1):65–72. https://doi.org/10.1016/j.ijrobp.2013.09.021. Epub 2013 Oct 22
43. Meattini I, Cecchini S, Di Cataldo V, et al. Postmastectomy radiotherapy for locally advanced breast cancer receiving neoadjuvant chemotherapy. BioMed Res Int. 2014; Article ID 719175, 12 pages, 2014

44. Nagar H, Boothe D, Ginter PS, et al. Disease-free survival according to the use of postmastectomy radiation therapy after neoadjuvant chemotherapy. Clin Breast Cancer. 2015;15(2):128–34. https://doi.org/10.1016/j.clbc.2014.09.012. Epub 2014 Nov 11
45. Fowble B, Jairam AK, Wang F, et al. Indications for postmastectomy radiation after neoadjuvant chemotherapy in ypN0 and ypN1-3 axillary node-positive women. Clin Breast Cancer. 2018;18(1):e107–13. https://doi.org/10.1016/j.clbc.2017.07.016. Epub 2017 Aug 1
46. Krug D, Baumann R, Budach W, Dunst J, Feyer P, Fietkau R, Haase W, Harms W, Hehr T, Piroth MD, Sedlmayer F, Souchon R, Wenz F, Sauer R. Individualization of post-mastectomy radiotherapy and regional nodal irradiation based on treatment response after neoadjuvant chemotherapy for breast cancer: a systematic review. Strahlenther Onkol. 2018;194(7):607–18. https://doi.org/10.1007/s00066-018-1270-x. English. Epub 2018 Jan 30
47. Meattini I, Poortmans PMP, Marrazzo L, Desideri I, Brain E, Hamaker M, et al. Exclusive endocrine therapy or partial breast irradiation for women aged >/=70 years with luminal A-like early stage breast cancer (NCT04134598 - EUROPA): proof of concept of a randomized controlled trial comparing health related quality of life by patient reported outcome measures. J Geriatr Oncol. 2020;12:182.
48. The EXPERT trial (examining personalised radiation therapy for low-risk early breast cancer. https://clinicaltrials.gov/ct2/show/NCT02889874.
49. Partial breast vs no irradiation for women with early breast cancer at ClinicalTrials.gov; https://clinicaltrial.gov/ct2/show/NCT03646955.
50. The PRECISION Trial (profiling early breast cancer for radiotherapy omission): a phase II study of breast-conserving surgery without adjuvant radiotherapy for favorable-risk breast cancer. https://clinicaltrials.gov/ct2/show/NCT02653755.
51. Kirwan CC, Coles CE, Bliss J. It's PRIMETIME post-operative avoidance of radiotherapy: biomarker selection of women at very low risk of local recurrence cli. Oncologia. 2016;28:594–6.
52. The IDEA (Individualized Decisions for Endocrine therApy) study at ClinicalTrials.gov; https://clinicaltrials.gov/ct2/show/NCT02400190
53. A prospective cohort study evaluating risk of local recurrence following breast conserving surgery and endocrine therapy in low risk LUMINAL A Breast cancer (LUMINA) at ClinicalTrials.gov; https://clinicaltrials.gov/ct2/show/NCT01791829.
54. Scott JG, Berglund A, Schell MJ, et al. A genome-based model for adjusting radiotherapy dose (GARD): a retrosepective, cohort-based study. Lancet Oncol. 2016;18:202–11.
55. Mamounas EP, Bandos H, et al. NRG oncology/NSABP B-51/RTOG 1304: phase III trial to determine if chest wall and regional nodal radiotherapy (CWRNRT) post mastectomy (Mx) or the addition of RNRT to whole breast RT post breast-conserving surgery (BCS) reduces invasive breast cancer recurrence-free interval (IBCR-FI) in patients (pts) with pathologically positive axillary (PPAx) nodes who are ypN0 after neoadjuvant chemotherapy (NC). J Clin Oncol. 37(15_suppl) https://doi.org/10.1200/JCO.2019.37.15_suppl.TPS600.

46 Older Adult Patients

Isacco Desideri, Theodora Karnakis,
and Etienne Brain

46.1 Background

46.1.1 Older Adult Definition and Geriatric Assessment

The global population is not only growing rapidly but also ageing at an accelerated pace, projecting 434 million people over age 80 from 2040 [1]. This epidemiological transition comes with a rising number of older adults presenting with multi-morbidities including (other) cancer [2, 3]. Indeed, more than 60% of all cancers are diagnosed after the age of 65, displaying age-dependent intrinsic and extrinsic changes (e.g. inflammation, immunosenescence, environmental, psychosocial) responsible for frailty [4]. This multidimensional decline, poorly approached by chronological age alone, requires an in-depth, general, and holistic assessment of each single person to avoid the alleged and feared common under-treatment, but also the likely even more frequent overtreatment [5]. The Société Internationale d'Onco Gériatrie (SIOG, International Society of Geriatric Oncology, www.siog.org) strongly recommends the use of geriatric assessment to guide treatment decision in older patients with cancer [6].

Geriatric assessment is multidimensional; evaluates different domains including physical function, cognition, nutrition, comorbidities, psychological status, and social support; and allows stratifying patients between fit, frail, and vulnerable status, depending on the reversibility of deficits. It can unveil geriatric issues requiring specific geriatric interventions to make the treatment feasible [7], bringing prognostic information to consider in models of competing risks for outcome, and eventually improving the treatment benefit/risk ratio. However, geriatric assessment implementation in routine remains a challenge and requires important training and education, mixing the world of oncology and geriatrics to create a shared language and using a screening tool as the gateway or minimum starting point to any cancer treatment decision-making [8].

SIOG has published recommendations for breast cancer management in the older patient (last update accepted for publication 2021,

I. Desideri (✉)
Department of Experimental and Clinical Biomedical Sciences Mario Serio, University of Florence, Florence, Italy

Radiation Oncology Unit, Oncology Department, Azienda Ospedaliero Universitaria Careggi, Florence, Italy
e-mail: isacco.desideri@unifi.it

T. Karnakis
Instituto do Câncer do Estado de São Paulo- ICESP & Hospital Sírio-Libanês, São Paulo, Brazil
e-mail: dratheodora@karnakis.com.br

E. Brain
Department of Medical Oncology, Institut Curie, Saint-Cloud, France
e-mail: etienne.brain@curie.fr

© The Author(s), under exclusive license to Springer Nature Switzerland AG 2022
O. Kaidar-Person et al. (eds.), *Breast Cancer Radiation Therapy*,
https://doi.org/10.1007/978-3-030-91170-6_46

Lancet Oncology), from early-stage BC to metastatic setting [9].

46.1.2 Radiation Therapy

Following breast-conserving surgery (BCS), whole breast irradiation (WBI) remains the gold standard, as supported by the Oxford overview [10]. However, the CALGB 9343 trial randomised 636 women aged 70 and older after BCS between adjuvant tamoxifen alone or with WBI, showing no impact on overall survival of the omission of RT [11]. Therefore, many guidelines [e.g. National Institute for Care and Clinical Excellence (NICE), National Comprehensive Cancer Network (NCCN)] have now implemented such strategy in good prognosis luminal tumours at some expense of increased local relapse. However, the recently presented 10-year update of the PRIME-2 trial, randomising low-risk patients aged 65 or older between endocrine therapy with or without WBI, showed a continuing increase of local recurrences in the arm without WBI (9.8% vs. 0.9% at 10 years, $p = 0.00008$), a decreased risk of regional recurrences (0.5% with vs. 2.3% without WBI, $p = 0.014$), without any impact on the other endpoints. The benefit of WBI was especially pronounced in the ER-low (18.8% without WBI) subgroup, compared to ER-high (9.2% without WBI), $p = 0.007$ [I Kunkler, presented at the SABCS meeting 2020].

Shorter courses using hypofractionated schedules are very attractive alternatives to standard WBI, avoiding multiple burdensome transportations, especially in older patients. Although with no specific focus on this segment of the population, several randomised trials have demonstrated equivalent rates of local control and late toxicity (cosmesis) using various regimens, taken successfully to its next step of ultra-hypofractionated WBI as in the FAST Forward trial (26 Gy in 5 fractions over 1 week only) [12].

The boost of RT to the tumour bed after BCS is a matter of debate for older patients. Although it decreases local relapse [13], the absolute benefit decreases with age, while risks of late adverse effects such as fibrosis increase [14, 15]. Therefore, in most current guidelines, a boost is advised after age 60 only in case of a high risks of local recurrence.

Partial breast irradiation (PBI) combines increased dose per fraction and small target volume confined to the tumour bed, and may be intensified by shortening treatment duration, namely accelerated PBI (APBI). Although not studied specifically for older patients, it represents an attractive de-escalating strategy as found in several prospective phase III clinical trials (see Table 46.1) [16–21]. However, only one subgroup analysis focused on PBI for patients aged 70 and older with good prognosis early breast cancer [oestrogen receptor-positive (ER+), axillary node-negative, pT <3 cm, and clear margins], showing an improved quality of life profile and equivalent local relapse rates compared with WBI [22]. Therefore, the UK consensus recommends PBI for women aged 50 and older, with this favourable phenotype [23], as do the European Society for Therapeutic Radiology and Oncology (ESTRO) [24, 25] and the American Society for Radiotherapy and Oncology (ASTRO) [26].

The specific single fraction intra-operative RT (IORT) has also been tested in two large phase III randomised clinical trials with conflicting results, and different IORT techniques (electron vs. kV) making its recommendation specifically for older patients still controversial [16, 17]. In an attempt to further minimise the number of days of RT, others have investigated innovative hypofractionated brachytherapy-based schedules, showing promises with APBI in 2 days using HDR brachytherapy [27], single 18 Gy fraction with multi-catheter HDR brachytherapy [28], or a 3-fraction schedule [29]. Despite excellent local control and acceptable toxicity profiles compared with standard schedules, none again was studied in older patients. This stresses the need for specific research to fill in the gap of knowledge for the most prominent segment of our patients' population, deserving better than one retrospective analysis on older populations [30], or a small series (26 older patients) treated with HDR-brachytherapy [31].

Table 46.1 Main published phase 3 trials investigating partial breast irradiation

Trial	Study period	Study patients, overall (elderly)	Elderly patients %	RT technique, study design	OS rates	LR rates	Subgroup analysis in elderly
IMRT APBI Florence [21]	2005–2013	520 (117)	22.5 (>o = 70 years)	Accelerated IMRT APBI vs WBI	At 10-year: 91.9% (APBI) vs 91.9% (WBI); $p = 0.86$	At 10-year: 3.7% (APBI) vs 2.5% (WBI); $p = 0.40$	Yes
GEC-ESTRO [20]	2004–2009	1184 (190)	16 (>70)	Brachytherapy APBI vs WBI	At 5-year: 97.27% (APBI) vs 95.55% (WBI); $p = 0.11$	At 5-year: 1.44% (APBI) vs 0.92% (WBI); $p = 0.42$	No
TARGIT-A [16]	2000–2012	3451 (NR)	NR	IORT[a] IORT vs WBI	At 5-year: 96.1% (IORT) vs 94.7% (WBI); $p = 0.099$	At 5-year: 3.3% (IORT) vs 1.3% (WBI); $p = 0.042$	No
ELIOT [17]	2000–2007	1305 (137)	10.5 (>o = 70 years)	IORT[a] IORT vs WBI	At 5-year: 96.8% (IORT) vs 96.9% (WBI); $p = 0.59$	At 5-year: 4.4% (IORT) vs 0.4% (WBI); $p < 0.0001$	Yes
OCOG-RAPID [18]	2006–2011	2135 (NR)	NR	APBI vs WBI	No difference at 8 years	At 8-year: 3% (APBI) vs 2.7% (WBI)	No
NSABP-B39/RTOG 0413 [19]	2005–2013	4216 (515)	25 (> 70)	APBI vs WBI	No difference at 10-years	At 10-year: 4.6% (APBI) vs 3.9% (WBI) *[equivalence criteria not met]	No

APBI accelerated partial breast irradiation, *PBI*, partial breast irradiation; *IMRT* intensity modulated radiotherapy, *EBRT* external beam radiotherapy, *IORT* intraoperative radiotherapy, *WBI* whole-breast irradiation, *IBTR* Ipsilateral breast tumour recurrence, *CI* confidence interval, *NR* Not reported

[a]Experimental arm technique

46.2 Systemic Treatments

Perhaps the most provocative consideration regarding the missing information for the treatment of older patients derive from the systemic treatments. Indeed, there is a constant discrepancy between the lack of (or light) impact of age on treatment outcome read in drug labels and what is observed in real-life, where more than twice adjustments and compliance issues occur after an age of 65–70. This statement is not limited to chemotherapy but applies also to more recent targeted agents as anti-HER2 therapies [32] or other biologics as CDK4/6 inhibitors [33], underlining the limitations of scales that predict toxicity to chemotherapy as the CARG [34] and CRASH scores [35], or the more recent CARG-Breast Cancer to be used for adjuvant chemotherapy [36]. Even soft systemic treatments, with low-grade toxicity, affect compliance in more than 50% of older patients [37].

In both adjuvant and metastatic settings, main efforts are directed towards a stricter selection of patients requiring chemotherapy, exploiting optimisation of hormonotherapy for those with ER+ disease or of anti-HER2 therapies in case of HER2-positive phenotype. However, if adjuvant chemotherapy in older patients remains usually a challenge given the often severe, although acute and of short-duration, side effects overstretching functional reserves, adjuvant endocrine therapy may also be an issue with chronic musculoskeletal events and extended prolonged discomfort. This especially highlights the importance to reach the good treatment decision, balancing treatment duration, intensity, life expectancy, patients' willingness, and cancer prognosis.

This challenge is best epitomised by the EUROPA trial (NCT04134598) comparing in women aged 70 and older following BCS for luminal-like EBC endocrine therapy and no RT versus breast RT and non hormonotherapy, based on health related quality of life by patient reported outcome measures [38].

References

1. www.un.org/en/development/desa/population/publications/pdf/ageing/WorldPopulationAgeing2019-Report.pdf. Accessed March 1, 2021.
2. Kanesvaran R, Mohile S, Soto-Perez-de-Celis E, Singh H. The globalization of geriatric oncology: from data to practice. Am Soc Clin Oncol Educ Book. 2020;40:e107–15.
3. White MC, Holman DM, Goodman RA, et al. Cancer risk among older adults: time for cancer prevention to go silver. Gerontologist. 2019;59(suppl 1):S1–6.
4. Zhang X, Meng X, Chen Y, Leng SX, Zhang H. The biology of aging and cancer: frailty, inflammation, and immunity. Cancer J. 2017;23(4):201–5.
5. Soto-Perez-de-Celis E, Li D, Yuan Y, Lau YM, Hurria A. Functional versus chronological age: geriatric assessments to guide decision making in older patients with cancer. Lancet Oncol. 2018;19(6):e305–16.
6. Wildiers H, Heeren P, Karnakis T, Hurria A, et al. International Society of Geriatric Oncology Consensus on Geriatric Assessment in Older Patient with Cancer. J Clin Oncol. 2014;32:2595.
7. Puts MT, Santos B, Hardt J, Monette J, Atenafu EG, Girre V, et al. An update on a systematic review of the use of geriatric assessment for older adults in oncology. Ann Oncol. 2014;25(2):307–15.
8. Decoster L, Van Puyvelde K, Mohile S, Wedding U, Basso U, Colloca G, Rostoft S, Overcash J, Wildiers H, Steer C, Kimmick G, Kanesvaran R, Luciani A, Terret C, Hurria A, Kenis C, Audisio R, Extermann M. Screening tools for multidimensional health problems warranting a geriatric assessment in older cancer patients: an update on SIOG recommendations†. Ann Oncol. 2015;26(2):288–300. https://doi.org/10.1093/annonc/mdu210. Epub 2014 Jun 16
9. Biganzoli L, Wildiers H, Oakman C, et al. Management of elderly patients with breast cancer: updated recommendations of the International Society of Geriatric Oncology (SIOG) and European Society of Breast Cancer Specialists (EUSOMA). Lancet J Oncol. 2012;13:e148–60.
10. Early Breast Cancer Trialists' Collaborative Group (EBCTCG), McGale P, Taylor C, Correa C, Cutter D, Duane F, Ewertz M, et al. Effect of radiotherapy after mastectomy and axillary surgery on 10-year recurrence and 20-year breast cancer mortality: meta-analysis of individual patient data for 8135 women in 22 randomised trials. Lancet. 2014;383(9935):2127–35.
11. Hughes KS, Schnaper LA, Bellon JR, et al. Lumpectomy plus tamoxifen with or without irradiation in women age 70 years or older with early breast cancer: long-term follow-up of CALGB 9343. J Clin Oncol. 2013;31(19):2382–7.
12. Murray Brunt A, Haviland JS, Wheatley DA, Sydenham MA, Alhasso A, Bloomfield DJ, et al. Hypofractionated breast radiotherapy for 1 week

versus 3 weeks (FAST-forward): 5-year efficacy and late normal tissue effects results from a multicentre, non-inferiority, randomised, phase 3 trial. Lancet. 2020;395(10237):1613–26.
13. Bartelink H, Horiot JC, Poortmans PM, et al. Impact of a higher radiation dose on local control and survival in breast-conserving therapy of early breast cancer: 10-year results of the randomized boost versus no boost EORTC 22881-10882 trial. J Clin Oncol. 2007;25(22):3259–65.
14. Collette S, Collette L, Budiharto T, et al. Predictors of the risk of fibrosis at 10 years after breast conserving therapy for early breast cancer: a study based on the EORTC trial 22881-10882 'boost versus no boost'. Eur J Cancer. 2008;44(17):2587–99. https://doi.org/10.1016/j.ejca.2008.07.032.
15. Vrieling C, Collette L, Fourquet A, et al. The influence of patient, tumor and treatment factors on the cosmetic results after breast-conserving therapy in the EORTC 'boost vs. no boost' trial. EORTC Radiotherapy and Breast Cancer Cooperative Groups. Radiother Oncol. 2000;55(3):219–32. https://doi.org/10.1016/s0167-8140(00)00210-3.
16. Vaidya JS, Wenz F, Bulsara M, Tobias JS, Joseph DJ, Keshtgar M, Flyger HL, Massarut S, Alvarado M, Saunders C, Eiermann W, Metaxas M, Sperk E, Sütterlin M, Brown D, Esserman L, Roncadin M, Thompson A, Dewar JA, Holtveg HMR, Pigorsch S, Falzon M, Harris E, Matthews A, Brew-Graves C, Potyka I, Corica T, Williams NR, Baum M. Risk-adapted targeted intraoperative radiotherapy versus whole-breast radiotherapy for breast cancer: 5-year results for local control and overall survival from the TARGIT-A randomised trial. Lancet. 2014;383(9917):603–13.
17. Veronesi U, Orecchia R, Maisonneuve P, Viale G, Rotmensz N, Sangalli C, Luini A, Veronesi P, Galimberti V, Zurrida S, Leonardi MC, Lazzari R, Cattani F, Gentilini O, Intra M, Caldarella P, Ballardini B. Intraoperative radiotherapy versus external radiotherapy for early breast cancer (ELIOT): a randomised controlled equivalence trial. Lancet Oncol. 2013;14(13):1269–77.
18. Whelan TJ, Julian JA, Berrang TS, Kim DH, Germain I, Nichol AM, et al. External beam accelerated partial breast irradiation versus whole breast irradiation after breast conserving surgery in women with ductal carcinoma in situ and node-negative breast cancer (RAPID): a randomised controlled trial. Lancet. 2019;394(10215):2165–72.
19. Vicini FA, Cecchini RS, White JR, Arthur DW, Julian TB, Rabinovitch RA, et al. Long-term primary results of accelerated partial breast irradiation after breast-conserving surgery for early-stage breast cancer: a randomised, phase 3, equivalence trial. Lancet. 2019;394(10215):2155–64.
20. Polgar C, Ott OJ, Hildebrandt G, Kauer-Dorner D, Knauerhase H, Major T, et al. Late side-effects and cosmetic results of accelerated partial breast irradiation with interstitial brachytherapy versus whole-breast irradiation after breast-conserving surgery for low-risk invasive and in-situ carcinoma of the female breast: 5-year results of a randomised, controlled, phase 3 trial. Lancet Oncol. 2017;18(2):259–68.
21. Meattini I, Marrazzo L, Saieva C, Desideri I, Scotti V, Simontacchi G, Bonomo P, Greto D, Mangoni M, Scoccianti S, Lucidi S, Paoletti L, Fambrini M, Bernini M, Sanchez L, Orzalesi L, Nori J, Bianchi S, Pallotta S, Livi L. Accelerated partial-breast irradiation compared with whole-breast irradiation for early breast cancer: long-term results of the randomized phase III APBI-IMRT-Florence trial. J Clin Oncol. 2020;24:JCO2000650. https://doi.org/10.1200/JCO.20.00650. Epub ahead of print
22. Meattini I, Saieva C, Marrazzo L, et al. Accelerated partial breast irradiation using intensity-modulated radiotherapy technique compared to whole breast irradiation for patients aged 70 years or older: subgroup analysis from a randomized phase 3 trial. Breast Cancer Res Treat. 2015;153(3):539–47. https://doi.org/10.1007/s10549-015-3565-2.
23. Bloomfield DJ. Development of postoperative radiotherapy for breast cancer: UK Consensus Statements—a Model of Patient, Clinical and Commissioner Engagement? Clin Oncol (R Coll Radiol). 2017;29(10):639–41.
24. Polgár C, van Limbergen E, Pötter R, et al. Patient selection for accelerated partial-breast irradiation (APBI) after breast-conserving surgery: recommendations of the Groupe Européen de Curiethérapie-European Society for Therapeutic Radiology and Oncology (GEC-ESTRO) breast cancer working group based on clinical evidence (2009). Radiother Oncol. 2010;94(3):264–73.
25. Icro, Meattini Carlotta, Becherini Liesbeth, Boersma Orit, Kaidar-Person Gustavo Nader, Marta Angel, Montero Birgitte Vrou, Offersen Marianne C, Aznar Claus, Belka Adrian Murray, Brunt Samantha, Dicuonzo Pierfrancesco, Franco Mechthild, Krause Mairead, MacKenzie Tanja, Marinko Livia, Marrazzo Ivica, Ratosa Astrid, Scholten Elżbieta, Senkus Hilary, Stobart Philip, Poortmans Charlotte E, Coles. European Society for Radiotherapy and Oncology Advisory Committee in Radiation Oncology Practice consensus recommendations on patient selection and dose and fractionation for external beam radiotherapy in early breast cancer. The Lancet Oncology. 2022;23(1):e21–e31. https://doi.org/10.1016/S1470-2045(21)00539-8.
26. Correa C, Harris EE, Leonardi MC, et al. Accelerated partial breast irradiation: executive summary for the update of an ASTRO evidence-based consensus statement. Pract Radiat Oncol. 2017;7(2):73–9.
27. Wilkinson JB, Chen PY, Wallace MF, Shah CS, Benitez PR, Martinez AA, Vicini FA. Six-year results from a phase I/II trial for hypofractionated accelerated partial breast irradiation using a 2-day dose schedule. Am J Clin Oncol. 2018;41(10):986–91.
28. Latorre JA, Galdós P, Buznego LA, et al. Accelerated partial breast irradiation in a single 18 Gy frac-

tion with high-dose-rate brachytherapy: preliminary results. J Contemp Brachytherapy. 2018;10(1):58–63. https://doi.org/10.5114/jcb.2018.73994.
29. Jethwa KR, Park SS, Gonuguntla K, et al. Three-fraction intracavitary accelerated partial breast brachytherapy: early provider and patient-reported outcomes of a novel regimen. Int J Radiat Oncol Biol Phys. 2019;104(1):75–82.
30. Kinj R, Chand ME, Gal J, et al. Five-year oncological outcome after a single fraction of accelerated partial breast irradiation in the elderly. Radiat Oncol. 2019;14(1):234.
31. Hannoun-Lévi JM, Lam Cham Kee D, Gal J, et al. Accelerated partial breast irradiation in the elderly: 5-year results of the single fraction elderly breast irradiation (SiFEBI) phase I/II trial. Brachytherapy. 2020;19(1):90–6.
32. Brain E, Caillet P, de Glas N, Biganzoli L, Cheng K, Lago LD, et al. HER2-targeted treatment for older patients with breast cancer: an expert position paper from the International Society of Geriatric Oncology. J Geriatr Oncol. 2019;10(6):1003–13.
33. Howie LJ, Singh H, Bloomquist E, Wedam S, Amiri-Kordestani L, Tang S, Sridhara R, Sanchez J, Prowell TM, Kluetz PG, King-Kallimanis BL, Gao JJ, Ibrahim A, Goldberg KB, Theoret M, Pazdur R, Beaver JA. Outcomes of older women with hormone receptor-positive, human epidermal growth factor receptor-negative metastatic breast cancer treated with a CDK4/6 inhibitor and an aromatase inhibitor: an FDA pooled analysis. J Clin Oncol. 2019;37(36):3475–83.
34. Hurria A, Togawa K, Mohile SG, Owusu C, Klepin HD, Gross CP, et al. Predicting chemotherapy toxicity in older adults with cancer: a prospective multicenter study. J Clin Oncol. 2011;29(25):3457–65.
35. Extermann M, Boler I, Reich RR, Lyman GH, Brown RH, DeFelice J, et al. Predicting the risk of chemotherapy toxicity in older patients: the chemotherapy risk assessment scale for high-age patients (CRASH) score. Cancer. 2012;118(13):3377–86.
36. Magnuson A, Sedrak MS, Gross CP, Tew WP, Klepin HD, Wildes TM, Muss HB, Dotan E, Freedman RA, O'Connor T, Dale W, Cohen HJ, Katheria V, Arsenyan A, Levi A, Kim H, Mohile S, Hurria A, Sun CL. Development and validation of a risk tool for predicting severe toxicity in older adults receiving chemotherapy for early-stage breast cancer. J Clin Oncol. 2021;39(6):608–18.
37. Kalsi T, Babic-Illman G, Fields P, Hughes S, Maisey N, Ross P, Wang Y, Harari D. The impact of low-grade toxicity in older people with cancer undergoing chemotherapy. Br J Cancer. 2014;111(12):2224–8. https://doi.org/10.1038/bjc.2014.496. Epub 2014 Sep 30. PMID: 25268369; PMCID: PMC4264435
38. Meattini I, Poortmans PMP, Marrazzo L, Desideri I, Brain E, Hamaker M, Lambertini M, Miccinesi G, Russell N, Saieva C, Strnad V, Visani L, Kaidar-Person O, Livi L. Exclusive endocrine therapy or partial breast irradiation for women aged ≥70 years with luminal A-like early stage breast cancer (NCT04134598 - EUROPA): proof of concept of a randomized controlled trial comparing health related quality of life by patient reported outcome measures. J Geriatr Oncol. 2021;12(2):182–9. https://doi.org/10.1016/j.jgo.2020.07.013. Epub 2020 Jul 29. PMID: 32739355

47 Non-resectable Patients

Einav Gal-Yam and Philip Poortmans

47.1 Background

The term non-resectable (inoperable) breast cancer refers to the situation where upfront surgery will not achieve complete excision of all tumours with clear margins. These cancers can present as primary locally advanced tumours with no evidence of metastases, as locoregional recurrent tumours after an initial primary breast cancer, or in the context of recurring or newly diagnosed metastatic disease. Overall, the prognosis of non-resectable disease, even in the non-metastatic setting is poor [1]. As in other clinical presentations, optimal management requires involvement of a multidisciplinary team, balancing the options for cure and for care to discuss a personalised approach for each individual patient [2]. Even when cure cannot be obtained, patients with advanced locoregional disease may live for several years.

E. Gal-Yam
Breast Cancer Institute, Institute of Oncology, Sheba Medical Center, Ramat-Gan, Israel
e-mail: Einav.niligal-yam@sheba.gov.il

P. Poortmans (✉)
Faculty of Medicine and Health Sciences, University of Antwerp, Antwerp, Belgium

Department of Radiation Oncology, Iridium Netwerk, Antwerp, Belgium
e-mail: philip.poortmans@gza.be

47.2 Locoregional Non-resectable Disease in the Absence of Distant Metastases

Primary Non-Resectable Disease Locally and/or regionally advanced non-resectable breast cancer generally refers to stage III disease including T0-3/N2-3 tumours with involvement of either matted/fixed ipsilateral axillary, and/or ipsilateral infraclavicular, supraclavicular or IMNs, or T4 tumours extending to the chest wall structures or the skin. While primary locally advanced non-resectable tumours at presentation occur at a frequency of less than 10% in Europe and the USA, they are still common in developing countries and observed in up to 60% of cases [3]. HER2-positive and triple-negative locally advanced breast cancer (LABC) generally occur in younger patient populations, while hormone receptor positive locally advanced disease occurs more often in older or deprived patients [3].

Treatment should be delivered by a combined modality approach involving medical, radiation, and surgical oncologists. At presentation, systemic workup should be performed to rule out the presence of detectable distant metastases. If no metastatic disease is detected then primary systemic therapy (PST) incorporating standard protocols aimed at cure is warranted. In most HER2 positive and triple negative cases, 6–8 cylces of

© The Author(s), under exclusive license to Springer Nature Switzerland AG 2022
O. Kaidar-Person et al. (eds.), *Breast Cancer Radiation Therapy*,
https://doi.org/10.1007/978-3-030-91170-6_47

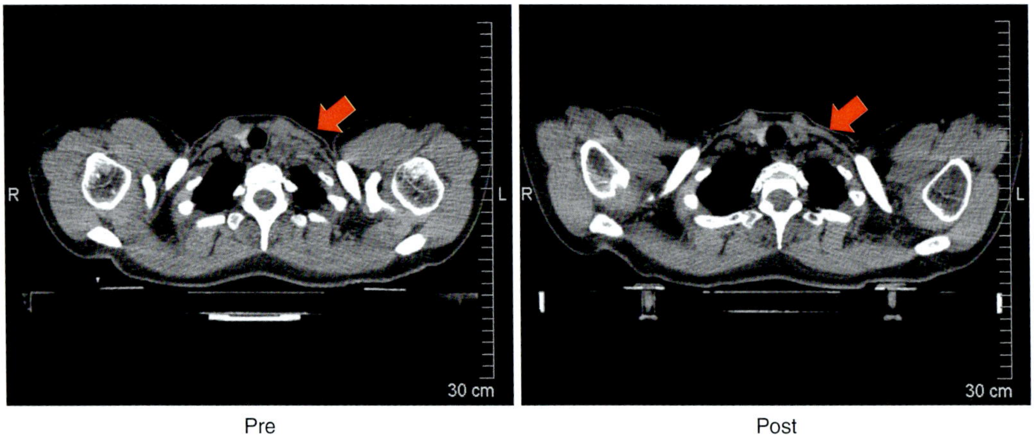

Fig. 47.1 CT imaging in RT position of a locoregionally advanced breast cancer patient pre (left) and post (right) systemic therapy. The initially pathological lymph nodes in axilla level 4 (supraclavicular) left disappeared completely

combination chemotherapy are used. In the case of HER2 positive disease dual HER2 blockade (usually with trastuzumab and, if available, pertuzumab) is added to the chemotherapy backbone. This treatment results in resectability of most tumours and in complete responses in 25–70% [4]. In triple-negative Programmed death-ligand (PDL-1) positive patients, recent trials have shown that addition of immunotherapy to the chemotherapy backbone significantly increased complete response rates up to ~65% [5, 6]. In stage IIIB, the benefit of addition of pembrolizumab was the greatest with pathologic complete responses in 48.6% of patients vs 23.1% in the placebo arm [7].

In the case of hormone receptor positive disease responses to systemic chemotherapy or endocrine therapy are much more modest with complete responses encountered in less than 10% of the cases [8]. Since endocrine treatment has not been amply examined in premenopausal patients, younger patients with higher grade luminal tumours will usually receive chemotherapy, while older patients with lower-proliferative tumours may receive endocrine treatment, usually with aromatase inhibitors. Trials comparing chemotherapy with endocrine therapy in these cases showed comparable efficacy [8]. Addition of targeted drugs such as CDK4/6 inhibitors to endocrine therapy in the preoperative setting is evaluated in ongoing trials and may eventually have a role in some luminal tumours [9]. In all cases in which non-resectable disease is reduced to resectable disease, surgery followed by postoperative locoregional RT is indicated, aiming at definitive cure [3]. For patients which are not rendered resectable by treatment, as occurs more often in luminal-like breast cancer, RT either preoperative with delayed surgical resection after 2–3 months or in a radical setting, followed by long-term endocrine therapy can lead to prolonged disease-free survival [10].

Patients presenting with regionally advanced disease should be seen by the radiation oncologist prior to initiation of therapy to carefully document the extent of initial nodal involvement, preferably using a CT-scan in the RT-treatment position for later image coregistration (Fig. 47.1).

Inflammatory breast cancer is a special entity of LABC with a characteristic oedema and redness of the breast caused by involvement of the dermal lymphatics by cancerous cells. Inflammatory breast cancer tends to be hormone receptor negative and to occur in younger patients often presenting without distant metastases at diagnosis but invariably evolving towards an ominous disease course including locoregional progression, if no response can be obtained with PST. Even in those cases, radical locoregional treatments are indicated to prevent the burden of locoregional progression. In case of a good response to PST, mastectomy with axillary dissection should be planned, without an immediate reconstruction and swiftly followed by locoregional RT. [3]

Locoregional recurrent disease refers to the ipsilateral recurrence of either breast/chest wall or regional nodal disease. Risk factors for locoregional recurrence include larger primary tumour size and positive nodes, negative hormone receptors, and younger age [11]. Again, systemic work up is required to exclude the presence of concomitant distant metastases. Most isolated ipsilateral local regional recurences are resectable and should be surgically excised, followed by postoperative RT and systemic therapy including re-administration of chemotherapy, which was shown to be beneficial in ER negative tumours and endocrine therapy in hormone positive tumours [12]. However, diffuse skin recurrence presenting as rash, or multiple skin papules, bulky chest wall or nodal recurrence involving musculoskeletal or neurological features, and supraclavicular or internal mammary nodes are generally not amenable to upfront resection. In these cases PST should be used as an approach to downsize recurrent disease. The choice of PST depends largely on which prior systemic treatment was given and the time that elapsed from the primary tumour until recurrence. Systemic protocols utilised usually resemble those in the metastatic setting. If the tumours become resectable then surgery may be attempted. However, extensive chest wall and supraclavicular/internal mammary resections are currently less performed and RT may be used instead. In the case where the disease is not amenable to surgery, systemic therapy is given continuously to reach a maximal response, followed by consolidation radiation.

In case of previous RT, re-irradiation can be considered, depending on the individual case presentation and the risk for subsequent locoregional recurrences. Hyperthermia can be added to re-irradiation for recurrences like at the chest wall (see sections "Reirradiation"and "Hyperthermia") [13].

Non-Resectability due to Medical Conditions Patients who are in a medical condition not allowing a major surgical intervention, or for those refusing surgery, radical RT can still offer durable disease control and—eventually—cure. However, doses required to obtain sustained tumour control are higher compared to elective post- or preoperative RT and thereby often go with side effects including fibrosis, skin changes, and, rarely, radiation necrosis and ulceration. Already in 1980, Pierquin et al. reported on 43 patients with T3 breast cancer that were treated with exclusive RT, leading to only 23% locoregional persistent or recurrent disease at 5 years, with an overall disease-free survival of 56% [14]. In another study, 187 patients with T2-T4 or N2 tumours treated between 1970 and 1984 underwent preoperative RT followed by mastectomy and axillary lymph node dissection. A pathological complete response was obtained overall in 10%, amounting to 26% in triple-negative breast cancer patients. After a follow-up of 32 years, the 25-year locoregional control rate was 89%, with DFS and OS rates both at 30%. Reassuringly, postoperative grade > 2 complication rate was only 19% [10]. Therefore, RT without surgery may be considered as an option for controlling disease symptoms and delaying or even preventing local progression (Fig. 47.2) [15].

47.3 Locoregional Non-resectable Disease in the Presence of Distant Metastases

Overall, about 5% of all new breast cancer diagnoses are made in stage IV. Additionally, up to 25% of all initial early breast cancer patients progress over time to incurable disease, most often due to distant metastases. Part of these metastatic patients present with synchronous non-resectable local or regional disease. While locoregional disease is not life-threatening, it may often lead to devastating symptoms for which effective treatments are required. Additionally, in specific cases of metastatic disease aggressive treatment to the local tumour may be beneficial.

In patients with metastatic disease, a careful evaluation should be made to estimate possible disease courses. Depending on factors including tumour burden, molecular tumour subtype, systemic therapy options, co-morbidity, and per-

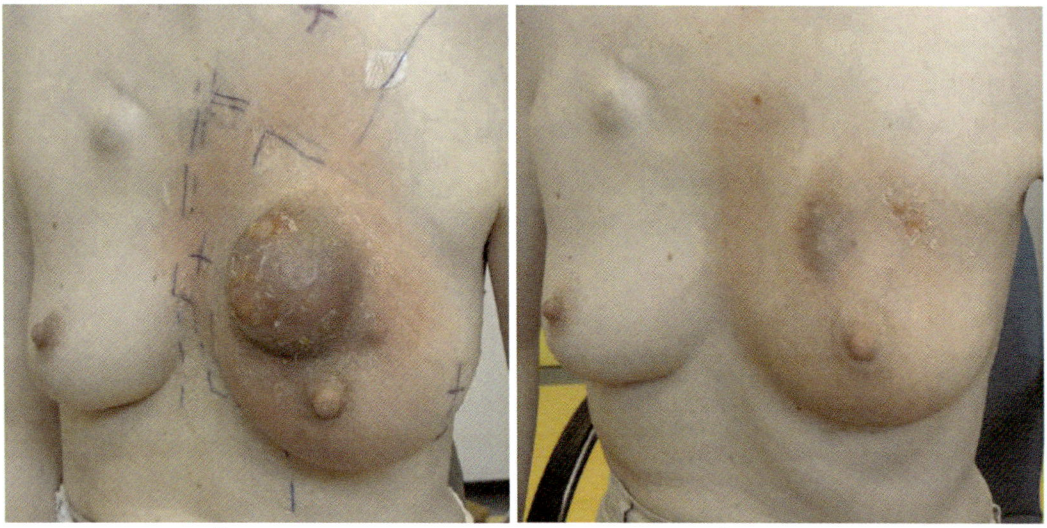

Fig. 47.2 Clinical image of a patient before and after radiation therapy combined with chemotherapy. She was originally not amenable to surgical therapy. Left: after induction chemotherapy and 1 day before starting RT. Right: 3 weeks after RT. Reproduced with permission from [15]

sonal preferences, several therapeutic approaches may be envisagable.

Local breast palliation: In patients who present with bulky, painful or ulcerated breast tumours in the context of diffuse metastatic disease, treatment objectives are usually of palliative intent. This can include local surgery *de propreté*, like already described in 1988 [16]. However, most often RT is used with schedules varying depending on the extent of locoregional tumour burden and estimated life expectancy. While satisfactory palliation can be obtained with short courses RT varying between single doses of 8–10 Gy and 20 Gy in 4 fractions, patients with a longer life expectancy might benefit longer from higher-doses schedules such as a total dose of 39–45 in 13–15 fractions [17]. Since the publication of the FAST-Forward Trial, 26 Gy in 5 fractions in 1 week should be considered as well, although experience in the advanced disease is still missing and results of the nodal substudy are awaited [18]. An additional dose of 6 Gy to the tumour bulk could be considered as well [19].

Locoregional treatment in the context of metastatic disease: The benefit of primary tumour resection and/or RT in stage IV breast cancer has been at the centre of debate for many years with mixed results coming mainly from retrospective trials [20]. The first reported randomised trial, including 350 stage IV breast cancer patients, failed to show an advantage from early initiation of locoregional treatments with a medias OS of just 20 months [21]. In the prospective multicentre phase III, randomised MF07–01 trial, a total of 274 treatment-naïve stage IV breast cancer patients were treated either with locoregional treatment (LRT) followed by systemic therapy or with systemic therapy alone. In a longer follow-up of median 40 months, median survival was significantly improved: 45 months after combined and 40 months after systemic treatment only. Moreover, an unplanned subgroup analyses showed that the risk of death was statistically lower in the LRT group than in the ST group for ER/PR positive patients (p = 0.01), for HER2 positive patients (p = 0.01), for patients younger than 55 years (p = 0.007) and for patients presenting with solitary bone-only metastases (p = 0.04) [22]. This may be explained by a synergistic interaction between biology and target treatments (endocrine and anti-HER2) with RT. In a recently reported randomised phase III

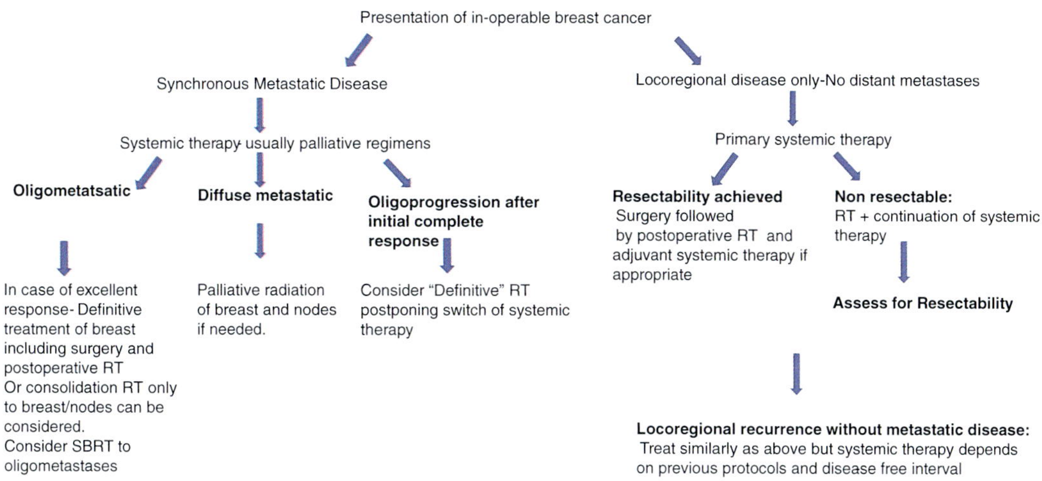

Fig. 47.3 Schematic algorithm for treatment in the various scenarios of presentation of inoperable breast cancer

trial of systemic therapy plus early local therapy (surgery and RT) versus systemic therapy alone in 256 women with de novo stage IV who responded to initial systemic therapy, median OS survival was 54 months and was not prolonged in the patients undergoing local treatment, nor was quality of life improved. Moreover, OS was worse among the patients with TNBC (n = 20) that received local treatment, possibly due to interruption of the chemotherapy [23]. In the same study, long-term QoL was evaluated in the cohort of patients who survived at least 3 years since randomisation. A total of 81 patients were analysed; 55 of whom had locoregional treatments together with systemic treatment. Locoregional treatment did not affect physical health, mental health, daily activities, or energy at 3 years compared to the time of diagnosis ($p > 0.05$). However, these variables were significantly better in stage I-III BC patients ($p < 0.001$) [23].

Thus, in selected cases, especially in low tumour burden and/or oligometastatic disease (often considered as less than five metastases detected by whole body imaging such as PET-CT, see ESTRO and EORTC consensus recommendations and taking into consideration biological factors as well, locoregional treatments identical to those in the non-metastatic disease can be considered, especially after achieving a good response to an initial course of systemic therapy [24]. Surgery and RT should be combined similarly to patients without metastases, except for withholding elective treatment of for example lymph node regions that were initially not involved. If surgery is not performed, consolidative RT may be indicated, including a boost dose to the sites of highest disease burden, using fractionation schedules as mentioned above.

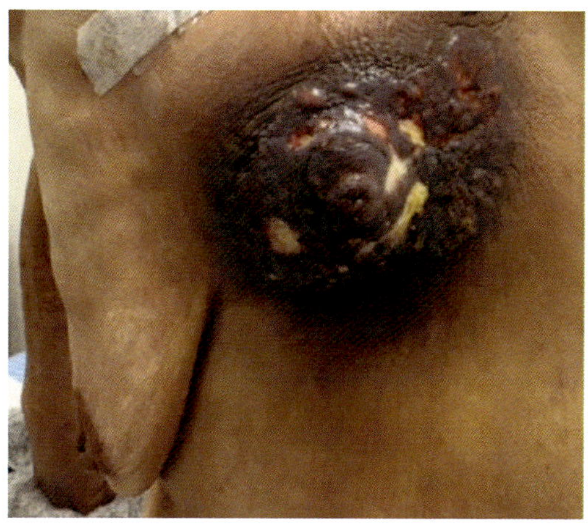

Fig. 47.4 Locally advanced inoperable breast cancer

Figure 47.3 summarises suggested clinical approach in cases of inoperable breast cancer. Figures 47.4 and 47.5 show cases of advanced chest wall disease, that treatment is aimed for palliation and local control.

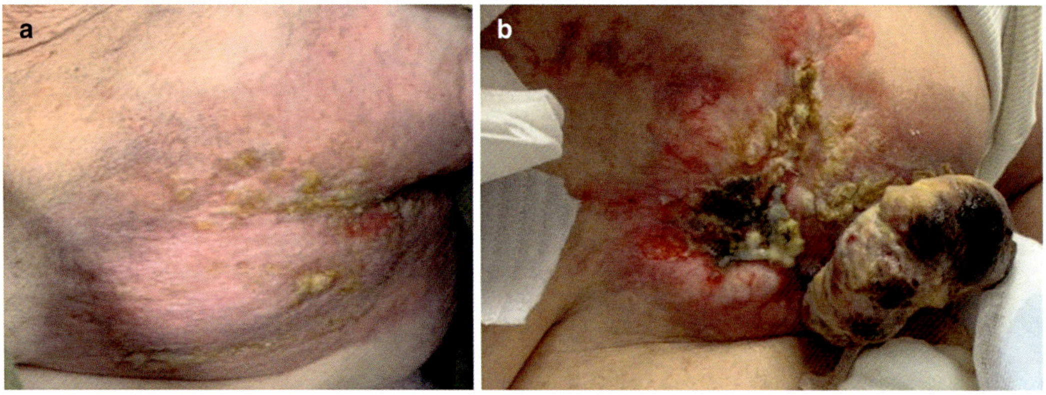

Fig. 47.5 (**a**, **b**) Locally advanced inoperable breast cancer, both cases resulted in self-amputation of the breast

47.4 Summary

We have described the various treatment options for patients presenting with inoperable breast cancer in different scenarios (see summary in Fig. 47.3). As systemic therapies are becoming more and more effective following the introduction of subtype specific and biologically targeted drugs, and RT techniques are evolving in parallel, their combined use in a well-concerted manner contributes to the prolongation of survival of breast cancer patients and improvement of their quality of life. The key remains a well-coordinated action of the entire multidisciplinary team who treat the breast cancer patients.

References

1. Garg PK, Prakash G. Current definition of locally advanced breast cancer. Curr Oncol. 2015;22:e409–10.
2. Cardoso F, et al. 5th ESO-ESMO international consensus guidelines for advanced breast cancer (ABC 5). Ann Oncol. 2020;31:1623–49.
3. Tryfonidis K, Senkus E, Cardoso MJ, Cardoso F. Corrigendum: management of locally advanced breast cancer—perspectives and future directions. Nat Rev Clin Oncol. 2015;12:312.
4. Wuerstlein R, Harbeck N. Neoadjuvant therapy for HER2-positive breast cancer. Rev Recent Clin Trials. 2017;12:81–92.
5. Mittendorf EA, et al. Neoadjuvant atezolizumab in combination with sequential nab-paclitaxel and anthracycline-based chemotherapy versus placebo and chemotherapy in patients with early-stage triple-negative breast cancer (IMpassion031): a randomised, double-blind, phase 3 trial. Lancet. 2020;396:1090–100.
6. Schmid P, et al. Pembrolizumab for early triple-negative breast cancer. N Engl J Med. 2020;382:810–21.
7. Suppan C, Balic M. Treatment options in early triple-negative breast cancer: update from the San Antonio Breast Cancer Symposium 2019. Memo Mag Eur Med Oncol. 2020;13:346–8.
8. Spring LM, et al. Neoadjuvant endocrine therapy for estrogen receptor-positive breast cancer a systematic review and meta-analysis. JAMA Oncol. 2016;2:1477–86.
9. Brandão M, Ignatiadis M. CDK4/6 inhibitors as neoadjuvant treatment in breast cancer-what can we learn? Ann Oncol. 2018;29:2274–8.
10. Riet FG, et al. Preoperative radiotherapy in breast cancer patients: 32 years of follow-up. Eur J Cancer. 2017;76:45–51.
11. Wapnir IL, Khan A. Current strategies for the management of locoregional breast cancer recurrence. Oncology (United States). 2019;33:19–25.
12. Wapnir IL, et al. Efficacy of chemotherapy for ER-negative and ER-positive isolated locoregional recurrence of breast cancer: final analysis of the CALOR trial. J Clin Oncol. 2018;36:1073–9.
13. Kaidar-Person O, Oldenborg S, Poortmans P. Re-irradiation and hyperthermia in breast cancer. Clin Oncol. 2018;30:73–84.
14. Pierquin B, et al. Radical radiation therapy of breast cancer. Int J Radiat Oncol Biol Phys. 1980;6:17–24.
15. Chargari C, Kirova YM, Cottu P, Salmon RJ, Fourquet A. Progressive inflammatory breast cancer in patient receiving chemotherapy: the importance of radiotherapy as a part of locoregional treatment. Radiother Oncol. 2009;90:160–1.
16. Meurette J, Leroy-Brasme T, Laurent JC, Cambier L, Depadt G. Ulcerated cancers of the breast: results of modified mastectomy. Apropos of 64 cases. J Chir (Paris). 1988;125:183–8.

17. Vempati P, et al. Palliation of ulcerative breast lesions with radiation. Anticancer Res. 2016;36:4701–5.
18. Murray Brunt A, et al. Hypofractionated breast radiotherapy for 1 week versus 3 weeks (FAST-forward): 5-year efficacy and late normal tissue effects results from a multicentre, non-inferiority, randomised, phase 3 trial. Lancet. 2020;395:1613–26.
19. Machiels M, et al. Accelerated adaptation of ultrahypofractionated radiation therapy for breast cancer at the time of the COVID-19 pandemic. Clin Oncol. 2020;33:e166.
20. Lee JS, Toktas O, Soran A. Role of locoregional treatment in de novo stage IV breast cancer. Clin Med Insights Oncol. 2020;14:1179554920942440.
21. Badwe R, et al. Locoregional treatment versus no treatment of the primary tumour in metastatic breast cancer: an open-label randomised controlled trial. Lancet Oncol. 2015;16:1380–8.
22. Soran A, et al. Randomized trial comparing resection of primary tumor with no surgery in stage IV breast cancer at presentation: protocol MF07-01. Ann Surg Oncol. 2018;25:3141–9.
23. Khan SA, et al. A randomized phase III trial of systemic therapy plus early local therapy versus systemic therapy alone in women with de novo stage IV breast cancer: a trial of the ECOG-ACRIN research group (E2108). J Clin Oncol. 2020;38:LBA2–LBA2.
24. Guckenberger M, et al. Characterisation and classification of oligometastatic disease: a European Society for Radiotherapy and Oncology and European Organisation for Research and Treatment of Cancer consensus recommendation. Lancet Oncol. 2020;21:e18–28.

Genetic Syndromes and RT for Breast Cancer

48

Rinat Bernstein-Molho, Bella Kaufman, and Lynda Wyld

48.1 Genetic Syndromes and Breast Cancer Risk

Most breast cancers are caused by somatic, non-hereditary, mutations acquired during the lifetime. However, some women are born with a germline mutation in one of their critical tumour suppressor genes. The majority of these women are heterozygotes and only when further somatic mutation occurs, does the function of the gene tumour suppressor gene decline (Knudson's two hit hypothesis [1, 2]) resulting in progression of the process of carcinogenesis. A number of key single gene mutations are linked to breast cancer development [3] and these account for up to 9% of all breast cancers [4]. These may be single gene mutations with variable penetrance that are classified according to the level of risk they confer (High risk: >four-fold increase; moderate: 2–four fold increase risk). *BRCA1* and *BRCA2* mutations together account for over 50% of all hereditary breast cancers [4], with *CHEK2* accounting for 11.7%, *ATM* for 9.7%, and *PALB2* for 9.3% [4] (Fig. 48.1) [5]. These genes are now widely and reliably tested for, either individually or via gene panels. There are also a range of low risk gene mutations [3] and over 100 single nucleotide polymorphisms (SNPs) linked to a slightly increased breast cancer risk [6]. These low-penetrance genes and SNPs are not routinely tested for at present and understanding their clinical impact is more challenging as their effects may be very small. Interactions between SNPs complicates matters further. Cumulative risk scores based on SNP profiles are currently being developed but are not yet in clinical use [7].

The characteristics of key gene mutations linked to breast cancer risk are shown in Table 48.1. For the majority of the listed mutations risk reducing strategies are now well described, including imaging surveillance starting at a young age (using an age stratified combination of MRI or mammography), and primary prevention with either pharmacological strategies such as use of selective oestrogen receptor modulators (SERMS, such as tamoxifen or raloxifene) or aromatase inhibitors [8, 9], and risk-reducing surgery [10], both of which are effective. Moreover, for women newly diagnosed with breast cancer, the presence of such mutations has implications for treatment.

R. Bernstein-Molho (✉) · B. Kaufman
Breast Cancer Unit, Oncology Institute, Chaim Sheba Medical Center, Tel-Hashomer, Israel

Sackler School of Medicine, Tel-Aviv University, Tel-Aviv, Israel
e-mail: rinat.bernstein@sheba.health.gov.il

L. Wyld
University of Sheffield, Sheffield, UK

Doncaster and Bassetlaw Teaching Hospitals NHS Foundation Trust, Doncaster, UK
e-mail: L.wyld@sheffield.ac.uk

© The Author(s), under exclusive license to Springer Nature Switzerland AG 2022
O. Kaidar-Person et al. (eds.), *Breast Cancer Radiation Therapy*,
https://doi.org/10.1007/978-3-030-91170-6_48

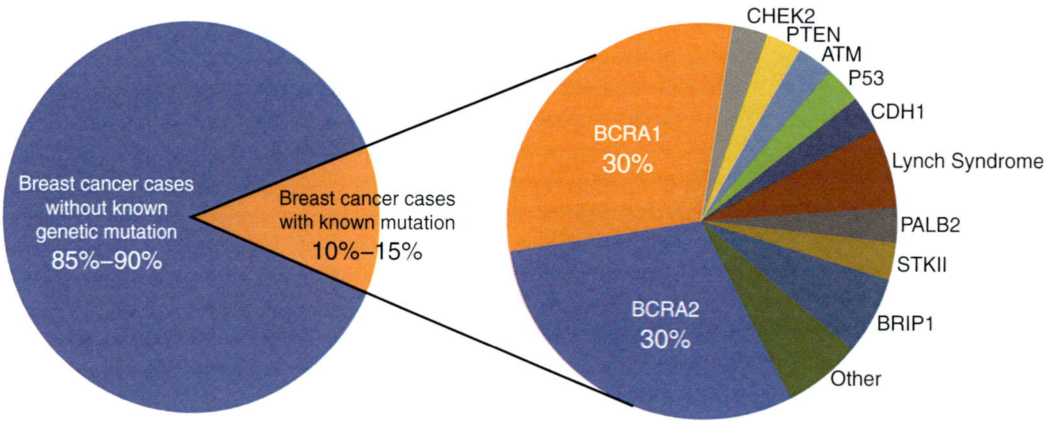

Fig. 48.1 Incidence of identifiable genetic mutations in patients with breast cancer (reproduced from Peleg Hasson et al., 2020 [5])

48.2 Genetic Syndromes and Breast Cancer Management

The main locoregional impact of carriage of these genes in woman with breast cancer is the increased risk of second primary cancers. While *BRCA1/2* mutation carriers with unilateral breast cancer have similar risk of ipsilateral recurrence after breast-conserving therapy (BCT) compared to sporadic cases, contralateral breast cancers are significantly greater in carriers versus controls, with reported 10- and 15-year estimates of 26% and 39% for carriers and 3% and 7% for controls, respectively (HR, 10.43; $P < 0.0001$) [62]. Many treating physicians and women therefore consider mastectomy as the primary treatment and may also propose and request contralateral risk reducing mastectomy. Data from several studies has shown that whilst risk reducing mastectomy in an unaffected carrier is associated with an extension of life expectancy [10], especially in *BRCA1* carriers, removal of the contralateral breast in carriers with breast cancer, at least in the short to medium term, carries little to no survival benefit [63]. This is due to the primary cancer having a predominant impact on life expectancy, with the highest risk of recurrence in the first 3 years. However, more nuanced analysis finds that for women with DCIS or good prognosis primary breast cancer there may be a benefit [64]. Longer-term studies looking at 10-year survivors of their primary cancer, also shows a beneficial impact as the effect to reduce second cancers becomes stronger [65]. Nevertheless, this approach should be based on individual considerations, including, apart from the prognosis of the primary cancer, also considerations including age, comorbidity, and patients' preferences. The 2021 NCCN Guidelines suggest that premenopausal carriers of BRCA mutations should consider additional risk reduction strategies, weighing up the potential risk reduction of contralateral mastectomy against the risk of tumour recurrence [66].

RT is standard after BCS and many women who are diagnosed with breast cancer and have their surgery before they know their carrier status may be faced with a genetic test result after they have had conservation surgery. They may then wish to review their surgical decision before they have RT. A woman may not wish to make an immediate decision to have mastectomy (and increasingly reconstruction in these younger women) for risk reduction purposes, especially considering what we know about the lack of short- and medium-term impact on survival.

Table 48.1 Characteristics of key gene mutations linked to breast cancer and evidence for RT-related complications

Gene mutation	Syndrome	Population gene frequency	Lifetime breast cancer risk	Breast cancer clinical characteristics	Increased risk for RT complications (level of evidence)
BRCA1 [11]	Breast and ovarian cancer, prostate cancer, pancreatic cancer	1/400–1/800 [12]	60% (confidence interval, CI, 40–75) [13]	Median age ~ 40–42 [13, 14] Basal epithelial triple-negative subtype ~65% [15, 16]	No (high) [17–25]
BRCA2 [26]	Breast and ovarian cancer, male breast cancer, prostate cancer, pancreatic cancer	1/400–1/800 [12]	55% (CI: 41–70) [13].	Median age 45 [13], range 55–64 [14]. Similar subtype distribution to sporadic breast cancer [27] although triple-negative slightly more likely in women over 50	No (high) [17–25]
PALB2 [28, 29]	Increased breast cancer risk and also pancreatic and prostate cancer but less certainty than for *BRCA* genes. Biallelic mutation carriers have Fanconi's anaemia	~1/900 [30, 31]	45% (CI: 31–56%) [32]	Less certainty than for *BRCA1/2* due to less data but probably an excess of triple-negative cancers [4, 32].	Unknown (no data)
CHEK2 [33]	Link to breast, colon, renal, sarcoma, and prostate cancer	1/160–1/235 [30, 31]	Odds ratio: ~2.5 (95% CI 2–3.1) [30, 31]	Tends to be associated with higher grade, larger cancers and inferior survival rates. Linked to ER-positive tumours [30, 34].	Unknown (very limited)
ATM [35]	Key gene regulating DNA damage response. Homozygotes (Louis Bar syndrome) have progressive ataxia, extreme radiation sensitivity, cutaneous telangiectasia, and high cancer risk (leukaemias, lymphomas and breast cancer). Heterozygotes have only increased cancer risk (mostly breast, and possibly prostate cancer).	1/242–1/338 [30, 31]	33% (24–40%) [36]	Linked to ER-positive tumours [30, 34]	Unknown (limited and inconsistent) [25, 37–41]
CDH1 [42]	Hereditary diffuse gastric cancer syndrome due to mutation of the intercellular adhesion molecule e-cadherin. Linked to early onset diffuse gastric cancer and breast cancer [43]	1/4225–1/5424 [30, 31]	39% (12–84%) by age 80 [44] 42% (23–68%) [45]	Lobular breast cancer, especially if bilateral. Median age 46 [46]	Unknown (no data)

(continued)

Table 48.1 (continued)

Gene mutation	Syndrome	Population gene frequency	Lifetime breast cancer risk	Breast cancer clinical characteristics	Increased risk for RT complications (level of evidence)
TP53 [47]	Li-Fraumeni syndrome. Key gene in DNA repair. Increased risk of breast cancer, brain cancer, adrenocortical carcinoma, lung cancer, sarcomas, lymphomas, and a range of other cancers.	1/5000 [47]–1/25000 [31]	75%, (50–100%), 6.4-fold increased risk (4.3–9.3) [48]	Median age 33 years. Excess of Her2-positive cancers [49]. Increased risk (30%) of second cancer within radiation field [50]. Approximately 5–8% of women under 30 with breast cancer will have LFS	Yes (limited) [25, 51–55]
STK11 [56]	Peutz–Jeghers syndrome: Skin pigmentation, GI hamartomas and increased risk of GI, gynae and breast cancers	1/10000–1/150,000 [31, 57]	45% (27–68%) by age 70 [57]	Median age for breast cancer diagnosis 44 [57].	Unknown (no data)
PTEN [58]	Cowden syndrome. Mutation of a tumour suppressor gene in the PI3K-AKT-mTOR pathway. Syndrome includes macrocephaly, mucocutaneous hamartomas, thyroid, breast, endometrial, renal, and colorectal cancers	1/8500–1/250,000 [31, 59]	39% age 70 (24–58%) [60]	Median age 42 for breast cancer	Unknown (very limited) [61]

However, if they complete their conservation therapy and have RT, this may make subsequent reconstruction more difficult. In particular, performing SSM/NSM on irradiated skin is associated with a higher risk of wound and nipple necrosis, which may place the reconstruction at risk, especially if implants are to be used. Similarly, there is a significantly higher rate of reconstruction complications if implant reconstruction is performed in an irradiated field [67]. The increasing use of PST (mostly due to stage and tumour biology) allows a helpful delay to permit the woman to choose the most suitable surgical option based on genetic test results. However, this option is only available for patients who have an indication for systemic treatment based on preoperatively available information.

48.3 RT-Related Complication in Patients with Hereditary Syndromes - Existing Data and Unmet Needs

Studies that investigated RT-related toxicity in *BRCA1/2* mutation carriers with early breast cancer found no evidence of a significant increase in acute and late radiation effects or contralateral breast cancer events related to radiation exposure compared to women with sporadic breast cancer [17–19]. Therefore, for mutation carriers who desire breast conservation, BCT should be offered if clinically appropriate. A number of studies evaluating the risk of contralateral breast cancer in women with a *BRCA1/2* mutation found that RT was not associated with an increase in contralateral breast cancer events [20–23]. Moreover, a study evaluating prophylactic contralateral breast RT in *BRCA1/2* carriers with early breast cancer found a significant reduction of subsequent contralateral breast cancers and a delay in their onset, with no increased toxicity at a median follow-up of 58 months [24].

For women with breast cancer who are carriers of a germline *TP53* mutation (who are expected to be unable to repair tissue damage from DNA-damaging RT and be at risk for significant RT-associated sequelae), there is limited evidence to inform the clinical question of the role of RT. The recommendations are based on a single case series by Heymann et al. [51]. In this study of six women, there were 11 events, consisting of three contralateral breast cancers, three ipsilateral breast recurrences, two RT-induced cancers, three new primary cancers. In contrast, only one event, (contralateral breast cancer), was reported among the two patients who had not received postoperative RT. Additional case reports support this observation [52–55]. Therefore, based on the expert panel opinions, irradiation of the intact breast in *TP53* mutation carriers is contraindicated and mastectomy is the recommended therapeutic option [25]. Postmastectomy RT should only be considered in patients with significant risks of locoregional recurrence.

For women with rare high-risk syndromes like *PTEN*-hamartoma tumour syndrome (which includes Cowden syndrome) or hereditary diffuse gastric cancer syndrome, there is no data on increased toxicity from RT. A single case report on increased toxicity in the setting of germline *PTEN* mutation was published in 2019 [61], however a causal relationship between Cowden syndrome and radiation sensitivity remains unclear, warranting further study in larger cohorts of Cowden syndrome patients.

Data regarding rates of toxicity in patients with moderate-penetrance breast cancer susceptibility genes (e.g. *PALB2*, *ATM*, and *CHEK2*) are limited or inconsistent (specifically in the case of *ATM* mutation carriers). Reassuring data about risks associated with *BRCA1/2* mutations should not be extrapolated when caring for these patients. High-quality data related to the risk of RT in carriers of a germline *ATM* mutation with breast cancer are missing. Since patients with ataxia telangiectasia (having biallelic *ATM* mutations) have an increased sensitivity to ionising radiation, with preclinical data confirming reduced ability of skin cells to replicate after x-ray exposure, concerns about the risk of RT in heterozygous *ATM* carriers were raised [37]. Case reports of radiation skin toxicity in heterozygous *ATM* mutation carriers exist [38, 39], but whether the incidence is higher than in other breast cancer populations is unclear. Data on the risk of contralateral breast cancers are also inconsistent, with some showing no increased risk [40, 41], and one showing significantly higher risk [38]. Potential absolute risks of ionising radiation for diagnostic purposes and RT at conventional doses for heterozygous carriers seem to be small [68]; however, more research is needed.

A single study suggested that patients with a specific polymorphism in *RAD50* gene who were exposed to ≥ 1 Gy to the contralateral breast had a fourfold greater contralateral breast cancer risk than unexposed carriers [69]. However, this observation requires replication, and the impact of rare variants and haplotypes in *RAD50* and other genes involved in the DNA double-strand break response on radiation-induced contralateral breast cancer warrants further investigation.

48.4 Current Recommendations/ Guidelines

A multidisciplinary joint ASCO-ASTRO-SSO Expert Panel including 52 members published guidelines based on a systematic review of the existing literature and a formal consensus process [25]. Several recommendations for local and systemic therapy were developed, though noticing the limited high-quality evidence available for the local therapy's clinical questions. The recommendations regarding RT are summarised here.

1. There is no evidence of increased toxicity or contralateral breast cancer events from radiation exposure in *BRCA1/2* carriers.
2. Radiation therapy should not be withheld in *ATM* carriers based on the currently available data. The risk-benefit ratio needs to be individually discussed.
3. For patients with germline *TP53* mutations, mastectomy is advised; RT is contraindicated except in those with significant risk of locoregional recurrence.

48.5 Summary

Although many genes associated with moderate to high risk for hereditary breast cancer are involved in DNA repair and radiation response pathways, data on adverse outcomes with the appropriate use of therapeutic radiation is limited or missing. Given the rarity of non–*BRCA1*-*BRCA2*–associated hereditary breast cancer, it is likely that data will continue to be limited to anecdotal experiences and retrospective series. Since most of the available data are derived from observational studies and data from RCTs are lacking, the recommendations provided here for locoregional management of early breast cancer in patients with hereditary predisposition are mostly based on expert panel consensus. For women with breast cancer who are treated with BCT or with mastectomy, for whom postmastectomy RT is considered, RT should not be withheld because of mutation status, except for mutations in *TP53*. For women with breast cancer who are carriers of a germline *TP53* mutation, irradiation of the intact breast is contraindicated. Mastectomy is the recommended therapeutic option. Postmastectomy RT in *TP53* mutation carriers should only be considered in patients with significant risk of locoregional recurrence. There is no evidence of a significant increase in toxicity or contralateral breast cancer related to radiation exposure among patients with a mutation in a *BRCA1/2* or a moderate-penetrance gene. Data regarding rates of toxicity between heterozygous *ATM* mutation carriers and noncarriers are limited and inconsistent. Potential absolute risks seem to be small; however, more research is needed.

References

1. Knudson AG Jr. Mutation and cancer: statistical study of retinoblastoma. Proc Natl Acad Sci U S A. 1971;68(4):820–3.
2. Knudson AG. Two genetic hits (more or less) to cancer. Nat Rev Cancer. 2001;1(2):157–62.
3. Apostolou P, Fostira F. Hereditary breast cancer: the era of new susceptibility genes. Biomed Res Int. 2013;2013:747318.
4. Buys SS, Sandbach JF, Gammon A, Patel G, Kidd J, Brown KL, et al. A study of over 35,000 women with breast cancer tested with a 25-gene panel of hereditary cancer genes. Cancer. 2017;123(10):1721–30.
5. Peleg Hasson S, Menes T, Sonnenblick A. Comparison of patient susceptibility genes across breast cancer: implications for prognosis and therapeutic outcomes. Pharmgenomics Pers Med. 2020;13:227–38.
6. Michailidou K, Lindstrom S, Dennis J, Beesley J, Hui S, Kar S, et al. Association analysis identifies 65 new breast cancer risk loci. Nature. 2017;551(7678):92–4.
7. Brentnall AR, van Veen EM, Harkness EF, Rafiq S, Byers H, Astley SM, et al. A case-control evaluation of 143 single nucleotide polymorphisms for breast cancer risk stratification with classical factors and mammographic density. Int J Cancer. 2020;146(8):2122–9.
8. Cuzick J, Sestak I, Bonanni B, Costantino JP, Cummings S, DeCensi A, Dowsett M, Forbes JF, Ford L, LaCroix AZ, Mershon J, Mitlak BH, Powles T, Veronesi U, Vogel V, Wickerham DL, SERM Chemoprevention of Breast Cancer Overview Group. Selective oestrogen receptor modulators in prevention of breast cancer: an updated meta-analysis of individual participant data. Lancet. 2013;381(9880):1827–34.
9. Cuzick J, Sestak I, Forbes JF, Dowsett M, Cawthorn S, Mansel RE, Loibl S, Bonanni B, Evans DG, Howell A, IBIS-II investigators. Use of anastrozole for breast cancer prevention (IBIS-II): long-term results of a randomised controlled trial. Lancet. 2020;395(10218):117–22.
10. Ingham SL, Sperrin M, Baildam A, Ross GL, Clayton R, Lalloo F, et al. Risk-reducing surgery increases survival in BRCA1/2 mutation carriers unaffected at time of family referral. Breast Cancer Res Treat. 2013;142(3):611–8.

11. Miki Y, Swensen J, Shattuck-Eidens D, Futreal PA, Harshman K, Tavtigian S, et al. A strong candidate for the breast and ovarian cancer susceptibility gene BRCA1. Science. 1994;266(5182):66–71.
12. Petrucelli N, Daly MB, Feldman GL. Hereditary breast and ovarian cancer due to mutations in BRCA1 and BRCA2. Genet Med. 2010;12(5):245–59.
13. Mavaddat N, Peock S, Frost D, Ellis S, Platte R, Fineberg E, et al. Cancer risks for BRCA1 and BRCA2 mutation carriers: results from prospective analysis of EMBRACE. J Natl Cancer Inst. 2013;105(11):812–22.
14. Wong-Brown MW, Meldrum CJ, Carpenter JE, Clarke CL, Narod SA, Jakubowska A, et al. Prevalence of BRCA1 and BRCA2 germline mutations in patients with triple-negative breast cancer. Breast Cancer Res Treat. 2015;150(1):71–80.
15. van der Groep P, van der Wall E, van Diest PJ. Pathology of hereditary breast cancer. Cell Oncol (Dordr). 2011;34(2):71–88.
16. Chen H, Wu J, Zhang Z, Tang Y, Li X, Liu S, et al. Association between BRCA status and triple-negative breast cancer: a meta-analysis. Front Pharmacol. 2018;9:909.
17. Park H, Choi DH, Noh JM, Huh SJ, Park W, Nam SJ, et al. Acute skin toxicity in Korean breast cancer patients carrying BRCA mutations. Int J Radiat Biol. 2014;90(1):90–4.
18. Shanley S, McReynolds K, Ardern-Jones A, Ahern R, Fernando I, Yarnold J, et al. Late toxicity is not increased in BRCA1/BRCA2 mutation carriers undergoing breast radiotherapy in the United Kingdom. Clin Cancer Res. 2006;12(23):7025–32.
19. Pierce LJ, Strawderman M, Narod SA, Oliviotto I, Eisen A, Dawson L, et al. Effect of radiotherapy after breast-conserving treatment in women with breast cancer and germline BRCA1/2 mutations. J Clin Oncol. 2000;18(19):3360–9.
20. Bernstein JL, Thomas DC, Shore RE, Robson M, Boice JD Jr, Stovall M, et al. Contralateral breast cancer after radiotherapy among BRCA1 and BRCA2 mutation carriers: a WECARE study report. Eur J Cancer. 2013;49(14):2979–85.
21. Drooger J, Akdeniz D, Pignol JP, Koppert LB, McCool D, Seynaeve CM, et al. Adjuvant radiotherapy for primary breast cancer in BRCA1 and BRCA2 mutation carriers and risk of contralateral breast cancer with special attention to patients irradiated at younger age. Breast Cancer Res Treat. 2015;154(1):171–80.
22. Metcalfe K, Gershman S, Lynch HT, Ghadirian P, Tung N, Kim-Sing C, et al. Predictors of contralateral breast cancer in BRCA1 and BRCA2 mutation carriers. Br J Cancer. 2011;104(9):1384–92.
23. Pierce LJ, Phillips KA, Griffith KA, Buys S, Gaffney DK, Moran MS, et al. Local therapy in BRCA1 and BRCA2 mutation carriers with operable breast cancer: comparison of breast conservation and mastectomy. Breast Cancer Res Treat. 2010;121(2):389–98.
24. Evron E, Ben-David AM, Goldberg H, Fried G, Kaufman B, Catane R, et al. Prophylactic irradiation to the contralateral breast for BRCA mutation carriers with early-stage breast cancer. Ann Oncol. 2019;30(3):412–7.
25. Tung NM, Boughey JC, Pierce LJ, Robson ME, Bedrosian I, Dietz JR, et al. Management of hereditary breast cancer: American Society of Clinical Oncology, American Society for Radiation Oncology, and Society of Surgical Oncology Guideline. J Clin Oncol. 2020;38(18):2080–106.
26. Wooster R, Bignell G, Lancaster J, Swift S, Seal S, Mangion J, et al. Identification of the breast cancer susceptibility gene BRCA2. Nature. 1995;378(6559):789–92.
27. Spurdle AB, Couch FJ, Parsons MT, McGuffog L, Barrowdale D, Bolla MK, et al. Refined histopathological predictors of BRCA1 and BRCA2 mutation status: a large-scale analysis of breast cancer characteristics from the BCAC, CIMBA, and ENIGMA consortia. Breast Cancer Res. 2014;16(6):3419.
28. Xia B, Sheng Q, Nakanishi K, Ohashi A, Wu J, Christ N, et al. Control of BRCA2 cellular and clinical functions by a nuclear partner, PALB2. Mol Cell. 2006;22(6):719–29.
29. Zhang F, Fan Q, Ren K, Andreassen PR. PALB2 functionally connects the breast cancer susceptibility proteins BRCA1 and BRCA2. Mol Cancer Res. 2009;7(7):1110–8.
30. Hu C, Hart SN, Gnanaolivu R, Huang H, Lee KY, Na J, et al. A population-based study of genes previously implicated in breast cancer. N Engl J Med. 2021;384:440.
31. Breast Cancer Association Consortium. Breast cancer risk genes—association analysis in more than 113,000 women. N Engl J Med. 2021;384:428.
32. Zhou J, Wang H, Fu F, Li Z, Feng Q, Wu W, et al. Spectrum of PALB2 germline mutations and characteristics of PALB2-related breast cancer: screening of 16,501 unselected patients with breast cancer and 5890 controls by next-generation sequencing. Cancer. 2020;126(14):3202–8. https://doi.org/10.1002/cncr.32905. Epub 2020 Apr 27
33. Naslund-Koch C, Nordestgaard BG, Bojesen SE. Increased risk for other cancers in addition to breast cancer for CHEK2*1100delC heterozygotes estimated from the Copenhagen general population study. J Clin Oncol. 2016;34(11):1208–16.
34. Bergstrom C, Pence C, Berg J, Partain N, Sadeghi N, Mauer C, et al. Clinicopathological features and outcomes in individuals with breast cancer and ATM, CHEK2, or PALB2 mutations. Ann Surg Oncol. 2020;28:3383.
35. Boder E. Ataxia-telangiectasia: an overview. Kroc Found Ser. 1985;19:1–63.
36. Marabelli M, Cheng SC, Parmigiani G. Penetrance of ATM gene mutations in breast cancer: a meta-analysis of different measures of risk. Genet Epidemiol. 2016;40(5):425–31.

37. Kastan M. Ataxia-telangiectasia--broad implications for a rare disorder. N Engl J Med. 1995;333(10):662–3.
38. Bernstein JL, Haile RW, Stovall M, Boice JD Jr, Shore RE, Langholz B, et al. Radiation exposure, the ATM gene, and contralateral breast cancer in the women's environmental cancer and radiation epidemiology study. J Natl Cancer Inst. 2010;102(7):475–83.
39. Varghese S, Schmidt-Ullrich RK, Dritschilo A, Jung M. Enhanced radiation late effects and cellular radiation sensitivity in an ATM heterozygous breast cancer patient. Radiat Oncol Investig. 1999;7(4):231–7.
40. Broeks A, Braaf LM, Huseinovic A, Nooijen A, Urbanus J, Hogervorst FB, et al. Identification of women with an increased risk of developing radiation-induced breast cancer: a case only study. Breast Cancer Res. 2007;9(2):R26.
41. Su Y, Swift M. Outcomes of adjuvant radiation therapy for breast cancer in women with ataxia-telangiectasia mutations. JAMA. 2001;286(18):2233–4.
42. Guilford P, Hopkins J, Harraway J, McLeod M, McLeod N, Harawira P, et al. E-cadherin germline mutations in familial gastric cancer. Nature. 1998;392(6674):402–5.
43. Blair VR, McLeod M, Carneiro F, Coit DG, D'Addario JL, van Dieren JM, et al. Hereditary diffuse gastric cancer: updated clinical practice guidelines. Lancet Oncol. 2020;21(8):e386–e97.
44. Pharoah PD, Guilford P, Caldas C, International Gastric Cancer Linkage C. Incidence of gastric cancer and breast cancer in CDH1 (E-cadherin) mutation carriers from hereditary diffuse gastric cancer families. Gastroenterology. 2001;121(6):1348–53.
45. Hansford S, Kaurah P, Li-Chang H, Woo M, Senz J, Pinheiro H, et al. Hereditary diffuse gastric cancer syndrome: CDH1 mutations and beyond. JAMA Oncol. 2015;1(1):23–32.
46. Corso G, Intra M, Trentin C, Veronesi P, Galimberti V. CDH1 germline mutations and hereditary lobular breast cancer. Familial Cancer. 2016;15(2):215–9.
47. Malkin D, Li FP, Strong LC, Fraumeni JF Jr, Nelson CE, Kim DH, et al. Germ line p53 mutations in a familial syndrome of breast cancer, sarcomas, and other neoplasms. Science. 1990;250(4985):1233–8.
48. Ruijs MW, Verhoef S, Rookus MA, Pruntel R, van der Hout AH, Hogervorst FB, et al. TP53 germline mutation testing in 180 families suspected of Li-Fraumeni syndrome: mutation detection rate and relative frequency of cancers in different familial phenotypes. J Med Genet. 2010;47(6):421–8.
49. Wilson JR, Bateman AC, Hanson H, An Q, Evans G, Rahman N, et al. A novel HER2-positive breast cancer phenotype arising from germline TP53 mutations. J Med Genet. 2010;47(11):771–4.
50. Bougeard G, Renaux-Petel M, Flaman JM, Charbonnier C, Fermey P, Belotti M, et al. Revisiting Li-Fraumeni syndrome from TP53 mutation carriers. J Clin Oncol. 2015;33(21):2345–52.
51. Heymann S, Delaloge S, Rahal A, Caron O, Frebourg T, Barreau L, et al. Radio-induced malignancies after breast cancer postoperative radiotherapy in patients with Li-Fraumeni syndrome. Radiat Oncol. 2010;5:104.
52. Ferrarini A, Auteri-Kaczmarek A, Pica A, Boesch N, Heinimann K, Schafer SC, et al. Early occurrence of lung adenocarcinoma and breast cancer after radiotherapy of a chest wall sarcoma in a patient with a de novo germline mutation in TP53. Familial Cancer. 2011;10(2):187–92.
53. Henry E, Villalobos V, Million L, Jensen KC, West R, Ganjoo K, et al. Chest wall leiomyosarcoma after breast-conservative therapy for early-stage breast cancer in a young woman with Li-Fraumeni syndrome. J Natl Compr Cancer Netw. 2012;10(8):939–42.
54. Limacher JM, Frebourg T, Natarajan-Ame S, Bergerat JP. Two metachronous tumors in the radiotherapy fields of a patient with Li-Fraumeni syndrome. Int J Cancer. 2001;96(4):238–42.
55. Salmon A, Amikam D, Sodha N, Davidson S, Basel-Vanagaite L, Eeles RA, et al. Rapid development of post-radiotherapy sarcoma and breast cancer in a patient with a novel germline 'de-novo' TP53 mutation. Clin Oncol (R Coll Radiol). 2007;19(7):490–3.
56. Hearle N, Schumacher V, Menko FH, Olschwang S, Boardman LA, Gille JJ, et al. Frequency and spectrum of cancers in the Peutz-Jeghers syndrome. Clin Cancer Res. 2006;12(10):3209–15.
57. Tchekmedyian A, Amos CI, Bale SJ, Zhu D, Arold S, Berrueta J, et al. Findings from the Peutz-Jeghers syndrome registry of Uruguay. PLoS One. 2013;8(11):e79639.
58. Georgescu MM. PTEN tumor suppressor network in PI3K-Akt pathway control. Genes Cancer. 2010;1(12):1170–7.
59. Nelen MR, Kremer H, Konings IB, Schoute F, van Essen AJ, Koch R, et al. Novel PTEN mutations in patients with Cowden disease: absence of clear genotype-phenotype correlations. Eur J Hum Genet. 1999;7(3):267–73.
60. Bubien V, Bonnet F, Brouste V, Hoppe S, Barouk-Simonet E, David A, et al. High cumulative risks of cancer in patients with PTEN hamartoma tumour syndrome. J Med Genet. 2013;50(4):255–63.
61. Tatebe K, Chmura SJ, Connell PP. Elevated radiation therapy toxicity in the setting of germline PTEN mutation. Pract Radiat Oncol. 2019;9(6):492–5.
62. Pierce LJ, Levin AM, Rebbeck TR, Ben-David MA, Friedman E, Solin LJ, et al. Ten-year multi-institutional results of breast-conserving surgery and radiotherapy in BRCA1/2-associated stage I/II breast cancer. J Clin Oncol. 2006;24(16):2437–43.
63. Carbine NE, Lostumbo L, Wallace J, Ko H. Risk-reducing mastectomy for the prevention of primary breast cancer. Cochrane Database Syst Rev. 2018;4:CD002748.
64. Heemskerk-Gerritsen BA, Rookus MA, Aalfs CM, Ausems MG, Collee JM, Jansen L, et al. Improved overall survival after contralateral risk-reducing mastectomy in BRCA1/2 mutation carriers with a history of unilateral breast cancer: a prospective analysis. Int J Cancer. 2015;136(3):668–77.

65. Metcalfe K, Gershman S, Ghadirian P, Lynch HT, Snyder C, Tung N, et al. Contralateral mastectomy and survival after breast cancer in carriers of BRCA1 and BRCA2 mutations: retrospective analysis. BMJ. 2014;348:g226.
66. National Comprehensive Cancer Network (NCCN) Clinical Practice Guidelines in Oncology https://www.nccn.org/store/login/login.aspx?ReturnURL=https://www.nccn.org/professionals/physician_gls/pdf/breast.pdf
67. Lee KT, Mun GH. Prosthetic breast reconstruction in previously irradiated breasts: a meta-analysis. J Surg Oncol. 2015;112(5):468–75.
68. van Os NJ, Roeleveld N, Weemaes CM, Jongmans MC, Janssens GO, Taylor AM, et al. Health risks for ataxia-telangiectasia mutated heterozygotes: a systematic review, meta-analysis and evidence-based guideline. Clin Genet. 2016;90(2):105–17.
69. Brooks JD, Teraoka SN, Reiner AS, Satagopan JM, Bernstein L, Thomas DC, et al. Variants in activators and downstream targets of ATM, radiation exposure, and contralateral breast cancer risk in the WECARE study. Hum Mutat. 2012;33(1):158–64.

Breast Cancer in Young Women

49

Elzbieta Senkus and Shani Paluch-Shimon

49.1 Background

Breast cancer in young women (≤40 years) is an uncommon disease, representing only a small proportion of all breast cancer patients in developed countries (4% of new estimated cases in the USA), with a cumulative risk of 0.4–0.45% of being diagnosed with breast cancer by age 40 [1, 2] and of 4.64% in the age group 15–39 in the Netherlands (https://iknl.nl/en/ncr). There is no effective screening tool for early detection of breast cancer in young women, and young women often have higher breast density and therefore imaging by mammography is often less effective; hence, MRI of the breast is often indicated as part of the diagnostic workup. Breast cancers arising in young women are characterised by higher proportion of grade 3, triple-negative phenotype or HER2 overexpression, lymphovascular invasion, lymphocytic infiltration and on gene expression profiling—by higher proportions of basal-like and HER2-enriched tumours, as compared with older women. Young women have less favourable outcomes than older women [3–6], particularly for Luminal-A like tumours, irrespective of stage at diagnosis [7].

Breast cancer at an early age is more likely to be associated with an increased familial risk and hereditary cancer syndrome, specifically germline mutations in *BRCA1* and *BRCA2* are more common in young women (see section about genetic syndromes). The presence of a germline mutation will impact therapeutic decisions and risk-reducing measures; thus, all women diagnosed with breast cancer ≤40 years should be offered genetic testing. The other significant risk factor for early onset breast cancer is mantle or chest wall radiation before the age of 25—these women have a cumulative risk of developing breast cancer by age 40–45 as do *BRCA1/2* mutation carriers [8, 9].

Young women with breast cancer face a multitude of unique challenges along the continuum of care—from concerns and risks to their fertility secondary to therapies they receive, dealing with the complexity of a hereditary cancer syndrome, psychosocial distress that is accentuated by the young age at diagnosis and numerous survivorship issues including premature menopause that may be induced by treatments they receive [10].

E. Senkus
Breast Unit, University Clinical Center, Department of Oncology & Radiotherapy, Medical University of Gdańsk, Gdańsk, Poland
e-mail: elsenkus@gumed.edu.pl

S. Paluch-Shimon (✉)
Breast Oncology, Sharett Institute of Oncology, Hadassah University Hospital, Jerusalem, Israel
e-mail: shanipal@hadassah.org.il

© The Author(s), under exclusive license to Springer Nature Switzerland AG 2022
O. Kaidar-Person et al. (eds.), *Breast Cancer Radiation Therapy*,
https://doi.org/10.1007/978-3-030-91170-6_49

49.2 Key Information for Clinical Practice

49.2.1 Special Considerations in Systemic Therapy

Historically young women were more likely to receive chemotherapy based on their age at diagnosis. However, it is now well established that systemic treatment decisions should be rather based on extent of disease and the biological characteristics of the tumour (including tumour size, nodal status, hormone receptor (HR) and HER2 overexpression or amplification, proliferation, and grade), patient's comorbidities and preferences. Young age alone is not a reason to give more aggressive therapy and the guidelines for choice of systemic therapy should follow those for women with breast cancer of all ages [11, 12]. The omission of adjuvant chemotherapy in young and very young women (≤35 years at diagnosis) with HR+ disease is appropriate in selected cases with favourable clinical and pathological features including low gene expression profiles, as for older women. It is important to note that young women were under-represented in both retrospective and prospective studies evaluating gene expression signatures as aids for deciding upon use of chemotherapy in hormone-positive (HR+) breast cancer. Unplanned subgroup analyses of the prospective studies have suggested that women under 50 may derive benefit from chemotherapy (or from the endocrine changes induced by chemotherapy) for genomic scores and clinical characteristics for which endocrine therapy would suffice in women over 50 [13]. Thus, while they may be used, this should be done with caution. Notably, commercially available prognostic genomic assays in HR+ early breast cancer have not been developed to predict which endocrine therapy is more appropriate according to genomic risk. For premenopausal with HR+ disease, choice of endocrine therapy includes tamoxifen or ovarian function suppression (OFS) in combination with tamoxifen or an aromatase inhibitor (in premenopausal women aromatase inhibitors can only be used if combined with ovarian function suppression). In women at higher risk of relapse, OFS with tamoxifen or an aromatase inhibitor (AI) is associated with a significant improvement in outcomes compared to tamoxifen alone [14, 15]. Notably, chemotherapy induced amenorrhea is not always indicative of ovarian function, so that when use of an AI is considered, OFS with monthly formulations of a GnRH analogue is imperative and ovarian function should be routinely monitored with serum hormonal profiles.

49.3 Unique Issues for Young Women

49.3.1 Fertility and Pregnancy

All young women diagnosed with breast cancer should be counselled about the potential impact of treatment on their fertility and should be offered fertility preservation [11, 16]. The use of a GnRH analogue as an ovarian protectant during chemotherapy should be offered but is not instead of fertility preservation [17]. Concerns about fertility are a major source of psychological distress and cause of nonadherence to therapy in young women and therefore addressing a young woman's fertility concerns is a critical to the success of her treatment and to her wellbeing [18, 19]. All retrospective available data demonstrate no detrimental effect of pregnancy after a breast cancer diagnosis in terms of breast cancer outcome [20–23], irrespective of subtype [24]. Results are awaited for the POSITIVE study which is the first prospective study evaluating endocrine therapy interruption and pregnancy in young women with HR+ breast cancer. Timing of pregnancy after breast cancer should be decided upon with the treating oncologist giving careful consideration to initial stage of disease and patient preference, with an understanding that when the woman has HR+ disease, endocrine therapy needs to be resumed and completed after delivery.

Breast cancer during pregnancy is uncommon. In the majority of cases, termination of the pregnancy is not indicated, and treatment of the breast cancer should follow existing guidelines [25, 26] and be managed by a multidisciplinary team with expertise in this area. Young women need to be counselled about nonhormonal contraceptive options.

49.3.2 Survivorship

Young women face a plethora of survivorship issues—many related to the side effects of endocrine therapy and the consequences of premature menopause. A significant proportion will suffer from sexual dysfunction and issues with body image and sexuality [27, 28]. Other key issues for young women will include neurocognitive symptoms ("onco-brain"), adverse impact on return to work and employment, and the consequences of a hereditary cancer syndrome including tailored screening and risk-reducing measures (such as risk-reducing salpingo-oophorectomy and risk-reducing mastectomy) [29]. Addressing all of these issues is imperative to ensuring quality of life and treatment adherence [30]. While not all survivorship issues can be prevented or resolved, many can be alleviated by early intervention.

49.4 Special Considerations in Local Therapy

49.4.1 Outcomes of Locoregional Therapies in Young Breast Cancer Patients

Breast cancer in young women is associated with higher risk of locoregional recurrence, even if corrected for stage and tumour characteristics. This phenomenon is observed in case of both breast-conserving therapy (BCT) and mastectomy [31–33].

Age was the only independent prognostic factor for local control ($P = 0.0001$) in the EORTC "boost versus no boost" trial (Fig. 49.1) and the largest absolute improvement from the use of additional radiation dose (boost) to the tumour bed was seen in patients aged ≤40 [34].

However, over the past four decades local recurrence rates decreased consistently thanks to improved diagnostics, and local as well as systemic treatments (Fig. 49.2). In three consecutive trials on breast conserving therapy accruing between 1980 and 2012, the 10-year local recurrence rate dropped from about 20% in one of the original mastectomy vs. BCT trials (EORTC 10801), to about 10% in the EORTC boost trial (patients between 40–50 years of age) to about 2% in the Dutch "Young Boost Trial" (patients below 50 years of age, about ¼ of them below 40 years of age) [35]. This led to selective omission of a boost dose to the primary tumour bed also in young patients without high-risk factors for local recurrence.

In women who have undergone mastectomy, young age is associated with poorer locoregional control [36]. Among patients enrolled in 13 International Breast Cancer Study Group (IBCSG) randomised trials, age <40 years, involvement of ≥4 lymph nodes, and inadequate axillary surgery were the key determinants of >15% risk of locoregional recurrence [37].

Importantly, similar or inferior long-term outcomes are observed in patients who have undergone mastectomy, compared to those undergoing BCT, although young BCT patients generally demonstrate higher locoregional recurrence rates, compared to those treated with mastectomy [32, 38–40]. In a systematic meta-analysis (22,598 patients ≤40 years from five population-based studies) and one pooled analysis of two clinical trials (10,898 BCT patients and 11,700 mastectomy patients), after adjustments for tumour stage, a nonsignificant trend for a lower risk of death was found in patients who underwent BCT (HR 0.9) (Fig. 49.3) [41]. Additionally, significantly higher breast cancer specific and overall survival rates were observed for stage IIB patients aged 20–34 years form the Surveillance, Epidemiology, and End Results (SEER) Program database, treated with BCS and radiation therapy, compared to mastectomy without RT [42]. The most plausible explanation for superior outcomes following BCT is the almost universal use of RT in this population. In contrast, in a large (129,692 patients) population-based Dutch study comparing BCT with mastectomy, in the long follow-up cohort (treated 1999–2005) the benefit of BCT

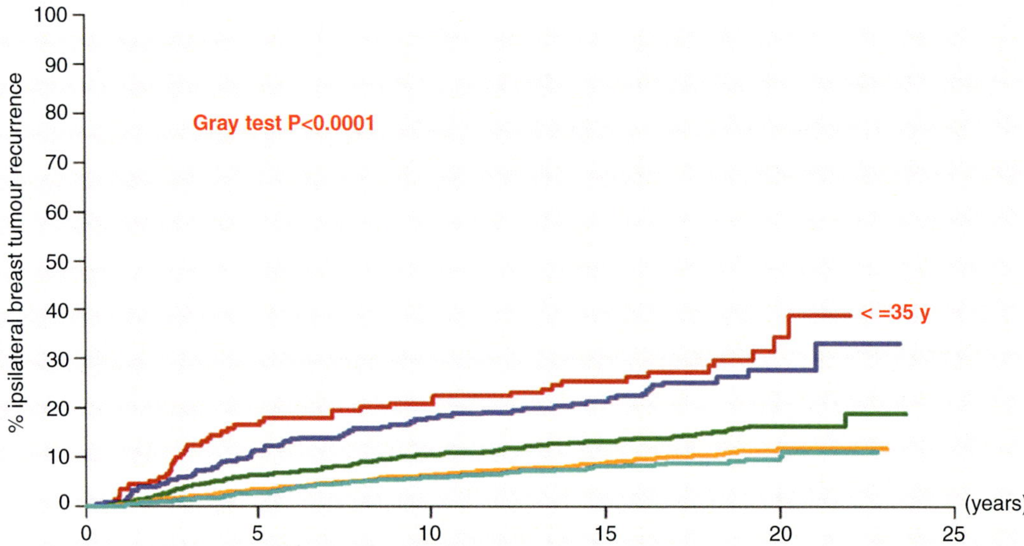

O	N	Number of patients at risk :					Age (years)
44	154	93	69	53	9		<=35 y
69	295	205	154	101	19		35 - 40
182	1334	1008	757	522	118		40 - 50
164	1803	1439	1079	706	109		50 - 60
132	1732	1339	933	558	68		>60

Fig. 49.1 Cumulative incidence of ipsilateral breast tumour recurrence for the whole study population by age. (Adapted with permission from: Bartelink H, Maingon P, Poortmans P, et al. Whole-breast irradiation with or without a boost for patients treated with breast-conserving surgery for early breast cancer: 20-year follow-up of a randomised phase 3 trial. Lancet Oncol. 2015 Jan;16(1):47–56)

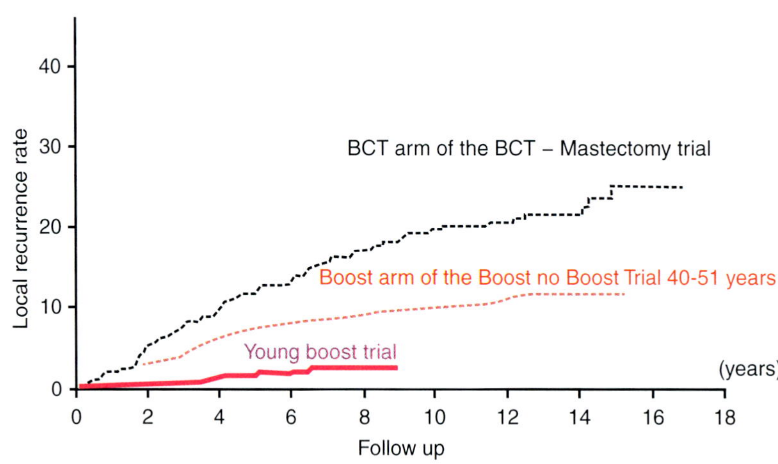

Fig. 49.2 Local breast recurrence rate in three consecutive trials on breast conserving therapy from 1980 till 2012 (Adapted with permission from: Poortmans PMP, Arenas M, Livi L. Over-irradiation. Breast. 2017 Feb;31:295–302, modified from Poortmans P, Aznar M, Bartelink H. Quality indicators for breast cancer: revisiting historical evidence in the context of technology changes. Semin Radiat Oncol 2012; 22: pp. 29–39)

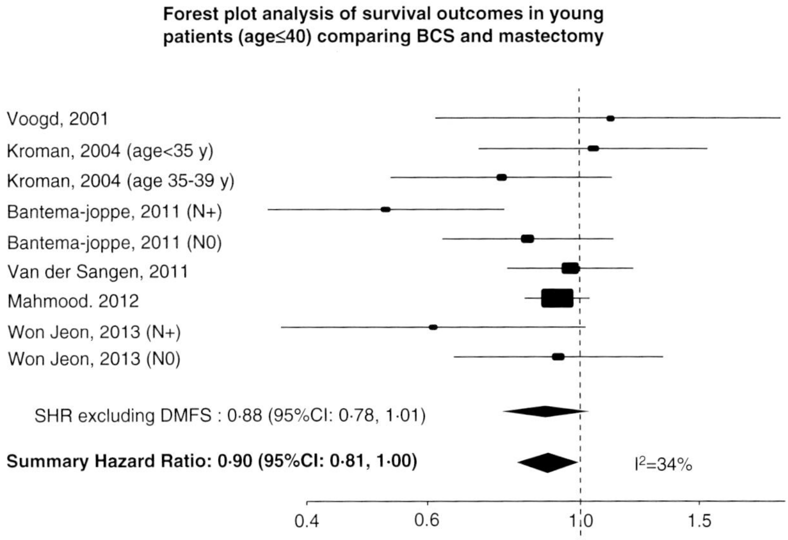

Fig. 49.3 Forest plot analysis of survival outcomes in young patients undergoing breast conservation surgery and mastectomy

was seen in all subgroups, except in patients <40 years with T1-2N0-1 disease [40]. Similarly, in the more recent cohort (2006–2012) from the same study, treated with contemporary adjuvant systemic therapy, the benefit of BCT was limited to T1-2N0-1 patients >50 years.

Additionally, a recent retrospective study reported that in BRCA1/2 mutation carrier breast cancer patients treated with skin-sparing/nipple-sparing mastectomies without PMRT there was a higher rate of local recurrences than those who underwent mastectomy and PMRT or BCT, despite earlier stage disease in the non-PMRT group. The authors attributed the higher local recurrence rate to the residual breast tissue and potential residual disease in such skin-sparing/nipple-sparing mastectomies [43] . These data provide strong support for offering BCT to all suitable patients, regardless of age. Younger patients are at higher risk of locoregional failure, but more extensive surgery does not reduce the risk of distant failure or death.

Interestingly, although young patients develop local failures more often than older patients, their prognosis following local recurrence and overall survival seem to be better, compared to the older population [44, 45]. Importantly, the age at diagnosis matters even among "young" patients: in a series of 167 women with T1-2 tumours, aged 26–45, treated with BCT, including brachytherapy boost, age ≤ 35 was associated with a three-fold increase in the risk of local failure, together with high tumour grade and negative hormone receptor status [46].

49.4.2 Role and Technical Aspects of RT in Young Breast Cancer Patients

Increased risk of local recurrence after BCT in younger women provides a rationale for the use of more "aggressive" RT. Indeed, the EORTC "boost versus no boost" trial demonstrated the largest absolute benefit from the tumour bed boost in patients aged <40, although the relative risk reduction was similar among all age groups [31]. As a result, this approach is uniformly recommended in women <50 by most guidelines [47–49]. As the local recurrence risk is higher in young patients, even with use of standard dose boost, there are attempts to improve these results by further radiation dose escalation. The optimal tumour bed dose in patients ≤50 has been tested in the "young boost" trial, comparing standard boost of 16 Gy to 26 Gy and the primary results are awaited, while the cosmetic impact of increasing the boost dose was clearly cumbersome [50].

Fractionation regimen in young breast cancer patients should not differ from those used in older patients. Further data waits for ultra-hypofractionation, as used in the FAST-Forward trial in the young population [51]. The 2018 American Society for Radiation Oncology (ASTRO) guidelines for whole breast irradiation (WBI) clearly states that there is no evidence of deleterious effects of moderately hypofractionated WBI in younger patients; thus, the decisions regarding its use should be made irrespective of age [52].

Young patients are not only at risk of true recurrence but also of second primary cancers within the conserved breast, therefore the policy of limiting the irradiation volume only to the tumour bed (partial breast irradiation—PBI) is generally not recommended in this population. According to the guidelines of the Groupe Européen de Curiethérapie-European Society for Therapeutic Radiology and Oncology (GEC-ESTRO) and ASTRO, PBI is considered appropriate and safe only in the age group >50 (without other defined risk factors), whereas, women ≤40 are clearly defined as "unsuitable" for PBI [53, 54].

Young patients who have undergone mastectomy share risk factors for locoregional failure with older age groups: primary tumour size and nodal stage, as well as lack of RT and appropriate adjuvant systemic therapy [55]. PMRT is indicated for the majority of young node-positive patients with some data suggesting benefit from irradiation in selected node-negative population. In a study of 502 patients with T1–2N0 tumours treated with mastectomy, after a median follow-up of 77 months, local recurrence rates in patients >40 and ≤40 were 1.7% and 7%, respectively; prognostic factors for locoregional recurrence in patients ≤40 included tumour size and presence of lymphovascular invasion [56].

Ductal carcinoma in situ (DCIS) is relatively infrequent in young women, being predominantly a screen-detected condition (most countries provide screening mammography from the age of 50), but if observed, is associated with high risk of local failure. Among 1607 women treated for DCIS in Ontario between 1994 and 2003 with breast conserving surgery and RT the 10-year cumulative local recurrence rate for patients younger than 45 years was 27%; for each year of increase in age the local recurrence rate decreased by 4%. In a Rare Cancer Network multicentre study of 373 DCIS patients ≤45, after median follow-up of 72 months, the local relapse-free survival was 63% for patients aged ≤39 years and 81% for those aged 40–45 years. In this study, conservative surgery without post-operative RT resulted in an unacceptable 10-year local recurrence rate of 54%, while irradiation without tumour bed boost was associated with reduction in local relapse (28% 10-year local recurrence rate) and further improvement was seen in those given the tumour bed boost (14% 10-year local recurrence rate)—$p < 0.0001$ (Fig. 49.4) [57].

49.4.3 Utilisation of Radiation Therapy in Young Breast Cancer Patients

In spite of generally higher risk of local failure, young patients seem to be the population most often exposed to suboptimal local treatments. In 317,596 patients from the US National Cancer Database, in the youngest age group (≤35 years) the adjusted odd ratio of having a mastectomy (versus patients aged 61–64) exceeded 2; higher frequency of mastectomy was also seen in other "younger" patients. Of concern, young women treated with conservative surgery were less likely to receive radiation (OR 0.69 for women ≤35). In contrast, the probability of receiving PMRT, both when indicated and when there were no indications for postoperative irradiation, was higher among younger patients [58].

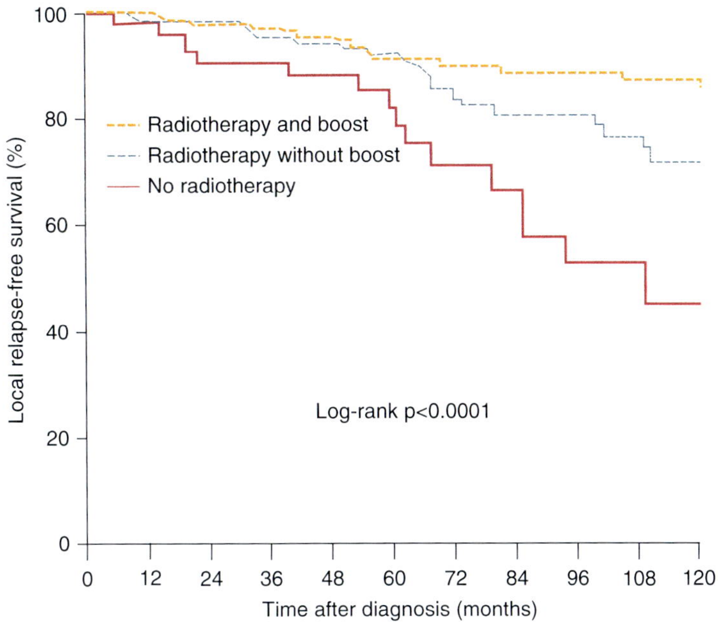

Number at risk

Radiotherapy and boost	150	143	133	126	115	99	90	78	64	51	44
Radiotherapy without boost	166	148	125	103	88	68	56	50	43	34	24
No radiotherapy	57	53	46	39	33	26	17	15	10	7	3

Fig. 49.4 Local relapse-free survival by treatment group (Adapted with permission from: Omlin A, Amichetti M, Azria D, et al. Boost radiotherapy in young women with ductal carcinoma in situ: a multicentre, retrospective study of the Rare Cancer Network. Lancet Oncol. 2006;7(8):652–6)

49.4.4 Complications of Radiation Therapy in Young Breast Cancer Patients

Young women, following the expected long post-treatment survival, are also at greater risk of long-term treatment toxicities. Indeed, among the participants of the Women's Environmental, Cancer, and Radiation Epidemiology (WECARE) study, women <40 who received >1.0 Gy of absorbed dose to the contralateral breast had a 2.5-fold greater risk for contralateral breast cancer (CBC) than unexposed women; this risk increase was not observed in women >40 [59]. A nonsignificant trend for increase in cardiovascular mortality among younger patient cohorts irradiated for cancer of the left breast was observed in the analysis of 308,861 women from the SEER database [60]. The issue of cardiac toxicity is, however, in the present time, largely obviated by the use of modern RT techniques, including deep inspiration breath hold. In contrast, in the EORTC "boost" study, the only cohort which did not experience increased risk of severe fibrosis related to boost administration were patients <41 years [34].

49.5 Conclusions

Young patients are at increased risk of locoregional recurrence irrespective of type of surgery. Long-term outcomes after BCT are at least equal and possibly superior to mastectomy, which may be related to lesser use of RT in patients that undergo mastectomy. Age, as a risk factor for locoregional failure, should be taken into account when considering indications for postmastectomy or regional irradiation. However, as young patients may be at increased risk of long-term treatment toxicities of RT in view of their longer life expectancy, meticulous care should be given to the use of optimal irradiation techniques.

References

1. DeSantis CE, Ma J, Gaudet MM, Newman LA, Miller KD, Goding Sauer A, et al. Breast cancer statistics, 2019. CA Cancer J Clin. 2019;69(6):438–51.
2. Bray F, Ferlay J, Soerjomataram I, Siegel RL, Torre LA, Jemal A. Global cancer statistics 2018: GLOBOCAN estimates of incidence and mortality worldwide for 36 cancers in 185 countries. CA Cancer J Clin. 2018;68(6):394–424.
3. Partridge AH, Gelber S, Piccart-Gebhart MJ, Focant F, Scullion M, Holmes E, et al. Effect of age on breast cancer outcomes in women with human epidermal growth factor receptor 2-positive breast cancer: results from a herceptin adjuvant trial. J Clin Oncol. 2013;31(21):2692–8.
4. Partridge AH, Hughes ME, Warner ET, Ottesen RA, Wong YN, Edge SB, et al. Subtype-dependent relationship between young age at diagnosis and breast cancer survival. J Clin Oncol. 2016;34(27):3308–14.
5. Fu J, Zhong C, Wu L, Li D, Xu T, Jiang T, et al. Young patients with hormone receptor-positive breast cancer have a higher long-term risk of breast cancer specific death. J Breast Cancer. 2019;22(1):96–108.
6. Keegan TH, Press DJ, Tao L, DeRouen MC, Kurian AW, Clarke CA, et al. Impact of breast cancer subtypes on 3-year survival among adolescent and young adult women. Breast Cancer Res. 2013;15(5):R95.
7. Zhong W, Tan L, Jiang WG, Chen K, You N, Sanders AJ, et al. Effect of younger age on survival outcomes in T1N0M0 breast cancer: a propensity score matching analysis. J Surg Oncol. 2019;119:1039.
8. Mulder RL, Kremer LC, Hudson MM, Bhatia S, Landier W, Levitt G, et al. Recommendations for breast cancer surveillance for female survivors of childhood, adolescent, and young adult cancer given chest radiation: a report from the International Late Effects of Childhood Cancer Guideline Harmonization Group. Lancet Oncol. 2013;14(13):e621–9.
9. Monticciolo DL, Newell MS, Moy L, Niell B, Monsees B, Sickles EA. Breast cancer screening in women at higher-than-average risk: recommendations from the ACR. J Am Coll Radiol. 2018;15(3 Pt A):408–14.
10. Ruggeri M, Pagan E, Bagnardi V, Bianco N, Gallerani E, Buser K, et al. Fertility concerns, preservation strategies and quality of life in young women with breast cancer: baseline results from an ongoing prospective cohort study in selected European Centers. Breast. 2019;47:85–92.
11. Paluch-Shimon S, Cardoso F, Partridge AH, Abulkhair O, Azim HA Jr, Bianchi-Micheli G, et al. ESO-ESMO 4th international consensus guidelines for breast cancer in young women (BCY4). Ann Oncol. 2020;
12. Cardoso F, Paluch-Shimon S, Senkus E, Curigliano G, Aapro MS, Andre F, et al. 5th ESO-ESMO international consensus guidelines for advanced breast cancer (ABC 5). Ann Oncol. 2020;31(12):1623–49.
13. Sparano JA, Gray RJ, Ravdin PM, Makower DF, Pritchard KI, Albain KS, et al. Clinical and genomic risk to guide the use of adjuvant therapy for breast cancer. N Engl J Med. 2019;380(25):2395–405.
14. Pagani O, Francis PA, Fleming GF, Walley BA, Viale G, Colleoni M, et al. Absolute improvements in freedom from distant recurrence to tailor adjuvant endocrine therapies for premenopausal women: results from TEXT and SOFT. J Clin Oncol. 2019;38:JCO1801967.
15. Francis PA, Pagani O, Fleming GF, Walley BA, Colleoni M, Lang I, et al. Tailoring adjuvant endocrine therapy for premenopausal breast cancer. N Engl J Med. 2018;379(2):122–37.
16. Lambertini M, Peccatori FA, Demeestere I, Amant F, Wyns C, Stukenborg JB, et al. Fertility preservation and post-treatment pregnancies in post-pubertal cancer patients: ESMO clinical practice guidelines(dagger). Ann Oncol. 2020;31(12):1664–78.
17. Lambertini M, Ceppi M, Poggio F, Peccatori FA, Azim HA Jr, Ugolini D, et al. Ovarian suppression using luteinizing hormone-releasing hormone agonists during chemotherapy to preserve ovarian function and fertility of breast cancer patients: a meta-analysis of randomized studies. Ann Oncol. 2015;26(12):2408–19.
18. Wassermann J, Gelber SI, Rosenberg SM, Ruddy KJ, Tamimi RM, Schapira L, et al. Nonadherent behaviors among young women on adjuvant endocrine therapy for breast cancer. Cancer. 2019;125:3266.
19. Ruddy KJ, Gelber SI, Tamimi RM, Ginsburg ES, Schapira L, Come SE, et al. Prospective study of fertility concerns and preservation strategies in young women with breast cancer. J Clin Oncol. 2014;32(11):1151–6.
20. Azim HA Jr, Santoro L, Pavlidis N, Gelber S, Kroman N, Azim H, et al. Safety of pregnancy following breast cancer diagnosis: a meta-analysis of 14 studies. Eur J Cancer. 2011;47(1):74–83.
21. Pagani O, Partridge A, Korde L, Badve S, Bartlett J, Albain K, et al. Pregnancy after breast cancer: if you wish, ma'am. Breast Cancer Res Treat. 2011;129(2):309–17.
22. V DES, Pagani O. Pregnancy after breast cancer: hope after the storm. Minerva Ginecol. 2017;69(6):597–607.
23. Kroman N, Jensen MB, Wohlfahrt J, Ejlertsen B, Danish Breast Cancer Cooperative G. Pregnancy after treatment of breast cancer—a population-based

study on behalf of Danish Breast Cancer Cooperative Group. Acta Oncol. 2008;47(4):545–9.
24. Lambertini M, Kroman N, Ameye L, Cordoba O, Pinto A, Benedetti G, et al. Long-term safety of pregnancy following breast cancer according to estrogen receptor status. J Natl Cancer Inst. 2018;110(4):426–9.
25. Loibl S, Schmidt A, Gentilini O, Kaufman B, Kuhl C, Denkert C, et al. Breast cancer diagnosed during pregnancy: adapting recent advances in breast cancer care for pregnant patients. JAMA Oncol. 2015;1(8):1145–53.
26. Amant F (Ed.) Textbook of cancer in pregnancy: https://www.esgo.org/explore/textbooks/textbook-of-cancer-in-pregnancy/
27. Rosenberg SM, Tamimi RM, Gelber S, Ruddy KJ, Bober SL, Kereakoglow S, et al. Treatment-related amenorrhea and sexual functioning in young breast cancer survivors. Cancer. 2014;120(15):2264–71.
28. von Hippel C, Rosenberg SM, Austin SB, Sprunck-Harrild K, Ruddy KJ, Schapira L, et al. Identifying distinct trajectories of change in young breast cancer survivors' sexual functioning. Psycho-Oncology. 2019;28(5):1033–40.
29. Rosenberg SM, Vaz-Luis I, Gong J, Rajagopal PS, Ruddy KJ, Tamimi RM, et al. Employment trends in young women following a breast cancer diagnosis. Breast Cancer Res Treat. 2019;177:207.
30. Rosenberg SM, Partridge AH. New insights into non-adherence with adjuvant endocrine therapy among young women with breast cancer. J Natl Cancer Inst. 2015;107:10.
31. Laurberg T, Alsner J, Tramm T, Jensen V, Lyngholm CD, Christiansen PM, et al. Impact of age, intrinsic subtype and local treatment on long-term local-regional recurrence and breast cancer mortality among low-risk breast cancer patients. Acta Oncol. 2017;56(1):59–67.
32. de Bock GH, van der Hage JA, Putter H, Bonnema J, Bartelink H, van de Velde CJ. Isolated loco-regional recurrence of breast cancer is more common in young patients and following breast conserving therapy: long-term results of European Organisation for Research and Treatment of Cancer studies. Eur J Cancer. 2006;42(3):351–6.
33. Kim SW, Chun M, Han S, Jung YS, Choi JH, Kang SY, et al. Young age is associated with increased locoregional recurrence in node-positive breast cancer with luminal subtypes. Cancer Res Treat. 2017;49(2):484–93.
34. Bartelink H, Maingon P, Poortmans P, Weltens C, Fourquet A, Jager J, et al. Whole-breast irradiation with or without a boost for patients treated with breast-conserving surgery for early breast cancer: 20-year follow-up of a randomised phase 3 trial. Lancet Oncol. 2015;16(1):47–56.
35. Poortmans PMP, Arenas M, Livi L. Over-irradiation. Breast. 2017;31:295–302.
36. Kent C, Horton J, Blitzblau R, Koontz BF. Whose disease will recur after mastectomy for early stage, node-negative breast cancer? A systematic review. Clin Breast Cancer. 2015;15(6):403–12.
37. Karlsson P, Cole BF, Chua BH, Price KN, Lindtner J, Collins JP, et al. Patterns and risk factors for locoregional failures after mastectomy for breast cancer: an International Breast Cancer Study Group report. Ann Oncol. 2012;23(11):2852–8.
38. van der Sangen MJ, van de Wiel FM, Poortmans PM, Tjan-Heijnen VC, Nieuwenhuijzen GA, Roumen RM, et al. Are breast conservation and mastectomy equally effective in the treatment of young women with early breast cancer? Long-term results of a population-based cohort of 1,451 patients aged ≤40 years. Breast Cancer Res Treat. 2011;127(1):207–15.
39. van der Sangen EJ, van den Heuvel ER, de Munck L, de Bock GH, Smit WG, Timmer PR, et al. Impact of primary local treatment on the development of distant metastases or death through locoregional recurrence in young breast cancer patients. Breast Cancer Res Treat. 2013;140(3):577–85.
40. Lagendijk M, van Maaren MC, Saadatmand S, Strobbe LJA, Poortmans PMP, Koppert LB, et al. Breast conserving therapy and mastectomy revisited: breast cancer-specific survival and the influence of prognostic factors in 129,692 patients. Int J Cancer. 2018;142:165–75.
41. Vila J, Gandini S, Gentilini O. Overall survival according to type of surgery in young (≤40 years) early breast cancer patients: a systematic meta-analysis comparing breast-conserving surgery versus mastectomy. Breast. 2015;24(3):175–81.
42. Ye JC, Yan W, Christos PJ, Nori D, Ravi A. Equivalent survival with mastectomy or breast-conserving surgery plus radiation in young women aged < 40 years with early-stage breast cancer: a National Registry-based Stage-by-Stage Comparison. Clin Breast Cancer. 2015;15(5):390–7.
43. Bernstein-Molho R, Laitman Y, Galper S, Jacobson G, Boursi B, Gal-Yam EN, et al. Locoregional treatments and ipsilateral breast cancer recurrence rates in BRCA1/2 mutation carriers. Int J Radiat Oncol Biol Phys. 2020;109:1332.
44. Courdi A, Doyen J, Gal J, Chamorey E. Local recurrence after breast cancer affects specific survival differently according to patient age. Oncology. 2010;79(5–6):349–54.
45. Miles RC, Gullerud RE, Lohse CM, Jakub JW, Degnim AC, Boughey JC. Local recurrence after breast-conserving surgery: multivariable analysis of risk factors and the impact of young age. Ann Surg Oncol. 2012;19(4):1153–9.
46. Guinot JL, Baixauli-Perez C, Soler P, Tortajada MI, Moreno A, Santos MA, et al. High-dose-rate brachytherapy boost effect on local tumor control in young women with breast cancer. Int J Radiat Oncol Biol Phys. 2015;91(1):165–71.
47. Cardoso F, Kyriakides S, Ohno S, Penault-Llorca F, Poortmans P, Rubio IT, et al. Early breast cancer: ESMO clinical practice guidelines for diagnosis, treatment and follow-up. Ann Oncol. 2019;30:1194–220.

48. https://www.nccn.org/professionals/physician_gls/pdf/breast.pdf (accessed 29/Nov/2020).
49. Meattini I, Lambertini M, Desideri I, De Caluwé A, Kaidar-Person O, Livi L. Radiation therapy for young women with early breast cancer: current state of the art. Crit Rev Oncol Hematol. 2019;137:143–53.
50. https://clinicaltrials.gov/ct2/show/NCT00212121 (accessed 19/Oct/2020).
51. Brunt AM, Haviland JS, Wheatley DA, Sydenham MA, Alhasso A, Bloomfield DJ, et al. Hypofractionated breast radiotherapy for 1 week versus 3 weeks (FAST-forward): 5-year efficacy and late normal tissue effects results from a multicentre, non-inferiority, randomised, phase 3 trial. Lancet. 2020;395:1613–26.
52. Smith BD, Bellon JR, Blitzblau R, Freedman G, Haffty B, Hahn C, et al. Radiation therapy for the whole breast: executive summary of an American Society for Radiation Oncology (ASTRO) evidence-based guideline. Pract Radiat Oncol. 2018;8(3): 145–52.
53. Polgár C, Van Limbergen E, Pötter R, Kovács G, Polo A, Lyczek J, et al. Patient selection for accelerated partial-breast irradiation (APBI) after breast-conserving surgery: recommendations of the Groupe Européen de Curiethérapie-European Society for Therapeutic Radiology and Oncology (GEC-ESTRO) breast cancer working group based on clinical evidence (2009). Radiother Oncol. 2010;94(3):264–73.
54. Correa C, Harris EE, Leonardi MC, Smith BD, Taghian AG, Thompson AM, et al. Accelerated partial breast irradiation: executive summary for the update of an ASTRO evidence-based consensus statement. Pract Radiat Oncol. 2017;7(2):73–9.
55. Lammers EJ, Huibers P, van der Sangen MJ, van de Poll-Franse LV, Poortmans PM, Ernst MF, et al. Factors contributing to improved local control after mastectomy in patients with breast cancer aged 40 years or younger. Breast. 2010;19(1):44–9.
56. Yildirim E, Berberoglu U. Can a subgroup of node-negative breast carcinoma patients with T1-2 tumor who may benefit from postmastectomy radiotherapy be identified? Int J Radiat Oncol Biol Phys. 2007;68(4):1024–9.
57. Omlin A, Amichetti M, Azria D, Cole BF, Fourneret P, Poortmans P, et al. Boost radiotherapy in young women with ductal carcinoma in situ: a multi centre, retrospective study of the Rare Cancer Network. Lancet Oncol. 2006;7(8):652–6.
58. Freedman RA, Virgo KS, Labadie J, He Y, Partridge AH, Keating NL. Receipt of locoregional therapy among young women with breast cancer. Breast Cancer Res Treat. 2012;135(3):893–906.
59. Stovall M, Smith SA, Langholz BM, Boice JD Jr, Shore RE, Andersson M, et al. Dose to the contralateral breast from radiotherapy and risk of second primary breast cancer in the WECARE study. Int J Radiat Oncol Biol Phys. 2008;72(4):1021–30.
60. Darby SC, McGale P, Taylor CW, Peto R. Long-term mortality from heart disease and lung cancer after radiotherapy for early breast cancer: prospective cohort study of about 300,000 women in US SEER cancer registries. Lancet Oncol. 2005;6(8):557–65.

50 Oligometastatic and Oligoprogression Disease

Cynthia Aristei, Melanie Machiels, Laura Torres Royo, and Meritxell Arenas Prat

50.1 Background

First reported in 1995, oligometastatic disease (OMD) was identified as intermediate between local and diffuse metastatic disease, with lesions limited in number and extent [1]. This led to changing the treatment paradigm, on the basis of the hypothesis that "if the primary cancer site was controlled, and the metastatic sites ablated by metastasis-directed therapy, a prolonged disease-free interval, and perhaps even cure, may be achieved" [2].

In early 2020, given such a broad spectrum of different OMD presentations, a joint ESTRO and EORTC document discriminated between induced OMD, that is, a history of poly-metastatic disease and genuine OMD, with the latter being sub-divided into recurrent or de novo OMD. Furthermore, the de novo form was differentiated into synchronous (occurring simultaneously with the primary tumour) and metachronous (occurring at least 3 months after diagnosis). *Oligorecurrence* is metachronous, repeat, OMD in patients not under active systemic therapy; *Oligoprogression* is progressive OMD on imaging in patients under active systemic therapy and *Oligopersistence* is stable OMD or a partial response on imaging in patients under active systemic therapy [3] (Fig. 50.1). A few months later the ESTRO-ASTRO consensus document defined OMD as 1–5 metastatic lesions, with a controlled primary tumour being optional, but where all metastatic sites must be safely treatable [4].

Oligometastatic breast cancer treatment varies with type of oligometastatic state and case. Metastasis-directed therapy is facilitated by recent advances in anatomical and functional imaging, surgical and ionising as well as non-ionising ablative techniques. Local ablative therapy may include local treatments such as surgery, radiation therapy, radiofrequency ablation, or cryoablation. Stereotactic ablative radiation therapy, is a valid option for OMD, and includes administration of high-dose irradiation to a limited target volume. The steep dose gradient around the target ensures maximum sparing of surrounding healthy tissues which are at risk of toxicity. It is less invasive than surgery and can be applied to up to more lesions in diverse organs

C. Aristei
Radiation Oncology Section, Department of Medicine and Surgery, University of Perugia and Perugia General Hospital, Perugia, Italy
e-mail: cynthia.aristei@unipg.it

M. Machiels
Iridium Kankernetwerk and University of Antwerp, Faculty of Medicine and Health Sciences, Wilrijk-Antwerp, Belgium
e-mail: Melanie.machiels@gza.be

L. T. Royo · M. A. Prat (✉)
Department of Radiation Oncology, Universitat Rovira I Virgili, Institut d'Investigació Sanitària Pere Virgili, Hospital Universitari de Sant Joan, Reus, Spain

© The Author(s), under exclusive license to Springer Nature Switzerland AG 2022

O. Kaidar-Person et al. (eds.), *Breast Cancer Radiation Therapy*,
https://doi.org/10.1007/978-3-030-91170-6_50

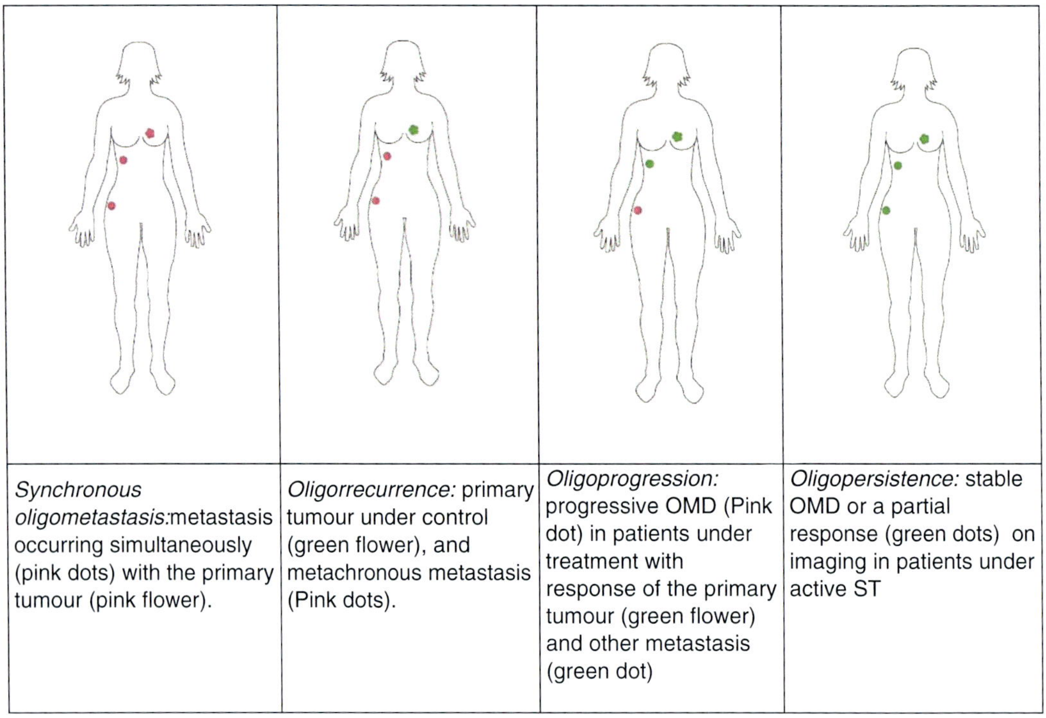

Fig. 50.1 Different presentations of OMD are represented graphically with the definition below them

[5–8]. There are different definitions for SBRT, in some countries it is defined as RT given in up to 5 to 8 large fractions, while in other countries it is defined by the dose size of the fraction and total dose and treatment intent (e.g. ablative versus one large fraction for palliation).

Advances in RT techniques enabled most RT departments to adopt SBRT for metastatic directed therapy in OMD safely over recent years (Fig. 50.2).

This chapter provides a critical appraisal of oligometastatic breast cancer treatment in clinical practice and its perspectives.

50.2 Existing Literature

As several systemic therapy options are available for metastatic breast cancer, fewer series have focused on SBRT in oligometastatic breast cancer than in oligometastases from other primary cancers such as lung, colorectal and prostate. Several dose and fractionation schemes as well as techniques to control organ motion (i.e. gating, dampening, tracking) were described, each more or less appropriate for specific metastatic locations. Use of appropriate equipment for high-precision RT is generally recommended together with delivery of high biological equivalent doses (BED). The few available retrospective studies were flawed by significant heterogeneity such as different types of primary tumours, number, size and location of metastases, RT techniques, doses and fractionation schemes. Furthermore, they were often restricted to patients who were not candidates for surgery. All these variables precluded drawing firm conclusions. Despite these limitations, SBRT provided local control of metastases ranging from 67% to 95% [5], which was long-lasting in most patients. Several single arm studies reported it was safe and well-tolerated with few side effects [8–11].

The results from the SABR-COMET Phase II Randomised Trial were encouraging [12]. In this trial 99 oligometastatic patients (only 13 patients with breast cancer in the SBRT group) with up to 5 metastases were randomised to receive either palliative standard of care treatments alone

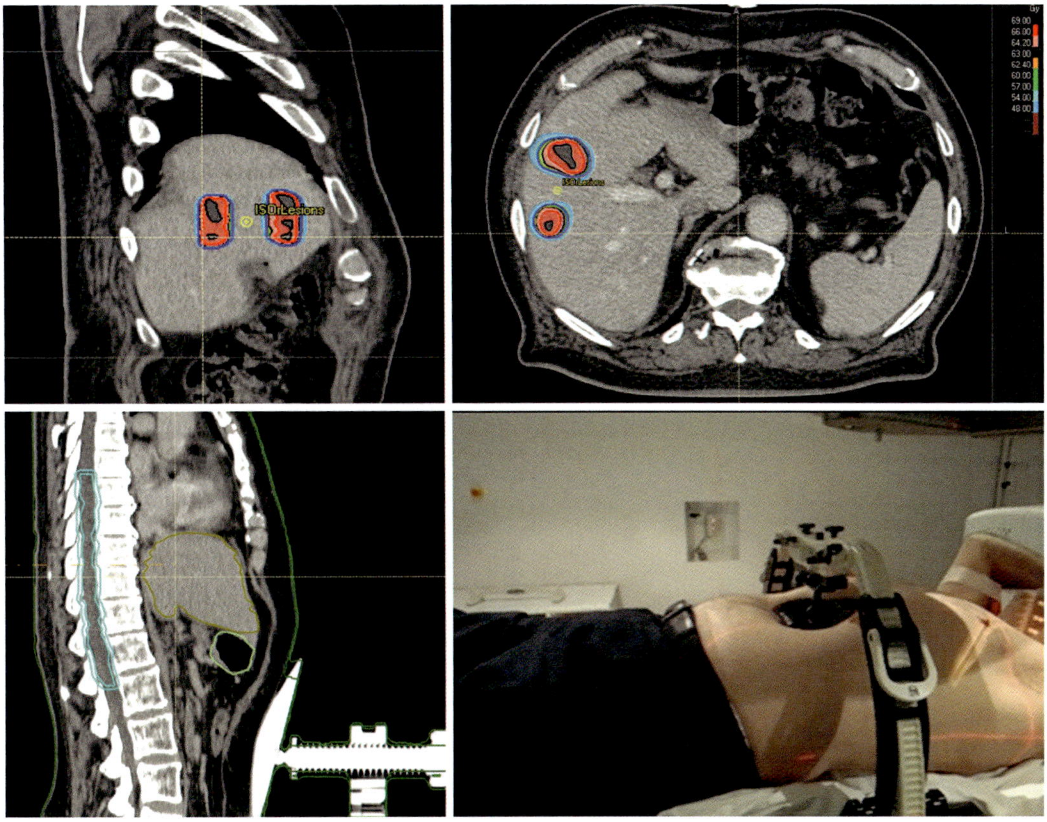

Fig. 50.2 Example of a patient treated with SBRT for liver metastases. Top row illustrates the dose distribution, and bottom row illustrates the abdominal compression used to reduce treatment uncertainties (e.g. inter- and intra-fractional motion)

(control group), or standard of care plus SBRT to all metastatic lesions. Median overall survival (OS) in the SBRT arm significantly improved from 28 to 41 months. The NRG-BR002 phase IIR/III trial of standard of care systemic therapy with or without SBRT for newly oligometastatic breast cancer (NCT02364557) was presented at ASCO annual meeting 2022. Metastatic directed therapy failed to show signal for improved PFS for patients with oligometastatic breast cancer at a median follow up of 35 months. Therefore, the phase III OS study will not start. Patients with oligometastatic breast cancer as defined by NRG-BR002 have long PFS and OS; high dose SBRT was safe with low rates of treatment-related adverse events, like the standard of care arm of the study. Local therapy for metastatic breast cancer enters a rapidly evolving landscape; there is the need for disease specific and biology-driven trials investigating ablative treatments for oligometastases.

Several ongoing clinical trials, with some including a range of primary tumours and metastasis locations, explore the role of SBRT in combination with systemic therapy in the management of oligometastatic breast cancer patients (Table 50.1)

50.3 Practical Guidelines

Planning for SBRT should be according to RT quality assurance treatment guidelines, according to the site, size, and proximity to OARs, regardless of tumour histology. Every effort should be made to ensure precise delivery of an adequate

Table 50.1 Ongoing clinical trials that explore the role of SBRT in combination with systemic therapy in the management of oligometastatic breast cancer

Trial/Identifier/Principal investigator/Country/Accrual time	Population and study summary	Estimated enrolment/ Phase	Primary end-point (P)/Secondary end-point (S)
SABR/SBRT trials			
[a]**SABR BC (STEREO-SEIN)** NCT02089100 France 2014–2023	SABR vs no specific treatment HHRR+ BC ≤ 5 M1 lesions, ≤ 10 cm or ≤ 500 mL; liver M1 ≤ 7 cm	280 Phase 3	P: PFS (minimal follow-up 3 years) S: Cumulative rate of LR and OS
SABR for spinal M1 tumours NCT03392233 China 2017–2027	Single group assignment BC, PC, NSCLC SABR spinal M1 (3 fx 24 Gy or 3 fx 30 Gy)	100 Phase 2	P: The rate of relief pain (1 week after RT to 2 years later) S: Degree and duration of pain relief, toxicity incidence.
[a]**SOC± SABR ± SURGERY M1 BC** NCT02364557 USA 2014–2022	SBRT (1–3-5 fx) or surgery at the discretion of treating physician vs SOC without intervention BC ≤ 4 M1 lesions, ≤ 5 cm	402 Phase 2–3	P: PFS (up to 3 years), OS (up to 8 years) S: New M1, adverse effects incidence, CTCs previous and after treatment in blood, ctDNA levels in plasma.
SOC ± SABR for M1 CANCER NCT03808337 USA 2019–2022	SOC + SABR vs SOC TNBC, NSCLC 1–5 M1 SABR (lung: 5 fx 50 Gy, 4 fx 48 Gy, 3 fx 54 Gy / others: 3 fx 27–30 Gy, bone: 1 fx 24 Gy)	142 Phase 2	P: PFS (up to 2 years) S: OS
SABR vs SOC breast and lung M1 NCT03808662 USA 2019–2022	SOC + SABR vs SOC TNBC, NSCLC 1–5 M1 SBRT (3 fx 27/30 Gy, 5 fx 50 Gy)	160 Phase 2	P: PFS (up to 52 weeks) S: OS (up to 100 months)
[a]**SABR for inoperable lung and liver M1 from BC** NCT02581670 De rose/ Italy 2015–2020	Single group assignment BC with lung and liver M1 SBRT <5 M1; < 5 cm	58 Phase 2	P: Toxicity, LC (2 years) S: PFS, OS, QoL
[a]**Intervention to liver and pulmonary M1 BC (IMET)** NCT02251353 Turkey 2014–2022	BC with lung and liver M1 Resection +/− radiofrequency ablation, transcatheter arterial chemoembolization, CyberKnife radiosurgery vs no intervention	300 Cohort	P: OS (3 years) S: PFS (3 years), Morbidity due to Treatment modality (6 months)
Standard treatment ± SABR in solid tumours with BONE M1 (STEREO-OS) NCT03143322 France 2018–22	SOC+ SABR vs SOC +/− palliative RT BC, PC, lung cancer 1–3 bone M1 SBRT (7 fx 27 Gy, 5 fx 35 Gy)	196 Phase 3	P: PFS (1 year) S: PFS, bone PFS, local control, cancer specific survival, SBRT toxicities, QoL, pain and cost utility (1, 2 and 3 years)
Immunological effects of Cyclophosphamide in MBC NCT02441270 Belgium 2015–2016	Single group assignment SABR +cyclophosphamide BC with ≥2 M1 (skin, subcutaneous, lymph node, superficial lesions)	5 Phase 1	P: Immunological effects In blood and tumour Biopsies S: Clinical/radiographical response of irradiated and non-irradiated M1

Table 50.1 (continued)

Trial/Identifier/Principal investigator/Country/Accrual time	Population and study summary	Estimated enrolment/ Phase	Primary end-point (P)/Secondary end-point (S)
SABR + ANTI-PD1 in TNBC M1 NCT03151447 China 2017–2018	Anti-PD1 (JS001) + SABR TNBC at least 1 M1 > 1 cm (liver, lung, bone, brain, or lymph nodes)	18 Phase 1	P: Adverse events related to treatment
SABR + Atezolizumab in advanced TNBC (AZTEC) NCT03464942 Australia 2018–2022	SABR + Atezolizumab vs SBRT TNBC ≥1 M1 measurable SBRT (1 fx 20 Gy or 3 fx 24 Gy)	52 Phase 2	P: PFS (24 months) S: Best objective response, adverse events incidence, PFR between different regimens, duration of response, disease control rate, time to treatment failure, OS between different regimens
Vaccination with FIt3L, RT and poly-ICLC NCT03789097 USA 2019–2023	Single group assignment Pembro + FIt3L + RT + poly-ICLC MBC, NHL, HNSCC	56 Phase 1–2	P: Dose limiting toxicity (63 days) S: Overall response rate (6 months)
SABR and oncolytic virus therapy before Pembrolizumab for M1 TNBC and NSCLC NCT03004183 USA 2017–2022	Single group assignment ADV/HSV-tk + Valacyclovir + SBRT + Pembrolizumab TNBC, NSCLC SABR (5fx 30Gy)	57 Phase 2	P: Objective response rate (30 days after last Pembrolizumab) S: Duration response, OS, PFS, adverse events, antitumour activity, clinical benefit rate (30 days after last pembrolizumab)
Single dose SABR (SRS) trials			
[a]**SRS in BC with brain M1** NCT04061408 China 2019–21	Single group assignment HER2+ BC with brain M1 (1–10) SRS (3–5 fx of 8 Gy) +/− anti-HER2 (allowed)	170 Phase 2	P: Intracranial LC (2 years) S: Intracranial distant M1 rate, PFS, OS, adverse events
[a]**Local therapy for brain M1 HER2+ BC (local HER-O)** NCT02898727 Australia 2017–2020	Single group assignment Neurosurgery +/− SRS or SRS alone (1 fx 20 Gy to 3 fx 24 Gy) + anti-HER2 HER2+ BC with brain M1 (1–5)	50 Phase 2	P: Percentage of WBRT 12 months after local therapy S: Distant failure, LC, extra-cranial failure, pattern of first failure, OS and cause of death, adverse events, neurocognitive function
[a]**T-DM1 alone vs T-DM1+ TMZ following SRS or surgery brain M1 HER2+ BC** NCT03190967 USA 2018–2022	T-DM1 vs T-DM1 + TMZ Previous SRS, surgery or WBRT HER2+ BC with brain M1	125 Phase 1–2	P: MTD of TMZ used with T-DM1, median time to progression S: Adverse event, time to WBRT, median survival
[a]**SRS + Pembrolizumab Brain M1 BC** NCT03449238 USA 2018–2024	Single group assignment Pembrolizumab + SRS BC with brain M1 (2–10, 5 mm - 4 Cm)	41 Phase 1–2	P: Tumour response non-irradiated 8 weeks, abscopal response, OS S: Abscopal effect elsewhere in the body

(continued)

Table 50.1 (continued)

Trial/Identifier/Principal investigator/Country/Accrual time	Population and study summary	Estimated enrolment/ Phase	Primary end-point (P)/Secondary end-point (S)
[a]**SRS + Atezolizumab Brain M1 TN BC** NCT03483012 USA 2018–2021	Single group assignment Atezolizumab (anti-PD-L1) + SRS TNBC with brain M1 (≤ 5)	45 Phase 2	P: PFS (24 weeks) S: Extracranial objective response, clinical benefit, OS, toxicity, radiation necrosis, patient outcome, abscopal response rate
[a]**SRS + Nivolumab BRAIN M1 BC** NCT03807765 USA 2019–2022	Single group assignment Nivolumab + SRS BC with brain M1 (≤ 10, ≤ 4 cm)	14 Phase 1	P: DLT up to 8 weeks) S: Intracranial local/distant brain tumour treatment (3, 6, 12 months), PFS (12 months), OS (24 months)

***P* Primary end-point, *S* Secondary end-point,** *BC* Breast Cancer, *fx* fraction, *ctDNA* Circulating Tumour DNA, *CTCs* Circulating tumour Cells, *DLT* Dose Limiting Toxicities, *HHRR* Hormonal Receptors, *HNSCC* Head and Neck cancer Squamous Cell Carcinoma, *LC* Local Control, *LR* Local Recurrence, *MBC* Metastatic Breast Cancer, *MTD* Maximum Tolerated Dose, *M1* metastases, *NHL* Non-Hodgkin Lymphoma, *NSCLC* Non–Small Cell Lung Cancer, *OS* Overall Survival, *PC* Prostate Cancer, *PFS* Progression-Free Survival, *QoL* Quality of Life, *RT* Radiation therapy, *SABR/SBRT* Stereotactic Ablative Radiation Therapy, *SOC* Standard of Care, *TMZ* Temozolamide, *TNBC* Triple-Negative Breast Cancer, *WBRT* Whole Brain Radio-Therapy

[a] Exclusively oligometastatic breast cancer

RT dose using advanced technologies and/or techniques that facilitate smaller set-up margins, all without compromising tumour coverage and limiting dose to normal tissues. At present, no evidence limits SBRT use to a maximal number of metastases, or a maximal lesion size. The only limitation is the ability to deliver curative intent SBRT safely, which can vary case-by-case. In fact, the primary goal of SBRT is to maximise tumour control and minimise short and long-term side effects. No firm recommendations can be made for SBRT in breast cancer.

In clinical practice, input is required from a multidisciplinary team that considers all options including metastatic-directed therapy as well as systemic therapy. Decision-making should take into account that oligometastatic treatment varies with type of oligometastatic state and case. To maximise long-term remission all OMD sites should be treated as progression often occurs at mapped metastatic locations. Tailoring therapy is the goal when safe delivery of SBRT is indicated and feasible. Risks and benefits must be assessed, bearing in mind lesion location and adjacent organs, volume of the lesion, length of systemic therapy interruption, and expected clinical benefit.

In synchronous and metachronous metastasis, prognosis, treatment options and risk of occult disseminated metastases can differ, with the length of the disease-free interval appearing to have a prognostic impact in the latter form [13]. Locoregional control of the primary tumour is not mandatory but should be taken into account as a prognostic factor when treating metachronous OMD. Whether SBRT is of benefit or not to patients with oligometastatic breast cancer requires further investigation as no studies have, as yet assessed its efficacy in the different histological subtypes. Molecular breast cancer subtypes impact upon prognosis and may be linked to an intermediate oligometastatic breast cancer status with limited metastatic capacity. Metastatic patterns in breast cancer patients with different subtypes are well-known [14]. HER2-positive and triple-negative tumours usually metastasize to visceral sites and luminal tumours to the bones. All subtypes, other than triple-negative, are more likely to metastasize into intermediate oligometastatic breast cancer and might consequently benefit more from SBRT. Furthermore, receptor-positive lesions were associated with better outcomes than receptor-negative metastases [10, 15]. Although young patients with hormone receptor-positive bone or subcutaneous oligometastatic breast cancer are ideal candidates for SBRT, patients with other molecular subtypes should not be excluded from SBRT. SBRT should be administered to patients with HER2-positive tumours who are receiving systemic anti-HER2 therapies and to triple-negative patients, particularly if they are receiving immunotherapy, as it should improve response and extend survival. Finally, in selected cases, SBRT may serve to delay systemic therapy.

50.4 Unmet Needs

Although SBRT use is increasing, many issues need to be clarified and many open questions need to be answered.

First of all, a "true" oligometastatic state should be defined together with the appropriate imaging tools and type of follow-up. Indeed, conventional imaging (CT, bone scan) seems to play a limited role in the detection of oligometastatic breast cancer. New metabolic and functional imaging tools have a higher sensitivity and specificity [16], but the information they provide is not always sufficient for the diagnosis of a "true" oligometastatic state. Furthermore, issues arise with the follow-up after breast cancer treatment. Although a more intensive approach than clinical examination and annual mammography seems required, what should constitute it still remains to be established. Risk factors including disease stage, biopathology and other features should be taken into account [17] .

Little information is available on efficacy and toxicity when SBRT is combined with systemic therapy [18]. As timing remains unclear, several ongoing studies are investigating outcome, safety and when to deliver SBRT during treatment with new drugs such as checkpoint inhibitors or targeted-therapies [19]. As most Radiation Oncology Centres do not administer systemic therapy, close collaboration is crucial between radiation and medical oncologists who should be aware of SBRT potentialities. SBRT should be considered as a valid option that should not be reserved for patients who do not respond to systemic therapy schedules.

To meet these needs, attempts are being made to understand the immunomodulating effect of SBRT and to identify molecular biomarkers and imaging patterns that detect OMBC and predict response to therapy [20]. Depending on the molecular subtype and gene profile, single and total doses might need to vary. These approaches fit in with the overall goal of precision medicine which is to define a unique disease phenotype and to tailor therapy so as to cure each single patient. Big data mining is expected to draw a new scenario in oligometastatic breast cancer [21, 22] and, in fact, the ESTRO and the EORTC joined in the OligoCare study, that is, a pragmatic observational basket study in order to evaluate outcomes after radical RT for oligometastatic patients [NCT03818503].

50.5 Summary

Oligometastatic breast cancer impacts disease outcome and often requires systemic therapy which is inevitably associated with toxicity and worse QoL. SBRT is a valid, safe option whether administered alone or combined with systemic therapy as it controls disease progression and favourably influences survival and QoL. The associated issues and open questions which were explored in this chapter need investigation so as to identify patients most likely to benefit from it and to establish its place in current therapies for oligometastatic breast cancer.

References

1. Hellman S, Weichselbaum RR. Oligometastases. J Clin Oncol Off J Am Soc Clin Oncol. 1995;13:8–10.
2. Reyes DK, Pienta KJ. The biology and treatment of oligometastatic cancer. Oncotarget. 2015;6:8491–524.
3. Guckenberger M, Lievens Y, Bouma AB, et al. Characterisation and classification of oligometastatic disease: a European Society for Radiotherapy and Oncology and European Organisation for Research and Treatment of Cancer consensus recommendation. Lancet Oncol. 2020;21:e18–28.
4. Lievens Y, Guckenberger M, Gomez D, et al. Defining oligometastatic disease from a radiation oncology perspective: an ESTRO-ASTRO consensus document. Radiother Oncol. 2020;148:157–66.
5. Corbin KS, Hellman S, Weichselbaum RR. Extracranial oligometastases: a subset of metastases curable with stereotactic radiotherapy. J Clin Oncol Off J Am Soc Clin Oncol. 2013;31:1384–90.
6. Milano MT, Katz AW, Schell MC, Philip A, Okunieff P. Descriptive analysis of oligometastatic lesions treated with curative-intent stereotactic body radiotherapy. Int J Radiat Oncol Biol Phys. 2008;72:1516–22.
7. Norihisa Y, Nagata Y, Takayama K, et al. Stereotactic body radiotherapy for oligometastatic lung tumors. Int J Radiat Oncol Biol Phys. 2008;72:398–403.
8. Mercier C, Claessens M, Buys MSc A, et al. Stereotactic ablative radiation therapy to all lesions in patients with oligometastatic cancers: a phase 1 dose-escalation trial. Int J Radiat Oncol Biol Phys. 2020; https://doi.org/10.1016/j.ijrobp.2020.11.066. Online ahead of print. S0360-3016(20)34638-1
9. Salama JK, Kirkpatrick JP, Yin F-F. Stereotactic body radiotherapy treatment of extracranial metastases. Nat Rev Clin Oncol. 2012;9:654–65.
10. Scorsetti M, Comito T, Clerici E, et al. Phase II trial on SBRT for unresectable liver metastases: long-term outcome and prognostic factors of survival after 5 years of follow-up. Radiat Oncol. 2018;13:234.
11. Trovo M, Furlan C, Polesel J, et al. Radical radiation therapy for oligometastatic breast cancer: results of a prospective phase II trial. Radiother Oncol J Eur Soc Ther Radiol Oncol. 2018;126:177–80.
12. Palma DA, Olson R, Harrow S, et al. Stereotactic ablative radiotherapy for the comprehensive treatment of Oligometastatic cancers: long-term results of the SABR-COMET phase II randomized trial. J Clin Oncol Off J Am Soc Clin Oncol. 2020;38:2830–8.
13. Sutera P, Clump DA, Kalash R, et al. Initial results of a multicenter phase 2 trial of stereotactic ablative radiation therapy for Oligometastatic cancer. Int J Radiat Oncol Biol Phys. 2019;103:116–22.
14. Harbeck N, Gnant M, et al. Lancet (London, England). 2017;389:1134–50.
15. Milano MT, Katz AW, Zhang H, Huggins CF, Aujla KS, Okunieff P. Oligometastatic breast cancer treated with hypofractionated stereotactic radiotherapy: some patients survive longer than a decade. Radiother Oncol J Eur Soc Ther Radiol Oncol. 2019;131:45–51.
16. deSouza NM, Liu Y, Chiti A, et al. Strategies and technical challenges for imaging oligometastatic disease: recommendations from the European Organisation for Research and Treatment of Cancer imaging group. Eur J Cancer. 2018;91:153–63.
17. Moschetti I, Cinquini M, Lambertini M, Levaggi A, Liberati A. Follow-up strategies for women treated for early breast cancer. Cochrane Database Syst Rev. 2016;2016:CD001768.
18. Palma DA, Olson R, Harrow S, et al. Stereotactic ablative radiotherapy versus standard of care palliative treatment in patients with oligometastatic cancers (SABR-COMET): a randomised, phase 2, open-label trial. Lancet (London, England). 2019;393:2051–8.
19. Hammers HJ, Vonmerveldt D, Ahn C, et al. Combination of dual immune checkpoint inhibition (ICI) with stereotactic radiation (SBRT) in metastatic renal cell carcinoma (mRCC) (RADVAX RCC). J Clin Oncol. 2020;38:614.
20. Muraro E, Furlan C, Avanzo M, et al. Local high-dose radiotherapy induces systemic Immunomodulating effects of potential therapeutic relevance in Oligometastatic breast cancer. Front Immunol. 2017;8:1476.
21. Quon H, McNutt T, Lee J, et al. Needs and challenges for radiation oncology in the era of precision medicine. Int J Radiat Oncol Biol Phys. 2019;103:809–17.
22. McNutt TR, Benedict SH, Low DA, et al. Using big data analytics to advance precision radiation oncology. Int J Radiat Oncol Biol Phys. 2018;101:285–91.

Re-irradiation

51

Sabine Oldenborg
and Jean-Michel Hannoun-Levi

51.1 Background

Postoperative breast cancer RT is crucial for reducing the risk of the occurrence of local relapse [1–5]. However, despite an optimal therapeutic approach, some patients may experience a local ipsilateral breast tumour recurrence (IBTR) or a new primary tumour in the same breast, with a 20-year cumulative incidence rate of 15% in older series, which is reduced significantly over the last four decades [2, 5, 6].

For second-IBTR or new primary breast cancer occurring in a previously irradiated area (i.e. Hodgkin disease, thoracic irradiation, BCT), salvage mastectomy was historically considered as the standard treatment, with no other alternative of care. However, advances in screening programmes and early detection, with effective treatments including locoregional and systemic therapies, decreased 5-year and 10-year rates of LRR with overall survival increasing [6]. Prolonged survival increases the chances for LR and LRR and/or second ipsilateral breast cancer, enforcing the need for re-treatment, including reirradiation, especially for the approximately half of recurrent breast cancer patients that present with isolated LR or regional only or LRR. Therefore, as RT is an integral part of breast conserving approach and is increasingly used in the postmastectomy setting for the first occurrence of breast cancer, re-irradiation as part of definitive treatment for locoregional recurrence gained more interest over the years.

Understanding of the fundamental principles of reirradiation is essential for the management of these patients. The current section aims to provide clinicians tools to manage the different scenarios of LRR with the limitation that most published data about reirradiation comes from animal studies, retrospective cohorts, with only limited data from prospective multicentre early phase trials.

51.2 Second Breast-Conserving Surgery

Historically the standard therapeutic approach of ipsilateral in-breast recurrence after BCT is mastectomy with rates of second recurrence after salvage mastectomy of approximately 10% [7, 8]. In selected cases, especially late-onset limited in-breast recurrence (including second primaries) or patients who refuse mastectomy, a second BCS can be considered [8–13]. Salvage BCS without reirradiation is not the recommended approach as it is associated with poor outcome and increased

S. Oldenborg
Department of Radiation Oncology, Amsterdam UMC, Amsterdam, The Netherlands

J.-M. Hannoun-Levi (✉)
Radiation Therapy Department, Antoine-Lacassagne Cancer Center, Nice, France
e-mail: jean-michel.hannoun-levi@nice.unicancer.fr

© The Author(s), under exclusive license to Springer Nature Switzerland AG 2022

O. Kaidar-Person et al. (eds.), *Breast Cancer Radiation Therapy*,
https://doi.org/10.1007/978-3-030-91170-6_51

mortality, however it can be offered in selected low risk patients who refuse mastectomy or BCS and reirradiation [14]. In general, local recurrence rates following repeat BCS without RT range from 10 to 50%, with most reports in the 30–35% range [8–13]. It seems that local control rates of salvage lumpectomy was similar those in prospective trials of newly diagnosed breast cancer patients treated with BCS alone [8–13] and the addition of repeat irradiation in LR significantly decreased local failure after salvage lumpectomy similar to that seen at primary diagnosis. Therefore, reirradiation should be offered in case of second BCS. Even though over the years RT planning and delivery significantly improved to optimise therapy and reduce OAR exposure, the use of 3D-CRT, DIBH and particle therapy in reirradiation to reduce RT-related toxicity and increase the therapeutic ratio is not well described in the literature. Today, the largest multicentre trial evaluating second BCT approach was conducted by the GEC-ESTRO Breast Cancer Working Group [10, 15] treated with salvage BCT including APBI with interstitial brachytherapy. Additionally, the RTOG 1014 phase II trial reported second BCT approach with EBRT-PBI [16]. Nevertheless, little is known about second-BCS and whole-breast irradiation [17]. As reirradiation is often offered in case of LRR after salvage mastectomy for non-metastatic recurrence much can be learned about the risks for OAR toxicity in case of whole breast reirradiation [18, 19]. Therefore, patients who have an explicit wish for breast conservation could be considered for salvage breast-conserving surgery followed by reirradiation, preferably partial breast irradiation to reduce potential toxicity. Moreover, as most of the data comes from the GEC-ESTRO Breast Cancer Working Group work [10, 15].

51.3 Challenges of Reirradiation and Maximal Cumulative Dose

Patients who have second LR or LRR without evidence of metastatic disease have a potential curative disease. Therefore, the two key principles of RT should not be compromise in this setting especially when considering treatment approach: disease control while minimising potential RT related toxicity. Treatment protocols for locoregional recurrence vary from country to country, in some the standard locoregional treatment approach is salvage mastectomy with/without reirradiation with/without hyperthermia while in others, second BCS and interstitial brachytherapy is the preferred approach. The OAR in case of reirradiation may change according to the technique (e.g. interstitial brachytherapy versus EBRT), and may include the skin, subcutis and lymphatic basins, heart, lungs, ribs, shoulder joint and brachial plexus and any other uninvolved tissue that might by exposed to RT dose. Depending on the RT volumes and treatment planning (e.g. vIMRT), other organs such as liver and thyroids gland should be considered. Efforts should be made to reduce potential RT dose to these organs including considering DIBH also for right-side RT if it provides dosimetric advantage for OARs and reduce the irradiated volumes if possible (e.g. by PBI, brachytherapy).

Reirradiation of the axillary lymph node areas should be avoided as it can lead to injury to the brachial plexus and lymphoedema; both lymphatics and nerves are slowly proliferative tissues with a higher risk for residual sub-clinical damage. Late osseous damage was estimated to have a α/β ratio of 1.8–2.8 Gy, indicating that the bone is behaving like a late responding tissue [20]. This complication can be a result of fractures, also associated with menopause, systemic treatments including aromatase inhibitors and osteoporosis. Additionally, osteonecrosis, which may result from radiation or from prolonged bisphosphonate treatment can also be the underlining process leading to rib fractures [21]. Rib fracture was reported in 7% of the patients at 5-year after reirradiation and hyperthermia [18]. Factors that are associated with increased risks for rib fracture include high RT doses (dose inhomogeneity resulting from multiple overlapping fields in the reirradiation setting and areas receiving 140% of the planned dose), high dose per fraction (e.g. 4 Gy per fraction), large RT volumes and older 2D techniques [18]. However, these data are from reirradiation of salvage mastectomy patients, thus little distance from the body surface to the rib cage and close proximity to lungs and heart. In case of second BCS, depending on the case, the breast glandular tissue and the pectoralis muscles might allow to reduce the dose near the rib cage. Additionally, with current TPS and 3DCRT planning, reirradiation can be done with homogenous planning with limited volumes receiving over 105% of the dose. Therefore, in these cases PBI, brachytherapy can have an advantage.

There is less data regarding the tolerance of the heart and/or lungs to reirradiation, therefore the dose should be limited as possible. Table 51.1 lists the normal tissue constraints in a prospective phase II trial of PBI-reirradiation. Additionally, the study by Fattah et al. [17] of whole breast reirradiation summarised the dose to OARs in case of breast/chest wall with/without regional lymphatics reirradiation which can be used for clinical reference. However, due to the lack of data on OAR tolerance to reirradiation, there is no consensus for normal tissue dose constraints in case of breast/chest wall reirradiation. Patients with comorbidities or previous sequela from previous irradiation, the tolerance for reirradiation can be reduced. A publication summarising studies of reirradiation for breast cancer [19] reported that the RT cumulative dose (EDQ2) in these studies ranges from less than 80 Gy to more than 130 Gy without significant toxicities. However, it is important to emphasise that these values are retrieved from small cohorts, using various RT schedules (per fraction, number of fractions per week and total dose), volumes and techniques, and toxicity not well reported [22, 23].

Table 51.1 Normal tissue dose constraints used in the NRG Radiation Therapy Oncology Group (NRG/RTOG), 1014 prospective phase II trial of 3D-external beam partial breast reirradiation, 1.5 Gy x 30 (twice a day), to a total dose of 45 Gy

Normal tissue	Constraints
Uninvolved ipsilateral breast	<60% of whole breast receive ≥ of prescribed dose <35% of whole breast receive prescribed dose
Contralateral breast	<3% receive prescribed dose
Ipsilateral lung	<15% receive 30% of the prescribed dose
Contralateral lung	<15% receive 5% of the prescribed dose
Heart Right side RT Left side RT	<5% receive 5% of the prescribed dose <5% receive 5% of the prescribed dose
Thyroid	Maximum point dose of 3% of the prescribed dose

51.4 General Principals when Considering Reirradiation

As the two key principals of RT of not compromising disease control while minimising potential RT related toxicity should lead the decision for selecting the patients who are good candidates for second BCS and reirradiation. Patients who have aggressive disease, radioresistant tumours or potentially reduced normal tissue tolerance should not be considered for second BCS. Therefore, the fundamental points to take into consideration for reirradiation should include [24] the following.

- Full evaluation of the previous irradiation course, guiding subsequent treatment planning.
- Careful consideration of the clinical benefit of reirradiation.
- Careful evaluation of other potential contributors to poor tolerance of reirradiation including comorbidities and systemic therapy.
- Careful evaluation of current disease and the possibility to reduce the irradiated volumes and doses to normal tissues; including omission of elective volumes, using radiosensitizers, such as chemotherapy and/or hyperthermia to reduce the radiation dose.

As of today, the choice between second BCS and salvage mastectomy remains under debate but both options can be discussed with the patient. The GEC-ESTRO Breast Cancer Working Group [10, 15] analysed 754 patients who experience a IBTR treated either by salvage mastectomy (377 patients) or second BCT (reirradiation was PBI with interstitial brachytherapy) (377 patients), the salvage treatment was not considered as prognostic factor in univariate analysis for any type of oncological items including third IBTR. However, time length between primary and salvage surgery (<36 months) and tumour size (≥30 mm) were both considered as prognostic factors in multivariate analysis for cumulative incidence of distant metastasis, disease-free, specific and overall survival (Table 51.2) [15]. Consequently, it appears that the impact of a second BCT is more systemic than local whatever the performed salvage local treatment (salvage mastectomy versus second BCT) while early local relapse (<36 months) could be candidate to adjuvant systemic therapies.

Basically, facing to IBTR, the first step is to consider the guidelines regarding the tumour features (Fig. Decision tree): if there is an indication of mastectomy (which remains the same whether it is a first or an IBTR: large tumour size, multifocality/centricity, extensive intraductal component), second BCT is definitely ruled out. If salvage mastectomy is not mandatory, technical feasibility of a second BCT has to be carefully evaluated. Indeed, the cutaneous and subcutaneous consequences of the first surgery and irradiation, the total delivered dose for the primary, the resultant breast size and the cosmetic impact have to be taken into consideration. Finally, patient's choice remains crucial after a full and detailed explanation of the risk and benefits of each salvage treatment.

Table 51.2 Multivariate analyses for prognostic factors of oncological outcomes performed on the matched (1:1) dataset (754 patients).

Patient selection for second BCS and reirradiation is highly important. Figure shows an example for decision tree for second conserving therapy (2ndCT) with reirradiation APBI (APBrI).

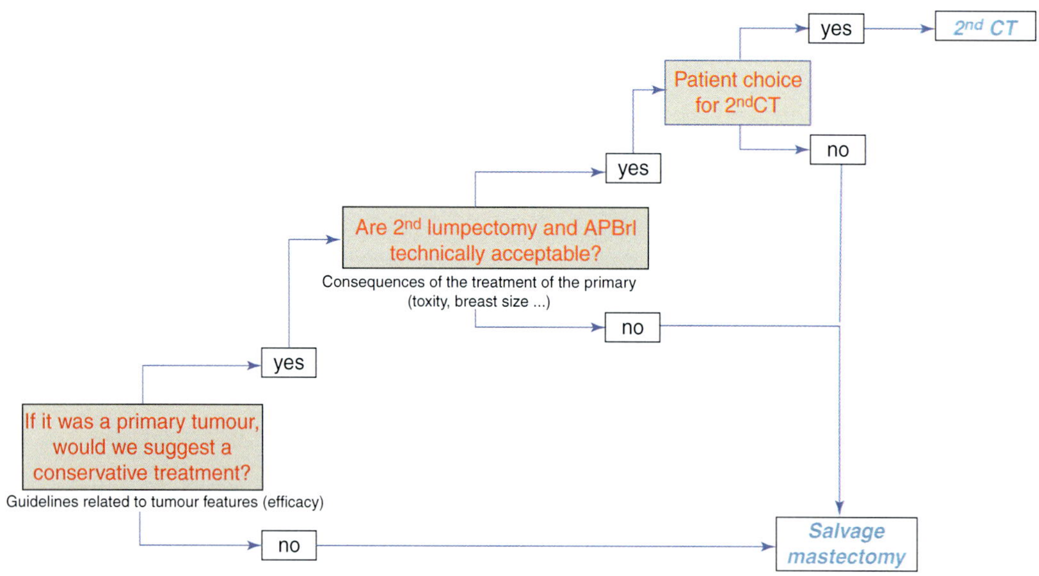

Table 51.2 Multivariate analyses for prognostic factors of oncological outcomes performed on the matched (1:1) dataset (754 patients)

	Multivariate analysis			
Oncological outcomes	Data	Hazard ratio	Confidence interval 95%	p value
Cumulative incidence of third ipsilateral breast tumour event	No			
Cumulative incidence of regional relapse	No			
Cumulative incidence of distant metastasis	Time length between primary and salvage surgery (<36 months) Period of salvage surgery ≤31.12.2001 ≥01.01. 2002/≤31.12.2009 ≥01.01. 2010 Tumour size (≥30 mm)	1.78 1 0.58 0.35 2.89	(1.02–3.08) – (0.34–0.94) (0.17–0.68) (1.70–4.87)	0.035 – 0.026 0.001 <0.001
Disease-free survival	Time length between primary and salvage surgery (<36 months) Period of salvage surgery ≤31.12.2001 ≥01.01. 2002/≤31.12.2009 ≥01.01. 2010 Tumour size (≥30 mm)	1.92 1 0.61 0.42 1.89	(1.23–3.00) – (0.40–0.91) (0.24–0.71) (1.16–3.06)	0.003 - 0.014 0.001 0.008
Specific survival	Age (<48 year) Time length between primary and salvage surgery (<36 months) Tumour size (≥30 mm) Tumour grade 1 2 3	1.78 1.71 2.09 1 2.22 2.51	(1.08–2.93) (0.94–3.10) (1.14–3.82) – (1.06–4.64) (1.20–5.29)	0.019 0.050 0.014 – 0.029 0.012
Overall survival	Time length between primary and salvage surgery (<36 months) Tumour size (≥30 mm)	2.01 1.67	(1.23–3.28) (0.96–2.90)	0.004 0.048

51.5 Reirradiation Protocols After Second BCS

51.5.1 Partial Breast Irradiation

At this time, there has been no phase III trial directly comparing these two therapeutic approaches. Nevertheless, encouraging results in terms of oncological and cosmetic outcomes after second BCS with additional partial breast reirradiation have been provided by the GEC-ESTRO Breast Cancer Working Group and the RTOG 1014 [10, 15, 16]. The initial report by the GEC-ESTRO Breast Cancer Working Group [10], included 217 patients reported that at a median follow-up of 3.9 years, local control rates were encouraging with 5- and 10-year actuarial second LRR rates of 5.6% and 7.2%, respectively. Distant metastases rates are 9.6% and 19.1% and overall survival 88.7% and 76.4%, respectively. In the multivariate analysis, histological grade was a prognostic factor for a second local relapse ($p = 0.008$) and for overall survival ($p = 0.02$), while tumour size was a prognostic factor for distant metastases ($p = 0.03$). The rate of grade 3–4 complications was 11% and an excellent to good cosmetic result was obtained in 85% of the patients [10]. A recent publication by the Breast cancer working group of the GEC-ESTRO reported the results of a matched-pair analysis between salvage mastectomy and BCS and brachytherapy of 1327 patients [15]. Data were collected from 15 centres in 7 European countries. Among the 1327 analysed patients (mastectomy, 945; conservative treatment, 382), 754 were matched by propensity score (mastectomy, 377; second BCS, 377). The analysis included patients of all ages presented no evidence of skin involvement or distant metastatic disease, had no history of contralateral breast cancer, had a tumour staged T1–2, and had at least 12 months between primary and salvage surgery. The median follow-up was 75.4 months (95% confidence interval [CI], 65.4–83.3) and 73.8 months (95% CI, 67.5–80.8) for mastectomy and second BCS, respectively (P = 0.9). In the matched analyses, no differences in 5-year overall survival and cumulative incidence of third breast event were noted between mastectomy and conservative treatment (88% [95% CI, 83.0–90.8] vs 87% [95% CI, 82.1–90.2], P = 0.6 and 2.3% [95% CI, 0.7–3.9] vs 2.8% [95% CI, 0.8–4.7], P = 0.4, respectively). The 5-year cumulative incidence of salvage mastectomy in the second BCS group was 3.1% (95% CI, 1.0–5.1).

The RTOG 1014 Phase 2 trial recently published short term outcomes of EBRT-PBI reirradiation in case of second BCS [16]. Eligible patients were those with unifocal, in-breast recurrences of less than 3 cm, and at least 1 year after primary BCT. The reirradiation protocol was of 1.5 Gy twice daily for 30 treatments during 15 days to a total dose of 45 Gy. The trial included a total of 65 patients but only 58 were included in the published analysis. The actual patient population were low risk patients including only 60% invasive cancer and over 90% of the lesions were less than 2 cm with predominantly ER positive tumours. The 5-year cumulative of local recurrence was 5% (95% CI, 1%–13%). Seven patients underwent ipsilateral mastectomies for a 5-year cumulative incidence of 10% (95% CI, 4%–20%) [16].

Therefore, conservative treatment could be considered a viable option for salvage treatment in selected cases indicated above [15].

Recently, new reirradiation techniques have emerged in combination with salvage lumpectomy, mimicking the process of a first breast conservative treatment, such as 3DCRT (Table 51.3), balloon-based brachytherapy and IORT (Table 51.4). The most used and well documented reirradiation technique is accelerated and partial breast reirradiation using multicatheter interstitial brachytherapy (Tables 51.5) [24].

Table 51.3 Partial breast reirradiation with external beam radiotherapy [11]

Authors	# pts	MFU (months)	Irradiation techniques	Dose (Gy) Total (Gy)	Dose/f	3rd IBTE rate (%)	5-y OS (%)	≥ G3 tox. (%)
Mullen et al. [12]	17	75	Cobalt + E-	50	2	–	–	–
Deutsch et al. [13]	39	51.5	E-	50	2	–	–	–
Janssen et al. [14]	83	35	3D CRT	45	1.8	14.5[a]	76	0
Thorpe et al. [10]	50	12.7	Proton	45–76	–	–	97	16
Arthur et al. [6]	58	12	3D CRT	45	1.5 (BID)	–	–	2

 # pts. number of patients, *MFU* median follow-up, *E-* electron, *Dose/f* dose per fraction, *3rdIBTE* third ipsilateral breast tumour event rate, *OS* overall survival, *≥G3 tox.* grade 3 and higher toxicity rate, *3DCRT* 3D conformal radiation therapy

[a]@ 21 m

Table 51.4 Partial breast reirradiation with IORT [11]

Authors	# pts	MFU (months)	Irradiation technique	Median Dose (Gy)	3rdIBTE-FS (%)	5-y OS (%)	≥ G3 tox. (%)
Kraus-Tiefenbacher et al. [15]	17	26	X 50 kV	20	100	–	–
Chin et al. [16]	12	14	X 50 kV	20	100	–	0
Thangarajah et al. [17]	41	58	X 50 kV	20	89.7	82	0
Blandino et al. [18]	30	47	E-	18	92.3	91.2	21

 # pts. number of patients, *MFU* median follow-up, *X 50 kV* X photons of 50 kV, *E-* electron beam, *3rdIBTE-FS* third ipsilateral breast tumour event free survival rate, *OS* overall survival, *≥ G3 tox.* grade 3 and higher toxicity rate

As these treatments are becoming widely available, and as opposed to multicatheter brachytherapy, require less specialised expertise, we recommend that these cases will be documented in prospective cohorts and close follow up to allow for careful evaluation before widely adopting this approach.

51.5.2 Whole Breast Re-irradiation

Mastectomy is the recommended treatment approach in patients who are not candidates for partial breast reirradiation. However, some patients received previous whole breast RT but were not exposed to a full dose and/or the RT volume included the entire breast volume (e.g. Hodgkin lymphoma patients). These patients often can be safely reirradiation to the whole breast up to the same doses as for other breast cancer patients. Moreover, in cases that patients refuse mastectomy and are not candidates for PBI because of high risk for recurrence, reirradiation of the whole breast can be considered after discussing with the patient the lack of data to support this approach and the risk of long-term toxicity. Reports of whole breast reirradiation are scarce and with limited number of patients, and toxicity data mainly comes from reirradiation of the chest wall [17, 22, 24]. A recent publication by a group from the Mayo Clinic [17] reported their experience with reirradiation for locoregional recurrent or second primary breast cancer. The study included 72 patients underwent reirradiation for second BCS or mastectomy. Median time between RT courses was 73 months and the median cumulative dose of both RT courses was 103.54 Gy (EDQ2). Sixty one percent of the patients were treated in a curative intent, and 47% had gross residual disease at time of reirradiation. Fifty-two patients (72%) were treated with photons with/without electrons and 20 (28%) with protons. The most common acute toxicity was radiation dermatitis grade 1 in 60%, grade 2 in 31% and grade 3 in 8% based on the CTCAE scale. One additional patient experienced grade 3 skin necrosis during treatment. However, it was not clear from the publication if it was progressive disease or due to radiation planning (e.g. bolus) as the authors noted that the patient had diffuse dermal lymphovascular invasion and indicated that it was a probable contributor to acute toxicity. Reirradiation volumes (breast/chest wall only or with regional lymphatics), and concurrent capecitabine at reirradiation were the only variables significantly associated with the development of acute grade 3 adverse events. Late grade 1 toxicity included brachial plexopathy in one patient, osteonecrosis in one, soft tissue necrosis in two patients (3%), decreased range of shoulder motion in 10%, chest wall and soft tissue fibrosis in 15%, and lung fibrosis in 18%. Osteonecrosis of the anterior second rib was experienced by a patient treated with curative intent using photons initially and at reirradiation. The irradiated volumes completely overlap, and courses were 46 months apart with cumulative dose 100.4 Gy (50 Gy to the breast followed by 50.4 Gy to the chest wall and nodes

Table 51.5 Partial breast reirradiation with brachytherapy [11]

Authors	# pts	MFU (months)	Irradiation techniques	Dose (Gy)		3rdIBTE-FS (%)	3rdIBTE (%)	OS		≥ G3 tox. (%)
				Total (Gy)	Dose/f			@	(%)	
Maulard et al. [19]	38	48	MIB LDR	30	–	–	21	5 y	55	8
Resch et al. [20]	17	50	MIB PDR EBRT	12.5 30	0.5–1	–	24	4 y	70	0
Hannoun-Levi et al. [21]	69	50	MIB LDR	30–50	–	77.4	–	5 y	91.8	10.2
Niehoff et al. [22]	19	19	MIB HDR PDR EBRT	28 30 58	2.5 1 2	62.5	37.5	1.5 y	68.7	3
Chadha et al. [23]	15	36	MIB LDR	30–45	–	89	–	3 y	100	0
Guix et al. [24]	36	89	MIB HDR	30	2.5	89.4	–	10 y	96.7	0
Hannoun-Levi et al. [25]	42	21	MIB HDR	34	3.4	97	–	–	3	
Kauer-Dorner et al. [26]	39	57	MIB PDR	50.1	0.6–1	93	–	5 y	87	17
GEC-ESTRO [5]	217	47	MIB LDR	46		94.4	–	5 y	88.7	11
			PDR	50.4				10 y	76.4	
			HDR	32	4					
Trombetta et al. [27]	18	40	Balloon HDR	34	3.4	88.9	–	–	–	
Smanyko et al. [28]	39	59	MIB HDR	22	4.4	94	–	5 y	69	8
Montagne et al. [29]	159	71	MIB HDR LDR	28–34 30–55	–	97.4	–	6 y	91.2	–
Forster et al. [30]	19	65	MIB PDR	49.8–50.4	0.5–0.7	100	–	5 y	100	0
			HDR		3.4–3.8					
GEC-ESTRO [7]	37	74	LDR/PDR/HDR	34.2–32	–/–/4	97.2	–	5 y	87	9.5
	7			46/50.4/32						

 # pts. number of patients, *MFU* median follow-up, *Dose/f* dose per fraction, *3rdIBTE-FS* third ipsilateral breast tumour event free survival rate, *3rdIBTE* third ipsilateral breast tumour event rate, *OS* overall survival, *≥ G3 tox.* grade 3 and higher toxicity rate, *MIB* Mutlicatheter interstitial brachytherapy, *LDR* low-dose rate, *PDR* pulsed-dose rate, *HDR* High-dose rate, *EBRT* external beam radiation therapy

Modified from Montagne L, Hannoun A, Hannoun-Levi JM. Second conservative treatment for second ipsilateral breast tumour event: A systematic review of the different re-irradiation techniques. Breast. 2020;49:274–280 at reirradiation). Late grade 2 toxicity included brachial plexopathy 3%, lymphoedema in 3%, soft tissue necrosis in 3%, wound complication in 4%, decreased range of shoulder motion in 6%, skin infection in 8%, new chest wall and soft tissue fibrosis in 13% and telangiectasia in 13%. However, both patients with brachial plexopathy the axilla was not retreated, and the plexopathy was noted with subsequent axillary recurrence with plexus involvement. Importantly, the investigators indicate that the time between RT courses and reirradiation was significant for toxicity at any time and overall a rate of 13% of patients experiencing grade 3 toxicity at any point (10% acute skin toxicity and 3% late skin necrosis), with none of the patients experiencing grade 4 or 5 toxicities. At 2 years, locoregional recurrence-free survival was 93.1% and overall survival was 76.8% among curative intent patients treated without gross disease [17].

If such an approach is planned, we recommend meticulous RT planning, homogenous RT plans with minimising areas of doses over 100% and reducing the doses to the ribs and costochondral junction. Minimising OAR exposure as possible. Patients treated with this approach need to be follow up carefully to evaluate and document any RT-related toxicity. Prospective databases and reporting these cases will allow for further data of the outcome of whole breast reirradiation with/without regional node using new RT techniques. Documenting and reporting RT related toxicity in daily practice is discussed in other sections.

51.5.2.1 Technical Considerations for Multicatheter Image-Guided Brachytherapy

The GEC-ESTRO published practical guidelines for multicatheter image-guided brachytherapy for breast cancer patients [25, 26]. The implantation of plastic tubes or more rarely rigid needles can be performed during or after the lumpectomy time. Each procedure has its own advantages and disadvantages [27]. Whatever the timing of the implant, it must be built according to the square/triangle geometric rules of the Paris System. During the implant, once the needle is inserted in the proximal entrance-skin point, it is crucial to target with the highest precision the expected exit-skin point and to push the needle in one (or two) gesture to keep the needle/catheter as straight as possible. The objective is to provide an implant with at least 2 plans (avoiding single plan except for very thin target volume with very few breast tissue) and keeping in mind that it is simpler to place a tube which will be not used to properly cover the target rather than to insert an extra tube after the post-implant CT-scan. The planification should be based of 3D-imaging analysis (CT-scan). Target (CTV) delineation modalities regarding the type of surgery (open or closed cavity) were already described by the Breast Cancer Working Group of GEC-ESTRO [25, 28]. The CTV must consider safety margins which are defined as the sum of "size of existing surgical resection margins" plus, "size of the added safety margins" [25, 28]. The presence of 4–6 clips marking the borders of the lumpectomy should be a prerequisite for brachytherapy but must be differentiated from those which were implanted at the time of lumpectomy performed for the primary breast cancer. The prescribed dose for APBrI is the same compared to its used for APBI: 34 Gy in 10 fractions (twice daily), 32 Gy in 8 fractions, 30.1 Gy in 7 fractions [25, 29]. The dose distribution optimisation must follow and respect the recommended dose-volume limits for implant, CTV and organs at risk (ipsilateral non-target breast, skin, rib, heart and ipsilateral lung) (Table 51.5) [25]. The dose distribution will be checked in each view (frontal, sagittal and transversal) in order to avoid $V_{200} > 1$ cm and confluence of 2 V_{200} isodoses.

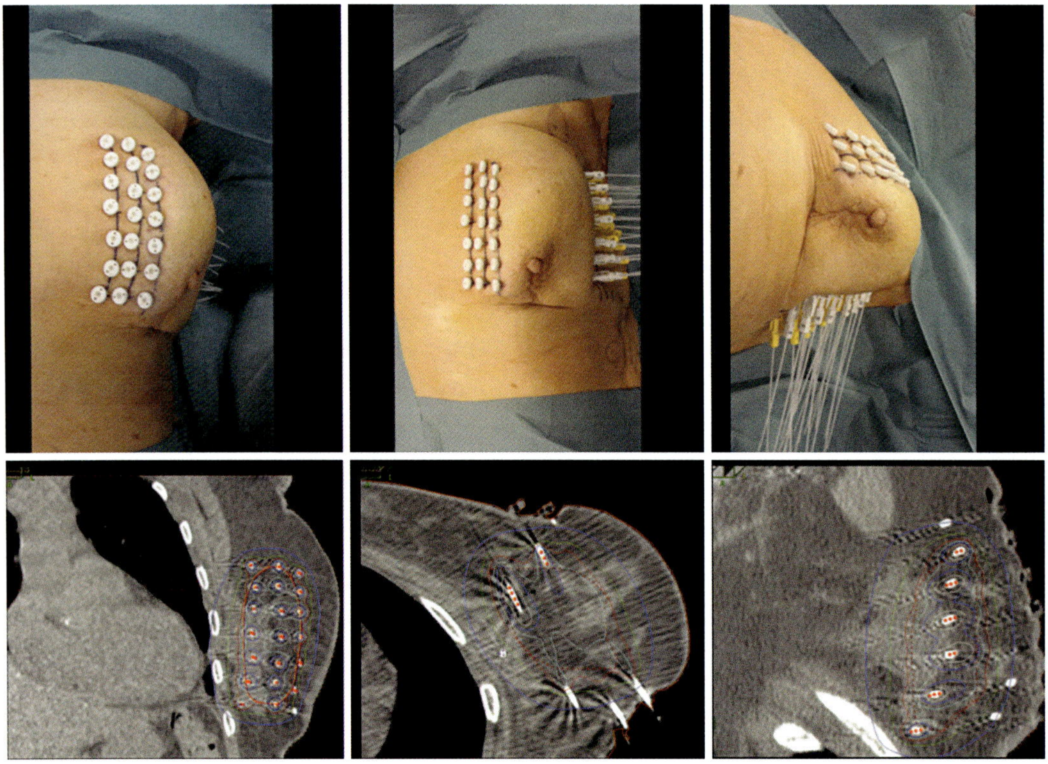

A: surgical margin

B: Irradiation margin

Final margin = A + B = 2 cm

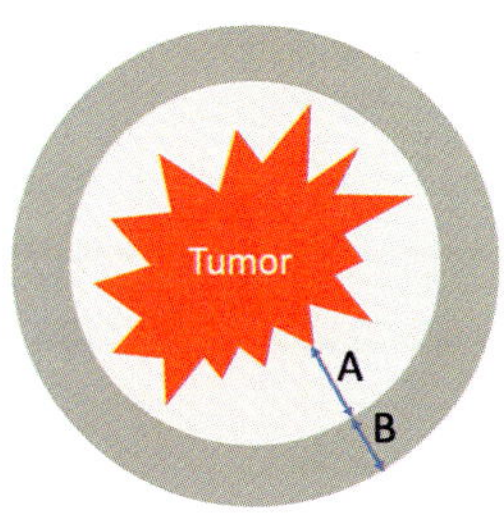

During the daily treatment it is essential to check before each fraction:

- the appearance of the skin: infection, flow, colour, deformation with potential haematoma (a daily disinfection around the puncture holes is warranted).
- the position of the catheters by verifying that the distal part remains in contact to the skin. In case of major displacement of the catheter, a new planification should be performed.

At the end of the treatment (after the last fraction), all catheters can be removed without any local anaesthesia. There is no need of systematic antibiotic prescription.

51.6 Summary

For IBTR or new primary breast cancer occurring in a previously irradiated area salvage mastectomy with/without reirradiation with/without hyperthermia was historically considered as the standard locoregional treatment approach. However, recent data suggest that in selected cases, second BCS and reirradiation can be offered to patients who opt for breast preservation. A multidisciplinary discussion should be associated with the shared decision-making process and informing the patient for pro and cons of each approach. In view of the potential long-term disease-free survival, meticulous target volume delineation and selection of the most appropriate techniques should be used to decrease the risk of toxicity. Data should be recorded and long-term follow is needed before adopting these treatments as the main approach in case of recurrence.

References

1. Fisher B, Dignam J, Wolmark N, et al. Lumpectomy and radiation therapy for the treatment of intraductal breast cancer: findings from National Surgical Adjuvant Breast and bowel project B-17. J Clin Oncol. 1998;16:441–52.
2. Veronesi U, Cascinelli N, Mariani L, et al. Twenty-year follow-up of a randomized study comparing breast-conserving surgery with radical mastectomy for early breast cancer. N Engl J Med. 2002;347:1227–32.
3. Leonardi MC, Maisonneuve P, Mastropasqua MG, et al. Accelerated partial breast irradiation with intraoperative electrons: using GEC-ESTRO recommendations as guidance for patient selection. Radiother Oncol. 2013;106:21–7.
4. Fastner G, Gaisberger C, Kaiser J, et al. ESTRO IORT task force/ACROP recommendations for intraoperative radiation therapy with electrons (IOERT) in breast cancer. Radiother Oncol. 2020;149:150–7.
5. Fisher B, Anderson S, Bryant J, et al. Twenty-year follow-up of a randomized trial comparing total mastectomy, lumpectomy, and lumpectomy plus irradiation for the treatment of invasive breast cancer. N Engl J Med. 2002;347:1233–41.
6. Poortmans PM, Arenas M, Livi L. Over-irradiation. Breast. 2016;31:295–302.
7. Abner AL, Recht A, Eberlein T, et al. Prognosis following salvage mastectomy for recurrence in the breast after conservative surgery and radiation therapy for early-stage breast cancer. J Clin Oncol. 1993;11:44–8.
8. Alpert TE, Kuerer HM, Arthur DW, et al. Ipsilateral breast tumor recurrence after breast conservation therapy: outcomes of salvage mastectomy vs. salvage breast-conserving surgery and prognostic factors for salvage breast preservation. Int J Radiat Oncol Biol Phys. 2005;63:845–51.
9. Hannoun-Levi JM, Ihrai T, Courdi A. Local treatment options for ipsilateral breast tumour recurrence. Cancer Treat Rev. 2013;39:737–41.
10. Hannoun-Levi JM, Resch A, Gal J, et al. Accelerated partial breast irradiation with interstitial brachytherapy as second conservative treatment for ipsilateral breast tumour recurrence: multicentric study of the GEC-ESTRO breast cancer working group. Radiother Oncol. 2013;108:226–31.
11. Kurtz JM, Jacquemier J, Amalric R, et al. Is breast conservation after local recurrence feasible? Eur J Cancer. 1991;27:240–4.
12. Salvadori B, Marubini E, Miceli R, et al. Reoperation for locally recurrent breast cancer in patients previously treated with conservative surgery. Br J Surg. 1999;86:84–7.
13. Aebi S, Gelber S, Anderson SJ, et al. Chemotherapy for isolated locoregional recurrence of breast cancer (CALOR): a randomised trial. Lancet Oncol. 2014;15:156–63.
14. Su Y, Guo R, Xue J, et al. Increased mortality with repeat lumpectomy alone after ipsilateral breast tumor recurrence. Oncologist. 2019;24:e818–27.
15. Hannoun-Levi JM, Gal J, Van Limbergen E, et al. Salvage mastectomy versus second conservative treatment for second ipsilateral breast tumor event: a propensity score-matched cohort analysis of the GEC-ESTRO breast cancer working group database. Int J Radiat Oncol Biol Phys. 2020;110(2):452–61.
16. Arthur DW, Winter KA, Kuerer HM, et al. Effectiveness of breast-conserving surgery and 3-dimensional conformal partial breast Reirradiation for recurrence of breast cancer in the ipsilateral breast: the NRG oncology/RTOG 1014 phase 2 clinical trial. JAMA Oncol. 2019;6:75–82.
17. Fattahi S, Ahmed SK, Park SS, et al. Reirradiation for Locoregional recurrent breast cancer. Adv Radiat Oncol. 2021;6:100640.
18. Oldenborg S, Valk C, van Os R, et al. Rib fractures after reirradiation plus hyperthermia for recurrent breast cancer: predictive factors. Strahlenther Onkol. 2016;192:240–7.
19. Kaidar-Person O, Oldenborg S, Poortmans P. Re-irradiation and hyperthermia in breast cancer. Clin Oncol (R Coll Radiol). 2018;30:73–84.
20. Overgaard M. Spontaneous radiation-induced rib fractures in breast cancer patients treated with post-mastectomy irradiation. A clinical radiobiological analysis of the influence of fraction size and dose-response relationships on late bone damage. Acta Oncol. 1988;27:117–22.
21. Harris SR. Differentiating the causes of spontaneous rib fracture after breast cancer. Clin Breast Cancer. 2016;16:431–6.
22. Harkenrider MM, Wilson MR, Dragun AE. Reirradiation as a component of the multidisciplinary management of locally recurrent breast cancer. Clin Breast Cancer. 2011;11:171–6.
23. Wagman R, Katz M. Re-irradiation of the chest wall for recurrent breast cancer. Int J Radiat Oncol Biol Phys. 2002;54:237–8.
24. Binkley MS, Hiniker SM, Chaudhuri A, et al. Dosimetric factors and toxicity in highly conformal thoracic Reirradiation. Int J Radiat Oncol Biol Phys. 2016;94:808–15.
25. Montagne L, Hannoun A, Hannoun-Levi JM. Second conservative treatment for second ipsilateral breast tumor event: a systematic review of the different re-irradiation techniques. Breast. 2020;49:274–80.
26. Strnad V, Major T, Polgar C, et al. ESTRO-ACROP guideline: interstitial multi-catheter breast brachytherapy as accelerated partial breast irradiation alone or as boost - GEC-ESTRO breast cancer working group practical recommendations. Radiother Oncol. 2018;128:411–20.

27. Polgar C, Van Limbergen E, Potter R, et al. Patient selection for accelerated partial-breast irradiation (APBI) after breast-conserving surgery: recommendations of the Groupe Europeen de Curietherapie-European Society for Therapeutic Radiology and Oncology (GEC-ESTRO) breast cancer working group based on clinical evidence (2009). Radiother Oncol. 2010;94:264–73.
28. Sumodhee S, Strnad V, Hannoun-Levi JM. Multicatheter interstitial brachytherapy for breast cancer. Cancer Radiother. 2018;22:341–4.
29. Major T, Gutierrez C, Guix B, et al. Recommendations from GEC ESTRO Breast Cancer Working Group (II): target definition and target delineation for accelerated or boost partial breast irradiation using multicatheter interstitial brachytherapy after breast conserving open cavity surgery. Radiother Oncol. 2016;118:199–204.
30. Strnad V, Ott OJ, Hildebrandt G, et al. 5-year results of accelerated partial breast irradiation using sole interstitial multicatheter brachytherapy versus whole-breast irradiation with boost after breast-conserving surgery for low-risk invasive and in-situ carcinoma of the female breast: a randomised, phase 3, non-inferiority trial. Lancet. 2016;387:229–38.

52 Re-irradiation Combined with Hyperthermia

Sabine Oldenborg and Jean-Michel Hannoun-Levi

52.1 Background

There is a strong biological and clinical rationale for the application of hyperthermia as an adjunct to RT and/or chemotherapy, as its biological working mechanism are complementary to, and synergistic with both treatment modalities. First of all, hyperthermia (temperatures up to 41–45 °C) alone induces protein denaturation leading to cytotoxicity. This process is limited and predominantly takes places in hypoxic, acidotic and nutrient-deprived cells, in parts of the tumour where chemotherapy and RT are less effective [1, 2]. In contrast, normal tissue is not affected as it is protected by perfusion through organised vascular structures. This effect of hyperthermia it too limited to be used as a single treatment modality. However, hyperthermia has also proven to interfere with the DNA repair mechanisms [3, 4], enhance perfusion and re-oxygenate tumour tissue [2, 5–11]. Thus, when combined, hyperthermia can enhance the effect of RT and/or chemotherapy. This enables using lower doses of these treatments to achieve the same cytotoxic effect, while potentially reducing the side effects of re-treatment.

S. Oldenborg (✉)
Amsterdam, The Netherlands

J.-M. Hannoun-Levi
Radiation Therapy Department, Antoine-Lacassagne Cancer Center, Nice, France
e-mail: jean-michel.hannoun-levi@nice.unicancer.fr

52.1.1 Indications

Indication for re-irradiation plus hyperthermia: combined DEGRO [12] and Dutch Institute for Healthcare Improvement guidelines [13]:

1. Adjuvant
   - Locoregional recurrence (LRR)/second primary tumour, in previously irradiated area in, the presence of one or more risk factors listed below.
   - If possible, it should be given after salvage ablation/resection ± systemic therapy.
   - Curative intention with M0 or M1 oligometastases.
   - Axilla recurrence without local recurrence: presence of recurrent LN, excised LN or elective regional re-irradiation.

   The following risk factors are considered when counselling the patient: LVI, grade 3, age ≤40 years, triple-negative tumour, tumour size >3 cm, resection margins (close vs. R1 vs. R2), multi-centricity, diffuse tumour growth, history of ≥1 previous LRR, nodal involvement, distant metastases, remaining options (and response to) systemic therapy. High-grade DCIS, if incompletely resected, could be considered as well.

© The Author(s), under exclusive license to Springer Nature Switzerland AG 2022
O. Kaidar-Person et al. (eds.), *Breast Cancer Radiation Therapy*,
https://doi.org/10.1007/978-3-030-91170-6_52

2. Palliative/Symptomatic (please see also the section about inoperable breast cancer).
   - Inoperable LRR in previously irradiated area (± neoadjuvant systemic therapy).
   - Individual determination of curative or palliative intention.

In case of areas of overlap with previous radiation fields ≤50%, consider re-irradiation without hyperthermia.

52.1.2 Clinical Results

Clinical evidence comes from the combined results of 5 phase III trials demonstrated a significant 26% increase of complete clinical response rates and a 20% improvement of the 3-year local control (LC) rate to 43%, when hyperthermia was added to re-irradiation for patients with non-resectable locoregional recurrent breast cancer in previously irradiated areas [14]. Toxicity was not affected by the addition of hyperthermia. A recent meta-analysis by Datta et al. [15] supported the combined results of the 5 phase III trials, published in 1996 [14]. In 16 studies (779 patients from single-arm studies and 83 patients from two-arm studies) complete response was improved from 38% for re-irradiation alone to 66.6% for re-irradiation with hyperthermia. A mean ERBT re-irradiation dose of 36.7 Gy (range 29.4–50.5 Gy) was delivered at an average dose per fraction of 2.7 Gy (2–4 Gy). Soon after the results of the 5 randomised trials became known, the Dutch National guidelines adopted the combination of re-irradiation plus hyperthermia as standard of care for recurrent breast cancer in previously irradiated area, preferably preceded by surgery [13]. As a consequence, over time, more patients with LRR breast cancer were treated with re-irradiation plus hyperthermia than anywhere else in the world. To get more insight in the long-term results of this treatment and variables that could affected these results, data form two Dutch hyperthermia institutes, using the same hyperthermia devices, were collected from 1988 up to 2006. In the one institute patients were irradiated with 4 Gy X 8 fractions, twice a week to a total dose of 32 Gy, using abutted photon and electron fields, whereas in the other institute patients were irradiated with 3 Gy X 12 fractions, four times a week to a total dose of 36 Gy, using either one single small electron field, or an alternating combination of electron fields. The clinical complete response rate was 30–58% for 583 treated patients depending on tumour size [16–18]. These rates were lower than expected based on the results from the prospective studies. The inclusion of small, single, easily treatable lesions in prospective studies shifted to including patients whose tumours even covered the whole chest wall, in daily practice. This was done to reduce local tumour burden as no other treatment options were left.

For the patient group that received re-irradiation plus hyperthermia as adjuvant treatment after surgery, the 5-year LC rate was 70%. The most important factor that affected duration of LC was time interval to recurrence. In the randomised trials late toxicity reports and analyses were hampered by different scoring criteria, lack of data and limited follow-up time. In the retrospective analysis, the fact that patient inclusion criteria in all daily practice allowed for treatment of patients with stigmata from previous treatment modalities still present, resulted in a higher cumulative ≥ grade 3 toxicity rate (33%) than expected. Whereas the difference in re-irradiation schedule and technique had no influence on tumour control, it did significant influence late toxicity. The 3-year risk on ≥grade 3 late toxicity doubled after 4 Gy X 8 fractions with large, abutted photon/electron fields [19, 20]. The re-irradiation schedule and inclusion criteria are now adapted to these results. What happens if re-irradiation plus hyperthermia precedes surgery is not known.

52.1.3 Techniques: Re-irradiation Plus Hyperthermia

For adjuvant intent, the core target volume encompasses the high-risk part of the mastectomy area (in case of ablatio for recurrence with indication for re-RT) or the area of re-resection (in case of resected chest wall recurrence after previous mastectomy). The CTV encompasses this area with a generous margin, generally 3 cm circular on the skin and the subcutis up to the underlying muscles or chest wall. If possible, margins can be individualised, among others based on patient's anatomy, tumour size and resection margins. For palliative/symptomatic intent, the CTV encompasses the chest wall area recurrent disease with a margin of ±3 cm circular on the skin and the subcutis up to the underlying muscles or chest wall. The dose schedule used in The Netherlands is 2 Gy X 23 fractions given, in 5 fractions a week to a total dose of 46 Gy, unless physical condition requires otherwise. Once a week this is combined with hyperthermia. The RT technique depends on the size and shape of the target volume. The dose constraints for OARs are determined individually, based on size and site of target volumes, and location and extend of areas overlapping with earlier RT. The DEGRO guidelines also recommend a total re-irradiation dose of 45–50 Gy, with the addition that cumulative doses should not exceed 100–110 Gy (2 Gy equivalent dose), time interval between primary radiation and re-irradiation should be >1 year, and severe radiogenic stigmata, caused by late radiation effects from previous RT, should be absent.

International quality assurance guidelines exist for both the application of hyperthermia as well as for the technical requirements for heating devices [21, 22]. Local hyperthermia, also referred to as superficial hyperthermia, is applied to superficially located target volumes and therefore commonly used to treat LRR of breast cancer. Although different devices exist Contact Flexible Microstrip Applicators (CFMA), connected to a 434 MHz generator are frequently used. For maximum effect on tumour tissue and limited effect on normal tissue, hyperthermia treatments are given, preferably, within 1 h before or after re-irradiation. This is done once a week, for the duration of the re-irradiation schedule. To be able to monitor temperatures during treatment, thermometry is to be placed on the skin at representative locations across the treatment volume. Special attention should be paid to locations with a high risk of hot or cold spots, for example, scars and shallow depth bones. For target volumes extending >1 cm deep invasive thermometry is performed using closed end Teflon catheters. After thermometry is installed, the CFMA is placed in such a way that its intrinsic water bolus matches with the irregular contours of the skin surface, to provide efficient coupling of the electromagnetic energy into the patient (Fig. 52.1). The minimal goal of the treatment is to reach a minimum of ≥41 °C for 60 mins throughout the re-irradiation volume, while skin temperatures of 43–44 °C for 60 mins must be avoided, due to the risk of blistering. With the tools currently available (water-bolus temperature, power, isolation material) it remains quite challenging to reduce local hotspots and/or pain while retaining therapeutic temperatures in the gross of the re-irradiation volume.

52.1.4 Specific Clinical Situations and Contraindications

Though there are temperature constraints to avoid local overheating, it appears that temperature ranges and time intervals for blistering to occur, differ per patient, and are not predictable. Probably, they depend on pre-treatment individual patient characteristics like skin sensitivity, stigmata from previous RT, chemotherapy and / or surgery. These may include extensiveness of previous surgery, scar dehiscence, postoperative infection, age, smoking history, diabetics, interval from last treatment to current re-irradiation plus hyperthermia. Skin flaps and scars are not a contraindication for hyperthermia, but as physiology is disturbed in these areas, they require additional monitoring [23–25]. In case of a seroma pocket in the treatment volume invasive thermometry inside as well as along the wall of the cavity is necessary, as electromagnetic heating of the fluid can cause extensive temperature rises. Catheters need to be removed after every treatment, and replaced before the start of a new treatment, because of infection risk (Table 52.1).

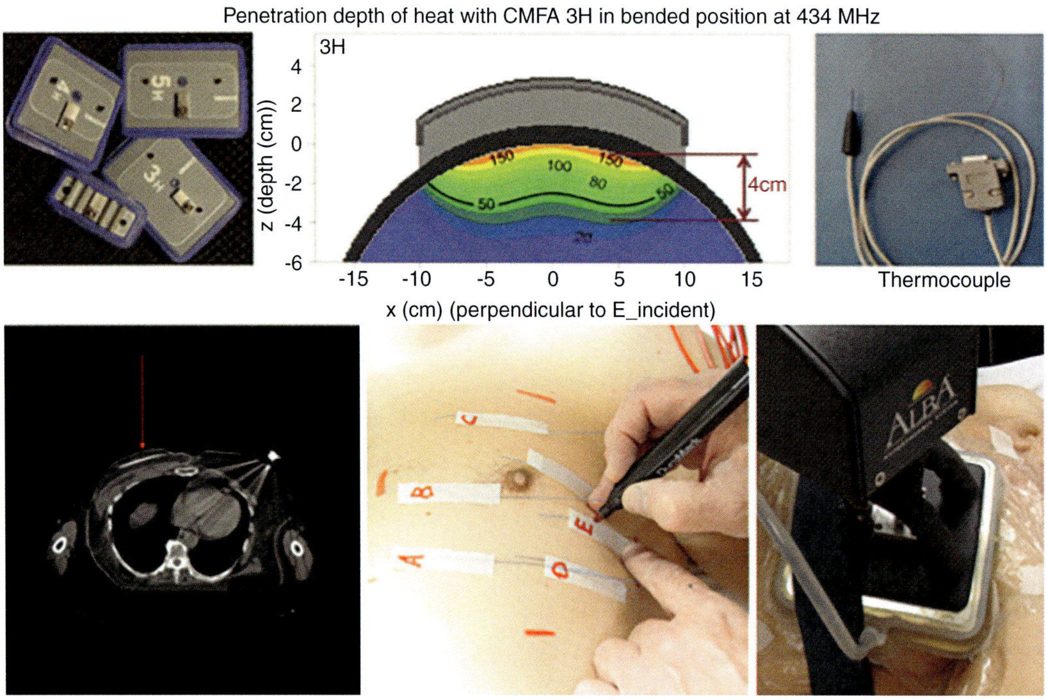

Fig. 52.1 Materials and Methods for treatments set-up (With courtesy of P.J. Zum Vörde Sive Vording, P. Pavoni, MD ALBA Medical System)

Table 52.1 Contraindications and relative contraindications for hyperthermia

Contraindications	Relative contraindications
1. Pregnancy 2. Pacemaker/ICD in the hyperthermia field, as the EM electromagnetic field might cause disturbances. The cardiologist should be consulted about the PM/ICD-dependency of the patient, similar to RT without hyperthermia. If non-dependent, the PM/ICD can be switched off before and re-initiated after treatment. If the patient is PM/ ICD-dependent, treatment should take place in presence of a cardiologist/pacemaker technician and crash trolley	1. Silicone implants in the hyperthermia field. The risk of leakage, hotspots, or deformations on the long-term are not clear. 2. Saline-filled implants in the hyperthermia field. The risk of leakage, hotspots, or deformations on the long-term are not clear. 3. Tissue expanders filled with saline in the hyperthermia field. If the patient and surgeon are prepared to empty the tissue expander, the treatment could take place. 4. Surgical stents and/or clips in the hyperthermia field might cause hotspots and overheating. It depends on their size, direction and whether treatment can take on the heating device place or not. 5. Other protheses or implants in the hyperthermia field. **For all prosthesis, it is dependent on location and depth.

52.1.5 Improvements

RT and hyperthermia characteristics may contribute to long-term tumour control and side-effects. A comparative study compared two different reRT regimens: either 4 Gy X 8 fractions, two times per week (once with hyperthermia) based on abutting photon-electron fields or 3 Gy X 12 fractions, four times per week (twice with hyperthermia) based on single or multiple electron fields. Hyperthermia was delivered within 1 h after RT using the same system to heat the tumour area to 41–43 °C. While

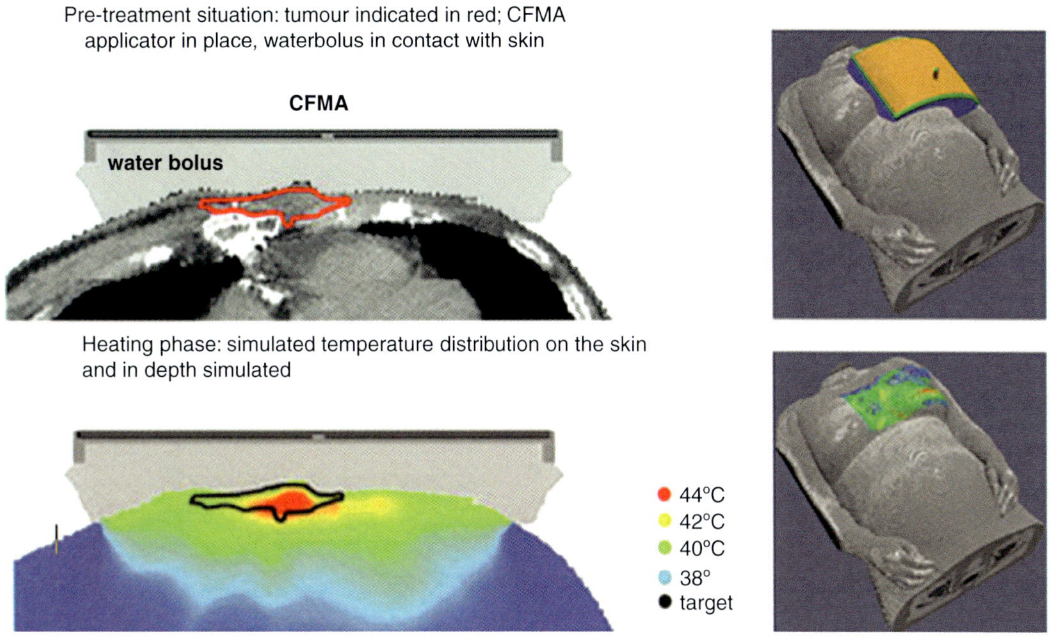

Fig. 52.2 Preliminary example of HT treatment planning system: PLAN2HEAT (with courtesy of P. Pavoni, MD ALBA Medical System)

the 5-year infield local control rates were similar, the 5-year overall survival rates were 13% lower and 5-year ≥ grade 3 toxicity was more than twice after the 4 Gy X 8 fractions schedule using limited-sized electron fields.

Apart from RT techniques, which are continuously improving, hyperthermia devices are being adjusted and updated too. For instance, multi-element systems are being built to allow for detailed 2D steering. In this way, heat can be steered away from unwanted hot-spots, while maintaining high temperatures in the target area. Also, hyperthermia treatment planning systems are being developed, using the dielectric properties of different tissues in combination with perfusion parameters. In the future this will enable predicting hotspot on forehand and help to decide how to obtain the most homogenous heating pattern. Invasive thermometry will then no longer be necessary. In addition, this system will be developed to allow for real-time adaptive planning for real time correction (Fig. 52.2).

In addition to a handful high quality hyperthermia institutes throughout Europa, Asia, and the US, there are a lot of private clinics offering "alternative hyperthermia" at high costs (both financially and ethically). These private practices do not comply to the international clinical and technical guidelines developed by the European Society for Hyperthermic Oncology (ESHO). It would, therefore, be extremely useful for patients, and oncology professionals to be able to gain access to an interactive map, with only HT clinics, working according to the ESHO guidelines. Both patient and professionals could then be able to locate the nearest reliable hyperthermia centre and obtain the right information and advice. Unfortunately, such a map does currently not exist, nor do audits. Members of the ESHO are working on displaying an updated list of centres working together on clinical studies on their website, as a surrogate option. An alternative might be offered here, by contacting institutes that participated in studies listed in the reference list.

52.2 Summary

Hyperthermia added to reirradiation improves clinical outcomes. Though not intrinsically toxic the combination of hyperthermia with reirradiation can lead to an accumulation of $\geq$ grade 3 toxicities, especially in patients presenting with stigmata from prior treatments. Therefore, a careful selection of patients, techniques and doses is needed, preferably based on individual situations. Biological research will hopefully aid this process in the future. However, clinical data should continuously be updated to reflect upon current and new protocols. While hyperthermia has proven its value in pre-clinical and clinical studies, it is still not widely used.

References

1. Horsman MR, Overgaard J. Hyperthermia: a potent enhancer of radiotherapy. Clin Oncol (R Coll Radiol). 2007;19:418–26.
2. Kampinga HH. Cell biological effects of hyperthermia alone or combined with radiation or drugs: a short introduction to newcomers in the field. Int J Hyperth. 2006;22:191–6.
3. Kampinga HH, Dynlacht JR, Dikomey E. Mechanism of radiosensitization by hyperthermia (> or = 43 degrees C) as derived from studies with DNA repair defective mutant cell lines. Int J Hyperth. 2004;20:131–9.
4. Krawczyk PM, Eppink B, Essers J, et al. Mild hyperthermia inhibits homologous recombination, induces BRCA2 degradation, and sensitizes cancer cells to poly (ADP-ribose) polymerase-1 inhibition. Proc Natl Acad Sci U S A. 2011;108:9851–6.
5. Jones EL, Prosnitz LR, Dewhirst MW, et al. Thermochemoradiotherapy improves oxygenation in locally advanced breast cancer. Clin Cancer Res. 2004;10:4287–93.
6. Overgaard J. The heat is (still) on--the past and future of hyperthermic radiation oncology. Radiother Oncol. 2013;109:185–7.
7. Sun X, Xing L, Ling CC, et al. The effect of mild temperature hyperthermia on tumour hypoxia and blood perfusion: relevance for radiotherapy, vascular targeting and imaging. Int J Hyperth. 2010;26:224–31.
8. Vujaskovic Z, Song CW. Physiological mechanisms underlying heat-induced radiosensitization. Int J Hyperth. 2004;20:163–74.
9. Winslow TB, Eranki A, Ullas S, et al. A pilot study of the effects of mild systemic heating on human head and neck tumour xenografts: analysis of tumour perfusion, interstitial fluid pressure, hypoxia and efficacy of radiation therapy. Int J Hyperth. 2015;31:693–701.
10. Hildebrandt B, Wust P. Interactions between hyperthermia and cytotoxic drugs. Cancer Treat Res. 2007;134:185–93.
11. Urano M, Kuroda M, Nishimura Y. For the clinical application of thermochemotherapy given at mild temperatures. Int J Hyperth. 1999;15:79–107.
12. Harms W, Budach W, Dunst J, et al. Breast cancer expert panel of the German Society of Radiation Oncology (DEGRO). Radiother Oncol. 2013;109:185–7.
13. Rutgers EJ, Nortier JW, Tuut MK, et al. Dutch Institute for Healthcare Improvement guideline, "treatment of breast cancer". Ned Tijdschr Geneeskd. 2002;146:2144–51.
14. Vernon CC, Hand JW, Field SB, et al. Radiotherapy with or without hyperthermia in the treatment of superficial localized breast cancer: results from five randomized controlled trials. International collaborative hyperthermia group. Int J Radiat Oncol Biol Phys. 1996;35(4):731–44.
15. Datta NR, Puric E, Klingbiel D, et al. Hyperthermia and radiation therapy in Locoregional recurrent breast cancers: a systematic review and meta-analysis. Int J Radiat Oncol Biol Phys. 2016;94(5):1073–87.
16. Oldenborg S, Rasch CRN, van Os R, et al. Reirradiation + hyperthermia for recurrent breast cancer en cuirasse. Strahlenther Onkol. 2018;3:206–14.
17. Oldenborg S, Griesdoorn V, van Os R, et al. Reirradiation and hyperthermia for irresectable locoregional recurrent breast cancer in previously irradiated area: size matters. Radiother Oncol. 2015;117(2):223–8.
18. Kaidar-Person O, Oldenborg S, Poortmans P. Re-irradiation and hyperthermia in breast cancer. Clin Oncol (R Coll Radiol). 2018;30:73–84. https://doi.org/10.1016/j.clon.2017.11.004.
19. Oldenborg S, Valk C, van Os R, et al. Rib fractures after reirradiation plus hyperthermia for recurrent breast cancer: predictive factors. Strahlenther Onkol. 2016;192:240–7.
20. Oldenborg S, van Os R, Oei SB, et al. Impact of technique and schedule of reirradiation plus hyperthermia on outcome after surgery for patients with recurrent breast cancer. Cancers. 2019;11(6):782.
21. Trefna HD, Crezee H, Schmidt M, et al. Quality assurance guidelines for superficial hyperthermia clinical trials: I. clinical requirements. Int J Hyperth. 2017;33(4):471–82.
22. Trefna HD, Crezee H, Schmidt M, et al. Quality assurance guidelines for superficial hyperthermia clinical trials II. Technical requirements for heating devices. Strahlenther Onkol. 2017;193:351–66.
23. Linthorst M, van Geel AN, Baaijens M, et al. Re-irradiation and hyperthermia after surgery for recurrent breast cancer. Radiother Oncol. 2013;109:188–93.

24. Linthorst M, Baaijens M, Wiggenraad R, et al. Local control rate after the combination of re-irradiation and hyperthermia for unresectable recurrent breast cancer: results in 248 patients. Radiother Oncol. 2015;117:217–22.
25. Linthorst M, van Rhoon GC, van Geel AN, et al. The tolerance of reirradiation and hyperthermia in breast cancer patients with reconstructions. Int J Hyperth. 2012;28:267–77.

53 Concomitant Radiation and Systemic Therapy in the Adjuvant and Metastatic Setting

Ivica Ratosa and Luca Visani

53.1 Concomitant Radiation and Chemotherapy (Fluoropyrimidines, Anthracyclines, Taxanes)

53.1.1 Background

Standard of care, when combining adjuvant treatment following surgery for early breast cancer, is postoperative chemotherapy followed by RT. Concomitant administration of chemotherapy and RT is a point of concern both for the adjuvant and advanced disease setting and it remains controversial. Consequently, concurrent administration is commonly avoided in clinical practice, as recommended by several international guidelines.

I. Ratosa (✉)
Division of Radiotherapy, Institute of Oncology Ljubljana, Ljubljana, Slovenia

Faculty of Medicine, University of Ljubljana, Ljubljana, Slovenia
e-mail: iratosa@onko-i.si

L. Visani
Radiotherapy Unit, Oncology Department Azienda Ospedaliero-Universitaria Careggi, University of Florence, Florence, Italy
e-mail: luca.visani@unifi.it

53.1.1.1 Fluoropyrimidines

Early breast cancer

- Fluoropyrimidines are a class of antimetabolites anticancer drugs represented by floxuridine and fluorouracil (5-FU), and capecitabine [1].
- Adjuvant capecitabine for 6–8 triweekly cycles currently represents the recommended adjuvant regimen in patients with triple-negative breast cancer whose tumours did not achieve a pathologic full response after primary systemic therapy, having demonstrated a significant advantage in terms of both DFS and OS in the phase III CREATE-X trial [2].
- Anyway, a major point of discussion is represented by the safety of the concomitant administration of capecitabine together with RT, since in the study the two treatments were given sequentially to avoid increased toxicity [2], and most international guidelines recommend giving adjuvant capecitabine after the completion of RT [3].
- In a recently published retrospective matched analysis, conducted on 64 patients with residual triple-negative breast cancer after preoperative chemotherapy with anthracyclines and taxanes, including 16 patients who received capecitabine-RT and 48 who received RT alone, radiation dermatitis was not significantly different between the two groups, but the capecitabine-RT group was more likely to

© The Author(s), under exclusive license to Springer Nature Switzerland AG 2022
O. Kaidar-Person et al. (eds.), *Breast Cancer Radiation Therapy*,
https://doi.org/10.1007/978-3-030-91170-6_53

require modifications in the RT schedule, including RT treatment breaks [4].
- In another matched cohort retrospective study, combined capecitabine/RT was associated with worse OS in clinical and matched controls, after adjusting for clinical size, pathological stage, and lymphovascular invasion [5].

Locoregionally advanced and metastatic breast cancer
- Small phase I/II studies have shown some benefit in pCR rate and local control with 5-FU-based chemoradiation therapy in locally advanced breast cancer without significant additional toxicity [6, 7].
- In a single-centre phase II prospective trial, the capecitabine-RT combination showed a 53.9% rate of at least grade 3 non-dermatitis toxicity (gastrointestinal and hand–foot skin reaction) and a 50% rate of grade 3 or higher treatment-related skin toxicity in patients with inoperable disease after chemotherapy, residual nodal disease after definitive surgery, unresectable chest wall or nodal recurrence after a prior mastectomy or oligometastatic disease. After a median follow-up of 12.9 months, 19 out of 32 (73%) included patients had partial or complete response [8]. Compared to non–triple-negative breast cancer phenotypes, patients with triple-negative phenotype had poorer median OS (22.8 vs 5.1 months; $p = 0.001$) and 1-year locoregional recurrence-free survival (63% vs 20%; $p = 0.007$) [8].

53.1.1.2 Anthracyclines

Early breast cancer
- Concurrent chemoradiation therapy after breast surgery was investigated in limited series and remains controversial, because of concerns of toxicity with anthracyclines and RT [9].
- A retrospective single institution cohort study conducted on 400 patients treated with concomitant adjuvant chemoradiation with either anthracyclines or CMF, after mastectomy or BCS, demonstrated that anthracyclines and concurrent RT reduced breast cancer relapse rate, and significantly improved local relapse-free survival (LRFS), event-free survival, and OS in patients receiving more than one cycle, although leading to increased haematologic and non-haematologic toxicities [9].
- Sixty-seven patients treated with BCS followed by 3DCRT and concomitant anthracyclines-based regimens were compared in terms of compliance and acute toxicity with the same number of patients irradiated sequentially. Acute grade ≥2 skin toxicity was significantly higher in the concomitant group compared to the sequential group, although there were no differences regarding the incidence of grade 3 desquamation. Mean RT duration was longer in the concomitant group, and haematological toxicity represented the main cause of treatment discontinuation, with higher rate of grade 3–4 neutropenia in the concomitant group [10].
- In a study evaluating long-term cardiovascular toxicity of 600 breast cancer patients who received concomitant chemoradiation, the risk of cardiovascular events was further increased in case of concomitant left-sided irradiation and doxorubicin ≥250 mg/m^2 [11].
- The SECRAB trial was a phase 3 randomised controlled trial, comparing concomitant to sequential chemotherapy RT combination in 2297 patients with early breast cancer. Most patients (54.2%) received cyclophosphamide methotrexate and 5-FU (CMF), followed by anthracycline chemotherapy (45.3%). Three-quarters (75.5%) of patients received hypofractionated RT (40–42.5 Gy in 15–16 fractions). After a median follow-up of 10.7 years, the 10-year local recurrence rates were 4.6% and 7.1% (hazard ratio 0.62; $p = 0.012$), respectively, and the greatest benefit was seen for the anthracycline-CMF group. There was no significant difference in the median OS or DFS. With respect to toxicity, patients in the concomitant arm developed higher rates of moderate/severe acute skin reaction (24% versus 15%; $p < 0.0001$) and telangiectasia (3% versus 1.7%; $p = 0.03$), compared to sequential arm [12].

Locoregionally advanced and metastatic breast cancer

- The anthracyclines-RT combination was mainly explored before the early 1990s. Gastrointestinal toxicity was moderate, but bone marrow depression was marked in all cases in a study conducted on 107 advanced breast cancer patients treated with epirubicin–ifosfamide and concomitant RT [13].

53.1.1.3 Taxanes

Early breast cancer

- Most studies that explored the feasibility of the combination of taxanes and RT after surgery or in locally advanced disease were published in the 2000–2006 period, following the introduction of these drugs in the adjuvant treatment (Table 53.1) [14–22].
- Although several experiences have shown mild skin events, taxane-based concurrent chemoradiation demonstrated to lead to significant lung toxicity, for example, pneumonitis, especially using paclitaxel given at weekly and every-three-weeks at doses of 60 mg/m^2 and 175 mg/m^2, respectively [23].
- In the routine clinical practice, postoperative RT is typically delivered with a target interval of 3–4 weeks after taxane therapy, and this sequential administration does not appear to result in increased pulmonary toxicity.

Locoregionally advanced and metastatic breast cancer

- In a monocentric study conducted on 51 patients, concurrent RT delivered with 60 Gy in 2 Gy/fraction together with weekly paclitaxel demonstrated an acceptable toxicity profile. Another similar study with patients treated for locoregional recurrence, either inoperable or resected, showed that concur-

Table 53.1 Clinical studies on the combination of taxanes and radiation therapy after surgery or in locally advanced disease

Study	Patients (n)	Paclitaxel		RT dosing (Gy)	Toxicity (%)
		Dose (mg/m^2)	Schedule		
Elmongy et al., 1999 [14]	32	175–225	Every 3 weeks	50.4–63	G3 skin toxicity (28)
Bellon et al., 2000 [15]	8	20–35	Every 3 weeks	46.80–50.40 plus boost	Acute skin toxicity requiring Delay exceeding 5 days (35)
	9	135–175	Every 3 weeks		
Taghian et al., 2001 [16]	7	175	Every 3 weeks	40–46 plus 6–20 boost	Pneumonitis (14)
	14	60–100	Weekly		
Hanna et al., 2002 [17]	20	175	Every 3 weeks	BCS: 45 plus 16 boost Mastectomy: 50.4 plus 10 boost	G3 skin toxicity (35) Pneumonitis (25)
Formenti et al., 2003 [18]	44	30	Twice weekly	45–46	G3 skin toxicity (10)
Kao et al., 2005 [19]	16	20–30	Every 2 weeks	60	G3 or higher skin toxicity (24)
	17	80	Weekly		
Burstein et al., 2006 [20]	16	60	Weekly	Mastectomy: 45 plus 4–10 boost BCS: 45 plus 10–16 boost	Pneumonitis (19)
	24	135–175	Every 3 weeks		
Chakravarthy et al., 2006 [21]	38	30	Twice weekly	45 plus 14 boost	Skin toxicity (3)
Chen et al., 2010 [22]	44	175	Every 3 weeks	39.60 plus 14 boost	G3 skin toxicity (5)

Abbreviations: *RT* radiation therapy, *BCS* breast conserving surgery, *G* grade rent taxanes-RT, particularly with paclitaxel, showed radiation dermatitis in the treatment field as the most prominent toxicity, and also mucositis with dysphagia occurred frequently. No patients had grade 3 radiation pneumonitis, and only 2% experienced grade 2 radiation pneumonitis [24, 25].

- Concomitant taxanes and RT outcomes were explored only anecdotally in case reports in the setting of metastatic disease, showing acceptable toxicity profile [26].
- In clinical practice, a short time interval before and after taxane-based chemotherapy administration is proposed for the metastasis-directed RT delivery (2–3 weeks, depending on the treated volume, total RT dose, and fractionation).

53.2 Concomitant Radiation Therapy and New Drugs

Combining RT with new systemic agents can be challenging in everyday clinical practice, as data on the treatment combination from the key randomised controlled trials, that lead to the new drug approval, are often lacking. In the era of the precision medicine, the concurrent combination of the new (targeted) drugs and RT will also require adaptation of the drug to the specific tumour biology, alongside with the redefining of the total radiation dose prescription, fractionation, treated volume, and dose to the organs at risk. Technical innovations in radiation oncology, allowing to deliver extremely high dose per fraction with a high precision to a small anatomical volume, might help to facilitate the improvement of the therapeutic index in the future.

53.2.1 Cyclin-Dependent Kinase 4/6 Inhibitors

Cyclin-dependent kinase 4/6 inhibitors (palbociclib, ribociclib, and abemaciclib have a median half-life of 29, 32, and 55 h, respectively) represent the standard of care for ER-positive HER2-negative advanced breast cancer [27]. Selective inhibition of cyclin-dependent kinase 4/6 affects the cell cycle by interfering with the transition from the G1 phase of the cell cycle to the S phase, reducing retinoblastoma protein phosphorylation and inducing G1 cell-cycle arrest [28]. Irradiation of the normal cells results in delayed progression through the G1, S, and G2 phases of the cell cycle [29]. Cells are most resistant to irradiation in G0, in early G1, and in the late S phase of the cycle. Conversely, cells are most radiosensitive in late G1, G2 and throughout the M phase of the cell cycle [30]. Concomitant cyclin-dependent kinase 4/6 inhibitor and RT could result in a higher percentage of G2/M cells, higher proportion of apoptotic cells, and lower proportion of S2 cells [31].

- There is minimal available information addressing the efficacy and toxicity of concurrent RT and cyclin-dependent kinase 4/6 inhibitors. Limited data from retrospective studies (Table 53.2) suggest that concurrent administration of cyclin-dependent kinase 4/6 inhibitors with RT is well tolerated, with a modest increase of grade 3 or higher AEs, haematological toxicity being the most common. However, grade 2–3 oesophagitis (dysphagia, odynophagia) and radiodermatitis were reported with concomitant administration of palbociclib and RT [32–34], as well as lung toxicity and grade 3 enterocolitis [35–37]. Enhanced toxicity was mainly reported with 2-dimensional RT and with larger target volumes. In selected cases with smaller metastases-directed RT volumes, RT may be carried out with low toxicity, without stopping systemic treatment such as cyclin-dependent kinase 4/6 inhibitors (depending on the vicinity of the organs at risk, especially gastrointestinal organs) [32, 38–44].
- In clinical practice, RT is typically delivered during the „off cycle week “(palbociclib and ribociclib), or the cyclin-dependent kinase 4/6 inhibitors are withheld 1–3 days before and 1–3 days after treatment.

Table 53.2 Relevant retrospective studies of concurrent radiation therapy and cyclin-dependent kinase 4/6 inhibitors

Study	Type of CDK4/6I (%)	RT site (%)	RT techniques	Median total RT dose (range)	Patients (treated sites)	Timing with RT (%)	≥G3 toxicity (%)
Hans et al, 2018 [38]	Palbociclib (100)	Bone (80)	3DCRT, SBRT	20 Gy and 60 Gy	5 (5)	Concomitant (100)	Neutropenia (40) Anaemia (20) Thrombocytopenia (40)
Meattini et al, 2018 [39]	Ribociclib (100)	Bone (100)	VMAT, 3DCRT	20 Gy (20–30)	5 (5)	Concomitant (100)	Neutropenia (20) Vomiting and diarrhoea (20)
Figura et al, 2019 [40]	Palbociclib (67) Abemaciclib (33)	Brain (100)	SRS	21 Gy (18–30)	15 (42)	RT before or concomitant (43)	None ≥G3 toxicity Radio-necrosis (2 lesions)
Ippolito et al, 2019 [41]	Palbociclib (79.2) Ribociclib (20.8)	Bone (91.6)	VMAT, IMRT, 3DCRT	30 Gy (8–36)	16 (21)	Concomitant (>80)	Neutropenia (31.3)
Chowdhary et al, 2019 [42]	Palbociclib (100)	Bone (78.2)	3DCRT, SBRT, IMRT	30 Gy (18–37.5)	16 (16)	RT before, after or concomitant (31.3)	No ≥G3 toxicity
Beddok et al, 2020 [32]	Palbociclib (100)	Bone (75)	HT, VMAT, SRS	Schedules: 20 Gy/5 fr 30 Gy/10 fr 8 Gy/1 fr 18 Gy/1 fr	30 (35)	Concomitant (100)	Neutropenia (3)
Guerini et al, 2020 [43]	Palbociclib (50) Ribociclib (33.3) Abemaciclib (16.7)	Bone (100)	3DCRT, HT, VMAT	Schedules: 20 Gy/5 fr 30 Gy/10 fr 8 Gy/1 fr 30 Gy/3 fr	18 (32)	Concomitant (100)	Ileitis (5) Neutropenia within 3 months after RT (61)
Ratosa et al, 2020 [44]	Palbociclib (65.2) Ribociclib (32.6) Abemaciclib (2.2)	Bone (80.7)	3DCRT, SBRT, HT	20 (8–63) Gy	46 (62)	RT before, after or concomitant (34.8)	Before the start of RT (6.5) During RT (4.3) 2-weeks after RT completion (15.2) 6-weeks after RT completion (23.9)

Abbreviations: *CDK4/6I* cyclin-dependent kinase 4/6 inhibitor, *RT* radiation therapy, *G3* grade 3, *3DCRT* 3-dimensional conformal radiation therapy. *SBRT* stereotactic body radiation therapy, *VMAT* volumetric modulated arc therapy, *IMRT* intensity modulated radiation therapy, *SRS* stereotactic radiosurgery, *HT* helical tomotherapy

53.3 Anti-HER2 Therapy

53.3.1 Monoclonal Antibodies (Pertuzumab, Trastuzumab)

Pertuzumab and trastuzumab are humanised recombinant monoclonal antibodies used in a conjunction with chemotherapy for the (neo) adjuvant treatment of early [45, 46] and advanced [27] breast cancer with HER2-overexpression. Trastuzumab, with or without pertuzumab is also used in one-year long maintenance therapy in the adjuvant setting for HER2-positive breast cancer [47]. Due to small to modest risk of development of congestive heart failure or decline in ejection fraction (LVEF), patients, receiving trastuzumab are undergoing routine heart monitoring during treatment.

Early breast cancer

- Trastuzumab in combination with adjuvant breast RT does not appear to increase any heart or skin toxicity [48]. Use of modern CT-based treatment planning and heart-sparing RT techniques may further lower the risk.

Advanced breast cancer

- Very limited data originating from small retrospective studies do not show increased toxicity in the setting of palliative metastasis-directed RT, SBRT, SRT or whole brain irradiation and concomitant use of trastuzumab or pertuzumab [49, 50].

53.3.2 Dual Tyrosine Kinase Inhibitor (Lapatinib)

- Lapatinib, a small molecule with a median half-life of 24 h, acts as a reversible inhibitor of HER1 and HER2, by acting on the catalytic site of the tyrosine kinase domain in the intracellular domain of the HER1/2 [49] and it is used as a treatment option in patients with metastatic HER2-overexpressing breast cancer [27]. Preclinical data suggest that lapatinib can potentiate radiation-induced cell death by increasing radiation-induced apoptosis and senescence when used in a combination with RT [51].
- Limited data from small retrospective studies are supporting the efficacy and safety of the administration of concurrent lapatinib and SRS. Two studies demonstrated improved local control rates post-SRS and no increased risk of radio-necrosis (1–1.3% vs. 3.5–6.3%) for patients undergoing concurrent administration of lapatinib and SRS compared to patients undergoing SRS-alone [52, 53].

53.3.3 Trastuzumab Emtansine (T-DM1)

The antibody-drug conjugate T-DM1 uses the trastuzumab antibody to deliver a cytotoxic agent mysantine (DM1) to HER2 expressing tumours. Mysantine induces apoptosis by interfering with microtubules in a dividing cell [54]. Trastuzumab emtansine (T-DM1) improves DFS in the post-primary systemic therapy setting for patients with residual invasive HER2-positive disease [55]. It is also a preferred choice after first line trastuzumab-based therapy in HER2-positive advanced breast cancer, providing OS benefit for those patients [27].

Early breast cancer

- Following the *KATHERINE* trial, postoperative RT was delivered concurrently with T-DM1 in the post-primary systemic therapy setting [55].
- T-DM1 seem to be safely administered together with RT. For patients receiving trastuzumab only vs T-DM1 in the adjuvant setting, reported grade 2 (9.9% vs 10.8%) and grade 3 (1.0 vs 1.4%) radiation skin injuries were comparable. Radiation pneumonitis (of any grade) occurred in 0.7% patients receiving trastuzumab compared to 1.5% patients in the trastuzumab emtansine group [55].

Advanced breast cancer

- Prospectively collected data on T-DM1 and palliative RT are lacking. In the phase 3 *EMILIA* trial, patients who received RT within 14 days of randomisation were excluded [56].
- The concurrent or sequential administration of T-DM1 and SRS is feasible. However, AEs in patients treated with T-DM1 and concomitant or sequential RT (interruption of T-DM1 for ≥1 week before SRS) included higher rates of clinically significant radio-necrosis (50–57% vs 28.6%), alopecia (25% vs 14.3%) and brain oedema (25% vs 28.6%). Cases were reported as developing intracranial haemorrhage with parenchymal brain metastases while on T-DM1, although the relationship with RT is not well established and seems not to be dependent on the timing of the drug administration [57–59].
- Small series of patients with metastatic HER2 disease treated for bone metastases concurrently with T-DM1 and palliative RT showed no increased toxicity [60].

53.4 Poly-Adenosine Diphosphate Ribose Polymerase Inhibitors

53.4.1 Olaparib, Talazoparib

Poly-adenosine diphosphate ribose polymerase (PARP) inhibitors such as olaparib and talazoparib are a preferred treatment option for patients with triple-negative breast cancer and known germline BRCA mutations [27]. Olaparib and talazoparib interfere with posttranslational modification of proteins involved in many cellular mechanisms, particularly DNA repair. As such, these drugs are potential radiosensitizers, based on their ability to enhance unrepaired DNA damage [61].

- The combination with palliative RT may lead to an increased rate of AEs, especially haematological, which could be amplified following pelvic or large-field spinal RT [62].
- In a single institutional dose-escalating phase I study, evaluating the combination of concurrent olaparib and 50 Gy in 25 fractions of RT delivered to the breast or chest wall in patients with locoregionally advanced or metastatic triple-negative breast cancer, the authors reported grade 3 radiodermatitis in 8.3% and grade 3 or higher lymphocytopenia in 45.8% patients [63]. In another phase I study of concomitant veliparib and postmastectomy RT, the absolute rate of any grade 3 AEs was 10% at 1-year and 46.7% at 3-year. Most common AEs were skin fibrosis, induration, and lymphoedema [64].

53.5 The Phosphatidylinositol 3-Kinase-AKT (PI3K) and Mammalian Target of Rapamycin (mTOR) Pathway

53.5.1 Everolimus

Everolimus (in combination with exemestane) is used as a treatment alternative beyond first line in selected patients with advanced ER-positive/HER2-negative breast cancer [27]. Everolimus belongs to a class of drugs that inhibit *mammalian target of rapamycin* (mTOR) and has been shown to be a potent radiosensitizer drug [65].

- Everolimus, an oral drug, is in general well tolerated, but its usage can be complicated with a serious AE. The combination of everolimus and RT may enhance AEs, especially lung toxicities, including grade 3 or 4 interstitial pneumonitis and lung fibrosis [66, 67].
- Cases of an inflammatory reaction within a previously irradiated volume occurring months after RT (a radiation recall phenomenon), resulting in enhanced radiodermatitis or colitis were also reported with everolimus administration [68, 69].

53.5.2 Alpelisib

Alpelisib, with a half-life of 7.6 hours, is an oral inhibitor of phosphatidylinositol-4,5-bisphosphate 3-kinase, catalytic subunit alpha (*PIK3CA*). It is approved as a treatment option in a combination with fulvestrant for patients with ER-positive/HER2-negative *PIK3CA*-mutated breast cancer, showing a progression-free survival benefit [27, 70].

- Alpelisib monotherapy is correlated with increased toxicity profile. Typical AEs include hyperglycemia, maculopapular rash, fatigue, and gastrointestinal symptoms (i.e. nausea, mucositis, and diarrhoea), which can lead to dose reductions, interruptions, or discontinuation in most patients (≈70%) receiving the drug [27, 70]. These AEs are reversible and manageable with appropriate monitoring and supportive medications [71].
- Data on efficacy and safety of alpelisib and RT combination are lacking. Preliminary data suggest that concomitant use of alpelisib an RT may enhance toxicity profile [72]. Highly conformal RT techniques are recommended for all patients undergoing metastasis-directed palliative RT to minimise radiation exposure of organs-at-risk. Until more data become

available, stopping the drug few days before and after RT is believed to be reasonable to avoid enhanced toxicity, taking into consideration the drug half-life.

53.5.3 Eribulin Mesylate

Eribulin (eribulin mesylate), an inhibitor of cell's microtubule dynamics, is a potential treatment option for selected pretreated group of patients with metastatic breast cancer [27]. Overall, grade ≥ 3 AEs include neutropenia (54.2%), alopecia (34.6%), leukopenia (31.4%), global peripheral neuropathy (27.4%), nausea (22.2%), and anaemia (19.1%) [73].

- Extremely limited data exist evaluating toxicity profile of an eribulin and RT combination. However, few small studies reported an acceptable toxicity profile. The most common AEs grade 3 or 4 being neutropenia (22.4–53.1%) and anaemia (35.4%) [74, 75].

53.5.4 Concomitant Radiation Therapy and Immunotherapy

The combination of immune checkpoint inhibitors (anti-programmed cell death protein 1, PD-1; pembrolizumab, nivolumab or anti-programmed death ligand, PD-L1; atezolizumab, avelumab, durvalumab) and RT is an emerging treatment strategy in patients with early or advanced breast cancer. A high level of evidence is now available, showing that RT could act as a as a potent immune response modulator and can trigger a systemic response in specific situations of a highly immunogenic tumour, especially when combined with systemic immunomodulatory agent [76]. Appropriate patient selection, the ideal dosing and fractionation, the optimal sequencing (concurrent, sequential) are still a matter of uncertainty, in part because of a lack of mechanistic insights [76]. Some of the directions, that will foster the safety and efficacy of the radioimmunotherapy combinations in the near future would include revisiting doses and fractionation schedules (including dose de-escalation and non-ablative personalised doses), reducing treatment volumes, sparing organs at risk such as draining lymph nodes and the intestine (immune cells, gut microbiome optimisation), redefining dose-volume histograms, minimising concomitant administration of chemoradiation, employing radiomics (by longitudinal, noninvasive monitoring of the tumour microenvironment), and clarifying the therapeutic values of the particle therapy [77].

Early breast cancer

- In the phase 3 KEYNOTE 522 study it was demonstrated that the percentage of patients with stage II or III triple-negative breast cancer and pCR was significantly higher among those receiving pembrolizumab in addition to standard of care-neoadjuvant chemotherapy (64% vs 51.2%; $p < 0.001$). In the postoperative phase, patients received RT as indicated and pembrolizumab or placebo every 3 weeks for up to 9 cycles. The incidence of treatment related grade 3 or higher AEs was 78.0% with pembrolizumab-chemotherapy group compared to 73.0% in the placebo-chemotherapy group. No AEs specifically related to the postoperative RT delivery were reported [78].

Advanced breast cancer

- Based on the data from phase 3 clinical trials, the combination of chemotherapy and immune checkpoint inhibitors is approved in the first-line treatment for patients with PD-L1 positive ($\geq 1\%$) metastatic triple-negative breast cancer [27].
- In the Impassion130 phase 3 clinical study, 451 patients with untreated metastatic triple-negative breast cancer were randomly assigned to receive atezolizumab with nab-paclitaxel and 451 were assigned to receive placebo plus nab-paclitaxel. In the intention-to treat patient population, median OS was 21.0 months with atezolizumab and 18.7 months in the placebo group ($p = 0.078$). A clinically meaningful OS benefit with atezolizumab plus nab-paclitaxel was seen in patients with PD-L1 immune cell-positive disease (41% of all patients) with the median OS of 25 vs 18 months with placebo.

Palliative RT was administered in 32 patients (7.1%) in the atezolizumab nab-paclitaxel group and in 24 (5.3%) patients in the placebo nab-paclitaxel group. It was not required to hold atezolizumab or placebo during palliative RT, whereas nab-paclitaxel was interrupted per institutional policy/standard of care. The most common grade 3 or higher AEs in the atezolizumab group were neutropenia (8%), peripheral neuropathy (6%), decreased neutrophil count (5%), and fatigue (4%). No increase in grade 3 or higher AEs with palliative RT (brain RT included) was reported [79, 80].

- In a phase 2 clinical study assessing the efficacy and safety of pembrolizumab and RT in patients with metastatic triple-negative breast cancer ($n = 17$, unselected for programmed death-ligand 1 expression), patients received 30 Gy in 5 fractions of 6 Gy over 5–7 days with 3DCRT technique. Pembrolizumab was administered 1–3 days after the first RT fraction and given triweekly thereafter until progressive disease or unacceptable toxicity. Irradiated sites were lymph nodes, bone, breast/chest wall or lung. The overall response rate for the whole cohort was 17.6%. The most common grade 3 or higher AEs reported were lymphopenia (12%), soft-tissue infection (6%) and fatigue (6%). No patient discontinued treatment due to treatment related AEs [81].
- The concurrent combination of immune checkpoint inhibitors and brain SRS appears to be safe and efficacious, with 1-year OS 64.6% and 51.6% ($p < 0.001$) for concurrent and sequential therapy, respectively, and with overall incidence rate of radio-necrosis for all studies of 5.3% [82].

53.5.5 Concomitant Radiation Therapy and Endocrine Therapy

The relationship between RT and endocrine therapy is not completely understood and still controversial—in the absence of the high-quality data—regarding the potentially increased toxicity (dermatitis, pneumonitis, skin and lung fibrosis) due to enhanced radiosensitivity, and/or reduced efficacy when RT and endocrine therapy are administered concurrently [83, 84].

- Data from retrospective studies and systematic reviews suggest that the therapeutic regimens of tamoxifen or aromatase inhibitors given concurrently or sequentially with postoperative RT both appear to be reasonable options with no statistically meaningful difference in terms of 10-year local control, OS, and RFS [84–86].
- Tamoxifen may potentiate post-radiation tissue retraction and fibrosis in the skin and lung, via the induction of the transforming growth factor (TGF)-β signalling. Tamoxifen may, if given in combination with RT, slightly increase the incidence of the pulmonary fibrosis, irrespective of the tamoxifen-RT sequencing or fractionation regimen [84].
- There is no evidence of increased treatment-related toxicity (radiation dermatitis or pulmonary toxicity) with concurrent aromatase inhibitors and RT regimens [84].
- Fulvestrant, used as a single agent or, even more commonly, combined with the novel drugs (i.e. cyclin-dependent kinase 4/6 inhibitors or alpelisib) in the first or second line in de novo or recurrent advanced breast cancer, does not appear to increase AEs when combined with RT [87].
- In clinical practice, both concurrent or sequential endocrine therapy-RT regimens are accepted and often based on the local clinical practice patterns.

53.6 Summary

Technical improvements, including 3D-based postoperative RT for breast cancer, the use of IMRT/VMAT for more complex target volumes, SBRT/SRS for metastasis and the use of IGRT, allow to deliver RT with a high anatomical precision, and reduce the doses to non-target volumes. Additionally, new systemic therapies are constantly introduced into daily use, in the adjuvant or metastatic setting. Data for the safety and efficacy of combing these new systemic treatments is often lacking. Therefore, we advise that centres create predefined protocols and prospective database to evaluate toxicity and efficacy of these new protocols.

References

1. NCI Dictionary of Cancer Terms. https://www.cancer.gov/publications/dictionaries/cancer-terms.
2. Masuda N, Lee SJ, Ohtani S, Im YH, Lee ES, Yokota I, Kuroi K, Im SA, Park BW, Kim SB, Yanagita Y, Ohno S, Takao S, Aogi K, Iwata H, Jeong J, Kim A, Park KH, Sasano H, Ohashi Y, Toi M. Adjuvant Capecitabine for breast cancer after preoperative chemotherapy. N Engl J Med. 2017;376:2147–59. https://doi.org/10.1056/NEJMoa1612645.
3. NCCN breast cancer guidelines, v4.2020. https://www.nccn.org/guidelines/category_1.
4. Sherry AD, Mayer IA, Ayala-Peacock DN, Abramson VG, Rexer BN, Chakravarthy AB. Combining adjuvant radiotherapy with Capecitabine in chemotherapy-resistant breast cancer: feasibility, safety, and toxicity. Clin Breast Cancer. 2020 Aug;20(4):344–52. https://doi.org/10.1016/j.clbc.2020.02.010.
5. Liu YL, Chin C, Catanese B, Lee SM, Zhan S, Kalinsky K, Connolly EP. Concurrent use of capecitabine with radiation therapy and survival in breast cancer (BC) after neoadjuvant chemotherapy. Clin Transl Oncol. 2018;20(10):1280–8. https://doi.org/10.1007/s12094-018-1859-7.
6. Bollet MA, Sigal-Zafrani B, Gambotti L, Extra JM, Meunier M, Nos C, Dendale R, Campana F, Kirova YM, Diéras V, Fourquet A, on behalf of the Institut Curie Breast Cancer Study Group. Pathological response to preoperative concurrent chemo-radiotherapy for breast cancer: results of a phase II study. Eur J Cancer. 2006;42:2286–95.
7. Kosma L, Koukourakis M, Skarlatos J, Zambatis C, Ardavanis A, Beroukas K, Yannakakis D. Hypofractionated radiotherapy with 5-fluorouracil radiosensitization for locally "far advanced" breast cancer. Am J Clin Oncol. 1997;20:562–6. https://doi.org/10.1097/00000421-199712000-00005.
8. Woodward WA, Fang P, Arriaga L, Gao H, Cohen EN, Reuben JM, Valero V, Le-Petross H, Middleton LP, Babiera GV, Strom EA, Tereffe W, Hoffman K, Smith BD, Buchholz TA, Perkins GH. A phase II study of preoperative Capecitabine and concomitant radiation in women with advanced breast cancer. Int J Radiat Oncol Biol Phys. 2017;99(4):777–83. https://doi.org/10.1016/j.ijrobp.2017.04.030.
9. Ismaili N, Elmajjaoui S, Lalya I, Lamia Boulaamane L, Belbaraka R, Abahssain H, Aassab R, Benjaafar N, El Guddari BEK, El Mesbahi O, Sbitti Y, Ismaili M, Errihani H. Anthracycline and concurrent radiotherapy as adjuvant treatment of operable breast cancer: a retrospective cohort study in a single institution. BMC Res Notes. 2010;3:247. https://doi.org/10.1186/1756-0500-3-247.
10. Leonardi MC, Morra A, Santoro L, Balduzzi A, Ivaldi GB, Vischioni B, Ferrari A, Fodor C, Dell'Acqua V, Cardinale DM, Cipolla C, Luini A, Colleoni M, Jereczek-Fossa BA, Orecchia R. Nonrandomized comparison between concomitant and sequential chemoradiotherapy with anthracyclines in breast cancer. Tumori. 2015;101(1):64–71. https://doi.org/10.5301/tj.5000218.
11. Kim DY, Youn JC, Park MS, Lee S, Choi SW, Ryu KH, Kim LS, Shim MS, Lee JJ, Han S. Cardiovascular outcome of breast cancer patients with concomitant radiotherapy and chemotherapy: a 10-year multi-center cohort study. J Cardiol. 2019 Aug;74(2):175–81. https://doi.org/10.1016/j.jjcc.2019.02.001.
12. Fernando IN, Bowden SJ, Herring K, et al. Synchronous versus sequential chemo-radiotherapy in patients with early stage breast cancer (SECRAB): a randomised, phase III, trial. Radiother Oncol. 2020;142:52–61. https://doi.org/10.1016/j.radonc.2019.10.014.
13. Lange OF, Scheef W, Haase KD, Heckmann M, Leyendecker R, Urban G, Zegners G. Palliative chemo-radiotherapy with ifosfamide and epirubicin as first-line treatment for high-risk metastatic breast cancer. Results of a prospective multicenter trial. Cancer Chemother Pharmacol. 1990;26(Suppl):S74–7. https://doi.org/10.1007/BF00685427.
14. Elmongy M, Stolier A, Linares L, Seiler M. Concurrent use of paclitaxel and radiation therapy for the adjuvant treatment of cancer of the breast [abstract]. Breast Cancer Res Treat. 1999;57:57.
15. Bellon JR, Lindsley KL, Ellis GK, Gralow JR, Livingston RB, Austin Seymour MM. Concurrent radiation therapy and paclitaxel or docetaxel chemotherapy in high-risk breast cancer. Int J Radiat Oncol Biol Phys. 2000;48:393–7. https://doi.org/10.1016/S0360-3016(00)00636-2.
16. Taghian AG, Assaad SI, Niemierko A, et al. Risk of pneumonitis in breast cancer patients treated with radiation therapy and combination chemotherapy with paclitaxel. J Natl Cancer Inst. 2001;93:1806–11. https://doi.org/10.1093/jnci/93.23.1806.
17. Hanna YM, Baglan KL, Stromberg JS, Vicini FA, Decker A, D. Acute and subacute toxicity associated with concurrent adjuvant radiation therapy and paclitaxel in primary breast cancer therapy. Breast J. 2002;8:149–53. https://doi.org/10.1046/j.1524-4741.2002.08306.x.
18. Formenti SC, Volm M, Skinner KA, et al. Preoperative twice-weekly paclitaxel with concurrent radiation therapy followed by surgery and postoperative doxorubicin-based chemotherapy in locally advanced breast cancer: a phase i/ii trial. J Clin Oncol. 2003;21:864–70. https://doi.org/10.1200/JCO.2003.06.132.

19. Kao J, Conzen SD, Jaskowiak NT, et al. Concomitant radiation therapy and paclitaxel for unresectable locally advanced breast cancer: results from two consecutive phase i/ii trials. Int J Radiat Oncol Biol Phys. 2005;61:1045–53. https://doi.org/10.1016/j.ijrobp.2004.07.714.
20. Burstein HJ, Bellon JR, Galper S, et al. Prospective evaluation of concurrent paclitaxel and radiation therapy after adjuvant doxorubicin and cyclophosphamide chemotherapy for stage ii or iii breast cancer. Int J Radiat Oncol Biol Phys. 2006;64:496–504. https://doi.org/10.1016/j.ijrobp.2005.07.975.
21. Chakravarthy AB, Kelley MC, McLaren B, et al. Neoadjuvant concurrent paclitaxel and radiation in stage ii/iii breast cancer. Clin Cancer Res. 2006;12:1570–6. https://doi.org/10.1158/1078-0432.CCR-05-2304.
22. Chen WC, Kim J, Kim E, et al. A phase ii study of radiotherapy and concurrent paclitaxel chemotherapy in breast-conserving treatment for node-positive breast cancer. Int J Radiat Oncol Biol Phys. 2012;82:14–20. https://doi.org/10.1016/j.ijrobp.2010.08.051.
23. Ellerbroek N, Martino S, Mautner B, Tao ML, Rose C, Botnick L. Breast-conserving therapy with adjuvant paclitaxel and radiation therapy: feasibility of concurrent treatment. Breast J. 2003;9:74–8. https://doi.org/10.1046/j.1524-4741.2003.09203.x.
24. Cai G, Cao L, Kirova YM, Feng Y, Chen JY. Prospective results of concurrent radiation therapy and weekly paclitaxel as salvage therapy for unre sectable locoregionally recurrent breast cancer. Radiat Oncol. 2019;14:115. https://doi.org/10.1186/s13014-019-1321-1.
25. Semrau S, Gerber B, Reimer T, Klautke G, Fietkau R. Concurrent radiotherapy and Taxane chemotherapy in patients with Locoregional recurrence of breast cancer. Strahlenther Onkol. 2006;182(10)):596–603. https://doi.org/10.1007/s00066-006-1549-1.
26. Kokufu I, Tanei T, Taniguchi H, Kimura F, Fukuda K, Yamamoto M, Yano T, Yamada K, Tamaoka K, Hosono M. Two cases of effective weekly paclitaxel administration and concurrent radiation for metastatic breast cancer. Gan To Kagaku Ryoho. 2003 Jan;30(1):111–4.
27. Cardoso F, Paluch-Shimon S, Senkus E, Curigliano G, Aapro MS, André F, et al. 5th ESO-ESMO international consensus guidelines for advanced breast cancer (ABC 5)†. Ann Oncol. 2020;31(12):1623–49. https://doi.org/10.1016/j.annonc.2020.09.010.
28. Xu H, Yu S, Liu Q, Yuan X, Mani S, Pestell RG, et al. Recent advances of highly selective CDK4/6 inhibitors in breast cancer. J Hematol Oncol. 2017;10 https://doi.org/10.1186/s13045-017-0467-2.
29. Bernhard EJ, Maity A, Muschel RJ, McKenna WG. Effects of ionizing radiation on cell cycle progression - a review. Radiat Environ Biophys. 1995;34:79–83. https://doi.org/10.1007/BF01275210.
30. Sharda N, Yang C-R, Kinsella T, Boothman D. Radiation Resistance. Encycl Cancer. 2002:1–11. https://doi.org/10.1016/b0-12-227555-1/00519-0.
31. Hashizume R, Zhang A, Mueller S, Prados MD, Lulla RR, Goldman S, et al. Inhibition of DNA damage repair by the CDK4/6 inhibitor palbociclib delays irradiated intracranial atypical teratoid rhabdoid tumor and glioblastoma xenograft regrowth. Neuro-Oncology. 2016;18:1519–28. https://doi.org/10.1093/neuonc/now106.
32. Beddok A, Xu HP, Henry AA, Porte B, Fourquet A, Cottu P, et al. Concurrent use of palbociclib and radiation therapy: single-Centre experience and review of the literature. Br J Cancer. 2020;123:905–8. https://doi.org/10.1038/s41416-020-0957-9.
33. Messer JA, Ekinci E, Patel TA, Teh BS. Enhanced dermatologic toxicity following concurrent treatment with palbociclib and radiation therapy: a case report. Reports Pract Oncol Radiother. 2019;24:276–80. https://doi.org/10.1016/j.rpor.2019.03.001.
34. Nasir UM, Mozeika AM, Sayan M, Jan I, Kowal N, Haffty B, et al. Severe gastrointestinal mucositis following concurrent palbociclib and palliative radiation therapy. Anticancer Res. 2020;40:5291–4. https://doi.org/10.21873/anticanres.14534.
35. Kawamoto T, Shikama N, Sasai K. Severe acute radiation-induced enterocolitis after combined palbociclib and palliative radiotherapy treatment. Radiother Oncol. 2019;131:240–1. https://doi.org/10.1016/j.radonc.2018.09.020.
36. Dasgupta A, Sahgal A, Warner E, Czarnota GJ. Safety of palbociclib concurrent with palliative pelvic radiotherapy: discussion of a case of increased toxicity and brief review of literature. J Med Radiat Sci. 2020:1–7. https://doi.org/10.1002/jmrs.435.
37. Kalash R, Iarrobino NA, Beriwal S, Sun M, Glaser SM, Champ CE. Palbociclib enhances pulmonary fibrosis in patients undergoing thoracic radiation therapy: a case series and review of the literature. Int J Radiat Oncol. 2018;102:e610. https://doi.org/10.1016/j.ijrobp.2018.07.1673.
38. Hans S, Cottu P, Kirova YM. Preliminary results of the association of Palbociclib and radiotherapy in metastatic breast cancer patients. Radiother Oncol. 2018;126:181. https://doi.org/10.1016/j.radonc.2017.09.010.
39. Meattini I, Desideri I, Scotti V, Simontacchi G, Livi L. Ribociclib plus letrozole and concomitant palliative radiotherapy for metastatic breast cancer. Breast. 2018;42:1–2. https://doi.org/10.1016/j.breast.2018.08.096.
40. Figura NB, Potluri TK, Mohammadi H, Oliver DE, Arrington JA, Robinson TJ, et al. CDK 4/6 inhibitors and stereotactic radiation in the management of hormone receptor positive breast cancer brain metastases. J Neuro-Oncol. 2019;144:583–9. https://doi.org/10.1007/s11060-019-03260-6.
41. Ippolito E, Greco C, Silipigni S, Dell'Aquila E, Petrianni GM, Tonini G, et al. Concurrent radiotherapy with palbociclib or ribociclib for metastatic breast cancer patients: preliminary assessment of toxicity. Breast. 2019;46:70–4. https://doi.org/10.1016/j.breast.2019.05.001.

42. Chowdhary M, Sen N, Chowdhary A, Usha L, Cobleigh MA, Wang D, et al. Safety and efficacy of Palbociclib and radiation therapy in patients with metastatic breast cancer: initial results of a novel combination. Adv Radiat Oncol. 2019;4:453–7. https://doi.org/10.1016/j.adro.2019.03.011.
43. Guerini AE, Pedretti S, Salah E, Simoncini EL, Maddalo M, Pegurri L, et al. A single-center retrospective safety analysis of cyclin-dependent kinase 4/6 inhibitors concurrent with radiation therapy in metastatic breast cancer patients. Sci Rep. 2020;10 https://doi.org/10.1038/s41598-020-70430-2.
44. Ratosa I, Orazem M, Scoccimarro E, Steinacher M, Dominici L, Aquilano M, et al. Cyclin-dependent kinase 4/6 inhibitors combined with radiotherapy for patients with metastatic breast cancer. Clin Breast Cancer. 2020; https://doi.org/10.1016/j.clbc.2020.05.013.
45. Moja L, Tagliabue L, Balduzzi S, Parmelli E, Pistotti V, Guarneri V, D'Amico R. Trastuzumab containing regimens for early breast cancer. Cochrane Database Syst Rev. 2012;4:CD006243. https://doi.org/10.1002/14651858.
46. Denduluri N, Chavez-MacGregor M, Telli ML, Eisen A, Graff SL, Hassett MJ, et al. Selection of optimal adjuvant chemotherapy and targeted therapy for early breast cancer: ASCO clinical practice guideline focused update. J Clin Oncol. 2018;36(23):2433–43. https://doi.org/10.1200/JCO.2018.78.8604.
47. Piccart-Gebhart MJ, Procter M, Leyland-Jones B, Goldhirsch A, Untch M, Smith I, et al. Herceptin adjuvant (HERA) trial study team. Trastuzumab after adjuvant chemotherapy in HER2-positive breast cancer. N Engl J Med. 2005;353(16):1659–72. https://doi.org/10.1056/NEJMoa052306.
48. Mignot F, Ajgal Z, Xu H, Geraud A, Chen JY, Mégnin-Chanet F, Kirova Y. Concurrent administration of anti-HER2 therapy and radiotherapy: systematic review. Radiother Oncol. 2017;124(2):190–9. https://doi.org/10.1016/j.radonc.2017.07.006.
49. Segovia-Mendoza M, González-González ME, Barrera D, Díaz L, García-Becerra R. Efficacy and mechanism of action of the tyrosine kinase inhibitors gefitinib, lapatinib and neratinib in the treatment of HER2-positive breast cancer: preclinical and clinical evidence. Am J Cancer Res. 2015;5(9):2531–61.
50. Kroeze SG, Fritz C, Hoyer M, Lo SS, Ricardi U, Sahgal A, et al. Toxicity of concurrent stereotactic radiotherapy and targeted therapy or immunotherapy: a systematic review. Cancer Treat Rev. 2017;53:25–37. https://doi.org/10.1016/j.ctrv.2016.11.013.
51. Yu T, Cho BJ, Choi EJ, Park JM, Kim DH, Kim IA. Radiosensitizing effect of lapatinib in human epidermal growth factor receptor 2-positive breast cancer cells. Oncotarget. 2016;7(48):79089–100. https://doi.org/10.18632/oncotarget.12597.
52. Parsai S, Miller JA, Juloori A, Chao ST, Kotecha R, Mohammadi AM, et al. Stereotactic radiosurgery with concurrent lapatinib is associated with improved local control for HER2-positive breast cancer brain metastases. J Neurosurg. 2019;132(2):503–11. https://doi.org/10.3171/2018.10.JNS182340.
53. Kim JM, Miller JA, Kotecha R, Chao ST, Ahluwalia MS, Peereboom DM, et al. Stereotactic radiosurgery with concurrent HER2-directed therapy is associated with improved objective response for breast cancer brain metastasis. Neuro-Oncology. 2019;21(5):659–68. https://doi.org/10.1093/neuonc/noz006.
54. Lewis Phillips GD, Li G, Dugger DL, Crocker LM, Parsons KL, Mai E, et al. Targeting HER2-positive breast cancer with trastuzumab-DM1, an antibody-cytotoxic drug conjugate. Cancer Res. 2008;68:9280–90. https://doi.org/10.1158/0008-5472.CAN-08-1776.
55. von Minckwitz G, Huang C-S, Mano MS, Loibl S, Mamounas EP, Untch M, et al. Trastuzumab Emtansine for residual invasive HER2-positive breast cancer. N Engl J Med. 2019;380:617–28. https://doi.org/10.1056/nejmoa1814017.
56. Diéras V, Miles D, Verma S, Pegram M, Welslau M, Baselga J, et al. Trastuzumab emtansine versus capecitabine plus lapatinib in patients with previously treated HER2-positive advanced breast cancer (EMILIA): a descriptive analysis of final overall survival results from a randomised, open-label, phase 3 trial. Lancet Oncol. 2017;18:732–42. https://doi.org/10.1016/S1470-2045(17)30312-1.
57. Stumpf PK, DiM C, Robin TP, Carlson JA, Stuhr KA, Contreras-Zarate MJ, et al. Combination of trastuzumab emtansine and stereotactic radiosurgery results in high rates of clinically significant radionecrosis and dysregulation of aquaporin-4. Clin Cancer Res. 2019;25:3946–53. https://doi.org/10.1158/1078-0432.CCR-18-2851.
58. Carlson JA, Nooruddin Z, Rusthoven C, Elias A, Borges VF, Diamond JR, et al. Trastuzumab emtansine and stereotactic radiosurgery: an unexpected increase in clinically significant brain edema. Neuro-Oncology. 2014;16:1006–9. https://doi.org/10.1093/neuonc/not329.
59. Geraud A, Xu HP, Beuzeboc P, Kirova YM. Preliminary experience of the concurrent use of radiosurgery and T-DM1 for brain metastases in HER2-positive metastatic breast cancer. J Neuro-Oncol. 2017;131:69–72. https://doi.org/10.1007/s11060-016-2265-z.
60. Géraud A, Xu HP, Beuzeboc P, Kirova YM. Preliminary results of the concurrent use of radiotherapy for bone metastases and trastuzumab emtansine in patients with HER2-positive metastatic breast cancer. Cancer/Radiotherapie. 2016;20:312–3. https://doi.org/10.1016/j.canrad.2016.03.010.
61. Dulaney C, Marcrom S, Stanley J, Yang ES. Poly(ADP-ribose) polymerase activity and inhibition in cancer. Semin Cell Dev Biol. 2017;63:144–53. https://doi.org/10.1016/j.semcdb.2017.01.007.
62. Césaire M, Thariat J, Candéias SM, Stefan D, Saintigny Y, Chevalier F. Combining PARP inhibition, radiation, and immunotherapy: a possible strat-

egy to improve the treatment of cancer? Int J Mol Sci. 2018;19 https://doi.org/10.3390/ijms19123793.
63. Loap P, Loirat D, Berger F, Ricci F, Vincent-Salomon A, Ezzili C, et al. Combination of Olaparib and radiation therapy for triple negative breast cancer: preliminary results of the RADIOPARP phase 1 trial. Int J Radiat Oncol Biol Phys. 2021;109(2):436–40. https://doi.org/10.1016/j.ijrobp.2020.09.032.
64. Jagsi R, Griffith KA, Bellon JR, Woodward WA, Horton JK, Ho A, et al. Concurrent veliparib with chest wall and nodal radiotherapy in patients with inflammatory or locoregionally recurrent breast cancer: the TBCRC 024 phase I multicenter study. J Clin Oncol. 2018;36:1317–22. https://doi.org/10.1200/JCO.2017.77.2665.
65. Manegold PC, Paringer C, Kulka U, Krimmel K, Eichhorn ME, Wilkowski R, et al. Antiangiogenic therapy with mammalian target of rapamycin inhibitor RAD001 (Everolimus) increases radiosensitivity in solid cancer. Clin Cancer Res. 2008;14(3):892–900. https://doi.org/10.1158/1078-0432.CCR-07-0955.
66. Deutsch E, Le Péchoux C, Faivre L, Rivera S, Tao Y, Pignon JP, et al. Phase I trial of everolimus in combination with thoracic radiotherapy in non-small-cell lung cancer. Ann Oncol. 2015;26(6):1223–9. https://doi.org/10.1093/annonc/mdv105.
67. Willemsen AE, Grutters JC, Gerritsen WR, van Erp NP, van Herpen CM, Tol J. mTOR inhibitor-induced interstitial lung disease in cancer patients: comprehensive review and a practical management algorithm. Int J Cancer. 2016;138(10):2312–21. https://doi.org/10.1002/ijc.29887.
68. Bourgier C, Massard C, Moldovan C, Soria JC, Deutsch E. Total recall of radiotherapy with mTOR inhibitors: a novel and potentially frequent side-effect? Ann Oncol. 2011;22(2):485–6. https://doi.org/10.1093/annonc/mdq741.
69. Ioannidis G, Gkogkou P, Charalampous P, Diamandi M, Ioannou R. Radiation-recall dermatitis with the everolimus/exemestane combination ten years after adjuvant whole-breast radiotherapy. Radiother Oncol. 2014;112(3):449–50. https://doi.org/10.1016/j.radonc.2014.08.030.
70. André F, Ciruelos E, Rubovszky G, Campone M, Loibl S, Rugo HS, et al. SOLAR-1 study group. Alpelisib for PIK3CA-mutated, hormone receptor-positive advanced breast cancer. N Engl J Med. 2019;380(20):1929–40. https://doi.org/10.1056/NEJMoa1813904.
71. Rugo HS, André F, Yamashita T, Cerda H, Toledano I, Stemmer SM, et al. Time course and management of key adverse events during the randomized phase III SOLAR-1 study of PI3K inhibitor alpelisib plus fulvestrant in patients with HR-positive advanced breast cancer. Ann Oncol. 2020;31(8):1001–10. https://doi.org/10.1016/j.annonc.2020.05.001.
72. Day D, Prawira A, Spreafico A, Waldron J, Karithanam R, Giuliani M, et al. Phase I trial of alpelisib in combination with concurrent cisplatin-based chemoradiotherapy in patients with locoregionally advanced squamous cell carcinoma of the head and neck. Oral Oncol. 2020;108:104753. https://doi.org/10.1016/j.oraloncology.2020.104753.
73. Kaufman PA, Awada A, Twelves C, Yelle L, Perez EA, Velikova G, et al. Phase III open-label randomized study of eribulin mesylate versus capecitabine in patients with locally advanced or metastatic breast cancer previously treated with an anthracycline and a taxane. J Clin Oncol. 2015;33(6):594–601. https://doi.org/10.1200/JCO.2013.52.4892.
74. Meattini I, Desideri I, Di Cataldo V, Francolini G, De Luca CC, Scotti V, et al. Safety of eribulin mesylate and concomitant radiotherapy for metastatic breast cancer: a single-center experience. Future Oncol. 2016;12(9):1117–24. https://doi.org/10.2217/fon-2015-0059.
75. de Bono JS, Molife LR, Sonpavde G, Maroto JP, Calvo E, Cartwright TH, et al. Phase II study of eribulin mesylate (E7389) in patients with metastatic castration-resistant prostate cancer stratified by prior taxane therapy. Ann Oncol. 2012;23(5):1241–9. https://doi.org/10.1093/annonc/mdr380.
76. Chargari C, Levy A, Paoletti X, Soria JC, Massard C, Weichselbaum RR, et al. Methodological development of combination drug and radiotherapy in basic and clinical research. Clin Cancer Res. 2020;26(18):4723–36. https://doi.org/10.1158/1078-0432.CCR-19-4155.
77. Deutsch E, Chargari C, Galluzzi L, Kroemer G. Optimising efficacy and reducing toxicity of anticancer radioimmunotherapy. Lancet Oncol. 2019;20(8):e452–63. https://doi.org/10.1016/S1470-2045(19)30171-8.
78. Schmid P, Cortes J, Pusztai L, McArthur H, Kümmel S, Bergh J, et al. KEYNOTE-522 investigators. Pembrolizumab for early triple-negative breast cancer. N Engl J Med. 2020;382(9):810–21. https://doi.org/10.1056/NEJMoa1910549.
79. Schmid P, Adams S, Rugo HS, Schneeweiss A, Barrios CH, Iwata H. IMpassion130 trial investigators. Atezolizumab and nab-paclitaxel in advanced triple-negative breast cancer. N Engl J Med. 2018;379(22):2108–21. https://doi.org/10.1056/NEJMoa1809615.
80. Schmid P, Rugo HS, Adams S, Schneeweiss A, Barrios CH, Iwata H. IMpassion130 investigators. Atezolizumab plus nab-paclitaxel as first-line treatment for unresectable, locally advanced or metastatic triple-negative breast cancer (IMpassion130): updated efficacy results from a randomised, double-blind, placebo-controlled, phase 3 trial. Lancet Oncol. 2020;21(1):44–59. https://doi.org/10.1016/S1470-2045(19)30689-8.
81. Ho AY, Barker CA, Arnold BB, Powell SN, Hu ZI, Gucalp A, et al. A phase 2 clinical trial assessing the efficacy and safety of pembrolizumab and radiotherapy in patients with metastatic triple-negative

breast cancer. Cancer. 2020;126(4):850–60. https://doi.org/10.1002/cncr.32599.
82. Lehrer EJ, Peterson J, Brown PD, Sheehan JP, Quiñones-Hinojosa A, Zaorsky NG, et al. Treatment of brain metastases with stereotactic radiosurgery and immune checkpoint inhibitors: an international meta-analysis of individual patient data. Radiother Oncol. 2019;130:104–12. https://doi.org/10.1016/j.radonc.2018.08.025.
83. Chargari C, Toillon RA, Macdermed D, Castadot P, Magné N. Concurrent hormone and radiation therapy in patients with breast cancer: what is the rationale? Lancet Oncol. 2009;10(1):53–60. https://doi.org/10.1016/S1470-2045(08)70333-4.
84. McGee SF, Mazzarello S, Caudrelier JM, Lima MAG, Hutton B, Sienkiewicz M, et al. Optimal sequence of adjuvant endocrine and radiation therapy in early-stage breast cancer - a systematic review. Cancer Treat Rev. 2018;69:132–42. https://doi.org/10.1016/j.ctrv.2018.06.015.
85. Harris EE, Christensen VJ, Hwang WT, Fox K, Solin LJ. Impact of concurrent versus sequential tamoxifen with radiation therapy in early-stage breast cancer patients undergoing breast conservation treatment. J Clin Oncol. 2005;23(1):11–6. https://doi.org/10.1200/JCO.2005.09.056.
86. Pierce LJ, Hutchins LF, Green SR, Lew DL, Gralow JR, Livingston RB, et al. Sequencing of tamoxifen and radiotherapy after breast-conserving surgery in early-stage breast cancer. J Clin Oncol. 2005;23(1):24–9. https://doi.org/10.1200/JCO.2005.01.198.
87. Ding J, Guo Y, Jiang X, Li K, Fu W, Cao Y. Concomitant fulvestrant with reirradiation for unresectable locoregional recurrent estrogen receptor positive (ER+) breast cancer: a case report and narrative review. Medicine (Baltimore). 2020;99(30):e21344. https://doi.org/10.1097/MD.0000000000021344.

Part X

Risk Assessment and Radiation Quality Assurance

Risk Assessment and Quality Management in Radiation Oncology

54

Gustavo Nader Marta, Wellington F. P. Neves-Junior, and Núria Jornet

54.1 Background

Over the last decades, quality management has been of unique importance in modelling the structure of modern radiation oncology departments. Quality management programmes set benchmarks related to personnel, equipment, procedures and policies and have been a valuable conductor for the proper and safe functioning of the radiation oncology process [1]. Risk management is a core part of any quality management programme and includes prospective risk assessments before implementing any new technique or before any modification of processes, incident reporting and incident learning systems and risk mitigation strategies. In 2013, Council Directive 2013/59/Euratom of 5 December 2013 [2] laying down basic safety standards for protection against the possible dangers arising from exposure to ionising radiations, recognised prospective risk assessment as mandatory before implementing any new technique or equipment.

G. N. Marta (✉) · W. F. P. Neves-Junior (✉)
Department of Radiation Oncology, Hospital Sírio-Libanês, Sao Paulo, Brazil

N. Jornet
Núria Jornet Hospital de la Santa Creu i Sant Pau, Barcelona, Spain
e-mail: NJornet@santpau.cat

54.2 Risk Assessment

RT is a complex process where distinct specialists such as radiation oncologists, medical physicists, RTTs and/or nurses work in close cooperation to prepare and deliver treatment. Safe delivery of RT is a complex task that has become even more challenging due to last years' advances in techniques and technologies that are worldwide quickly adopted by all radiation oncology departments. A number of accidents, among others in France [3, 4] and in the USA [5–9], brought RT safety into the media front pages. Thus, in early 2010, after these mediatic accidents and following the report "To Err is Human" from the Institute of Medicine (IOM) [10], we observed a growing interest in incident learning as a key tool to ensure the safety and quality of care in radiation oncology, with more than 40 publications on incident learning systems (ILS). Several reports on ILS focusing on radiation oncology, issued by international organisations [11–15], highlighted the importance on reporting not only incidents but also "near misses". While incidents are defined as unwanted or unexpected changes from normal system behaviour which cause an adverse effect to persons or equipment, a "near miss" (or "good catch") would be defined as an event or situation that could have resulted in an accident, injury, or illness but did not either by chance or through timely intervention.

© The Author(s), under exclusive license to Springer Nature Switzerland AG 2022
O. Kaidar-Person et al. (eds.), *Breast Cancer Radiation Therapy*,
https://doi.org/10.1007/978-3-030-91170-6_54

Almost 20000 patients per year have their treatment impaired to some unidentified level by poor-quality RT procedures in the USA [16]. Although it is difficult to estimate the error rates associated with radiation oncology, Eric Ford et al. suggested a rate of misadministration of 0.2% [17], even if this rate may be an underestimation. According to US Nuclear Regulatory Commission, more than 60% of radiation oncology incidents are due to human errors [18, 19]. The activities and failures of individual people is the central issue of the problem, but their rationale and behaviour is greatly induced and controlled by their working setting and by larger structural processes. Foremost RT errors often include combinations of several individuals and a sum of broader contributing aspects [20].

The prospective risk assessment differs from ILS in its setting in time. Indeed, the purpose is to prospectively search for possible error pathways, before any incident has occurred, aiming to prevent further accidents in radiation oncology. Even if there are different methodologies to perform prospective risk analyses, all coincide in the definition of potential adverse events (initiating event) and score the risk as a combination of occurrence probability of the event, the probability of detection (safety barriers in place) and the severity of the consequence. The latter range from irrelevant or inconvenient incidents to catastrophic events (including the patient death).

As recognised by the British Institute of Radiology, Institute of Physics and Engineering in Medicine National Patient Safety Agency, Society and College of Radiographers and The Royal College of Radiologists report, in any structure errors are to be expected; nonetheless, by understanding why they happen, it is possible to reduce their incidence and increase detection before harm occurs [12].

The purpose of a risk assessment and quality management platform is to safeguard the patient from accidents, recognising factors that contribute to incidents and creating strategies to manage and mitigate errors. See also "Quality Assurance Programmes in Radiation Oncology" section.

54.3 Tools to Assess and Mitigate Risks

Traditionally, in radiation oncology, quality improvement was mainly achieved through technological advances. As such, quality assurance (QA) has mainly been equipment-based following guidelines on the tests, tolerances and frequencies issued by scientific societies. This approach is often referred as "prescriptive" QA, with many documents prescribing all sorts of tests with different periodicities. An example is the American Association of Medical Physics (AAPM) task group 142 [21] regarding QA of medical linear accelerators, that recommends the routine tests including daily, monthly and annual tests with associated tolerance levels. In the last years it has been difficult to keep the pace with new technology, so that the early adopters have faced the challenge of its implementation and at the same time developing QA guidelines. In order to streamline QA of new technologies and techniques is important to prospectively perform a risk analysis of not only the technology but the entire process which will most probably be affected by its implementation. This will help to identify the issues in which we should focus from a quality and safety perspective. When focusing only on prescriptive equipment QA, many resources are spent on testing parts that can remain stable for long periods of time whilst almost no effort is dedicated to address inadequate process design, information flow, deficient training, documentation, miscommunication, misunderstanding and human errors. This is in contrast with the lessons learned from ILS, showing that most incidents are not due to failures in the equipment but in the process itself.

Therefore, a change in paradigm was needed. The adoption of prospective risk analysis methods allows to better "think systems" and design more efficient and effective allocation of resources, enhancing quality and safety together. A turning point towards risk assessment was the publication of the AAPM task group 100 (TG 100) report [22] that presented a structured methodology based on Failure Mode and Effect Analysis (FMEA) to analyse clinical processes, identifying and ranking risks in order to develop prioritised actions to mitigate them. The FMEA analysis must be performed by a multidisciplinary team and starts from a process map describing each step or the process or workflow. The first part of the analysis is an exercise of possibilities, where for each step as many possible potential failure modes need to be identified. Next, for each of these modes, one or more potential causes that may lead to it are also identified—and for this task, incident learning systems can be useful, bearing in mind that each failure mode can, and usually does, have several causes. There is no single cause/person responsible, and there should be safety circle of care to prevent medical errors (at different layers) to stop an error to occur and identify it prior to its occurrence ("good catch"). Finally, for each failure mode, assuming it occurs, the potential effect or impact on the outcome of the process is to be determined.

The second part of FMEA consists of scoring the list of failure modes, causes and effects, considering the likelihood of affecting the outcome of the process and the impact on it. The multidisciplinary team must assign numerical values (from 1 to 10) to three parameters that describe [1] the following.

1. "O" (occurrence): how likely a given cause for the specific failure can occur;
2. "D" (lack of detectability): how likely the failure will not be detected in time to be prevented;
3. "S" (severity): how severe the effect of the failure might be.

Although previous institutional experience or studies might be available to help choosing those values, its selection will largely depend on expert opinion. The TG 100 has developed scales and terminologies for O, S and D parameters that are specifically related to RT outcomes and observations and are recommended to be used [1]. Finally, these three parameters are multiplied to result on a single quantity called *risk priority number* (RPN = O × D × S). This metric is then used to rank each failure and drive the quality management programme to prioritise resources and efforts on higher RPN value, or higher risk failures. On the same lines el Foro Iberoamericano de Organismos Reguladores Radiológicos y Nucleares developed a prospective risk evaluation methodology based on risk matrices [22]. They have developed a software tool (SEVRRA) [23] with the purpose of facilitating the evaluation of the risk level of radiation oncology departments. The different potential failure modes will be classified in four categories: very high, high, medium and low risk.

While new quality control tests can be designed to tackle specific process failure modes that deal with equipment malfunctioning, an effective quality management programme should also deal with failure modes related to human errors. In order to minimise the probability of occurrence and maximise the detectability different actions can be taken [13].

1. Automation: May help in reducing human errors, it can also be used for QA.
2. Peer review: double checks of clinical decisions, contours, treatment plans, in-room imaging checks and so on.

3. Checklists: utmost importance on standardisation of practices, procedures and on ensuring compliance. Helps prevent humans on relying solely on memory on performing multiple tasks.
4. Audits: independent evaluation of critical processes or implementation of new technologies.
5. Staff training and competency: continuing education on operational and safety procedures.
6. Policies and procedures: careful and clear description and documentation, readily available to everyone to ensure standardisation and compliance. Clear distribution of tasks and responsibilities between staff groups.
7. Communication: clear lines of communication among the team with objectivity and completeness of information to fulfil tasks. Methods of flagging non-standard situations or dissemination of warning of non-standard behaviours.
8. Incident learning system: a formalised system, method or organisation for logging, reporting and evaluating incidents and near-misses. This needs to be accessible to all teams and periodically re-evaluated by a commission.
9. Converting the data collected from the learning system to change policies, department procedures, training, checklists and so on.

All these processes should be known/transparent to the team members and be part of RT department daily routine. It is human to err and for machines to malfunction, but it is our responsibility to learn, prevent and make appropriate modifications to prevent the next incident. As it is very tempting to apportion blame to just one issue or person, however such an approach will drive to additional errors and problems and is not part of the safety and quality management. Moreover, there is no place for seeking blame, as there is no single process/person responsible. It should be a team effort to create a friendly and safe environment for reporting errors, or "near miss". All should be part of the culture of safety and excellence.

54.4 Summary

RT department should adopt the quality control measures according to the national (if available) and international QA programmes, but also adopt quality control tests according to department workflow. Special care should be given when changing RT protocols/techniques, and appropriate training is advised. Implementation incident and near misses reporting and learning systems, is utmost important for risk assessment and quality management. Regular feedback to the staff members will improve the quality culture of the organisation which is the key for any success of a quality management programmes. Our goal should be to adopt strategies to improve patient care reducing any non-compliance to protocols that could lead to an adverse event. Medical errors have an impact on the lives the patients their relatives and also on medical staff that were involved in the incident and may threaten trust in the healthcare system. It is in our ability, as a team, to welcome a quality culture which should include patient safety, and therefore provide not only a good quality treatment but a safe one.

Figure 54.1 illustrates the essential aspects of process control.

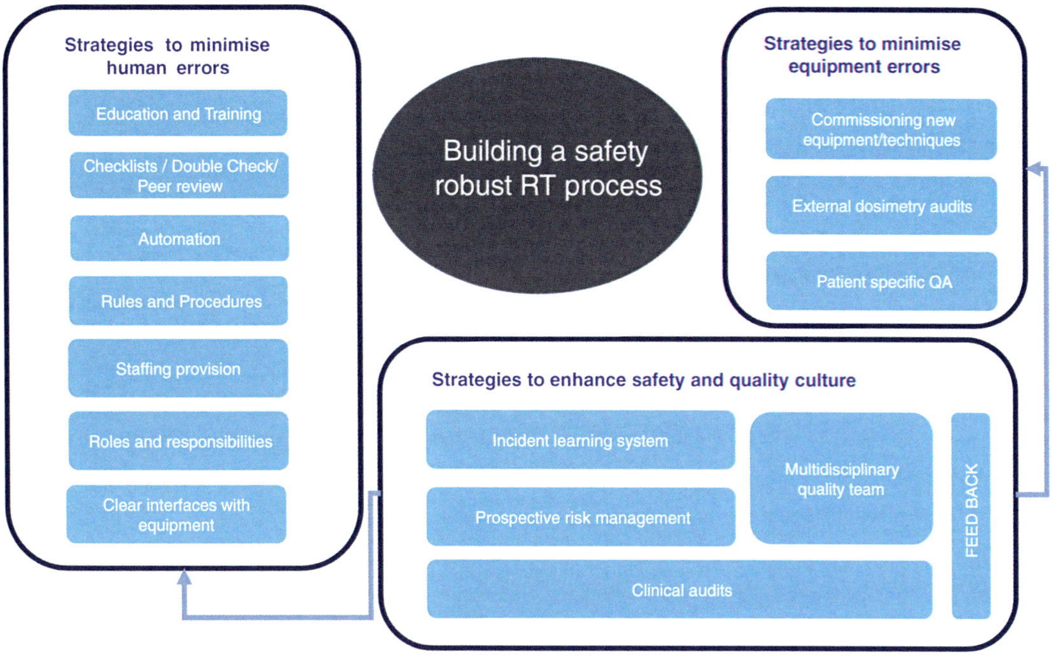

Fig. 54.1 Highlight the importance of keeping workload moderate; this needs a good staffing provision with a clear definition of roles and responsibilities. The interface with the equipment has to be clear, preferably in the national language; and keep the alerts strictly to what is necessary with clear codes on the severity of the alert

References

1. Huq MS, Fraass BA, Dunscombe PB, Gibbons JP Jr, Ibbott GS, Mundt AJ, et al. The report of Task Group 100 of the AAPM: Application of risk analysis methods to radiation therapy quality management. Med Phys. 2016;43:4209.
2. Official Journal of the European Union. European Council Directive 2013/59/Euratom on basic safety standards for protection against the dangers arising from exposure to ionising radiation and repealing directives 89/618/Euratom, 90/641/Euratom, 96/29/Euratom, 97/43 Euratom and 2003/122/Euratom. OJ of the EU. 2014;L13(57):1–73. Available at https://eur-lex.europa.eu/LexUriServ/LexUriServ.do?uri=OJ:L:2014:013:0001:0073:EN:PDF
3. Peiffert D, Simon JM, Eschwege F. L'accident d'Epinal: passé, présent, avenir [Epinal radiotherapy accident: passed, present, future]. Cancer Radiother. 2007;11(6–7):309–12. https://doi.org/10.1016/j.canrad.2007.09.004. Epub 2007 Oct 24
4. Borius PY, Debono B, Latorzeff I, Lotterie JA, Plas JY, Cassol E, Bousquet P, Loubes F, Duthil P, Durand A, Caire F, Redon A, Berry I, Sabatier J, Lazorthes Y. Traitement des métastases cérébrales par radiochirurgie stéréotaxique : étude de 33 cas liés à un accident de "surexposition" [Dosimetric stereotactic radiosurgical accident: Study of 33 patients treated for brain metastases]. Neurochirurgie. 2010;56(5):368–73. https://doi.org/10.1016/j.neuchi.2010.07.002. Epub 2010 Aug 12
5. Bogdanich W. Radiation offers new cures, and ways to do harm. New York, NY: New York Times; 2010. p. 1.
6. Bogdanich W. As technology surges, radiation safeguards lag. New York, NY: New York Times; 2010. p. A1.
7. Bogdanich W, Rebelo K. A pinpoint beam strays invisibly, harming instead of healing. New York, NY: New York Times; 2010.
8. Bogdanich W, Ruiz RR. Radiation errors reported in Missouri. New York, NY: New York Times; 2010. p. A17.

9. Oved MC. Radiotherapy error could affect thundreds. USA Today. 2007. Health & Behavior.
10. Kohn LT, Corrigan JM, Donaldson MS, editors. To Err is Human: Build-ing a Safer Health System. Washington DC: 2000 by the NationalAcademy of Sciences; 2000.
11. Donaldson L. Radiotherapy Risk Profile: Technical Manual. Geneva: World Health Organization; 2008.
12. Donaldson L. Towards safer radiotherapy. London: British Institute of Radiology, Institute of Physics and Engineering in Medicine, National Patient Safety Agency, Society and College of Radiographers, The Royal College of Radiologists; 2007. https://www.rcr.ac.uk/system/files/publication/field_publication_files/Towards_saferRT_final.pdf
13. American Society for Radiation Oncology. Safety is no accident - A framework for quality radiation oncology care 2019. https://www.astro.org/ASTRO/media/ASTRO/PatientCare and Research/PDFs/Safety_is_No_Accident.pdf. Accessed 28 Aug 2020.
14. Ortiz LP, Cossett JM, Dunscombe P, et al. ICRP Report No. 112: pre- venting accidental exposures from new external beam radiation therapy technologies. ICRP; 2009. p. 112.
15. European Commission. Radiation Protection. General guidelines on risk management in external beam radiotherapy. https://ec.europa.eu/energy/sites/ener/files/documents/RP181web.pdf. Accessed 25 Sept 2020.
16. Dunscombe P, Evans S, Williamson J, et al. Introduction to quality. In: Thomadsen B, editor. Quality and safety in radiotherapy. Madison, WI: Medical Physics Publishing; 2013. p. 1–30.
17. Ford EC, Terezakis S. How safe is safe? Risk in radiotherapy. Int J Radiat Oncol Biol Phys. 2010;78:321–2.
18. World Health Organization. International agency for research on cancer. Globocan; 2012.
19. Duffey RB, Saull JW. Know the risk: Learning from errors and accidents: Safety and risk in today's technology. Waltham, MA: Butterworth-Heinemann Publications; 2003.
20. Marks LB, Rose CM, Hayman JA, Williams TR. The need for physician leadership in creating a culture of safety. Int J Radiat Oncol Biol Phys. 2011;79:1287–9.
21. Klein EE, Hanley J, Bayouth J, Yin F-F, Simon W, Dresser S, et al. Task Group 142 report: Quality assurance of medical accelerators. Med Phys. 2009;36(9):4197.
22. APLICACIÓN DEL MÉTODO DE LA MATRIZ DE RIESGO A LA RADIOTERAPIA OIEA, VIENA, 2012 IAEA-TECDOC-1685/S ISBN 978-92-0-332510-3 ISSN 1011-4289 © OIEA, 2012
23. https://www.foroiberam.org/sevrra

55 Treatment-Related Quality Assurance

Angelo Filippo Monti and Maria Grazia Brambilla

55.1 Background

Treatment-related quality assurance in breast RT is complex and requires a thorough understanding of all steps to produce a final clinical acceptable treatment plan. Not only would these steps be grounded on dosimetry and RT planning, but they have also to take account of simulation and interaction with boundary conditions, such as patient's individual anatomy and ancillary devices and conditions that might be able to influence the planned treatment's delivery or outcomes. This chapter focuses on some key elements of treatment-specific QA, in order to present an overview of the main factors that could compromise treatment preparation and delivery itself. Clear procedures in terms of prescription, techniques, dose calculation and delivery are illustrated; hints and practical advice are reported.

55.2 Methods for Treatment-Related Quality Assurance

Naming A standardised volumes' naming (nomenclature) in target volumes and OARs during delineation is strongly suggested; this will help to prevent confusion among clinicians and facilitate treatment plan quality control. Consistent language and terminology are known to have an impact on workflow management and to reduce errors [1, 2], for example bilateral breast irradiation needs attention, in order to avoid serious misunderstandings during treatment. Additionally, it is encouraged to use consistent naming recommended by the Global Harmonization papers. This will allow automation of reports and pooling or data capturing in national or international registries [2]. For breast cancer, the recommended nomenclature for CTVs is used in ESTRO delineation guidelines [3].

Geometry The inter- and intra-observer variability in volume delineation should be evaluated and prevented or at least minimised. Particularly, the correct shape and location of the CTV and nearby located OARs are important parameters in ensuring optimal plans to minimise the side effects of RT [4, 5]. Automatic contouring can be a very useful aid to assist clinical practice to reduce variability and improve consistency, but clinicians have to be carefully cultured regarding its functioning in order to avoid unpredictable errors [6].

Patient positioning is also a concern, it should be supportive and comfortable to be tolerated by the patient and maintained during the whole treatment thus its variability should be always evaluated and controlled (see section on patient positioning) [7, 8].

A. F. Monti (✉) · M. G. Brambilla
ASST GOM Niguarda, Milan, Italy
e-mail: angelofilippo.monti@ospedaleniguarda.it; mariagrazia.brambilla@ospedaleniguarda.it

© The Author(s), under exclusive license to Springer Nature Switzerland AG 2022
O. Kaidar-Person et al. (eds.), *Breast Cancer Radiation Therapy*,
https://doi.org/10.1007/978-3-030-91170-6_55

Several techniques that can help to reduce the OARs exposure exist (see section on Techniques to reduce OAR dose). These include DIBH [9], gating techniques, CPAP [10], or four-dimensional CT [11] to reduce the heart dose in case of left-sided breast RT as well as of lung dose in any side and possibly heart dose in case of right IMN-RT. Yet these techniques require patients and staff training and cooperation for a successful clinical application, so a QA programme should be instituted as well [12, 13].

Breathing is a concern when considering changes in body shape. In case of IMRT based on tangential fields, in which the beam is tightly fitted to the target, it is a common practice to extend the photon fluence outside the limit of the body contour to account for changes in shape and position of the target (CTV) due to respiration or to potential breast oedema. This situation, however and in contrast to what is often claimed, is not an issue in VMAT treatments thanks to the rotation of the beam that thereby does not skim off at a constant area. Moreover, the skin itself is not part of the target volume, except for T4b,c,d disease, and treatment series are becoming shorter following the introduction of moderate and now ultra-hypofractionation. Nevertheless, various strategies are available in the TPS, including auto expansion of the beam fluence outside of the body contour, to avoid underdosage of the section of the target moving outside the body borders in case this might be an issue [14–16].

Techniques and TPS Different RT techniques can be used for breast cancer RT. Conventional tangential wedge fields, field-in-field, IMRT, VMAT, tomotherapy, and several hybrid techniques that combine for example tangential fields with VMAT [17]. Each of them may provide different dose distributions even when planning the same case. Among these, intensity modulated techniques are growing in their utilisation because of their superior dose shaping and homogeneity or, in the case of for examples SIB, a desired dose inhomogeneity [15, 18]. Whichever the technique used, QA in the RT treatment planning process is essential to ensure that the calculation algorithms can correctly reproduce the delivered dose [19, 20]. Independent dose audits found that TPS errors in dose calculations are possible, especially with complex techniques, highlighting the need for careful beam modelling in the TPS [21]. An independent software for MU recalculation can help to identify the presence of TPS errors [22]. But, pure recalculation is not an exhaustive substitute for dose delivery QA. Especially in complex modulated plans with lots of MLC segments, a second dose engine check cannot prevent failures in dose delivery due to LINAC malfunctioning. Absolute dose should be measured at the treatment machine preferably in more than one single point; this can be done with pre-treatment measurements with dedicated dosimetric phantoms or the on-board EPID (Fig. 55.1), which can be used in vivo measurements too [23, 24]. Pre-treatment verification should be executed in advance for each patient, whenever a new technique is introduced; once the technique is consolidated and an acceptable confidence is reached, weekly or monthly QA can be implemented on reference plans [20].

Another issue concerning the TPS is the dose prediction in inhomogeneous tissues, such as lung, in which some outdated pencil beam-based TPSs are known to fail. Improvements in the calculated dose have been shown when the TPS algorithm considers photon scatter and changes in electron transport properly. For this reason, whenever possible, a modern type-b (i.e. Collapsed Cone) or Monte Carlo algorithm should be preferred for dose calculation [25–27]. This suggestion is also valid for dose prediction in superficial and build-up regions, in which type-a and fast hybrid algorithms (such as AAA) are proved to be inaccurate. When one of this algorithms is used to calculate the dose, to partially minimise the inaccuracy related to the dose interpolation between calculated points in the TPS, a small dose grid size ($\leq$2 mm), should be used [28].

Other Considerations Care should be taken when additional devices are involved in breast treatment as in the following.

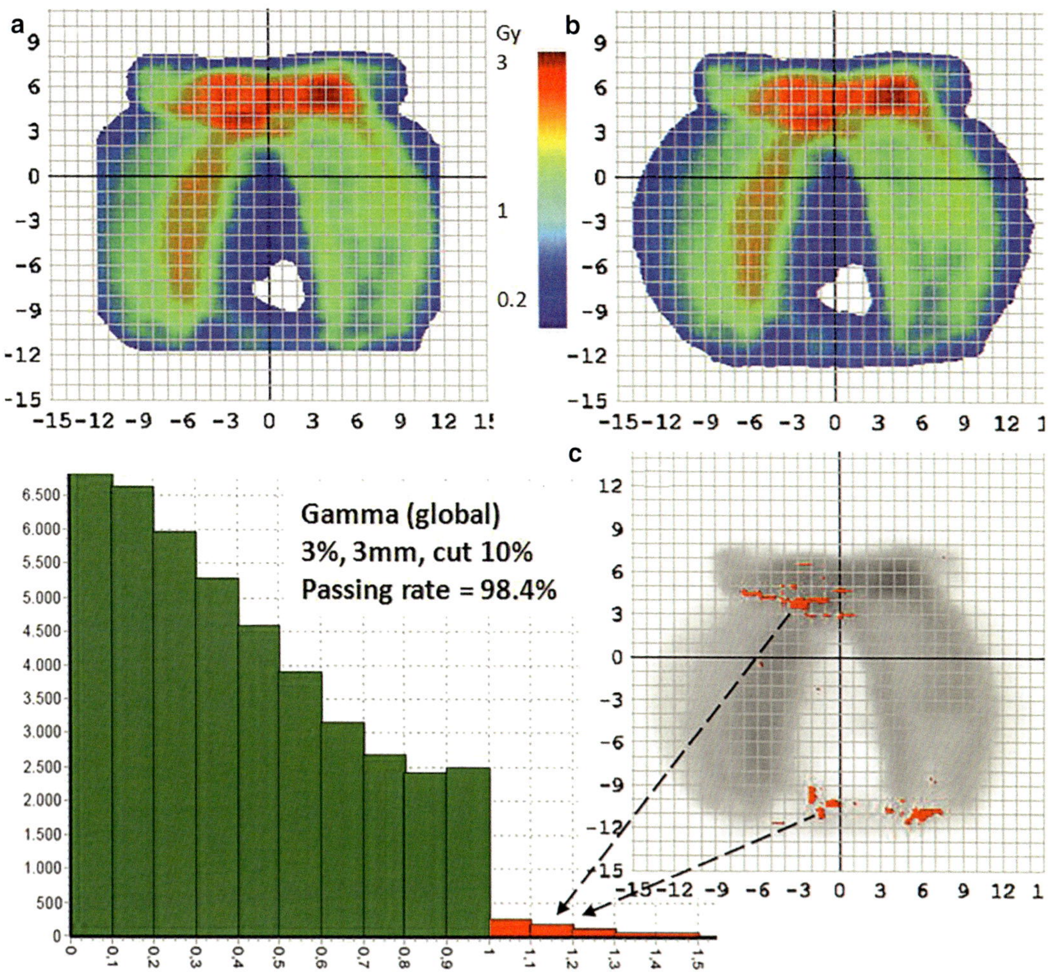

Fig. 55.1 Pre-treatment QA with an on-board EPID in a breast treatment: (**a**) EPID dose measurements; (**b**) TPS dose prediction at EPID surface, (**c**) Comparison with a gamma metrics with a 3% dose-difference, a 3 mm distance-to-agreement and a 10% dose cut-off. Results are summarised in the histogram: the percentage of points satisfying the gamma requirements (in green) is 98.4, dotted lines highlight areas of discrepancies

Bolus material is widely used in PMRT or in cases that the skin is intentionally part of the target volume (see section "chest wall bolus"). The primary goal of using a bolus is to serve as a "tissue equivalent" slice over the build-up region to overcome the skin sparing effects of a megavoltage photon beam, therefore, to allow for a sufficient and uniform dose to the subcutis and skin (if it is part of the CTV). Although, a bolus can improve the PTV coverage at the surface (if indicated to do so), and may homogenise the dose distribution, care must be given to accurate fit of the bolus to the chest wall. This should be verified during every sessions, because inadvertent air gaps between the bolus and the skin can reduce the delivered dose, compromising the target coverage, especially in high risk patients with skin involvement (e.g. for ESTRO recommendations skin is part of CTV in case of T4b,c,d tumours only) [29].

CIEDs (Cardiac implantable electronic device) are a particular concern in breast cancer as they are often located close to the target volumes. If direct or scattered dose can reach the CIED, its cumulative dose should be estimated prior the treatment. Due to the variety of models in literature there are examples of some devices that have suffered deleterious effects at a dose of 0.15 Gy, while others exhibited dose tolerance above 20 Gy. Therefore, the manufacturer should declare the maximum admissible dose of their device. Modern CIED are less sensitive to accumulated dose and safer, especially during imaging procedures. Anyhow international protocols agree to keep the cumulative dose at <5 Gy level [30]. Even if out of the primary beam, CIEDs can be exposed to magnetic and radiofrequency fields or neutrons, which may be considered. Over the course of neutron-producing therapy (15 and 18 MV photon or proton therapy), the risk of device malfunction has been found to be between 12% and 29% per course of treatment. It is preferred to avoid use of protons, and limit photon use to energies less than (or equal to) 10 MV in order to reduce such risks.

The presence of either prostheses or tissue expanders is not generally a problem in the technique choice, because of their near tissue-equivalence. The implanted material does not strictly form part of the CTV and should therefore not be irradiated per se, anyway it has lack of radiation sensitivity for doses up to 60 Gy [31]. Care should be taken if metal or high-density material is part of the prostheses. In these cases, their artefact should be managed in order to avoid dose miscalculation; this can be done by assigning a bulk density to the artefact itself or adapting the electron densities inside the TPS [32]. Capsular contracture, which rates are increased after RT, and which can compromise the surface dose and the consequent breast reconstruction, can be limited by lowering the dose to the non-target volumes that are surrounding the implanted material such as the pectoral muscles and the chest wall [33].

55.3 Summary

Breast radiation treatment is a complex procedure, it requires highly specialised equipment, trained professionals as well as specified protocols. Treatment-related quality assurance includes control and measurement procedures strictly connected to the technical part of the treatment process, involving all acting devices and steps, and a constant improvement should be always pursued.

References

1. Mayo CS, et al. American Association of Physicists in Medicine task group 263: standardizing nomenclatures in radiation oncology. Int J Radiat Oncol Biol Phys. 2018;100(4):1057–66. https://doi.org/10.1016/j.ijrobp.2017.12.013.
2. Mir R, et al. Organ at risk delineation for radiation therapy clinical trials: global harmonization group consensus guidelines. Radiother Oncol. 2020;150:30–9. https://doi.org/10.1016/j.radonc.2020.05.038.
3. Offersen BV, et al. ESTRO consensus guideline on target volume delineation for elective radiation therapy of early stage breast cancer. Radiother Oncol. 2015;114:3–10. https://doi.org/10.1016/j.radonc.2014.11.030.
4. Winfield E, et al. Survey of UK breast radiotherapy techniques: background prior to the introduction of the quality assurance Programme for the START (standardisation of radiotherapy) trial in breast cancer. Clin Oncol. 2002;14(4):267–71. https://doi.org/10.1053/clon.2002.0053.
5. Pitkänen MA, et al. Quality assurance in radiotherapy of breast cancer variability in planning target volume delineation. Acta Oncol. 2001;40(1) https://doi.org/10.1080/028418601750071055.
6. Chen X, et al. CNN-based quality assurance for automatic segmentation of breast cancer in radiotherapy. Front Oncol. 2020;10(524) https://doi.org/10.3389/fonc.2020.00524.
7. Xiang Q, et al. Which technique of positioning and immobilization is better for breast cancer patients in postmastectomy IMRT, single-pole or double-pole immobilization? J Appl Clin Med Phys. 2019;20(1):168–74. https://doi.org/10.1002/acm2.12506.
8. Haffty BG. Supine or prone breast radiation: upsides and downsides. Int J Radiat Oncol Biol Phys. 2018;101(3):510–2. https://doi.org/10.1016/j.ijrobp.2018.03.023.
9. Mast ME, et al. Left-sided breast cancer radiotherapy with and without breath-hold: does IMRT reduce the cardiac dose even further? Radiother Oncol. 2013;108(2):248–53. https://doi.org/10.1016/j.radonc.2013.07.017.
10. Reckhow J, et al. Continuous positive airway pressure with deep inspiration breath hold in left-sided breast radiation therapy. Med Dosim. 2020;20:30133. https://doi.org/10.1016/j.meddos.2020.09.006.
11. Yan Y, et al. Dosimetric comparison between three- and four-dimensional computerised tomography radiotherapy for breast cancer. Oncol Lett. 2019;2:1800–

14. https://doi.org/10.3892/ol.2019.10467. Epub 2019 Jun 12
12. Jiang SB, et al. Quality assurance challenges for motion-adaptive radiation therapy: gating, breath holding, and four-dimensional computed tomography. Int J Radiat Oncol Biol Phys. 2007;71(1):103–7. https://doi.org/10.1016/j.ijrobp.2007.07.2386.
13. Doebricha M, et al. Continuous breath-hold assessment during breast radiotherapy using portal imaging. phiRO. 2018;5:64–8. https://doi.org/10.1016/j.phro.2018.02.006.
14. Nicolini G, et al. Planning strategies in volumetric modulated are therapy for breast. Med Phys. 2011;38(7):4025–31. https://doi.org/10.1118/1.3598442.
15. Virén T, et al. Tangential volumetric modulated arc therapy technique for left-sided breast cancer radiotherapy. Radiat Oncol. 2015;8 https://doi.org/10.1186/s13014-015-0392-x.
16. Tyran M, et al. Safety and benefit of using a virtual bolus during treatment planning for breast cancer treated with arc therapy. J Appl Clin Med Phys. 2018;19(5):463–72. https://doi.org/10.1002/acm2.12398.
17. Kaidar-Person O, et al. Postmastectomy radiation therapy planning after immediate implant-based reconstruction using the European Society for Radiotherapy and Oncology-Advisory Committee in radiation oncology practice consensus guidelines for target volume delineation. Clin Oncol (R Coll Radiol). 2021;33(1):20–9. https://doi.org/10.1016/j.clon.2020.09.004.
18. Jin GH, et al. A comparative dosimetric study for treating left-sided breast cancer for small breast size usingfive different radiotherapy techniques: conventional tangential field, filed-in-filed, Tangential IMRT, Multi-beam IMRT and VMAT. Radiat Oncol. 2013;15 https://doi.org/10.1186/1748-717x-8-89.
19. Commissioning of Radiotherapy Treatment Planning Systems: Testing for Typical External Beam Treatment Techniques *IAEA TECDOC 1583*, 2008. http://www-pub.iaea.org/MTCD/Publications/PDF/te_1583_web.pdf
20. Ezzell GA, et al. IMRT commissioning: multiple institution planning and dosimetry comparisons, a report from AAPM task group 119. Med Phys. 2009;36(11):5359–73. https://doi.org/10.1118/1.3238104.
21. Kerns JR, et al. Treatment planning system calculation errors are present in Most imaging and radiation oncology Core-Houston phantom failures. Int J Radiat Oncol Biol Phys. 2017;98(5):1197–203. https://doi.org/10.1016/j.ijrobp.2017.03.049.
22. Al Amria I, et al. Radiotherapy pre-treatment dose validation: A second verification of monitor units (MU) with a commercial software. J Med Phys. 2012;37(4):235–9. https://doi.org/10.4103/0971-6203.103610.
23. Vazquez Quino LA, et al. Patient specific pre-treatment QA verification using an EPID approach. Technol Cancer Res Treat. 2014;13(1) https://doi.org/10.7785/tcrt.2012.500351.
24. Koo M, et al. Retrospective analysis of portal dosimetry pre-treatment quality assurance of hybrid IMRT breast treatment plans. J Radioth Pract. 2020:1–8. https://doi.org/10.1017/S1460396920000072.
25. Krieger T, et al. Monte Carlo- versus pencil-beam/collapsed-cone dose calculation in a heterogeneous multi-layer phantom. Phys Med Biol. 2005;50(5):859–68. https://doi.org/10.1088/0031-9155/50/5/010.
26. Fogliata A, et al. Critical appraisal of treatment techniques based on conventional photon beams, intensity modulated photon beams and proton beams for therapy of intact breast. Radiother Oncol. 2002;621(2):137–45. https://doi.org/10.1016/s0167-8140(01)00476-5.
27. T. Knöös at al. Comparison of dose calculation algorithms for treatment planning in external photon beam therapy for clinical situations. Phys Med Biol. 2006;51(22):5785–807. https://doi.org/10.1088/0031-9155/51/22/005.
28. Akino Y, et al. Evaluation of superficial dosimetry between treatment planning system and measurement for several breast cancer treatment techniques. Med Phys. 2013;40(1) https://doi.org/10.1118/1.4770285.
29. Robar JL, et al. Intrapatient study comparing 3D printed bolus versus standard vinyl gel sheet bolus for postmastectomy chest wall radiation therapy. Pract Radiat Oncol. 2018;8(4):221–9. https://doi.org/10.1016/j.prro.2017.12.008.
30. Miften M, et al. Management of radiotherapy patients with implanted cardiac pacemakers and defibrillators: a report of the AAPM TG-203. Med Phys. 2019;46(12):757–88. https://doi.org/10.1002/mp.13838.
31. Bachour Y, et al. The influence of radiotherapy on the mechanical properties of silicone breast implants. Plast Reconstr Surg Glob Open. 6(7):2018. https://doi.org/10.1097/GOX.0000000000001772.
32. Yoon J. Modeling of the metallic port in breast tissue expanders for photon radiotherapy. J Appl Clin Med Phys. 2018;19(3):205–14. https://doi.org/10.1002/acm2.12320.
33. Sithole ME. Depth dose enhancement in the presence of silicone gel breast prosthesis. Int. J. Radiat. Research. 2019;17(3):439–46. http://ijrr.com/article-1-2599-en.html

56 Patient-Specific Quality Assurance

Enrico Clementel and Coreen Corning

56.1 Introduction

The importance of QA in RT cannot be overstated: indeed, in most modern departments, quality and safety activities accompany the patient along their journey from referral to treatment. The aim of such activities is two-fold: minimise the risk of accidents and provide optimal quality of treatment (see section on quality assurance programmes in radiation oncology).

Patient-specific QA activities are part of a larger departmental risk management strategy which must cover both structural/systematic and human errors and their interplay [1]. Patient-specific QA addresses elements along the treatment path (Fig. 56.1) that are heavily dependent on specific features of the tumour, such as: delineation of targets and organs, beam arrangement, dose prescription and dose limitation to organs at risk. Patient-specific QA intervenes across the treatment chain and has a twofold aim: avoid continued reproduction of human and systematic errors to a patient's treatment and, with equal importance, ensure optimal quality of treatment, that is, maximise the therapeutic ratio. From a risk management perspective, patient-specific QA represents the last set of barriers to mitigate mistakes. It also represents an important quality improvement tool. This chapter focusses on key elements of patient-specific QA, in particular peer review, delivery QA and IGRT protocols.

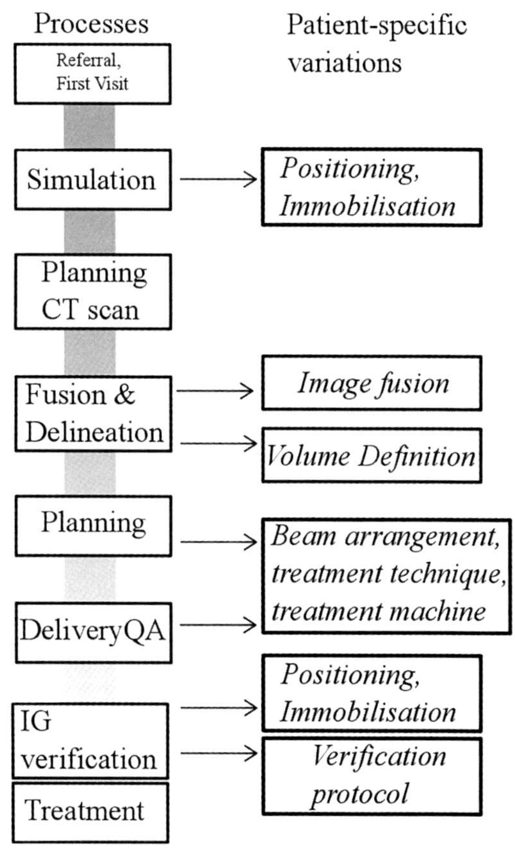

Fig. 56.1 Sources of patient-to-patient variations and errors across the treatment chain. *IG*, Image guided

E. Clementel (✉) · C. Corning
EORTC Headquarters, Brussels, Belgium
e-mail: enrico.clementel@eortc.org; coreen.corning@eortc.org

© The Author(s), under exclusive license to Springer Nature Switzerland AG 2022

O. Kaidar-Person et al. (eds.), *Breast Cancer Radiation Therapy*,
https://doi.org/10.1007/978-3-030-91170-6_56

Table 56.1 Example of a template protocol for peer review

Patient class-specific checklist—template	Acceptable	Acceptable variation	Unacceptable variation
Image co-registration (if applicable)			
Target delineation (margins, extension, anatomical barriers. Separate boost entry if required)			
Target coverage (prescription, uniformity, acceptable compromises. Separate boost entry if required)			
OAR delineation (extension, PRV margins)			
OAR dose constraints (provide priority and thresholds for all prescription doses, if multiple)			
Overall outcome			
Date and signatures			

Bold: radiation oncologist, *Italic*: medical physicist. Details from the actual clinical protocol for the selected patient class should be reported, including guidance on delineation borders, margins, and dose-volume thresholds.

56.2 Methods for Patient-Specific QA

Peer review is a process defined as a reassessment of the treatment plan by a multidisciplinary team of one or more radiation oncologists, medical physicists and dosimetrists/RTTs. According to an analysis of literature on peer review, 10% of peer-reviewed plans are modified and 2.5% undergo major modifications, averaged over mixed diseases sites. This study suggests that peer review is a valuable tool, albeit such rates may differ across different disease sites [2]. Furthermore, it has been observed that plans not conforming to established clinical protocols result in worse outcome for patients [3].

If departmental resources do not allow for peer review of all plans, the frequency of peer review should include a proper selection based on the disease prevalence, anatomical location, dose fractionation schedule and chosen treatment technique.

Peer review is primarily a tool to reduce inter-observer variability in the clinic: as such, the re-evaluation of the patient plan should not only be a "second opinion" but also a systematic evaluation based on a predefined protocol. Such protocols should ensure scoring of plans against the departmental protocol for the specific class of patients considered. For example, peer review of locoregional treatment of breast cancer patients should include an evaluation on target volume and organ at risk delineation and coverage; recognising that left vs right breast irradiation scoring might differ concerning dose constraints (e.g. for the heart). The peer-review protocol should list which elements of the plan should be evaluated, by which staff members, and against which criteria. We report an example in Table 56.1.

Measurement of delivery of the plan on a phantom, or delivery QA, can be considered part of the peer-review process. Delivery QA can be performed by a variety of techniques, a detailed breakdown of which is beyond the scope of this chapter. It is, however, important to sample the output dose distribution, preferably on several points, and compare with the planned distribution, for example by means of gamma analysis. Pure recalculation of dose distribution checks only the quality of the beam model so it must be coupled with absolute output measurements to offer a complete end-to-end delivery QA.

56.3 Recording Peer-Review Outcome

Recording peer-review outcome is as important as conducting peer review. Wet-ink signed paper records or digitally signed Electronic Health Records can be used. All peer-review parameters should be recorded in an electronic database or spreadsheet, preferably entered directly by the reviewers. If paper records are used, double data entry in an electronic spreadsheet is recommended, that is, data should be entered by two different personnel independently with a simple automated identity check to minimise the risk of input mistakes.

It is highly recommended to establish a proper taxonomy of peer-review outcomes for the records, and to use standard terminology for structures and dose-volume parameters. This standardisation effort greatly facilitates retrospective studies and inter-departmental data sharing. It is recommended to classify peer-review outcomes using the terminology suggested by the Global Harmonization Group as *Per Protocol* (green light), *Acceptable Variation* (yellow light), *Unacceptable Variation* (red light, replan) [4], to use AAPM TG 263 for structure naming and dose-volume parameters [5] and the Global Harmonization Group OAR consensus contouring guidance for delineation of organs at risk [4].

More importantly, recording peer-review feedback allows for observation of intra- and inter-departmental historical trends, a crucial tool for quality management. Plan elements which frequently perform poorly in peer review can prompt corrective actions to be taken, and intra-reviewer biases addressed to improve consistency of the peer-review process across the department. Frequent reports should be produced on the aggregated peer-review records by the departmental quality manager and discussed with the multidisciplinary team.

56.4 IGRT Methods

In room IGRT is an essential step for high-quality RT treatment delivery for breast cancer patients. It not only provides verification of target volume dose delivery which has been shown to increase overall survival [6, 7] but also allows for the adaption/individualisation of margins to reduce normal tissue toxicity. IGRT employs either 2D or 3D imaging and/or surface guidance. The type of image guidance used is dependent on locally available equipment, whereas the frequency and timing (online versus offline) is driven by the chosen treatment technique, dose/fractionation schedule, local practice of adaptive RT, target and normal tissue motion versus the possible detrimental effect of its dose to the patient [8]. Because of these variabilities strict guidance is left to national guidelines or, where these do not exist, up to the department itself.

56.5 Summary

Patient-specific QA is necessary to ensure high-quality standards of treatment and should be conducted according to pre-specified protocols. Its benefits not only affect the individual patient, but if organised correctly, the entire patient population. Outcomes should be recorded as part of a department's long-term quality improvement strategy.

References

1. Scalliet P. Risk, society and system failure. Radiother Oncol. 2006;80(3):275–81. https://doi.org/10.1016/j.radonc.2006.07.003.
2. Brunskill K, et al. Does peer review of radiation plans affect clinical care? A systematic review of the literature. Int J Radiat Oncol Biol Phys. 2017;97(1):27–34. https://doi.org/10.1016/j.ijrobp.2016.09.015.
3. Peters LJ, et al. Critical impact of radiotherapy protocol compliance and quality in the treatment of advanced head and neck cancer: results from TROG 02.02. J Clin Oncol. 2010;28(18):2996–3001. https://doi.org/10.1200/JCO.2009.27.4498.
4. Mir R, et al. Organ at risk delineation for radiation therapy clinical trials: global harmonization group consensus guidelines. Radiother Oncol. 2020; https://doi.org/10.1016/j.radonc.2020.05.038.
5. Mayo CS, et al. American Association of Physicists in Medicine task group 263: standardizing nomenclatures in radiation oncology. Int J Radiat Oncol Biol Phys. 2018;100(4):1057–66. https://doi.org/10.1016/j.ijrobp.2017.12.013.
6. Johnson-Hart CN, Price GJ, Faivre-Finn C, Aznar MC, van Herk M. Residual setup errors towards the heart after image guidance linked with poorer survival in lung cancer patients: do we need stricter IGRT protocols? Int J Radiat Oncol Biol Phys. 2018;102(2):434–42. https://doi.org/10.1016/j.ijrobp.2018.05.052.
7. FitzGerald TJ, et al. Processes for quality improvements in radiation oncology clinical trials. Int J Radiat Oncol Biol Phys. 2008;71(1 SUPPL):76–9. https://doi.org/10.1016/j.ijrobp.2007.07.2387.
8. https://www.acr.org/-/media/ACR/Files/Practice-Parameters/IGRT-RO.pdf?la=en.